FOURTH EDITION

Assessments in Occupational Therapy Mental Health

An Integrative Approach

T0321994

FOURTH EDITION

Assessments in Occupational Therapy Mental Health

An Integrative Approach

Edited by

Barbara J. Hemphill, DMin, OTR, FAOTA

Christine K. Urish, PhD, OTR/L, BCMH, FAOTA

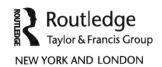

Routledge
Taylor & Francis Group

NEW YORK AND LONDON

First published in 2020 by SLACK Incorporated

Published 2024 by Routledge
605 Third Avenue, New York, NY 10017
4 Park Square, Milton Park, Abingdon, Oxon OX14 4RN

Routledge is an imprint of the Taylor & Francis Group, an informa business

Library of Congress Cataloging-in-Publication Data

Names: Hemphill, Barbara J., editor. | Urish, Christine, 1965- editor.
Title: Assessments in occupational therapy mental health : an integrative
  approach / edited by Barbara J. Hemphill, Christine K. Urish.
Description: Fourth edition. | Thorofare, NJ : SLACK Incorporated, [2020] |
  Includes bibliographical references and index.
Identifiers: LCCN 2020012056 (print) | ISBN 9781630918132 (hardcover)
Subjects: MESH: Occupational Therapy--methods | Mentally Disabled
  Persons--rehabilitation | Needs Assessment
Classification: LCC RM735.3 (print) | NLM WM
  450.5.O2 | DDC 615.8/515--dc23
LC record available at https://lccn.loc.gov/2020012056

ISBN: 9781630918132 (hbk)
ISBN: 9781003522645 (ebk)

DOI:10.4324/9781003522645

Dedication

To Pat Pangburn, a very dear friend who assisted me over the past years and remains in my memory. I want to thank her for her expertise in computer language, and her ability to challenge my ideas in a soft and loving manner. She was knowledgeable in various writing styles, and I learned a great deal from her. During my association with her, she was able to learn and understand the profession of occupational therapy and became an asset to me while I was engaged in a variety of writing projects. I miss her very much.

—*Barbara J. Hemphill, DMin, OTR, FAOTA*

Contents

Acknowledgments

I would like to thank my friends and colleagues and my husband who gave me the courage and the support needed to accomplish this task. Without them, I could not have completed this project. I want to extend my appreciation to the authors who contributed to this endeavor. Through medical stresses, deaths, surgeries, heart attacks, and emotional turmoil, theses authors maintained their dedication and commitment to this project. This project could not have been completed without their steadfast tenacity. I am indebted to their patient and faithful trust. I want to thank Christine Urish for her contribution as secondary editor. Her editorial skills and knowledge added to the value of the manuscript.

—*Barbara J. Hemphill, DMin, OTR, FAOTA*

I would like to acknowledge the following individuals related to this work: Dr. Barbara Hemphill for the opportunity to collaborate and contribute in a significant manner to this exceptional scholarly work; Ms. Eliza Gillies, Ms. Mary Scheck, and Mr. Tom Crone for the support and assistance during the writing and editing process; and the occupational therapy students and clients over the years who provided ongoing motivation for me to continue engagement in life-long learning and pursuit of clinical excellence. Lastly, to my grandfather, Virgil Urish, who instilled a love for learning and reminded me I could "do anything" if I put my mind to it.

—*Christine K. Urish, PhD, OTR/L, BCMH, FAOTA*

About the Editors

Barbara J. Hemphill, DMin, OTR, FAOTA, received her Bachelor of Science degree in occupational therapy from the University of Iowa. She received her Master of Science degree in occupational therapy from Colorado State University. During her tenure as a therapist at Ft. Logan Mental Health Center, she was fortunate to work with Dr. Maxwell Jones, the founder of the Therapeutic Community Concept in mental health, and developed the B.H. Battery, a projective test based on analytical frame of reference. She began her teaching career at Cleveland State University. She became an associate professor and tenured in the department of occupational therapy at Western Michigan University. She retired emeritus after 19 years. In addition to her degrees, she has an earned Doctor of Ministry degree from the Ecumenical Theological Seminary in Detroit.

Dr. Hemphill has served on the editorial boards of the *Occupational Therapy Practice Journal* and the *American Journal of Occupational Therapy* and presently serves on the editorial board of the *Occupational Therapy in Mental Health* journal. She has written numerous international, national, and state peer-reviewed papers. Her papers include two at the World Federation for Occupational Therapy: one entitled "Holism in Occupational Therapy" and the second entitled "Occupational Therapy and Spirituality: A Global Perspective." She has presented numerous papers at national occupational therapy conferences. Among them are: "Methods in Spirituality: An Educational Experience," "Spirituality in the Treatment Setting," "Spirituality in the Health Care Setting," and "Spirituality as an Occupation." At the state level, she has presented papers at the Michigan Occupational Therapy conference, and her presentations have included "Spiritual Assessments in the Treatment Setting" and "Spirituality With the Intellectual Disabled."

Her publication record has spanned over 25 years. Her most proud accomplishment is having edited books on the topic of mental health assessment. Among them are *The Evaluative Process in Psychiatric Occupational Therapy*, which was translated into Japanese; *Mental Health Assessment in Occupational Therapy*; and *Assessments in Occupational Therapy Mental Health*. She has published in the *American Journal of Occupational Therapy* and *Occupational Therapy in Mental Health*. The topics range from marketing to depression to deinstitutionalization. Her most recent publication focused on social justice and spirituality in occupational therapy. She has been recognized for her contributions to education, research, and publications. She has served on state and national committees, most notably serving as chair of the Ethics Commission of the American Occupational Therapy Association. Her awards include Fellow of the American Occupational Therapy Association, as well as Fellow of the Michigan Occupational Therapy Association. She was recently named among the most 100 influential occupational therapists in the past century.

Dr. Hemphill continues to contribute to her profession after retirement. She has taught courses in spirituality to occupational therapy students online and in the classroom. Her ministry is in the community. She has taught spirituality courses at senior centers and retirement homes. She also taught a series of courses about C.S. Lewis and a PBS course entitled "A Question of God," a debate between Freud and C.S. Lewis.

Christine K. Urish, PhD, OTR/L, BCMH, FAOTA, graduated from Western Michigan University in 1989 with a Bachelor of Science degree in occupational therapy. She began her career working as an occupational therapist at an inpatient psychiatric setting and inpatient/outpatient addiction treatment providing treatment to clients across the lifespan. She completed her Master of Science degree in 1993 and returned to clinical practice. In 1994, she began her career in higher education at St. Ambrose University, teaching in occupational therapy until June 2018. At present, Dr. Urish is a professor of occupational therapy at Drake University. Christine completed her PhD from the University of Iowa in 2005. Along the way, she has worked with the most amazing mentors, including Dr. Barbara Hemphill, who was a motivating and encouraging force in her career from the early days at Western Michigan University, at the start of her clinical practice, throughout the completion of her PhD, and to the present day. Another mentor, Dr. Vilia Tarvydas, encouraged her early writing career. Dr. Urish continues to engage in clinical practice as an occupational therapist in behavioral health at the University of Iowa Hospitals & Clinics. Dr. Urish is Board certified as an occupational therapist in mental health by the American Occupational Therapy Association and is a Fellow of the American Occupational Therapy Association. Dr. Urish has served in the past as affiliate President for the National Alliance on Mental Illness and as President of the Iowa Occupational Therapy Association. Dr. Urish is a tireless advocate for individuals with mental illness, the profession of occupational therapy, and occupational therapy students.

Contributing Authors

Jennifer Allison, OTD, OTR/L (Chapter 21)
Assistant Professor
School of Occupational Therapy
College of Health Sciences
Brenau University
Gainesville, Georgia

Sue Baptiste, MHSc (Chapter 4)
Professor
School of Rehabilitation Sciences
Faculty of Health Sciences
McMaster University
Hamilton, Ontario, Canada

*Carolyn M. Baum, PhD, OTR/L, FAOTA
(Chapters 6 and 15)*
Professor
Occupational Therapy, Neurology, and
Social Work
Washington University
St. Louis, Missouri

*Marie-Louise F. Blount, AM, OT, FAOTA
(Foreword)*
Clinical Professor, Retired
New York University
New York, New York

*Brent Braveman, PhD, OTR/L, FAOTA
(Chapter 24)*
Occupational Therapist
Director of Rehabilitation Services
MD Anderson Cancer Center
Houston, Texas

*Catana Brown, PhD, OTR/L, FAOTA
(Chapters 25 and 26)*
Professor
Midwestern University
Glendale, Arizona

Ann Chapleau, DHS, OTR/L (Chapter 30)
Professor
Department of Occupational Therapy
Western Michigan University
Kalamazoo, Michigan

*Lisa Tabor Connor, PhD, MSOT, OTR/L
(Chapter 6)*
Elias Michael Executive Director and
Professor
Occupational Therapy and Neurology
Washington University
St. Louis, Missouri

Brock Cook, BA, OT (Chapter 9)
Lecturer (Occupational Therapy)
College of Health Sciences
James Cook University
Townsville, Queensland, Australia

*Mary V. Donohue, PhD, OT/L, FAOTA
(Chapter 5)*
Occupational Therapist
Associate Editor
Occupational Therapy in Mental Health

*Catherine A. Earhart, BA, OT Cert, OTR/L
(Chapter 11)*
Director of Development
Allen Cognitive Group/
ACLS and LACLS Committee
California

*Glen Gillen, EdD, OTR, FAOTA
(Chapter 10)*
Professor and Director
Programs in Occupational Therapy
Vice Chair
Department of Rehabilitation and
Regenerative Medicine
Assistant Dean
Vagelos College of
Physicians and Surgeons
Columbia University
New York, New York

*Kristine Haertl, PhD, OTR/L, FAOTA
(Chapter 7)*
Professor
Department of Occupational Therapy
St. Catherine University
St. Paul, Minnesota

Ashley Hartman, MS, OTR/L
(Chapter 13)
Occupational Therapist
Tender Touch Rehab Services
Spotswood, New Jersey

Barbara J. Hemphill, DMin, OTR, FAOTA
(Chapters 1 and 27)
Professor Emeritus Occupational Therapy
Western Michigan University
Kalamazoo, Michigan

Margo B. Holm, PhD, OTR/L, FAOTA,
ABDA (Chapter 20)
Professor Emerita
Occupational Therapy
University of Pittsburgh
Pittsburgh, Pennsylvania

Michael K. Iwama, PhD, MSc, BSc, BScOT
(Chapter 9)
Dean and Professor
School of Health and
Rehabilitation Sciences
MGH Institute of Health Professions
Boston, Massachusetts

Celeste Januszewski, OTD, OTR/L, CPRP
(Chapter 16)
Clinical Assistant Professor
University of Illinois at Chicago
Chicago, Illinois

Noomi Katz, PhD, OTR (Chapter 12)
Director
Research Institute for
Health and Medical Professions
Ono Academic College
Kiryat Ono, Israel
Professor Emeritus
Hebrew University
Jerusalem, Israel

Lisa Mahaffey, PhD, OTR/L, FAOTA
(Chapters 3 and 16)
Associate Professor of
Occupational Therapy
Occupational Therapy Program
Midwestern University
Downers Grove, Illinois

Kathleen Matuska, PhD, OTR/L, FAOTA
(Chapter 29)
Professor of Occupational Therapy
St. Catherine University
St. Paul, Minnesota

Deane B McCraith, MS, OT/L, LMFT
(Chapter 11)
Director of Education and Research
Allen Cognitive Group/
ACLS and LACLS Committee
California

Christine Raber, PhD, OTR/L
(Chapter 17)
Professor
Master of Occupational Therapy Program
Shawnee State University
Portsmouth, Ohio

Emily Raphael-Greenfield, EdD, OTR/L, FAOTA
(Chapters 10 and 13)
Special Lecturer
Programs in Occupational Therapy
Department of Rehabilitation and
Regenerative Medicine
Vagelos College of
Physicians and Surgeons
Columbia University
New York, New York

Nadine Revheim, PhD, OTR/L
(Chapter 22)
Licensed Psychologist
Private Practice

Joan C. Rogers, PhD, OTR, FAOTA
(Chapter 20)
Professor Emeritus
Occupational Therapy
University of Pittsburgh
Pittsburgh, Pennsylvania

Jane Ryan, MBA/CHM, LOTR, CLT
(Chapter 8)
Occupational Therapist
Denham Springs, Louisiana

Victoria Schindler, PhD, OTR, BCMH,
FAOTA (Chapter 18)
Professor of Occupational Therapy
Stockton University
Galloway, New Jersey

Emily Schulz, PhD, OTR/L, CFLE, ACUE
(Chapter 28)
Assistant Clinical Professor
Northern Arizona University
Phoenix, Arizona

Mary P. Shotwell, PhD, OT/L, FAOTA
(Chapter 21)
Professor and Program Director
Occupational Therapy Program
University of St. Augustine for the
Health Sciences
St. Augustine, Florida

Franklin Stein, PhD, OTR/L, FAOTA
(Chapter 31)
Editor
Annals of International Occupational Therapy
Professor Emeritus
Department of Occupational Therapy
University of South Dakota
Vermillion, South Dakota

Linda Kohlman Thomson, MOT, FAOTA
(Chapter 23)
Occupational Therapist
Bellingham, Washington

Joan Toglia, PhD, OTR/L, FAOTA
(Chapters 13 and 14)
Dean and Professor
School of Health & Natural Sciences
Mercy College
Dobbs Ferry, New York
Adjunct Clinical Professor of
Cognitive Sciences
Rehabilitation Medicine
Weill Cornell Medical College
New York, New York

Carolyn A. Unsworth, BAppSci(OccTher),
PhD, OTR (Chapter 19)
Professor of Occupational Therapy
School of Health, Medical and
Applied Sciences
Central Queensland University
Adjunct Professor
La Trobe University
Melbourne, Australia
Jönköping University
Jönköping, Sweden

Christine K. Urish, PhD, OTR/L, BCMH,
FAOTA (Chapters 1 and 2)
Professor of Occupational Therapy
Drake University
Des Moines, Iowa

Janet Watts, PhD, OTR Retired
(Chapter 17)
Emeritus Associate Professor
Department of Occupational Therapy
Virginia Commonwealth University
Richmond, Virginia

Suzanne White, MA, OTR/L, FAOTA
(Chapter 14)
Clinical Associate Professor
Occupational Therapy Program
SUNY Downstate Medical Center
New York, New York

Timothy J. Wolf, OTD, PhD, OTR/L, FAOTA
(Chapter 15)
Department Chair
Associate Professor
Occupational Therapy
University of Missouri
Columbia, Missouri

Preface

In 1982, the first edition of *The Evaluative Process in Psychiatric Occupational Therapy* was published. The purposes of this text were to provide occupational therapy students with knowledge about the evaluation process, to provide therapists with information about assessments that was current and accurate, and to generate research for developing assessment tools. The text was translated into Japanese, and subsequent editions were used in international occupational therapy programs. Other texts published were entitled *Mental Health in Occupational Therapy*, and two texts were entitled *Assessments in Occupational Therapy Mental Health*. All had the subtitle *An Integrative Approach*.

All texts have been focused on the original purpose. The common thread has been research, and each chapter was written by the assessment's originator or by an individual extremely well-versed with research on the assessment. There is no intent in the text to present or recommend any one assessment over another. There is no intent to endorse a particular theory or frame of reference. The editors did not impose criteria for each assessment's usefulness or level of research development. It is the belief of the editors that practitioners shall determine the usefulness and credibility of an assessment and encourage students to do further research in assessments.

In the present edition, an attempt was made to include assessments that were currently used and to include assessments from the previous editions. In order to be included in this text, an assessment had to have 75% new material within the chapter. This was accomplished either through updating the literature review, research development, or adding a case study. The chapters that are updated include "Client-Centered Assessment: The Canadian Occupational Performance Measure," "Writing as an Assessment Tool in Mental Health," "The Assessment of Occupational Functioning–Collaborative Version," "Role Assessments Used in Mental Health," "The Performance Assessment of Self-Care Skills," "The Comprehensive Occupational Therapy Evaluation," "Work-Related Assessments: The Worker Role Interview, Work Environment Impact Scale, and Assessment of Work Performance," and "The OT-QUEST: The Occupational Therapy Quality of Experience and Spirituality Assessment Tool." The summary chapters include "Performance-Based Assessments and Neuropsychological Assessments: A Comparison," "Assessments Used Within the Model of Human Occupation," and "Work-Related Assessments: The Worker Role Interview, Work Environment Impact Scale, and Assessment of Work Performance."

There are 15 new assessments in this text and 1 assessment that was not included in the second edition but is included in this edition. This assessment, the Kohlman Evaluation of Living Skills, has been revised, updated, and received additional research to warrant inclusion in this edition.

Each chapter includes the theoretical basis, including historical development, rationale, and a literature review; a presentation of the research, including the statistical analysis; the procedure about how the assessment is administered and materials needed; a presentation of a case study if there is no research; and suggestions for further research. Each author was asked to use language consistent with the current *Occupational Therapy Practice Framework: Domain and Process*.

Spirituality has become an important part of the evaluation process in occupational therapy. It is one of the client factors in developing client profiles and is a part of the holistic triad. The chapter entitled "The OT-QUEST: The Occupational Therapy Quality of Experience and Spirituality Assessment Tool" is updated, and a summary chapter on "Spiritual Assessments in Mental Health Occupational Therapy" was added.

Traditionally, the last section included a chapter on research. This content now appears as part of the Introduction in a chapter entitled "Evidence-Based Practice and Assessment in Occupational Therapy."

It has been 12 years since publication of the second edition. Since that time, there seems to be increased development of assessments and research on previous ones. An increased number of occupational therapists are practicing in mental health and are seeing the need to develop new assessments and revitalize ones that have stood the test of time. There have been assessments developed in the areas of interviewing; psychological, cognitive, and sensory learning; daily living; and behavior. Specifically, there has been a plethora of assessment development in psychological and cognitive areas. The Kawa (River) Model, Routine Task Inventory–Expanded, Weekly Calendar Planning Activity, and Executive Function Performance Test are just a few. One other assessment that has received attention and is new to this text is the Allen Cognitive Level Screen–5 and Allen Diagnostic Module (2nd Edition). This screening and assessment is one of those that was developed over the years and is now appearing for the first time.

The pressure to develop assessments specific to occupational therapy is ever expanding as a result of the need to demonstrate the effectiveness of practice. This is evident in the development of assessments and research being conducted on those that need further development. This is a compilation of current assessments that have appeared in journals, reported in workshops, presented at conferences, obtained from unpublished manuscripts, and observed through use. Like the previous texts, this is a book for occupational therapists by occupational therapists. It is hoped that practitioners will encourage students to conduct research to facilitate further development of assessments in mental health.

—*Barbara J. Hemphill, DMin, OTR, FAOTA*

Foreword

In this fourth edition of a classic work that has been used by occupational therapists over many years, Barbara J. Hemphill and Christine K. Urish have provided us with a comprehensive exploration of assessments used by professionals and students in mental health. Updating the previous editions and concentrating particularly on research into the validity, reliability, and applicability of the instruments discussed has provided us with a thorough and timely approach to the understanding of people coping with mental illness and the formulation of necessary efforts to aid these clients in moving toward more fulfilling lives. The text is primarily valuable for its practical usefulness to occupational therapists, students, and others who wish to select and use these instruments.

Thanks to the editors themselves, this essential update to our information about these mental health assessments will provide a guide to a range of available instruments and will lead necessarily to their informed and appropriate use. Barbara Hemphill has a long, ground-breaking, and honored career in teaching and publication in occupational therapy. Her record in these regards is clear, and she continues to contribute to our knowledge and understanding in valued ways. Christine Urish, a young leader in mental health occupational therapy, has contributed as writer and editor and has helped to make the current edition a thorough and useful work. Professor Urish is a member of the occupational therapy faculty at Drake University, Des Moines, Iowa.

This fourth edition introduces and provides a wider range of assessments and some changes in organization but is primarily valuable for its breadth of content and its integration of a range of approaches used in mental health today. The section on the interviewing process, a key beginning and important clinical skill, introduces new instruments and their utility and applicability. The section on psychological assessments adds much new material, including many cognitive assessments. These range from traditional and long-established instruments to new and updated measures. Sensory assessment, a new contribution to this work, reflects a long-established interest in how sensory competence adds to mental health. The section on learning assessments, in this edition a total of six chapters, represents new approaches and authors, as well as the latest version of the Kohlman Evaluation of Living Skills and pertinent research on that measure. A section on behavioral assessments also represents a new approach to this area, with some new authors and emphasis on the Model of Human Occupation, occupation itself (an important concept in current professional thinking), and assessments of life roles and the part they play in the attainment of personally satisfying mental health. Spiritual assessments are given greater attention in this edition, with a variety of approaches to investigating and incorporating spirituality into practice. The final section of the book presents measures on balance in life activities and attainment of life goals. Both of these approaches have been carefully studied among students and the general public. Altogether, a major advance in current thinking and its application are assembled in this work.

The features of the new edition, of this clear and polished work, that deserve the most attention are its thoroughness and strength, and particularly its emphasis on research findings as they apply to all included instruments. Occupational therapists, students, and others who use it will find its valuable assets to be its comprehensiveness and its clear applicability to their work.

—*Marie-Louise F. Blount, AM, OT, FAOTA*

Part I

Introduction

1

Assessment in Occupational Therapy

Christine K. Urish, PhD, OTR/L, BCMH, FAOTA
Barbara J. Hemphill, DMin, OTR, FAOTA

> *Man, through the use of his hands, as they are energized by mind and will,*
> *can influence the state of his own health.*
> (Reilly, 1962)

In 2017, the 100th year since the advent of the occupational therapy profession, the authors believe it is important to historically review how this text has evolved and how it has affected the occupational therapy profession. When *The Evaluative Process in Psychiatric Occupational Therapy* (Hemphill, 1982) was first published, the author proposed a method for assessing patients. It was a structure for selecting assessments based on the ability of the therapist to identify patient dysfunction and progress. This structure allowed the therapist to select and use assessments from a broad repertoire to achieve an integrative view of patients with emotional disorders.

In stepping back, one must consider how business was conducted in the 1970s and 1980s; there was no email, so networking occurred at professional conferences. Contracts were initially typed using a manual typewriter and then typed using an electronic typewriter; the U.S. Postal System was used to send and receive legal documents. Fast forward to 2017, and contracts are created via word processing software on a computer, sent to authors for their signatures, scanned, and returned—all electronically. For this edition of the text, the authors worked collaboratively with contributors from around the globe, often electronically, sharing the same computer screen to edit the work contained within this text.

Hemphill, B. J., & Urish, C. K. (Eds.). *Assessments in Occupational Therapy Mental Health: An Integrative Approach, Fourth Edition* (pp. 3-13). © 2020 Taylor & Francis Group.

This text has grown widely since the first edition was published in 1982 and has been called a motivator for other occupational therapy assessment texts, such as Asher's (2014) *Occupational Therapy Assessment Tools*, now in the fourth edition. In this chapter, we will provide a historical overview of the concept of assessment through the examination of several lectures by Eleanor Clarke Slagle, providing an overview of the occupational therapy process using the *Occupational Therapy Practice Framework: Domain and Process, Third Edition* (American Occupational Therapy Association [AOTA], 2014), which contains the official terminology of the profession, as a guide. Within this chapter, the ethics of evaluation and assessment are considered, the current practice in relation to occupational therapy assessment and reimbursement is examined, and an overview of the major sections contained within the text is provided.

Assessment and Slagle Lectures

Since the profession began in 1917, many things have changed; however, one component has remained consistent—the occupational therapist examines the client's level of function through the assessment of occupational performance limitations to plan effective treatment. In the 2017 compendium of the Eleanor Clarke Slagle Lectures from 1955 through 2016, several lecturers specifically addressed the role of assessment and the evaluative process in occupational therapy (Padilla & Griffiths, 2017), specifically, the 1983 Eleanor Clarke Slagle Lecture "Clinical Reasoning: The Ethics, Science, and Art" by Joan Rogers (as cited in Padilla & Griffiths, 2017). Occupational therapy practitioners are directed first to consider the assessment question "What is the patient's occupational status?" (Padilla & Griffiths, 2017, p. 267). In 1983, Rogers (as cited in Padilla & Griffiths, 2017) directed the profession to work toward the development of assessment instruments to use in clinical practice. This contributor's work can be found in Chapter 20, "The Performance Assessment of Self-Care Skills," developed with Dr. Margo Holm.

In the 2000 Eleanor Clarke Slagle Lecture "Our Mandate for the New Millennium: Evidence-Based Practice," Margo Holm (as cited in Padilla & Griffiths, 2017) directed occupational therapy practitioners to examine evidence-based practice. The mandate of evidence-based practice continues to be present within the profession. Occupational therapy practitioners must consider the best assessment tools to utilize during the evaluation process, as well as what strategies to utilize for collecting the best evidence to continue moving the occupational therapy profession forward. Practitioners and researchers/scholars must work collaboratively in the development of measurement tools to justify and further define occupational therapy services to the broader population. In Chapter 2, this text addresses the concept of evidence-based practice as it relates to assessments in occupational therapy in mental health.

Moving forward in the professional literature, the 2008 Eleanor Clarke Slagle Lecture "Embracing Ambiguity: Facing the Challenge of Measurement" by Wendy Coster (as cited in Padilla & Griffiths, 2017) reminded the profession of the significant importance of measurement in clinical practice as it relates to reimbursement implication; however, the profession must be mindful to not lose sight of the whole person. Coster (as cited in Padilla & Griffiths, 2017) directed the profession to "go beyond selecting instruments with the best reliability or predictive accuracy, or the application of modern methods such as Rasch analysis. We must also examine and challenge some of the assumptions underlying the current use of measures and the conclusions being drawn from this use" (p. 591). Coster (as cited in Padilla & Griffiths, 2017) further noted that occupational therapists must be willing to attempt different strategies to capture the client's story and offered the following assessments as options to accomplish this goal: Activity Card Sort (Chapter 6) and the Model of Human Occupation assessments, such as the Occupational Self-Assessment (Chapter 16). An additional assessment (although not suggested by Coster) for consideration is the Kawa (River) Model assessment (Chapter 9). Lastly, Coster (as cited in Padilla & Griffiths, 2017) encouraged occupational therapy practitioners to examine research or systematic reviews that concluded that therapeutic intervention "does not improve function" (p. 599) because practitioners need to critically consider the outcome measures utilized and determine whether the study examined more than basic physical function and to challenge study results due to the holistic nature of the occupational therapy profession.

Within the past decade, two Eleanor Clarke Slagle Lectures have addressed the impact of assessment on the profession of occupational therapy. Glen Gillen's (as cited in Padilla & Griffiths, 2017) 2013 lecture, "A Fork in the Road: An Occupational Hazard," challenged occupational therapy practitioners regarding how cognition was being measured. Clients' lives and occupations are complicated, and as such Gillen (as cited in Padilla & Griffiths, 2017) suggested that occupational therapists "stop trying to convince ourselves and our colleagues we can predict occupational performance from non-occupation based assessments" (p. 692). Gillen shares further insights into cognitive assessment in the current text in Chapter 10. The other Eleanor Clarke Slagle Lecture indirectly related to assessment was the 2014 address given by Maralynne Mitcham (as cited in Padilla & Griffiths, 2017) entitled "Education as Engine." Within this lecture, Mitcham (as cited in Padilla & Griffiths, 2017) directed the profession to consider "education as a product, learning as a process, and living as progress" (p. 708).

The current text embraces the notions purported by Mitcham (as cited in Padilla & Griffiths, 2017). This text never intended to suggest or direct occupational therapy practitioners toward one assessment over another. Rather, the text offers occupational therapy practitioners the opportunity to critically examine assessments that are utilized within the profession to foster education and best practice: the learning process. As occupational therapy practitioners, we can demonstrate benefits to society and our clients through the education process, lead change and learning in clients' lives through therapeutic intervention, demonstrate the power of the life journey when we engage in actions that improve conditions for our clients, create lives of meaning, and transform that which is within our hands. The occupational therapy process, which includes client assessment, is a key to the journey of positive occupational engagement, performance, and living.

Assessment and
Occupational Therapy Practice Framework

The start of the occupational therapy process begins with the evaluation. The *Framework* (AOTA, 2014) presents the professional terminology utilized by occupational therapy practitioners and defines the domain of concern within the profession: occupation. The occupational therapy practitioner begins by conducting an occupational profile. The *Framework* (AOTA, 2014) defines the occupational profile as "the initial step in the evaluation process, which provides an understanding of the client's occupational history and experiences, patterns of daily living, interests, values, and needs. The client's reasons for seeking services, strengths and concerns in relation to performing occupations and daily life activities, areas of potential occupational disruption, supports and barriers, and priorities are also identified" (p. S10). Chapter 3 in this text provides insights into the occupational profile.

Based on information gathered within the occupational profile, the occupational therapy practitioner moves to analyze the patient's occupational performance.

This [is the] step in the evaluation process during which the client's assets and problems or potential problems are more specifically identified. Actual performance is often observed in context to identify supports for and barriers to the client's performance. Performance skills, performance patterns, context or environment, client factors, and activity demands are all considered, but only selected aspects may be specifically assessed. Targeted outcomes are identified. (AOTA, 2014, p. S10)

The occupational therapy practitioner considers all areas of occupation. An assessment included in this text, Creative Participation Assessment, considers all areas across the occupational therapy process (Chapter 8). Although it may appear that the occupational therapy process is linear in nature, the evaluation process serves to direct the intervention plan and its implementation and to review its progress toward targeted outcomes; however, the occupational therapist may return to reassess an area of occupational performance at any time during treatment. Effective assessment of a client's occupational performance is essential to the planning and implementation of therapeutic intervention (AOTA, 2014). Within the analysis of occupational performance, the occupational therapy practitioner may use multiple methods to assess the client, environment or context, occupation and occupational performance. The *Framework* (AOTA, 2014) suggested that standardized assessments are preferred when available to facilitate the collection of objective data impacting various aspects of occupation and performance. The occupational therapist is directed to use valid and reliable instruments to facilitate identification of client needs and to justify and support the necessity of therapeutic intervention. Occupational therapy practitioners choose assessments taking into consideration the client needs and beliefs and potential assumptions that underlie occupational performance, in addition to the practitioner's theoretical approach and access to psychometrically sound standardized measures (AOTA, 2014).

Assessment and Ethics

Assessment in occupational therapy is utilized in clinical practice and in research. Assessment can impact reimbursement and occupational therapy services available to the client. As such, occupational therapy practitioners need to be aware of the ethics that govern the profession of occupational therapy (AOTA, 2015). The *Occupational Therapy Code of Ethics* (AOTA, 2015) is a document reviewed and updated by the AOTA on a regular basis. It is the responsibility of the occupational therapy practitioner to be aware of and follow the *Code of Ethics* (AOTA, 2015) at all times.

The standards of conduct within the *Code of Ethics* (AOTA, 2015) that relate to the evaluation process include the following: beneficence, autonomy, justice, veracity, and fidelity. In the area of beneficence, occupational therapy practitioners are directed to provide appropriate evaluation to meet client needs. Further, assessments are utilized that are evidence based, current, and relate to the current scope of occupational therapy practice (AOTA, 2015). The concept of autonomy directs the occupational therapy practitioner to allow the client choice. In the area of assessment, the client is free to participate or refuse to participate in any part of the assessment process. The occupational therapist should explain the nature and purpose of the evaluation process, as well as the necessity of the assessment being administered to the level of client understanding, to facilitate understanding of the process and the importance of assessment in effective treatment planning and intervention implementation (AOTA, 2015). Justice guides the occupational therapy practitioner to possess credentials necessary for the administration of specific assessments, such as the Assessment of Motor and Process Skills discussed in Chapter 10, as well as to refrain from engaging in duplication/copying of assessment materials that would infringe on copyright of the assessment materials. Within the area of veracity, occupational therapy practitioners are required to report assessment results in an accurate manner. Occupational therapists must communicate in a truthful manner at all times because the client has a right to accurate information regarding the results of the assessment(s) conducted. Furthermore, occupational therapy practitioners must represent credentials and/or qualifications to administer specific assessments in an accurate manner. Occupational therapy practitioners are required to maintain professional competence in all areas of occupational therapy practice, including assessment. From the perspective of fidelity, the occupational therapy practitioner is required to address incompetence or impaired clinical practice that could jeopardize the safety of the client(s). For example, if one occupational therapist observes a colleague who is impaired due to an addiction, has been administering assessments for which he or she does not possess the requisite credentials, or has been reporting assessment outcomes inaccurately, the occupational therapist has a responsibility to address the behavior of his or her colleague (AOTA, 2015). Nearly every standard of conduct can be addressed during the evaluation process and through the use of assessments in occupational therapy. Within the changing landscape of health care, occupational therapists need to be ever aware of professional roles and responsibilities and engage in ongoing professional activity to maintain clinical competence.

Assessment and Current Health Care Climate

Coding for occupational therapy evaluation and reevaluation was updated as of January 1, 2017. However, because health care is in a constant state of change, the occupational therapy practitioner is directed to the American Medical Association's *Current Procedural Terminology* (CPT) manual for current information (AOTA, 2017). The change in coding was designed to distinguish different levels of evaluation. This action was advocated by the AOTA to reflect current occupational therapy practice. The new evaluation codes (97165, 97166, 97167) reflect low, moderate, and high complexity. One reevaluation code, 97168, was also included in the updated coding system (AOTA, 2017). The CPT manual identified that occupational therapy evaluations must include an occupational profile (see Chapter 3). The updated coding system assists the occupational therapy practitioner in communicating the complete scope of occupational therapy practice and in promoting the distinct value of the profession (AOTA, 2017).

In determining which code to assign, the occupational therapy practitioner must critically examine three elements: (1) occupational profile and history, (2) assessment of occupational performance and identification of deficits, and (3) clinical decision making. The occupational therapist must ensure that the code chosen ethically represents the patient condition, the analysis of the occupational therapist, and the assessment/identification of the client's performance concerns and goals (AOTA, 2017). For the therapist to code the client at moderate level of complexity, all three areas must be moderate; if one area is low, then the client would be coded low.

First, the occupational therapist considers the occupational profile and history. The key words in choosing a level for this area are the following: brief (low), expanded (moderate), and extensive (high). When the occupational therapy practitioner conducts a brief history and review of medical or therapy records relating to the presenting problem, the code is considered low. An expanded history includes a review of the physical, cognitive, and psychosocial history related to current functional performance. An extensive history includes an additional review of these areas as related to current functional performance.

Second, the occupational therapy practitioner conducts an analysis of occupational performance of the client. An assessment that identifies one to three performance deficits that emanate in activity limitations or participation restrictions would be considered low complexity (AOTA, 2017), with three to five performance deficits indicative of moderate complexity and five or more performance deficits defined as high complexity. Levels of assessment are also considered related to the complexity of the assessment from the perspective of data collection and analysis. Analysis of data from problem-focused assessment is defined as low complexity, detailed assessment is moderate complexity, and comprehensive assessment is high complexity (AOTA, 2017). CPT defines performance deficits in this category as being physical, cognitive, and psychosocial in nature.

Last, the occupational therapy practitioner considers what skills were utilized and what aspects of the client affected the decision-making intensity. Within the area of clinical decision making, the following key words are considered: problem-focused assessment and limit number of treatment options. The finding that a modification of tasks or assistance was not necessary would yield a low complexity code. Moderate complexity relates to a detailed assessment and the consideration of several treatment options and a modification of the task or assistance with assessment was necessary; the client may or may not present with comorbidities. High complexity relates to a comprehensive assessment with consideration of multiple treatment options and a significant modification of tasks or assistance to facilitate the completion of the evaluation (AOTA, 2017).

Although it may appear the new coding system is complex and challenging, the process is clear, and requirements are provided for occupational therapists to identify and justify within documentation of the evaluation process (AOTA, 2017). Within the ever-changing health care climate, occupational therapy practitioners must utilize measures that are reliable and valid and must be able to assess the quality and value of therapeutic services across a variety of clinical practice settings (Leland, Crum, Phipps, Roberts, & Gage, 2015). The sections that follow describe how assessments are organized within the text.

Psychological Dimension

The psychological dimension, the first dimension, "is the ability to process information from past events and information currently available … to view one's self, others, and one's life situation realistically. The psychological dimension is influenced by and derived from the emotions and feelings of the human experience" (Krishnagiri, 2000). Krishnagiri (2000) would include the cognitive aspects of the human in this dimension, but this author prefers to include it in the learning dimension. This is an arbitrary division and only serves to describe testing procedures. In the psychological dimension, Azima and Azima (1959), Fidler (1982), and Mosey (1996) have proposed testing procedures. To support the assessment tool theoretically, theories of Freud (1976), Jung (1954), Maslow (1954), and Rogers (1951) are utilized.

Mosey (1996) coined the term *object relations* to describe a person's relationship to people and occupation—the person's ego function. This part of the patient's psyche helps therapists identify patient needs and body image and to gain insight. Other psychological functions, such as reality contact, intrinsic gratification, body concept, decision making, problem solving, and social relationships, are evaluated. The most effective methods for evaluating these occupational performances are with projective media, such as painting or pencil drawings. The occupational performances in the psychological dimensions can be measured with projective media. The focus is on completion of a task, not on analyzing symbolic content. Although the patient is able to project his or her unconscious needs into symbolic images, it is the responsibility of the therapist to observe the manner in which the task is completed. Viewing the patient in action is valuable when observing how patients express their innermost needs, feelings, and emotions onto the environment.

Projective assessments were developed previously by Azima and Azima (1959), Fidler (1982), Shoemyen (1982), and Hemphill-Pearson (1999), but little has been done to advance their use. Other assessments are the Goodman Battery (Evaskus, 1982), Lerner's (1982) Collage Scoring System, and Build a City (Clark, 1999).

Frequently, the use of projective media will facilitate the expression of religious content. Allowing the patient to express his or her faith tradition is a means by which the therapist can assess the patient's level of spiritual development and his or her concerns about the relationship between his or her disability and faith tradition. In evaluating a mentally ill patient where religious content is presented, it is important for the therapist to distinguish between a mystical experience and religious delusions. Mystics describe their experience as ecstatic and joyful. When they express their experience, the words *serenity, wholeness, transcendence,* and *love* are used. Persons with psychosis are often confused and frightened by the religious hallucinations, which are distressing and often accompanied by an angry God. Both mystics and persons with psychosis experience what appears to be a break from reality. For mystics, this period of withdraw is welcomed. However, when the period ends, they return to normal activity. For the person with psychosis, the withdrawal from reality is involuntary. Delusions can last for years and result in driving the individual into deeper distress. Mystics are often respected members of the community (Newberg, D'Aquili, & Rause, 2002). Another difference is in how each interprets his or her religious experience. Persons with psychosis may have feelings of religious grandiosity and an inflated egotistical importance. They may think they have messages from God or have some spiritual powers. In contrast, mystics experience a state of calm, a loss of pride, and the emptying of the self.

Behavioral Dimension

The second dimension is the behavioral dimension. It draws on the theories of cognitive, behavioral, social, and learning sciences. Techniques such as reinforcement, modeling, token economies, desensitization, biofeedback, and stress management are used as treatment principles. The body of knowledge from occupational therapy literature comes from the writings of Fidler and Velde (1999), Kielhofner (1999), Mosey (1996), and Reilly (1962). In the behavioral dimension, the therapist is concerned with the role the environment plays in the acquisition of behavior for occupational performance. It is important in this dimension to consider the patient's behavior in the context of the environment.

The patient's environment (life space) and the patient's lifestyle are analyzed (Chapter 29). The patient's life space includes the expected environment. For example, it is important to know if the patient is homeless, comes from the inner city, a rural area, or a middle-class neighborhood. The patient's lifestyle (race, ethnic background, value system) influences the assessment process. Combined, the patient's lifestyle and life space can influence the acquisition of behavior. For example, an assessment that is culturally biased will not give a true picture of the patient's disabilities or abilities.

Social interaction process, based on the principle that socialization is a developmental process that results from classical conditioning, is assessed in the behavioral dimension. In this dimension, socialization is not a skill but rather an occupation that an individual acquires through interaction with the environment. The occupations of communication and group interaction are attributes evaluated in this dimension. It is important to identify any environmental barriers that are prohibiting the performance of the activity.

The assessment is generally done by taking a patient's history using interviewing techniques and checklists. Assessments such as the Interest Checklist (Matsutsuyu, 1983), Occupational Role History (Florey & Michelman, 1982), Life Style Performance Profile (Fidler, 1982), Activity Configuration (Spahn, 1965), Adolescent Role Assessment (Black, 1976), History Interview (Henry & Mallinson, 1999), and The Barth Time Construction (Barth, 1988) are used to assess the behavioral dimension. The assessments based on the Model of Human Occupation are included in this dimension. Included in this text are chapters on "The Assessment of Occupational Functioning–Collaborative Version" (Chapter 17) and three summary chapters: "Assessment Used Within the Model of Human Occupation" (Chapter 16), "Role Assessments Used in Mental Health" (Chapter 18), and "Work-Related Assessments: The Worker Role Interview, Work Environment Impact Scale, and Assessment of Work Performance" (Chapter 24).

The behaviors that express the patient's spirituality are included in this dimension. Occupational performances such as religious attendance, praying, reading spiritual material, attending spiritual groups, volunteering, and engaging in activities that have deep spiritual meaning are expressions of a patient's spirituality. Chapter 28, "The OT-QUEST: The Occupational Therapy Quality of Experience and Spirituality Assessment Tool," assesses the spiritual performance of patients.

Learning Dimension

There are two differences between the behavioral and the learning dimension (the third dimension). The first difference is the method of administration. Behavioral assessments are administered by interview only or by interview and task performance. The therapist is interested in learning what is hindering the patient from performing the activity. Learning assessments are administered by task only. The therapist is interested in the performance of a skill. It is important to actually observe the skill in context and determine what is preventing the patient from performing the skill. The second difference is the method of assessment. Learning assessments use scales or some other form of measurement to compare scores, whereas behavioral assessments generally do not.

There are two factors that the therapist must be concerned with when using a learning assessment: the patient's cognitive function and the patient's level of skill development. Cognitive functions have a direct impact on the patient's performance—the ability to learn. However, the therapist is interested in the performance of a skill, not how the patient acquired the skill. Assessments that measure skill do not measure cognitive function; cognitive function is a biological dimension, not a skill function. Finally, the patient's developmental level must be related to the assessment or the task being performed. The therapist cannot ask a 2-year-old to tie his or her shoe when the child is not developmentally ready.

Functions that are assessed in the learning dimension are work skills, activities of daily living, leisure, and social skills. It is most important that the assessment involve a task that simulates a life skill. This is what distinguishes a learning assessment from all other occupational therapy assessments. Even though the same functions appear to be assessed in the behavioral dimension, learning assessments are used by actually performing or simulating the skill. "The Performance Assessment of Self-Care Skills" (Chapter 20), "The Comprehensive Occupational Therapy Evaluation" (Chapter 21), "The Independent Living Scales" (Chapter 22), "Kohlman Evaluation of Living Skills" (Chapter 23), and "The Test of Grocery Shopping Skills" (Chapter 25) are included in this dimension.

In the area of spirituality, the therapist needs to know the patient's faith tradition to understand the problems that might arise when teaching an occupational performance that is influenced by that faith, such as dressing. For example, in some Amish traditions, buttons are not used on clothing. Teaching a person who does not have buttons on his or her clothing how to button would require some creative maneuvering.

Biological Dimension

The fourth dimension is the biological dimension. This area of assessment has received the most attention and research. Its concepts can easily be observed and measured. In the psychological literature, it is referred to as the *biomedical model*. It asserts that abnormality is an illness of the body. The Allen Cognitive Level Screen–5 in Chapter 11 is an assessment that examines the level of cognition with the use of a leather-lacing project. It has been rigorously examined to determine its reliability and validity.

There has been a series of research reporting a connection between spirituality and the mind. The brain is a collection of "physical structures that gather and process sensory, cognitive, and emotional data: the mind is the phenomenon of thoughts, memories, and emotions that arise from the perceptual processes of the brain" (Newberg et al., 2002, p. 33). The brain makes the mind. "Science cannot demonstrate a way for the mind to occur except as a result of the neurological functioning of the brain" (Newberg et al., 2002, p. 33). All that is meaningful in human experience and spirituality happens in the mind. Studies have indicated that the limbic system is integral to religious and spiritual experience. It is the association between areas of the brain that is essential if the individual is going to have a meaningful and spiritual life.

The association areas of the brain are structures that gather together or associate neural information from various parts of the brain. The association areas eventually tap into memory and emotional centers to allow the person to organize and respond to the exterior world. For example, it has been suggested that the visual association area is active in individuals who use images to help facilitate meditation or prayer. There are several association areas in the cerebral cortex: visual, orientation, attention, and verbal. These four association areas are extremely important in patient assessment. They relate to each other and can affect the patient's sense of self, emotional response to activity, and the ability to express religious beliefs. If an area of the brain is affected by trauma, stroke, depression, alcoholism, or drugs, the therapist needs to know the relationship to the patient's faith tradition.

For example, if a patient has a strong religious tradition that believes in using images in worship, such as during communion, and the patient has an injury in the visual association area, he or she will have difficulty relating to these images in recovery. These patients will have trouble praying and using meditation. Damage in the orientation area will cause trouble relating to mystical and religious experiences. The verbal association will make it difficult for the patient to express his or her religious beliefs. This dimension within the text is addressed in a chapter on "Spiritual Assessments in Mental Health Occupational Therapy" (Chapter 27) as well as the "The OT-QUEST: The Occupational Therapy Quality of Experience and Spirituality Assessment Tool" (Chapter 28).

Summary

In developing a client's profile, the therapist gathers information from a wide variety of sources. This includes information obtained from the client, the family, and his or her medical, spiritual, and cultural history. This information can be obtained through standard and nonstandard testing, by interviewing the client, and from his or her environment. This chapter presented four dimensions that may be used to gather and integrate information about patients in order to develop a profile. The integrative approach to develop a client's profile is based on a holistic triad—mind, body, and spirit. In an attempt to present a holistic approach to assessments, spirituality was added to the discussion. There is a suggestion that more than one assessment from competing frames of reference can be used to achieve a holistic approach. Therefore, the integrative approach to patient assessment draws on the concepts and philosophy of occupational therapy. The principles in the *Framework* developed by the AOTA (2014) are the guidelines used during the assessment process, and this chapter utilizes the *Framework* and integrates the language of applying assessments to the evaluative process. Many of the assessments are currently being developed, and it cannot be overemphasized that ongoing assessment development and research in mental health is desirable.

References

American Occupational Therapy Association. (2014). Occupational therapy practice framework: Domain and process (3rd ed.). *American Journal of Occupational Therapy, 68*(Suppl. 1), S1-S48.

American Occupational Therapy Association. (2015). Occupational therapy code of ethics. *American Journal of Occupational Therapy, 69*(Suppl. 3).

American Occupational Therapy Association. (2017). *New occupational therapy evaluation coding overview.* Retrieved from https://www.aota.org/~/media/Corporate/Files/Advocacy/Federal/Evaluation-Codes-Overview-2016.pdf

Asher, I. E. (2014). *Occupational therapy assessment tools* (4th ed.). Bethesda, MD: AOTA Press.

Azima, H., & Azima, F. (1959). Outline of a dynamic theory of occupational therapy. *American Journal of Occupational Therapy, 8*, 215.

Barth, T. (1988). Barth time construction. In B. Hemphill (Ed.), *Mental health assessment in occupational therapy: An integrative approach to the evaluative process* (pp. 115-129). Thorofare, NJ: SLACK Incorporated.

Black, M. (1976). Adolescent role assessment. *American Journal of Occupational Therapy, 30*, 73-79.

Clark, E. (1999). Build a City. In B. Hemphill-Pearson (Ed.), *Assessments in occupational therapy mental health: An integrative approach* (pp. 155-170). Thorofare, NJ: SLACK Incorporated.

Evaskus, M. (1982). The Goodman Battery. In B. Hemphill (Ed.), *The evaluative process in occupational therapy* (pp. 85-125). Thorofare, NJ: SLACK Incorporated.

Fidler, G. (1982). The lifestyle performance profile: An organizational frame. In B. Hemphill (Ed.), *The evaluative process in psychiatric occupational therapy* (pp. 43-47). Thorofare NJ: SLACK Incorporated.

Fidler, G., & Velde, B. (1999). *Activities: Reality and symbol.* Thorofare, NJ: SLACK Incorporated.

Florey, L. L., & Michelman, S. M. (1982). Occupational role history: A screening tool for psychiatric occupational therapy. *American Journal of Occupational Therapy, 36*, 301-308.

Freud, S. (1976). Psychical (or mental) treatment. In J. Starchey (Ed.), *The complete psychological work.* New York, NY: W. W. Norton & Company.

Hemphill, B. J. (1982). *The evaluative process in psychiatric occupational therapy.* Thorofare, NJ: SLACK Incorporated.

Hemphill-Pearson, B. (1999). How to use the B.H. Battery. In B. Hemphill-Pearson (Ed.), *Assessments in occupational therapy mental health: An integrative approach* (pp. 139-152). Thorofare, NJ: SLACK Incorporated.

Henry, A., & Mallinson, T. (1999). The occupational performance history interview. In B. Hemphill-Pearson (Ed.), *Assessments in occupational therapy mental health: An integrative approach* (pp. 59-70). Thorofare, NJ: SLACK Incorporated.

Jung, C. (1954). *Man and his symbols.* Garden City, NY: Harper and Row.

Kielhofner, G. (1999). *A model of human occupation: Theory and application* (2nd ed.). Baltimore, MD: Williams & Wilkins.

Krishnagiri, S. (2000). Occupations and their dimensions. In J. Hinojosa & M. Blount (Eds.), *The texture of life: Purposeful activities in occupational therapy*. Bethesda, MD: AOTA Press.

Leland, N. E., Crum, K., Phipps, S., Roberts, P., & Gage, B. (2015). Advancing the value and quality of occupational therapy in health service delivery. *American Journal of Occupational Therapy, 69*(1), 1-7.

Lerner, C. (1982). The magazine picture collage. In B. Hemphill (Ed.), *The evaluative process in occupational therapy* (pp. 139-154). Thorofare, NJ: SLACK Incorporated.

Maslow, A. H. (1954). *Motivation and personality*. New York, NY: Harper and Row.

Matsutsuyu, J. (1983). The Interest Checklist. *American Journal of Occupational Therapy, 23*, 323-328.

Mosey, A. C. (1996). *Psychosocial components of occupational therapy*. New York, NY: Raven Press.

Newberg, A., D'Aquili, E., & Rause, V. (2002). *Why God won't go away*. New York, NY: Ballantine Books.

Padilla, R., & Griffiths, Y. (Eds.). (2017). *The Eleanor Clarke Slagle Lectures in occupational therapy 1955-2016: A professional legacy centennial edition*. Bethesda, MD: AOTA Press.

Reilly, M. (1962). Occupational therapy can be one of the great ideas of the 20th century medicine. *American Journal of Occupational Therapy, 16*, 1-9.

Rogers, C. (1951). *Client-centered therapy*. Boston, MA: Houghton-Mifflin.

Shoemyen, C. (1982). The Shoemyen Battery. In B. Hemphill (Ed.), *The evaluative process in psychiatric occupational therapy* (pp. 63-83). Thorofare, NJ: SLACK Incorporated.

Spahn, R. (1965). *The patient gets busy: Change or process*. Paper presented at the meeting of the American Orthopsychiatric Society, New York, NY.

Evidence-Based Practice and Assessment in Occupational Therapy

Christine K. Urish, PhD, OTR/L, BCMH, FAOTA

The conscientious, explicit and judicious use of current best evidence is making decisions about the care of individual patients.
(Sackett, Rosenberg, Gray, Haynes, & Richardson, 1996, p. 312)

During the 2000 Eleanor Clarke Slagle Lecture, lecturer Margo B. Holm directed occupational therapy practitioners toward a mandate of becoming evidence-based practitioners (Holm, 2000): "The fact that patient outcomes are improved with occupational therapy services is no longer sufficient to justify our services, unless we can also explain what we do and how we do it so that others can replicate our interventions and achieve similar outcomes with comparable patients with like needs, wants, and expectations" (Holm, 2000, p. 576). Although it has been nearly 2 decades since this lecture was given, occupational therapists are continuing to address the importance of utilizing best evidence to move the profession forward in research, education, and clinical practice. When engaging in clinical decision making within clinical practice, occupational therapy practitioners must consider their experience, the external scientific evidence available, and the client's situations and values (Brown, 2017). A study conducted in 2016 found that occupational therapists practicing in mental health settings had a positive attitude toward evidence-based practice (EBP); however, individuals with more clinical experience were less positive in their attitudes toward EBP (Hitch, 2016). Hitch (2016) stated that advanced qualifications (experience) may exert a more positive impact upon attitudes, but further research was suggested.

Several official documents exist within the profession of occupational therapy that illuminate the necessity for EBP. The *Standards of Continuing Competence*, developed by the Commission on Continuing Competence and Professional Development, state that occupational therapy practitioners are responsible for the integration of relevant evidence

Hemphill, B. J., & Urish, C. K. (Eds.). *Assessments in Occupational Therapy Mental Health: An Integrative Approach, Fourth Edition* (pp. 15-35). © 2020 Taylor & Francis Group.

for the patient populations they serve and should demonstrate the ability to meet clients' needs, as well as the demands of a dynamic profession (American Occupational Therapy Association [AOTA], 2015b). The *Standards of Continuing Competence* further indicate that practitioners are responsible for the synthesis and application of evidence from a variety of sources, including collaboration with the patient in making clinical decisions (AOTA, 2015b). Lastly, the *Standards of Continuing Competence* directs practitioners to continually update their performance based on the most current research and evidence available (AOTA, 2015b).

The AOTA's (2015a) *Occupational Therapy Code of Ethics* affirms the importance of EBP in providing the best care possible to the client related to the concept of beneficence (i.e., to do good). Further, the *Occupational Therapy Practice Framework: Domain and Process, Third Edition* (AOTA, 2014) directs practitioners to conduct analysis of occupational performance as an evaluative step within the occupational therapy process. During this phase of the occupational therapy process, the patient's assets, problems, or potential problems are identified. Performance skills, performance patterns, context or contexts, activity demands, and patient factors are taken into consideration, and the practitioner chooses areas of assessment based on these aspects. Specific patient outcomes are identified. On completion of the analysis of occupational performance, an intervention plan is developed. Intervention is implemented and a review of the intervention is conducted to ascertain progress toward targeted outcomes (AOTA, 2014). Therefore, assessment in the occupational therapy process is a mechanism to identify patient functional limitations and facilitate the development of an effective intervention plan, as well as to determine whether the intervention that was implemented was effective in the facilitation of improved function and change in occupational performance. During this process, practitioners are directed to use all available evidence from scientific, narrative, pragmatic, and ethical aspects of clinical reasoning to facilitate the selection of assessments and the gathering of evaluation data (AOTA, 2014). Assessments that are utilized during the evaluation process should be valid and reliable and should illuminate the areas of occupational performance in which the patient has limitations. Upon completion of assessment, intervention approaches are chosen based on best practice and evidence. The intervention plan is to be developed in collaboration with the patient, which is another aspect of the use of EBP in occupational therapy. In intervention review, the intervention plan is reexamined, and patient outcomes are considered to determine whether the plan should be modified and intervention should be continued or whether occupational therapy services should be discontinued or the patient referred elsewhere (AOTA, 2014).

What Is Evidence-Based Practice?

EBP in health care service delivery has been identified as an important consideration in psychiatric occupational therapy that should be strengthened (Tsang, 2002). Further, it has been suggested that occupational therapists speak up about their profession and voice the positive outcomes and evidence that exist within the profession (Dickinson, 2003). Through presentation of evidence-based information about the profession of occupational therapy, decision makers and patients may come to attach an increased value for the services occupational therapy practitioners provide (Dickinson, 2003). EBP has been defined within medicine by Sackett et al. (1996); however, the definition of EBP within occupational therapy differs somewhat from the definition proposed by Sackett et al. An evidence-based occupational therapy practice uses research evidence combined with clinical knowledge and reasoning to facilitate clinical decision making regarding what interventions are effective for specific clients (Law, Baum, & Dunn, 2017). The need for EBP has come from an increased demand for accountability combined with ongoing restraint in health care spending. These needs have facilitated an increased interest in the use of research evidence within the practice of occupational therapy.

The desire for documented outcomes in health care is not a new concept (Foto, 1996; Fuller, 2011). Payers and policy makers continue to demand objective evidence of treatment efficacy and cost effectiveness of occupational therapy services. Through the utilization of EBP in occupational therapy, assessment of patient outcomes can provide information regarding the outcomes of a variety of interventions and meet the needs of payers and policy makers (Foto, 1996). Occupational therapy practitioners have a responsibility to utilize an evidence-based perspective. Patients expect this kind of practice, and, as a profession, we have an obligation to ensure we are providing the best practice; furthermore, we need to demonstrate our ability to provide quality services that are of value and provide the best outcomes at minimum cost (Law et al., 2017). The goal of EBP in occupational therapy is to provide improved intervention to the patient that is supported by assessments that are based upon solid evidence (Brown, 2017). Occupational therapy outcomes in psychiatric occupational therapy need to be documented through research by professionals outside of the discipline (Tsang, 2002). The benefit of research-based EBP is that the knowledge obtained from critical review of research can facilitate change that has the potential to expand the body of occupational therapy knowledge (Brown & Rodger, 1999). EBP in occupational therapy focuses on therapeutic practice that is valid and that considers safety and value. EBP is not based solely on opinion, past clinical practice, or precedent (Brown & Rodger, 1999).

What Is Not Evidence-Based Practice?

One problem in this area is that EBP has not been well-defined from a universal perspective. As a result, confusion may be present among researchers, practitioners, and payers (LaGrossa, 2003). Different individuals may feel strongly about one aspect or another from an evidence-based perspective, and, as a result, subtle variations of terminology and how terminology is utilized are present within the health care arena (LaGrossa, 2003). EBP in occupational therapy does not mean that the practitioner sets aside his or her own professional knowledge or expertise. Rather, EBP means that the practitioner focuses on the integration and utilization of research knowledge in conjunction with clinical judgment, expertise, and patient choice (Law et al., 2017). EBP does not mean that all patients who come to receive occupational therapy services with similar occupational performance concerns will be provided with the same assessment and intervention (Lim, Frater, & Samaras, 2014). Another myth about EBP is that it is based entirely on research and fails to take into consideration the occupational therapy practitioner's knowledge, clinical judgment, or expertise. EBP relies on the clinical knowledge and judgment of the practitioner as one piece of the evidence in making clinical decisions (Lim et al., 2014). Research and patient contributions are the other essential elements. The goal of EBP is to provide the best care to the patient through thoughtful consideration and evaluation of all of the evidence available and does not deny the clinical judgment and expertise of the occupational therapy practitioner (Lim et al., 2014).

Goal of Evidence-Based Assessment in Mental Health

The goal of EBP is to include the best evidence available for the assessment, intervention planning, intervention implementation, and outcomes monitoring for each patient who receives occupational therapy services. Ultimately, the goal is to provide patients with the most appropriate intervention (Gutman, 2011). Improved function may follow when the occupational therapy practitioner uses evidence to choose appropriate areas to assess in each patient he or she is serving, plans interventions based on the outcomes of the assessment, and considers the patient's values, needs, and goals, along with the best evidence available. Occupational therapy practitioners who work in the adult mental health discipline were reported to be challenged integrating standardized assessment measures to document effectiveness of occupational therapy services within daily practice (Fuller, 2011). One study found that 68.4% of Canadian occupational therapists used one standardized assessment measure when working with individuals diagnosed with depression and schizophrenia while providing inpatient and community-based care (Rouleau, Dion, & Korner-Bitensky, 2015); this study also reported that the Canadian Occupational Performance Measure (Chapter 4) was utilized most frequently across clinical settings and diagnoses studied.

Improving Intervention Outcomes Through Assessment/Intervention

When assessments are selected that have proven to be valid and reliable and are used to facilitate the planning of intervention that has been proven to be effective, ongoing evidence can be generated and added to the body of knowledge within the profession of occupational therapy. This procedure would be described as best practice, and occupational therapy practitioners have an obligation to provide therapeutic intervention according to best practice (Law et al., 2017).

Best Practice in Measurement

One of the most essential considerations with regard to EBP in occupational therapy is the consistent use of outcome measures to evaluate services (Law et al., 2017). Information from outcome measures facilitates decision making as to which programs and services are most effective and adds to the body of knowledge, which builds evidence to support the ongoing provision of occupational therapy interventions. Occupational therapy practitioners are directed to "mine the gold" in considering what researchers in other disciplines have found regarding how individuals interact with their environment to perform tasks. This action can further the profession of occupational therapy through the development of advanced thinking and clinical practices based on the critical review and analysis of available research literature (Law et al., 2017).

Occupational therapy practitioners are directed to become systematic in the choice and utilization of measures that formalize observation and interview data collected within occupational therapy practice. Creating a systematic plan can assist other professionals in viewing the importance and necessity of occupational therapy services. When others cannot understand the how and why of occupational therapy assessment and intervention, our professional practice may be challenged as possibly unscientific or lacking evidence rather than viewed from a formal professional evidence-based perspective (Law et al., 2017).

The use of evidence in practice is essential due to the changes in service delivery, funding mechanisms, and increased pressure to demonstrate service efficacy (Law et al., 2017). Individuals who consume occupational therapy services are more informed regarding their choices through the use of the internet and various media. This raises the occupational therapy practitioner's need to be knowledgeable of and provide evidence-based assessment and intervention. Use of EBP provides a means for the occupational therapy practitioner to stay current with regard to what is known about specific conditions and problems. EBP offers the practitioner the opportunity to critique and apply relevant research knowledge to clinical practice. Further, the use of EBP can facilitate critical discussion with the service recipient and the patient's care provider with regard to various interventions. Through this action, the potential risks and benefits of various intervention choices can be discussed and analyzed. Effectiveness of interventions can be considered to determine whether changes should be instituted during the course of therapy (Law et al., 2017).

When occupational therapy practitioners utilize measures that were developed by or used within other disciplines, they must be extremely mindful of the need to articulate how occupational therapy views problems or solutions differently than the other disciplines that may utilize these measures (Law et al., 2017). When occupational therapy practitioners use measures that other professionals use but do not make explicit the significant contribution of occupational therapy from an occupation-focused perspective, others will be unaware of the important contribution that occupational therapists can make. An example would be when considering the context of environment. Social workers may consider environment but may be more concerned with addressing the social or cultural concerns within the environment, whereas from an occupational therapy perspective, the concern may be the physical and temporal features present within the environment that may facilitate or hinder an individual's performance (Law et al., 2017).

It is essential in the context of measurement that we practice from a patient-centered perspective (Law et al., 2017). What this means in terms of assessment is that occupational therapy practitioners need to identify assessments that illuminate the problems experienced by the patient. Occupational therapy practitioners need to direct their resources toward addressing specific concerns regarding the occupational performance raised by the patient and the patient's priorities. The assessments that occupational therapy practitioners choose need to facilitate this process (Law et al., 2017). In considering possible assessments to use, practitioners should first critique the measure in terms of its focus, sensitivity to change, standardization, reliability, validity, strengths, and weaknesses, as well as the overall relevance of the assessment to the problems the therapist wishes to address with the patient.

Assessment from an EBP perspective provides a means for the occupational therapy practitioner to provide information to the patient about what is known and what is not known about the effectiveness of assessments and interventions. Rapport can be facilitated through this use of EBP. The therapist is in active dialogue with the patient concerning the outcomes of an assessment and the appropriate interventions to be selected (Law et al., 2017). Utilization of EBP facilitates a change in the role of the occupational therapist. Occupational therapy practitioners are considered experts in their area of professional knowledge; however, patients need to be considered because the individual who lives the experience of functional limitation has an increased perspective and should not be discounted from the process (Law et al., 2017). When including the patient in the EBP process, information needs to be provided in a manner that the patient can easily understand. Extensive use of professional terminology or jargon is not suggested. When using an evidence-based approach, occupational therapy practitioners need to embrace the fact that interventions may evolve from dialogue with the patient. This differs from previous practice, which may not have included the patient in this discussion and in which the therapist selected interventions in advance and in isolation from the patient's input (Law et al., 2017).

Searching and Evaluating the Evidence in Assessment

Developing an effective search and evaluation strategy is an essential component of the utilization of EBP (Tickle-Degnen, 1998). Further, being able to understand and interpret different types of reviews (e.g., mixed methods review, systematic review, meta-analysis review, rapid review, scoping review) are important skills for the occupational therapy practitioner to possess (Unsworth, 2017).

How to Search for Best Evidence

The amount of professional literature available each month to occupational therapy practitioners can make it seem daunting to try to stay current (Law et al., 2017). Colleges or universities may offer assistance to clinicians by providing access to medical and health literature resources, including print journals, online journals, and computerized databases. Many resources exist on the internet to assist the occupational therapy practitioner in the development of effective searching strategies (Bennett, 2017). To manage the volume of resources available in the medical literature, occupational therapy practitioners should consider establishing a surveillance strategy (Hall-Flavin, 2005). This means that the practitioner chooses a small number of journals whose focus is central to his or her daily clinical practice and reviews a limited number of more general health-related areas (Hall-Flavin, 2005). Alternatively, if there are several therapists in a clinic who have an interest in different areas of clinical practice, but who wish to stay as current as possible with evidence-based literature, they could form a journal club. Using a journal club, occupational therapy practitioners would report on the findings from their own reviews of the literature and professional discussion could occur regarding the information obtained. Through the use of this mechanism, therapists may be able to better manage the plethora of information they are confronted with in their desire to seek out and consume research information to facilitate EBP.

Collaboration is key to EBP (Coster, 2004), and occupational therapy practitioners must collaborate. When a practitioner discovers a resource or new technique or procedure, the practitioner has a professional duty to share this information with colleagues. Active collaboration and sharing in this manner saves time and makes it so no one person feels as if he or she is reinventing the wheel (Coster, 2004). One suggestion for the sharing of knowledge is to develop an EBP tips sheet. When an individual identifies new information that could be shared with others, he or she could record it on a sheet or form and then this form is duplicated to share with all staff members.

Several EBP databases should be considered by occupational therapy practitioners when searching for best evidence regarding potential assessments and interventions

Table 2-1

Available Websites and Databases for Accessing Evidence-Based Research Literature

Name	URL
American Occupational Therapy Association Evidence Briefs Series (must be an AOTA member to access)	https://www.aota.org/Practice/Researchers/practice-guidelines.aspx
OTseeker (Occupational Therapy Systematic Evaluation of Evidence)	http://www.otseeker.com
PubMed	https://www.ncbi.nlm.nih.gov/pubmed/
University of York Centre for Reviews and Dissemination	http://www.york.ac.uk/inst/crd/crddatabases.htm#DARE
Cochrane	http://www.cochrane.org/index.htm
Bandolier	http://www.bandolier.org.uk
National Guideline Clearinghouse	https://www.thecommunityguide.org/resources/national-guideline-clearinghouse
Open Access Peer-Reviewed Journals (*The Open Journal of Occupational Therapy*; Physical Therapy and Rehabilitation Journals)	http://scholarworks.wmich.edu/ojot https://www.omicsonline.org/physicaltherapy-rehabilitation-journals.php
American Occupational Therapy Association Guidelines for Critically Appraised Paper	https://www.aota.org/Practice/Researchers.aspx
HighWire	http://highwire.stanford.edu/lists/browse.dtl

they may use with patients. These databases are divided into two basic categories—unscreened (unfiltered) and screened (filtered; Table 2-1). Unscreened databases contain articles from journals that have not been screened according to a predetermined quality standard. Each journal has a peer-review process, and these reviews provide a primary quality check. MEDLINE and the Cumulative Index to Nursing and Allied Health Literature (CINAHL) are databases that would fit into this category. Journal articles that are accessed through these sources should be scrutinized by the practitioner to determine the quality of the evidence contained within the article (Wong, Barr, Farina, & Lusardi, 2000). Screened databases are prefiltered, and articles are selectively chosen for inclusion based on a minimum rating on a scoring system that addresses the scientific rigor of the research. The Cochrane Library is an example of a screened database. Other databases provide a synthesis and/or summarization of evidence and provide recommendations related to clinical practice; OTseeker is an example. Clinical guidelines provide the occupational therapy practitioner with recommendations that can be used to assist in clinical decision making. Guidelines are developed by experts within any given field (Wong et al., 2000). Systematic reviews and randomized controlled trials are important sources of data utilized in the development of clinical guidelines. The Agency for Healthcare Research and Quality has developed clinical guidelines in a variety of clinical areas. EBP reports in psychiatry exist for mental health conditions and substance abuse (Agency for Healthcare

Research and Quality, 2017). When entering the phrase "occupational therapy and mental health" into the National Guidelines Clearinghouse database, 73 related items were identified (National Clearinghouse Guidelines, 2017). Advantages and disadvantages to the use of clinical guidelines exist (Roberts & Barber, 2001).

The usefulness of clinical practice guidelines in ongoing clinical practice should be critiqued by occupational therapy practitioners (Stergiou-Kita, 2010). Clinical practice guidelines may be easier to use with some areas of practice than with others. Guidelines are just that; they may not provide the specific, straightforward solution that the practitioner desires (Roberts & Barber, 2001). Most of the developed guidelines for medicine and nursing are for specific conditions. However, when providing intervention for individuals who present with complex and multiple disabilities, the use of clinical practice guidelines may not be as straightforward as the practitioner would like (Roberts & Barber, 2001).

Evaluating the Evidence

Once studies have been obtained or guidelines secured, occupational therapy practitioners are directed to ask specific questions that can facilitate the review and evaluation of information obtained (Tickle-Degnen, 1998). When researching the literature, if meta-analysis is available, one should attempt to secure research articles of this nature. A meta-analysis can potentially save time because it summarizes the statistical findings from a large number of individual research studies. Research participants in the studies selected for review need to be critically examined to determine whether they are similar to the patient for whom the occupational therapy practitioner will be assessing and providing intervention (Tickle-Degnen, 1998). Next, the assessment or intervention presented in the article needs to be considered. Would it address the functional concerns of the patient in the area of assessment or the needs and attributes of the patient in the area of intervention? Then, the assessment or intervention should be considered for practicality. Is the assessment practical to administer in the practitioner's setting in terms of resources of time, funding, personnel, and equipment? Does it possess good reliability and validity? Lastly, is the outcome obtained from the intervention one that the occupational therapy practitioner intends to work toward with the patient for whom he or she is providing intervention (Law et al., 2017)? In considering all of these areas, the occupational therapy practitioner must also consider the level of evidence provided by the research.

Because occupational therapy practitioners were concerned about the application of Sackett et al.'s (1996) levels of evidence related to occupational therapy research evidence, the AOTA developed a classification system to address these concerns. The classification system being used by the AOTA within the evidence-based literature review project includes a level of evidence coding format that takes into consideration the design, sample size, internal validity, and external validity of a study to assign a level of evidence (Liberman & Scheer, 2002). Level of evidence for research design is coded as follows:

- Randomized controlled trial is considered level of evidence I.
- Nonrandomized controlled trial with two groups is level of evidence II.
- Nonrandomized controlled trial with one group addressing one treatment condition, with a pre-test and post-test, is considered level of evidence III.
- A research study with a single subject design is level of evidence IV.
- Narratives and case studies are identified as NA in the level of evidence for the research design (Liberman & Scheer, 2002).

The sample size of a study also receives a rating. Studies with greater than 20 participants per condition (experimental and control) receive a level of evidence rating of A. Studies with fewer than 20 participants per condition receive a level of evidence rating of B. A 3-point system has been identified for rating internal validity within a study. Level I is assigned to studies with high internal validity that demonstrated no alternative explanation for the outcomes obtained within the study. Level II is assigned to studies with moderate internal validity in which the study attempted to control for a lack of randomization. Level III is assigned to studies that demonstrated low internal validity, as when two or more serious alternative explanations could be provided for the outcome obtained within the study (Liberman & Scheer, 2002).

External validity is evaluated as well. Studies that present a high level of external validity, in which participants represent the populations and interventions were representative of current practice, receive a level of evidence rating of a. Moderate external validity in a study is assigned a level of evidence rating of b. Low external validity rating, in which the sample was heterogeneous and one is not able to ascertain whether the outcomes presented within the study were similar for all diagnoses or the intervention provided does not reflect current practice, receives a level of evidence rating of c (Liberman & Scheer, 2002).

Therefore, a study with a level of evidence rating IA2a would be a randomized controlled trial with greater than 20 participants per conditions with a moderate level of internal validity and a high level of external validity. Although disagreements exist from a variety of different disciplines regarding levels of evidence, there are interventions being utilized widely within clinical practice in psychiatry that have not been supported by research (Torrey et al., 2001).

Process of Evidence-Based Practice

The ability to obtain research information to facilitate EBP can be developed through the formation of partnerships with patients, service providers, researchers, payers, and policy makers, as well as in the educational curriculum (Moyers & Finch-Guthrie, 2016; Stube & Jedlicka, 2007). The changing nature of mental health services places occupational therapy practitioners at a crossroads, needing to be able to clearly demonstrate the effectiveness of the services being provided. As a result, it is increasingly important for occupational therapists to know how to engage in the process of searching for best evidence to assist them in selecting and implementing the most effective interventions in practice (Lloyd, Bassett, & King, 2004). There are five steps to utilizing an evidence-based approach in occupational therapy practice. These steps, in conjunction with patient collaboration and the practitioner's clinical reasoning skills, form the basis for evidence-based occupational therapy practice (Bennett & Bennett, 2000; Brown, 2017):

1. Formulating clinical questions
2. Searching the literature and sorting the evidence
3. Critically reviewing and appraising the evidence
4. Applying applicable findings to practice
5. Evaluating the effect/outcomes: Reassessing the evidence-based practice process

Formulating Clinical Questions

Questions that arise from everyday clinical practice related to therapy, prevention, etiology and harm, diagnosis, prognosis, and economic analysis can become the basis of a clinical question. The key to effective searching of electronic evidence available on the internet and through electronic databases is the formulation of a clear question (Bennett & Bennett, 2000; Brown, 2017). Questions can relate to assessments or to intervention effectiveness or can be descriptive to the gathering of more information about patients with specific occupational performance limitations (e.g., what is the effectiveness of occupational therapy in the context of recovery model in the areas of community integration for adults with severe and persistent mental illness; AOTA, 2011). Another example question is "Do older adult women in the community with depression experience a difference in activity participation from those who are not diagnosed with depression?" (Tickle-Degnen, 2000). The occupational therapy practitioner may wish to gain information on a variety of different types of evidence in addition to the usefulness of an assessment. Other questions may include those related to the efficacy of an intervention, the description of a condition, the clinical outcome prediction, and the individual lived experience of a client (Brown, 2017). An effective method for the development of a clinical question is the use of patient/problem/population, intervention, comparison of intervention, and outcome (PICO). Examples of questions are:

P: How could a practitioner describe a group of patients similar to the patient I am interested in securing information about?

I: What intervention am I considering for use?

C: What is the alternative to the intervention I have identified, or what is another intervention for which I would like to make a comparison?

O: What is the outcome I would like to measure? What improvement is desired (UIC: University Library, 2017)?

An example of an intervention effectiveness question could be the following: "What are the most effective interventions for increasing participation in satisfying daily life activities among elderly women with depression who live in the community?" (Tickle-Degnen, 2000, p. 103). Another approach is a PICOTT (Medical University of South Carolina, 2017). The TT added at the end of PICO are acronyms for the type of question (i.e., diagnosis, therapy, prognosis, etiology/harm, prevention) and for the type of study design (e.g., randomized controlled trial, cohort study, case series). Therefore, instead of stopping at PICO, some occupational therapy practitioners may choose to be more specific with PICOTT.

Searching the Literature and Sorting the Evidence

Searching the literature was addressed earlier in this chapter. Planning a search strategy through development of a PICO or PICOTT and then keeping a record of the databases searched and the terms utilized is an effective strategy. If occupational therapy practitioners do not have access to medical and health databases through their place of employment, making connections with colleges and universities may yield access to these resources. Some colleges and universities may welcome partnering with practitioners (Moyers & Finch-Guthrie, 2016). Students enrolled in educational programs need to learn research strategies and may be available as a resource to access the resources desired and present their findings.

Considering the level of evidence and the type of research findings that relate to the PICO or PICOTT question posed is key. The occupational therapy practitioner needs to be able to effectively rank the research evidence that was available and the ability of the research to answer the PICO or PICOTT question. Secondary evidence through systematic reviews and meta-analysis studies can provide the practitioner with a good deal of information that has been summarized and possibly simplified to provide a trustworthy presentation of previously conducted research in a specific area of interest (Unsworth, 2017).

Critically Reviewing and Appraising the Evidence

To effectively critique the evidence obtained, occupational therapy practitioners may need to update their research knowledge. Understanding various research designs, methodologies, and statistics will facilitate the effective review and appraisal of available evidence. In appraising the available evidence, the power of a research study, randomization, and clinical significance need to be considered. To determine whether an intervention was effective, one must consider whether the number of participants who participated in the study was sufficient to determine statistical significance or the power to detect change (Bennett & Bennett, 2000; Brown, 2017). Random assignment is an important consideration when examining the causal relationship between the intervention and the outcome obtained. Statistical significance is most commonly established such that a 95% likelihood exists that the effects obtained were due to the intervention, with a 5% likelihood that the results were due to chance. Clinical significance assists the therapist in examining the results from a different perspective and may seem more practical to the occupational therapy practitioner. Results that do not indicate statistical significance may be deemed clinically significant if some change, but not a statistically significant change, occurred. Some occupational therapy practitioners have expressed concern with regard to the interpretation of statistics contained within research papers. The internet is a helpful resource, containing statistical tutorials. Journal articles such as "How to Read and Understand a Scientific Paper: A Step-by-Step Guide for Non-Scientists" (Raff, 2014), "How to Read a Paper: Statistics for the Non-Statistician I: Different Data Need Different Statistical Tests" (Greenhaigh, 1997a), and "How to Read a Paper: Statistics for the Non-Statistician II: Significance, Relations and Their Pitfalls" (Greenhaigh, 1997b) could be of great assistance. Critical examination of the rigor of the study design, outcome measures chosen to examine the variable of interest, level of evidence, sample size, and internal and external validity need to be considered when reviewing the evidence (Brown, 2017).

Occupational therapy practitioners can also ask themselves the following questions to facilitate review of literature (Bennett & Bennett, 2000; Tickle-Degnen, 1998):

- Were the participants in the research similar to the patient or patients for whom information is being reviewed?
- Did the intervention presented in the study meet the needs of the therapist and the patient?
- Was the intervention in the study practical to implement in terms of time, money, equipment, and required personnel in comparison to other intervention options?
- Was the outcome that was measured an outcome that was identified as important and desired by the patient?

Applying Applicable Findings to Practice

It is important that occupational therapy practitioners collaborate to collect and share research evidence and strategies that have proven successful to change practice. Success in this area will assist in ensuring good quality and effective services to patients (Roberts & Barber, 2001). Once research findings have been obtained and reviewed, application of these findings depends on patient factors and problems, practitioner clinical reasoning and expertise, and institutional factors (Brown, 2017). During this step of the process, ongoing and effective communication with the patient is significant. Information needs to relate to the patient's needs and concerns and be presented in a clear manner (Tickle-Degnen, 1998).

Evaluating the Effect/Outcomes: Reassessing the Evidence-Based Practice Process

The last step of the process is the evaluation of the entire process. Examination of the procedures undertaken and reflection on the effectiveness or ineffectiveness of the process can facilitate changes and improvements that could be implemented (Bennett & Bennett, 2000).

It was reported that education-based approaches that incorporated methods to improve the clinician's knowledge and skills, in addition to an organizational approach that facilitated collaboration, teamwork, and effective leadership, were effective for implementing EBP (Stube & Jedlicka, 2007). In considering professional development and to begin incorporating EBP into one's clinical repertoire, one should allocate time for reflection on the patients and current practice. Keeping a notebook of the clinical questions that arise during assessment and intervention can be one method of facilitating reflection regarding clinical practice. Ongoing search of the literature for information on trends in evidence for occupational therapy in mental health can be helpful and provide insight and significant overview for the future direction of the occupational therapy practitioner (Hitch, Pepin, & Stagnitti, 2015).

Collaboration with colleagues on setting clinic priorities and working with one another to share knowledge and research resources is a good suggestion to foster collaboration and interprofessional EBP (Finch-Guthrie, 2016). Practitioners are directed to access quality information and use their skills to critically appraise the information obtained. Some practitioners may need to attend continuing education courses to increase their knowledge of research design and bias to increase their ability to determine the quality of the information available.

Practitioners should identify their current practice and compare this practice with a benchmark (Menon, Korner-Bitensky, Kastner, McKinnon, & Straus, 2009). In considering where their practice is and where they would like it to be, practitioners are directed to develop an improvement plan that is reasonable and doable. In consideration of their plan for change, practitioners must identify barriers to making the change and determine how these barriers can be overcome. Development of a plan for ongoing education can include taking continuing education courses, participating in a clinic-based journal club, completing critically appraised topics on the most recently published research literature, and reviewing critically appraised topics and disseminating this information to clinic colleagues. Practitioners are encouraged to consistently and continually reassess their progress (Menon et al., 2009). Are the assessments chosen yielding valid and reliable results? Are the interventions planned and implemented proving to be effective based on outcomes data?

Evaluating Evidence Using the Canadian Occupational Performance Measure

Research for literature assessing the Canadian Occupational Performance Measure (COPM; Chapter 4) was conducted online via PubMed and CINAHL. This research yielded a clinical review of the instrument published in 2004 (Carswell, McColl, Baptiste, Law, Polatajko, & Pollock). In addition, a manual search was conducted to secure articles that addressed the COPM that were not included within the database. Articles were considered for this review if the COPM was identified in the article title or abstract and if the article addressed one of the following: (1) the psychometric properties, (2) contribution to research outcomes, or (3) contribution to occupational therapy practice. This review yielded 88 articles, of which 76 could be placed into one of the three categories previously mentioned (Carswell et al., 2004).

If this review were not available, the occupational therapy practitioner could access similar information regarding the COPM assessment by conducting individual searches using CINAHL or PubMed by entering the term "Canadian Occupational Performance Measure" and other descriptive terms, such as a population of individuals with whom they are working (i.e., patients with mental health concerns or homeless individuals; Carswell et al., 2004).

The review included articles on the use of the COPM published in 35 different journals (Carswell et al., 2004). In considering the psychometric properties of the COPM, 19 articles examined the reliability, validity, and responsiveness of the instrument. The studies reviewed indicated strong test-retest reliability. In general, the studies reviewed indicated the COPM was a valid measure of occupational performance. One study challenged the concurrent validity of the COPM relative to other functional measures. One would anticipate a low correlation with an objective functional measure because the COPM may not address functional items that would be considered within typical functional measures. The review found the COPM to be sensitive to changes in patient outcomes over time in the areas of perceived performance and satisfaction when examining other functional measures, such as the Health Assessment Questionnaire and the Short Form-36 (Carswell et al., 2004).

In considering occupational therapy research outcomes and the use of the COPM, articles presented in this review identified the use of the COPM as an outcome measure (Carswell et al., 2004). These studies included 6 randomized controlled trials, 16 quasi-experimental designs, 10 case studies, and 2 patient surveys. The studies found the COPM to be useful as an outcome measure when examining new therapeutic interventions or specific therapeutic devices. There was most often agreement that the use of the COPM was an effective method for engaging patients in the therapeutic process and setting goals. The review also provided information on the negative aspects or limitations of the COPM. Despite the limitations, the literature presented in this review indicated that the COPM has been utilized in a successful fashion with a variety of patients, from homeless individuals to outpatients, patients with mental health needs, patients in a neurorehabilitation unit, and older adults residing in a care facility. Thirty-three articles were reviewed and identified that described the use of the COPM in the provision of patient-centered occupational therapy services from an EBP perspective (Carswell et al., 2004).

Overall, this review suggested that the measurement properties of the COPM were repeatedly identified as satisfactory to excellent (Carswell et al., 2004). The review identified that interrater reliability is not testable, as each patient determines specific problems and assigns scores for the patient's own situation. Therefore, consistency of the responses was measured as test-retest reliability. This review presented information from studies that suggested the COPM was not appropriate for patients who lacked insight, who were diagnosed with dementia, or who relied on health care professionals to make decisions (Carswell et al., 2004).

As a measure, the COPM is effective in identifying patient occupational performance concerns and areas the patient wishes to address within occupational therapy services. Without such measures, how would an occupational therapy practitioner provide patient-centered therapy services? Therefore, the COPM is an assessment that facilitates the identification of performance concerns from the patient's perspective. The performance components that are causing the patient's concerns can then be further evaluated by the occupational therapy practitioner (Carswell et al., 2004).

The COPM can facilitate the occupational therapy practitioner's use of EBP as the measure gains information from the patient's perspective, an essential feature of EBP. Through use of this measure, occupational therapy practitioners can develop and implement meaningful patient intervention and measure changes that can be attributed to occupational therapy intervention (Carswell et al., 2004). This review of the COPM highlights the fact that the instrument has become an accepted outcome measure for occupational therapy practitioners.

A study of occupational therapy in acute mental health practice identified four core elements of clinical practice (Lloyd & Williams, 2010):

1. Individual assessment
2. Therapeutic groups
3. Individual treatment
4. Discharge planning

Assessments addressing occupational performance, roles, interests, communication and interaction, and work roles were most often cited within the study. These assessments were closely related to the Model of Human Occupation (MOHO; Chapter 16). The assessments were identified as assisting the occupational therapy practitioner through a holistic view of the client and facilitation of clinical reasoning incorporating a collaborative assessment process with the client (Lloyd & Williams, 2010).

Review of Outcome Measures

Evidence regarding the effectiveness of therapeutic services is most commonly described according to specific outcome measures (Laver-Fawcett, 2014). In considering outcome measures, the occupational therapy practitioner is concerned with precision and accuracy (Law et al., 2017).

Precision

Precision and the related concepts of reliability and validity are of concern when considering assessments from an EBP perspective. Reliability and validity are affected by random error. An assessment will be deemed less precise the greater the error (Helewa & Walker, 2000). In considering assessment, there are four major sources of error (Hulley & Cummings, 1988):

1. Observer variability
2. Subject variability
3. Instrument variability
4. Environmental variability

Observer variability consists of the variability in measurement that is attributable to the observer and the observer's involvement in the administration process. *Subject variability* is the differences in the participant that may be attributed to fatigue, time of day, mood, or other biological factors. *Instrument variability* is specific to the design of the instrument (e.g., rounding scores up). *Environmental variability* includes environmental factors that may change during the course of an assessment, such as noise, temperature, and lighting (Hulley & Cummings, 1988).

Five guidelines exist for critical evaluation of the precision of an assessment (Helewa & Walker, 2000):

1. Are the assessment methods standardized? If so, administration, scoring, and interpretation of the measure according to standardized procedures yields increased precision and accuracy of the assessment results and can facilitate the planning of an effective intervention that addresses the patient's functional limitations.

2. Are the individuals administering the assessment trained to perform this function? Appropriate training and qualifications can yield increased precision and accuracy.

3. Has the instrument been well-refined? Some assessments have been developed in a way that has reduced variability. Assessments that have been well-refined yield increased precision and accuracy.

4. Has automation been developed for the assessment? Measures that have been automated reduce the potential for variability and human error. As a result, the measure would be viewed as more precise.

5. Does evidence exist that variability is due to the order of the measurements administered? The order of measurements can influence precision by providing a training effect or fatiguing the patient. Considering the order of measurements can increase the precision of the measurements administered (Helewa & Walker 2000).

Occupational therapy practitioners should consider the strategies available to increase the precision of assessments. As a guide, the first two strategies are essential, whereas the fifth strategy is considered most likely to improve precision, if feasible, within the measurement process (Hulley & Cummings, 1988).

Accuracy

A measure is identified as accurate if it actually measures what it was intended to measure (Hulley & Cummings, 1988). Internal and external validity of research are considered relative to accuracy. If the findings of a research study lead to a specific set of inferences, the accuracy of the measure used for the phenomena addressed in the study must be considered. When a measure is accurate, it measures what it is intended to measure, with systematic error being minimal (Helewa & Walker, 2000). Having accuracy in measurements can increase the validity of the conclusions drawn from the assessment findings. Comparison of an instrument to a gold standard is the method to assess accuracy of an instrument.

Six guidelines exist for the critical evaluation of accuracy within a measure (Helewa & Walker, 2000):

1. Was the measurement utilized considered unobtrusive? Patients may bias their own results on a measure if they anticipate pain or other negative factors. Measurements that are designed so that the participant is not aware of the measure eliminate the chance for the participant to bias the assessment results and, therefore, increase the accuracy of the measure.

2. Were the administrators of the outcomes measures independent or masked to the treatment conditions? Individuals who implement the intervention and then assess the participant's progress may bias the results in efforts to make the experimental intervention appear favorable. In reviewing literature regarding intervention effectiveness, outcome measures that have been conducted by individuals who are trained and masked to the treatment conditions can increase the accuracy of the assessment.

3. Have instruments been appropriately calibrated? Appropriate calibration increases the accuracy of the assessment results.

4. Does the measure appropriately predict the outcome of concern? If a measure predicts change in the variable of concern, the measure is said to have good predictive validity, and accuracy of the prediction is an important consideration.

5. Does the assessment agree with other approaches available to measure the same variable of concern, and thereby display convergent validity or criterion-related validity? If so, this is another way the attribute measured can be considered from an accuracy perspective.

6. Does the assessment make sense and provide a reasonable approach for measuring the variable of concern? Face validity is the final consideration relative to accuracy.

Precision and accuracy are two important concerns when reviewing outcomes literature. Occupational therapy practitioners can learn about not only the assessments utilized but also the outcomes obtained in a particular study through close consideration of the precision and accuracy of the measures used within the study (Helewa & Walker, 2000). There are other guidelines that practitioners must consider in critical examination of measurements utilized in outcome studies. First, is the measurement sensitive? Does the measure identify differences when, in fact, differences exist? This is an important consideration when viewing the results of an outcome study. Another consideration in viewing the results of an outcome study is to ascertain whether the measurement was responsive to change that may have occurred. A responsive measure would measure change within the variable of interest when, in fact, a change had occurred. Lastly, is the characteristic of interest specific to the measurement chosen? Will the measure detect changes present due to occupational therapy intervention or would psychiatric intervention confound the potential results that could be obtained from the measure (Helewa & Walker, 2000)?

Occupational therapy practitioners are urged to read outcome studies with caution and to critically analyze the measures chosen in relation to the results (Mairs, 2003). One study reported a randomized controlled trial to examine the effectiveness of a community reentry program to facilitate effective community functioning in patients diagnosed with schizophrenia and schizoaffective disorder prior to discharge. Intervention groups were occupational therapy or the community reentry program. In this article, the researchers provided a significant description of the community reentry program and only a limited description of what was conducted within occupational therapy services. The outcome measure that was selected to determine the effectiveness of the two intervention groups was attendance at the patient's first scheduled outpatient appointment. As a result of this measure, the researchers reported a significant difference between individuals who participated in occupational therapy intervention and those who received community reentry services. Individuals in the community reentry program who attended the first outpatient appointment came to 85%, whereas individuals who received occupational therapy services and were considered the control group attended the first outpatient appointment at a rate of only 37%. Attendance at the first outpatient appointment, when considered as an outcome measure of the two interventions, was deemed a very limited indicator of community functioning; however, this was not addressed by the researchers. This illuminates the importance of the occupational therapy practitioner critically reading the entire journal article and critically analyzing the outcome measures that were utilized within the research to ascertain whether a change as a result of the intervention proposed within the study was valid (Mairs, 2003).

Advantages of Evidence-Based Assessment

Utilizing an EBP perspective in clinical practice provides the practitioner with information regarding specific interventions and services that have been proven effective. Selecting an assessment that has proven to be valid and reliable can enable the occupational therapy practitioner to state that the outcomes obtained from intervention were as a result of the intervention (Carswell et al., 2004). If services that have been provided are being challenged by a managed care system or other funding agency, use of an evidence-based assessment can provide justification that the results obtained from the assessment were valid and reliable and that treatment works (Carswell et al., 2004). Through the use of valid and reliable assessments, the occupational therapy practitioner is able to ascertain the functional performance limitations present within the patient and plan intervention according to the patient's values and goals. Including the patient in the implementation of goals and intervention is an important aspect of EBP. Therefore, assessments should be chosen that illuminate the patient's perceived concerns so that effective intervention can be planned and implemented.

Why Evidence-Based Practice May Not Be Used

Occupational therapy practitioners who wish to utilize EBP may encounter barriers to implementation of this practice within their clinic environment. Knowledge translation does not occur without significant effort from the clinicians or without intentional efforts from the entire clinical team (Menon et al., 2009). Some managers may not promote or foster EBP among their subordinates (Alsop, 1997). There may be misperceptions as to what EBP is and what it is not, in addition to a lack of understanding of the research that is a portion of EBP. This lack of understanding related to research can be remedied through participation in continuing professional development, such as coursework and self-study, which is mandated through AOTA's *Standards of Continuing Competence* (2015b) and *Code of Ethics* (2015a).

Some practitioners may be reluctant to utilize EBP because they are uncertain as to what constitutes evidence (Alsop, 1997). Another reason why practitioners may not use EBP is that some research that is conducted is not published or disseminated widely or adequately, and thus practitioners do not have access to the evidence resources that may exist. Some of the research that is published and accessible may be viewed by practitioners as not applicable to their current clinical practice setting due to the degree of research language utilized within the article. Even when research is written in a clearly applicable manner, some practitioners may resist utilizing the evidence because the research may be viewed as "too scientific" and a challenge to their professional artistry (Alsop, 1997).

Other factors that have been identified as to why EBP was not used by occupational therapy practitioners included factors present within clinical practice guidelines, the level of practitioner experience, perceptions, patient expectations and preferences, and clinical practice setting limitations (Stergiou-Kita, 2010).

Case Study

Lauren is an occupational therapist who works in an outpatient pediatric setting and in an inpatient behavioral health unit. Lauren's clinical population includes children diagnosed with autism spectrum disorders, adjustment disorder, conduct disorder, oppositional defiant disorder, and attention deficit hyperactivity disorder, as well as learning disabilities. Lauren searches the literature to determine what assessments exist for the clients she serves. She has identified significant concerns in the children she serves in the area of negative self-perceptions, which she believes is negatively impacting their occupational performance and engagement. Because Lauren works in both inpatient and outpatient settings, she would like an assessment that is flexible and can be clinically beneficial in either setting. Furthermore, Lauren is an occupation-based and client-centered practitioner, so she is searching for assessments that will address these areas. Through her comprehensive search of the literature, Lauren identifies the Child Occupational Self-Assessment (COSA) as a possibility. This is an outcome measure that is designed to address children and youth perceptions of sense of occupational competence related to everyday activities (Kramer, ten Velden, Kafkes, Basu, Fedrico, & Kielhofner, 2014). Lauren continues to search the literature to discover more regarding this assessment. She determines that the instrument she is interested in has good content, structural, and substantive validity (Kramer, Kielhofner, & Smith, 2010). Because Lauren realizes the importance of not only considering research evidence, she consults with other occupational therapists she has networked with at the recent AOTA annual conference regarding her consideration of beginning to utilize this assessment with the clients she provides services to. Upon review of research conducted on the assessment, Lauren gains increased insights into important considerations in administration of the assessment, as well as strategies for effective treatment planning upon completion of the assessment (Kramer et al., 2010). Because the assessment is based on the MOHO, Lauren decides to enroll in an upcoming continuing education event related to MOHO to assist in effectively interpreting the assessment and plan treatment for the clients she serves. Lauren values the choice of this assessment as it is not done to a child/youth, rather it is a collaborative assessment conducted with the child/youth.

After Lauren attended the continuing education course on MOHO and has been utilizing the COSA for 6 months, she reports back to the occupational therapists she met at the AOTA conference. She shares improved client engagement and participation in scheduled sessions she believes has occurred because she is more effectively connecting with the children/youth she serves, and she attributes some of this to the nature of the COSA, as well as being able to target intervention planning more specifically toward client-identified areas of concern. The occupational therapists network together to plan a research project utilizing the COSA to further demonstrate the benefits that can be obtained through the use of the assessment to occupational therapy practitioners and the clients they serve.

Summary

Despite challenges that may exist related to knowledge translation of research findings and application to clinical practice, in our ever-changing clinical and health care landscape, EBP appears here to stay. Practitioners, scholars, and educators are encouraged to continue a professional commitment to sharing mental health knowledge and practice through publication of clinical findings (D'Amico, Jaffe, & Gibson, 2010).

References

Agency for Healthcare Research and Quality. (2017). *EPC reports: Mental health conditions and substance abuse.* Retrieved from https://www.ahrq.gov/research/findings/evidence-based-reports/search. html?f%5B0%5D=field_evidence_based_reports%3A13970

Alsop, A. (1997). Evidence-based practice and continuing professional development. *British Journal of Occupational Therapy, 60,* 503-508.

American Occupational Therapy Association. (2011). *Critically appraised topic: Persons with serious mental illness.* Retrieved from https://www.aota.org/~/media/Corporate/Files/Secure/Practice/CCL/Mental%20 Illness%20Recovery%20CAT.pdf

American Occupational Therapy Association. (2014). Occupational therapy practice framework: Domain and process (3rd ed.). *American Journal of Occupational Therapy, 68*(Suppl. 1), S1-S48.

American Occupational Therapy Association. (2015a). Occupational therapy code of ethics. *American Journal of Occupational Therapy, 69*(Suppl. 3), 6913410030p1-6913410030p8. https://doi.org/10.5014/ajot.2015.696S03

American Occupational Therapy Association. (2015b). Standards of continuing competence. *American Journal of Occupational Therapy, 69*(Suppl. 3), 6913410055p1-6913410055p3. https://doi.org/10.5014/ajot.2015.696S16

Bennett, S. (2017). *OTseeker: Searching for evidence.* Retrieved from http://www.otseeker.com/resources/ evidencebasedpractice.aspx#3

Bennett, S., & Bennett, J. W. (2000). The process of evidence based practice in occupational therapy: Informing clinical decisions. *Australian Journal of Occupational Therapy, 47,* 171-180.

Brown, C. (2017). *The evidence based practitioner: Applying research to meet client needs.* Philadelphia, PA: F. A. Davis Company.

Brown, T. G., & Rodger, S. (1999). Research utilization models: Frameworks for implementing evidence based occupational therapy practice. *Occupational Therapy International, 6*(1), 1-23.

Carswell, A., McColl, M. A., Baptiste, S., Law, M., Polatajko, H., & Pollock, N. (2004). The Canadian Occupational Performance Measure: A research and clinical literature review. *Canadian Journal of Occupational Therapy, 71,* 210-222.

Coster, W. (2004). Facilitating transfer of evidence based practice into practice. *Education Special Interest Section Quarterly, 14*(2), 1.

D'Amico, M., Jaffe, L., & Gibson, R. W. (2010). Mental health evidence in the *American Journal of Occupational Therapy. American Journal of Occupational Therapy, 64,* 660-669.

Dickinson, R. (2003). Occupational therapy: A hidden treasure. *Canadian Journal of Occupational Therapy, 70,* 133-135.

Finch-Guthrie, P. L. (2016). Establishing partnerships and organizational readiness. In P. Moyers & P. Finch-Guthrie (Eds.), *Interprofessional evidence-based practice: A workbook for health professionals.* Thorofare, NJ: SLACK Incorporated.

Foto, M. (1996). Outcome studies: the what, why, how, and when. *American Journal of Occupational Therapy, 50,* 87-88.

Fuller, K. (2011). The effectiveness of occupational performance outcome measures within mental health practice. *British Journal of Occupational Therapy, 74,* 399-405.

Greenhaigh, T. (1997a). How to read a paper: Statistics for the non-statistician I: Different data need different statistical tests. *British Medical Journal, 315,* 364-366.

Greenhaigh, T. (1997b). How to read a paper: Statistics for the non-statistician II: Significance, relations and their pitfalls. *British Medical Journal, 315,* 422-425.

Gutman, S. A. (2011). Special issue: Effectiveness of occupational therapy services in mental health practice. *American Journal of Occupational Therapy, 65,* 235-237.

Hall-Flavin, D. K. (2005). *Resources for accessing evidence-based practice information—Symposium I: Translating research into practice.* Retrieved from http://www.aaap.org/meetings2001am/proceedings/symposium1. html

Helewa, A., & Walker, J. M. (2000). *Critical evaluation of research in physical rehabilitation: Towards evidence-based practice*. Philadelphia, PA: W. B. Saunders.

Hitch, D. (2016). Attitudes of mental health occupational therapists toward evidence-based practice. *Canadian Journal of Occupational Therapy, 83*(1), 27-32.

Hitch, D., Pepin, G., & Stagnitti, K. (2015). Evidence for mental health occupational therapy: Trends in the first decade of the new millennium (2000-2013). *Sage Open*, 1-12.

Holm, M. B. (2000). Our mandate for the new millennium: Evidence-based practice. *American Journal of Occupational Therapy, 54*, 575-585.

Hulley, S. B., & Cummings, S. R. (1988). *Designing clinical research: An epidemiological approach*. Baltimore, MD: Williams & Wilkins.

Kramer, J., Kielhofner, G., & Smith, E. (2010). Validity of child occupational self-assessment. *American Journal of Occupational Therapy, 64*, 621-632.

Kramer, J., ten Velden, M., Kafkes, A., Basu, S., Fedrico, J., & Kielhofner, G. (2014). *Child occupational self-assessment*. Chicago, IL: Model of Human Occupation Clearinghouse.

LaGrossa, J. (2003). A lesson in evidence based research and practice. *Advance for Occupational Therapy Practitioners, 43*, 17-18.

Laver-Fawcett, A. J. (2014). Routine standardized outcome measurement to evaluate the effectiveness of occupational therapy interventions: Essential or optional? *Ergoterpeuten, 4*, 28-37.

Law, M., Baum, C., & Dunn, W. (2017). *Measuring occupational performance: Supporting best practice in occupational therapy* (3rd ed.). Thorofare, NJ: SLACK Incorporated.

Liberman, D., & Scheer J. (2002). AOTA's evidence based literature review project: An overview. *American Journal of Occupational Therapy, 56*, 344-349.

Lim, K. H., Frater, T., & Samaras, L. (2014). *Examining the wider context of evidence based occupational therapy. 2014 ENOTHE Congress*. Retrieved from http://enothe.eu/Wordpress%20Documents/2014%20Powerpoints/Examining%20the%20wider%20context%20of%20evidence%20based%20occupational%20therapy.pdf

Lloyd, C., Bassett, H., & King, R. (2004). Occupational therapy and evidence-based practice in mental health. *British Journal of Occupational Therapy, 67*, 83-88.

Lloyd, C., & Williams, P. L. (2010). Occupational therapy in the modern adult acute mental health setting: A review of current practice. *International Journal of Therapy and Rehabilitation, 17*, 436-442.

Mairs, H. (2003). Evidence-based practice in mental health: A cause for concern for occupational therapists? *British Journal of Occupational Therapy, 66*, 168-170.

Medical University of South Carolina. (2017). *Occupational therapy: PICOTT*. Retrieved from http://musc.libguides.com/c.php?g=107912&p=699693

Menon, A., Korner-Bitensky, N., Kastner, M., McKinnon, K. A., & Straus, S. (2009). Strategies for rehabilitation professionals to move evidence based knowledge into practice: A systemic review. *Journal of Rehabilitation Medicine, 41*, 1024-1032.

Moyers, P., & Finch-Guthrie, P. (2016). *Interprofessional evidence-based practice*. Thorofare, NJ: SLACK Incorporated.

National Clearinghouse Guidelines. (2017). *Occupational therapy and mental health*. Retrieved from https://www.guideline.gov/search?q=occupational+therapy+and+mental+health

Raff, J. (2014). How to read and understand a scientific paper: A step-by-step guide for non-scientists. *Huffington Post*. Retrieved from https://www.huffingtonpost.com/jennifer-raff/how-to-read-and-understand-a-scientific-paper_b_5501628.html

Roberts, A. E. K., & Barber, G. (2001). Applying research evidence to practice. *British Journal of Occupational Therapy, 65*, 223-227.

Rouleau, S., Dion, K., & Korner-Bitensky, N. (2015). Assessment practices of Canadian occupational therapists working with adults with mental disorders. *Canadian Journal of Occupational Therapy, 82*, 181-193. https://doi.org/10.1177/0008417414561857

Sackett, D., Rosenberg, W., Gray, J., Haynes, R., & Richardson, W. (1996). Evidence-based medicine: What it is and what it isn't. *British Medical Journal, 312*, 71-72.

Stergiou-Kita, M. (2010). Implementing clinical practice guidelines in occupational therapy practice: Recommendations from research evidence. *Australian Journal of Occupational, 57*, 76-87. https://doi.org/10.1111/j.1440-1630.2009.00842.x

Stube, J. E., & Jedlicka, J. S. (2007). The acquisition and integration of evidence-based practice concepts by occupational therapy students. *American Journal of Occupational Therapy, 61*, 53-61.

Tickle-Degnen, L. (1998). Using evidence for planning treatment for the client. *Canadian Journal of Occupational Therapy, 65*, 152-159.

Tickle-Degnen, L. (2000). Gathering current research evidence to enhance clinical reasoning. *American Journal of Occupational Therapy, 54*, 102-105.

Torrey, W. C., Drake, R. E., Dixon, L., Burns, B. J., Flynn, L., Rush, A. J., … Klatzker, D. (2001). Implementing evidence-based practices for persons with severe mental illnesses. *Psychiatric Services, 52*(1), 45-50.

Tsang, H. W. H. (2002). Evidence-based practice in psychiatric occupational therapy should be strengthened. *American Journal of Occupational Therapy, 56,* 475.

University of Illinois—Chicago: University Library. (2017). *Evidence-based practice: PICO.* Retrieved from http://researchguides.uic.edu/c.php?g=252338&p=3954402

Unsworth, C. (2017). Review papers: Getting best occupational therapy evidence into practice. *British Journal of Occupational Therapy, 80,* 143-144.

Wong, R., Barr, J. O., Farina, N., & Lusardi, M. (2000). Evidence-based practice: A resource for physical therapists. *Issues on Aging, 23,* 19-26.

Part II
The Interviewing Process

Occupational Profile and Interviewing in Occupational Therapy

Lisa Mahaffey, PhD, OTR/L, FAOTA

Everyone is a story. When I was a child, people sat around kitchen tables and told their stories. We don't do that so much anymore. Sitting around the table telling stories is not just a way of passing time. It is the way the wisdom gets passed along. The stuff that helps us to live a life worth remembering ...
We may need to listen to each other's stories once again.
(Remen, 1996, p. xxxvii)

A person's story is an illustration of their life and occupations and the context for compelling therapy. When occupational therapy practitioners gather a person's story, they develop an insider's understanding of the meaning and consequence of living with and being treated for a psychiatric disability. The process of telling one's story to a helper who perceives the value of the information fosters a collaborative intervention process. Gathering a person's story to build the occupational profile goes beyond the person's presenting impairment and symptoms and considers all of the aspects of the social and physical environment, the consequences of conventional medical treatment, and the accumulation of a lifetime of both affirming and difficult experiences. Interviewing is one of the most effective and flexible ways to help someone tell their story and to identify significant goals. This chapter will focus on the power and skill of interviewing as a way to build an occupational profile and to contextualize treatment in meaningful and motivating ways.

The Occupational Profile

According to the *Occupational Therapy Practice Framework: Domain and Process, Third Edition*, the process of building an occupational profile begins during the initial contact with the person seeking occupational therapy service (American Occupational Therapy Association [AOTA], 2014). The occupational profile is defined as a "summary of a client's

Hemphill, B. J., & Urish, C. K. (Eds.). *Assessments in Occupational Therapy Mental Health: An Integrative Approach, Fourth Edition* (pp. 39-51). © 2020 Taylor & Francis Group.

occupational history and experiences, patterns of daily living, interests, values and needs" (AOTA, 2014, p. S13). The occupational profile is the part of the evaluation process in which the person constructs their stories. The *Framework* (AOTA, 2014) suggests that the profile include information about the person's occupational history, as well as information on their current occupations, such as their daily patterns and routines, leisure and productive interests, and social networks, as well as the meaningful occupations that they wish to participate in going forward. In addition, the *Framework* (AOTA, 2014) suggests gathering information on the person's daily environments because where they live, who they live with, and the policies that govern the services they receive can support or hinder their participation in valued occupations and ultimately impact intervention outcomes (AOTA, 2014). Developing the occupational profile helps practitioners construct a complex understanding of the person's needs and leads to a more considered approach to the analysis of performance. Collaboratively building an occupational profile places the person in the role of expert-on-themselves and strengthens the person-centered process in therapy. Developing the occupational profile together also sets the stage for a collaborative approach to the analysis of occupational performance and a problem-solving process that considers all the factors that influence occupational participation.

The Value of Interviewing

The construction a person's occupational profile can be done through formal or informal methods, such as reviewing the person's records, observing them during their participation in social interactions, and conducting formal evaluations, most of which include at least a brief interview. Interviewing is an engaging and flexible method for gathering information. An interview can be done formally, but it can also be conducted through a seemingly casual conversation while the person is engaged in an occupation. The process of conducting an interview can support the development of a therapeutic rapport and assist practitioners in determining the most effective ways to use themselves in the therapy process (Taylor, 2008). Through interviewing, practitioners gather information about the person's sense of efficacy, sense of empowerment, and self-determination, as well as other things that cannot be observed.

Research on the power of developing narratives in recovery indicates that interviewing may have a healing impact of its own (Roe & Davidson, 2005). A narrative interview, one that elicits persons' stories, can result in persons developing a better awareness of their situation, including both the positive influences and the barriers that keep them from achieving desired goals and outcomes (Mallinson, Kielhofner, & Mattingly, 1996; Mattingly & Lawlor, 2000). Narrative interviewing after the onset of disability can spark an important process of story reconstruction—a process that builds a new narrative by tapping into unused resources, defining their experiences as meaningful, and including their psychiatric disability as an important part of their personal identity (Egan, 2009; Roe & Davidson, 2005). The creation of a narrative story can assist people who have recently encountered the onset of a psychiatric disability establish a sense of continuity with the person they were before they experienced symptoms (Roe & Davidson, 2005). According to Roe and Davidson (2005), reauthoring one's story supports the reconstruction of self-agency, which is a key dimension of recovery, even for people with very severe psychiatric symptoms.

Conducting the Interview

Choosing the Interview Method

Choosing a method for interviewing someone is dependent on a variety of factors. The most important factor is the expected outcome, which in most cases is to create the occupational profile to guide further evaluation for the selection of areas to conduct an analysis of occupational performance and, ultimately, to plan intervention. Other considerations include the characteristics of the treatment setting, such as the length of time people remain in treatment and the resources available to the practitioner and the person seeking help. The practitioner must also consider investment in, and the capacity of, the person being interviewed. Practitioners can choose to use one of the many established interviews in the occupational therapy literature, but there is value in exploring a variety of resources. Oral history websites such as Story Corps (n.d.) provide collections of questions and helpful hints for gathering rich narrative information.

Interviews are identified as formal or informal and fall on a continuum related to the level of structure. For the purposes of this chapter, formal interviews will be identified as those interviews with a predetermined set of questions, instructions for conducting the interview, documentation, and psychometric properties. Conversely, informal interviews are not based on a set of predetermined questions, are often done when convenient, and tend to be more casual and conversational. Interviews fall on a continuum that runs from a high level of structure to semistructured to completely unstructured. Structured interviews are formal interviews in which there is a standardized set of questions designed to get specific answers. Structured interviews allow for quantifiable data, making it possible to compare responses across participants and to use the results as outcomes measures. In order for the data to be compared, the interviewer must not deviate from the established protocol. Although the data gathered are considered reliable, the restrictive nature of a structured interview can be insensitive to the person's need to express their ideas and beliefs, which may impact the validity of the responses (Keegan, n.d.).

Semistructured interviews are also formal interviews with a collection of optional questions and prompts that are meant to guide the data-gathering process and yield information on all aspects of occupation. Several semistructured, formal interviews are included in this text. Two such interviews are the Canadian Occupational Performance Measure and the second edition of the Occupational Performance History Interview. A semistructured interview allows the interviewee to express their views and take an expert role on their experiences. Although it is possible to quantify the results of a semistructured interview through rating scales, the occupation-related details will be unique to each interviewee, making comparisons less reliable (Keegan, n.d.).

Unstructured interviews are informal interviews that can be done anywhere or any time the opportunity arises. Informal interviews often come out of the here-and-now interaction between the practitioner and the person seeking help. This makes informal interviews a very flexible form of data gathering that allows for real-time updates to the profile and adjustments to the treatment outcomes throughout the intervention process. It is important to note that informal does not mean unskilled. Informal interviews are often the result of an attentive practitioner who is able to capitalize on an important moment in therapy by asking strategic questions and eliciting responses that are enlightening for both participants. Data gathered during these interviews are difficulty to quantify, so it cannot be compared to other interviews nor can it be used to measure outcomes by itself. Instead, this interview process is used to enhance rapport, obtain more details about the person's occupations, assess the impact of therapy, and adjust treatment in order to achieve the person's desired outcomes. Informal interviews can be instrumental in creating a collaborative intervention process and in encouraging a greater sense of empowerment and self-determination for the person seeking help (Keegan, n.d.).

Combining interviewing with other evaluation tools can be an effective method for building the occupational profile. Practitioners may want to use a self-report tool, such as the Role Checklist (Oakley, Kielhofner, Barris, & Reichler, 1986), to establish an inventory of important daily life roles. Having the person complete the checklist in advance of the interview allows the practitioner to use the interview time to gather more details about their roles. The length of stay in acute care settings can be extremely short. The intervention must center on treatment goals that impact the recovery process within the brief time frame. Wrapping an interview around a self-report, goal-setting tool such as the Occupational Self-Assessment (Baron, Kielhofner, Iyenger, Goldhammer, & Wolenski, 2006) facilitates a collaborative intervention planning process that prioritizes the most important and achievable goals within the expected length of stay. Using an interview procedure such as this shifts the balance of power from practitioner-driven to person-driven, allowing for informed decisions about their own intervention process and a greater sense of empowerment (Taylor, 2008).

When practitioners have a set of formal interviews that range from structured to semistructured and several helpful questions for informal, unstructured interviews available to them, they can choose a strategy that best fits the situation. Matching the interview process with the opportunities available in the setting and the needs of the person results in a more effective data gathering and a greater sense of satisfaction for both participants.

Setting Up the Interview

Once practitioners establish a set of resources and a method for choosing an interview approach, they can turn their attention to other factors that contribute to an effective interview process. One of the most important is the interview environment. It is helpful to establish a dedicated space that is comfortable and relatively private with few distractions. If there is no place set aside for interviewing, then a sign placed nearby that states "In session, do not disturb" may be helpful. It is valuable to plan time in the therapy schedule for interviews, preferably a time when there is less activity in the milieu or when people are most alert and responsive. Seating arrangements are often at the discretion of the interviewer and sometimes the person being interviewed, but many find that setting up the chairs at a 90-degree angle allows persons to choose whether they want to look straight at the interviewer or look away during the verbal exchanges (Sommers-Flannagan & Sommers-Flannagan, 2009).

The formal interview process will be more successful if the practitioner spends time in advance thinking about the different parts of the interview. It is important to have a plan for the beginning and for transitioning into the body of the interview, which is where the important details are gathered. In addition, many practitioners neglect to consider how an interview will end. Planning ahead will ensure a smooth process and make the interview feel less contrived. The practitioner may also want to discuss confidentiality with the person, such as when and what information is shared with team members and what, if any, information should be kept confidential.

Beginning the Interview

Interviewers should begin by establishing a positive relationship with the person so they believe that their story is of value. Most interviewers will start the conversation with small talk, which helps to establish the interactive process and sends the message that the practitioner is interested in them as a person. An introductory statement that reviews the interview topics and the expected time frame will send a signal to the person that the formal interview is starting. Interviewers often find it helpful to being the interview with a more global question, such as "Tell me about your typical day" or "What are the most important points in your life?" Questions such as these give the interviewer information about the person's roles, routines and patterns, interests and values, social interactions, and environments within which the person functions every day. The person's responses then set the stage for the body of the interview, during which the interviewer obtains the details that will inform the treatment goals. Many formal semistructured interviews begin this way. The Occupational Performance History Interview includes a section titled "Critical Life Events" in which the interviewer asks the person to share their beliefs about their successes, failures, and life turning points (Kielhofner et al., 2008). These events are plotted on a grid, and the narrative plot line is used as a visual guide for gathering the details around the person's occupations. Plotting the person's critical life events can reveal the metaphor the person uses to describe their life situation (Kielhofner et al., 2008). One common metaphor is of momentum, in which the person talks about their lives slowing down or speeding up. The other is one of being trapped in their life circumstances with no discernible way out (Kielhofner et al., 2008). Recognizing the dominant metaphor early in the interview can increase the person's awareness of how their belief system impacts their recovery process.

The Body of the Interview

The middle or body of the interview is where the person, with help from the practitioner, drills down to get at the detailed information about day-to-day participation. The details are important for two reasons: (1) the perceived supports for, and the barriers to, occupational participation are found in the small details that arise out of the person's narrative; (2) knowing those details helps the practitioner and the person establish interventions that utilize the supports while finding ways to overcome the perceived barriers. It is this process that has the potential to alter the person's narrative going forward, thus positively impacting their recovery process (Asaba & Jackson, 2011; Christiansen, 1999; Kielhofner et al., 2008). For example, an interview may reveal that a person with a diagnosis of schizophrenia has never lived by themselves and as a result has never learned the steps to cleaning a bathroom or how to store leftovers after a meal. The most meaningful intervention strategies become clear during this section of the interview.

Ending the Interview

An interview comes to an end for several reasons. Practitioners may have all of the information they need or they may reach the end of the time allotted for the interview; the person may reach a point where they cannot or do not want to continue with the interview. In any situation, it is beneficial for the interview process to end in a way that keeps the door open for further communication. One important task is to review the main points of the interview to be sure the practitioner and the person share a common understanding of the person's story. Agreeing on the most important barriers to participation allows the practitioner to link the interview to a collaborative treatment process. If the interview ends before sufficient information is gathered, the practitioner will want to work with the person to establish a plan for meeting again. Sometimes the person will be willing to meet again or may be willing to answer some questions during their treatment sessions. They may be willing to complete a self-report form or write out responses in their down time. Having options available to people will support the data-collecting process by meeting multiple needs. Often, people think of things that are important to them after the interview is over, so it behooves both the interviewer and the person to reconnect at a later time to clarify important points. Interviewers can end a longer interview by asking if the person has any questions for them. Asking the person if they have questions, or even for their feedback on their experience with the interview, can help them internalize their role as a partner in the intervention process.

Before ending the interview, the participants must agree on a preliminary intervention plan. The identification of the supports and barriers to participation during the body of the interview guides the collaborative intervention planning process. Supported by the practitioner, the person can use the profile information to establish long- and short-term goals, setting the stage for completing the analysis of performance. Together the practitioners and the person can review the benefits of doing additional performance-based evaluations and begin to negotiate on the intervention strategies that will help meet their goals. The occupational profile helps the person frame their recovery from an occupational participation perspective, a perspective that allows them to have hope for recovery and a sense of personhood.

Building Skills for Interviewing

Several resources are available for practitioners who are interested in developing stronger interview skills, some of which are listed in the reference section of the chapter. An extensive review of skills is beyond the scope of this chapter; however, there is value in talking about some key skills that will help practitioners gather profile data. By far, the most important, and sometimes the most challenging, skill is listening with compassion. Compassionate listening requires that the interviewer use questions that are non-adversarial and then listen to the responses with a mind that withholds judgment (Cohen, Green, & Partnow, 2011). The compassionate listener is open to understanding the person's story and accepts the right of the person to have their own perceptions (Egan, 2009). The skill of listening is much more than *not talking*. Communication is a complex process in which people send and receive messages in several ways. Interviewers who are skilled at listening are attentive to the person's body language and vocal tone and are aware of their own nonverbal communication when asking questions and when processing the person's responses (Sommers-Flannagan & Sommers-Flannagan, 2009). Artful listeners understand the interview as something like a dance, with actions and reactions, in which the interviewer can encourage the person to tell their story by responding compassionately through both verbal and nonverbal means (Black, 2013). There are important cultural considerations when attempting to assess the meaning of body language, eye contact, and vocal quality. It is important for the interviewer to do some research on culture before beginning an interview with anyone who has a different cultural background.

Prompting is another important interview skill. Prompting is the use of questions or comments meant to encourage the person to share more information or clarify a point they made. It is common for people to respond to interview questions with general statements about themselves, such as "I am unable to manage an apartment on my own" (Mattingly & Lawlor, 2000). Prompting for details will help practitioners generate a more nuanced understanding of the person's beliefs about their ability to engage in occupation, as well as the value and meaning behind their occupational choices. There are many effective prompts, and with experience interviewers will discover the prompts that work best for them. Some prompts are simply meant to encourage the person to provide greater detail, such as the following statement: "I am interested in knowing more about that." Other prompts move the interview from the broader, more abstract concepts and beliefs related to occupation down to the smaller actions that are cause for those beliefs. For example, when exploring their understanding of their life roles, interviewers may prompt the person by saying one of the following: "Describe the tasks that fill your work day" or "What sort of things do you do each day in your role as a mother?" Another helpful prompt is to repeat a portion of what the person said and then ask them to expand on it. For example, the interviewer may say "Earlier you said you quit your job because of some difficulty with your boss. Describe a time when your boss made things difficult for you." A prompt such as this can give the interviewer insight into the specific aspects of work or work relationships that create barriers to participating in that occupation. Without this information, practitioners are left to make assumptions that are often based on their own experiences or biases. Prompting for details identifies valuable supports and gets down to the exact barriers to participation. Once the details are ferreted out, the collaborative intervention process converges on solutions that are motivating and have the greatest chance for success.

Several techniques can be used when the person being interviewed becomes too detailed or tangential or for eliciting more information when the person responds with only brief sentences or remains quiet. In the first case, it may become necessary for the practitioner to interrupt the person and redirect them back to the topic of interest. An interruption that is hurtful can damage rapport or put a halt to the interview because the person becomes unwilling to risk responding again. A benign way of interrupting is to take a bit of verbiage from an earlier response and ask the person to expand on it. "Earlier you said something that I would really like to know more about" or "I don't want to forget something you said earlier. Can you tell me …"

The person who is quiet often poses the greater challenge. The interviewer may start by simply asking the person if they have concerns about sharing their information. Often, making a simple observation such as "I get the sense that you are uncomfortable telling me things" can change the dynamic. Positive or negative symptoms of schizophrenia, a cognitive impairment, or a physical impairment may put the person in a situation where they find it difficult to formulate an answer or they fear the answer will not be the "correct" one. People may be hesitant to share information because they have been in situations in which their responses resulted in consequences they did not want, such as upsetting interventions or even institutionalization. The practitioner will need to build trust and create an environment in which the quiet person feels it is safe to share their experiences. Being genuinely interested in their story and being nonjudgmental are critical. The practitioner might step away from the interview and ask themselves some self-reflective questions, such as what might this person have experienced in their life in the past? What experiences might they have had in the mental health system? What are the biases the practitioner brings to the situation related to the person's medical report, history, or appearance? A practitioner who is able to create a compassionate bridge, such as identifying times in their lives when they were hesitant to share personal information, will often communicate more genuine interest and openness in the interview.

In addition to developing rapport, there are some techniques that a practitioner might use to gather interview data with people who are quiet. It may be more effective to gather information in smaller bits throughout the therapy process. Narrowing the focus of the interview and using props can increase the quality of the information gathered. For example, the practitioner can use a sorting task to create a list of interests. Preparing the person for the interview by reviewing the interview topics or using a self-report tool can help the person generate some thoughts in advance of the verbal exchange. Activities such as the leisure interest sorting task and self-report tools yield useful information without requiring extensive verbal responses. Many sources in the occupational therapy literature suggest gathering information from other significant people in the person's life (AOTA, 2014). Although this information is helpful, the practitioner should never assume that the data represent the person's perspective. One way to use the evaluation data that are gathered from a significant other is to formulate specific questions that allow the person to clarify with shorter answers. This process yields needed information that is informed by the person's own perspective. As practitioners develop rapport and learn how to best communicate with the quiet person, they can refine that perspective and adjust their intervention accordingly.

Sometimes it helps to encourage stories. Stories often provide the practitioner with a greater understanding of the meaning that surrounds the person's occupational participation, meaning that is difficult to obtain when people respond with abstract generalizations (Mattingly & Lawlor, 2000). A simple request like "Give me an example" or "Tell me about a time when you really felt like an artist" can elicit a story that reveals rich and unique connections between meaning and action. These meanings are often not understood by the interviewee and therefore difficult for them to explain in any other way. The meanings associated with actions, particularly actions the person feels unable to perform, provide a powerful context for intervention.

When Techniques Become Ineffective

At this point, it is valuable to explore some of the most used ineffective listening and prompting techniques. Resources that teach active listening focus on aspects of the interview such as eye contact, head movement, and using verbalizations such as "uh huh," which are used to indicate to the person that the interviewer is listening (Mindtools, n.d.). The interviewer must pay attention to the verbal and nonverbal responses of the person being interviewed because there are times when these techniques backfire. For example, excessive eye contact can feel intense and intimidating for people, especially if they have been in dangerous power relationships. Too much head bobbing and too many "uh huh" statements can become distracting and uncomfortable, causing the person to stop talking to minimize the distraction. Much has been written about the power of empathy when caring for others (Mindtools, n.d.); however, many attempts at empathy are misguided. Making statements such as "I know how you feel" can be very off-putting, especially if the interviewer has not had the same experiences as the person. Even if the interviewer has had a similar experience, people often have very different emotional responses. Disclosing similar experiences can be validating; however, before the interviewer reveals anything, they must ask themselves: "Does revealing my story call attention to me, thereby distracting the person from the value of their own story?" and "Will learning my story really help the person gain knowledge or feel their experience is valid?" Another common mistake is using statements that sound like sympathy. "That must have been awful" or "You poor thing" are statements that pass judgment. Even statements like "You had to be a strong person to survive that experience" can come across as a judgment of their responses to traumatic events and to their decisions in their life, leaving them feeling too uncomfortable to share additional information (Sommers-Flannagan & Sommers-Flannagan, 2009).

Documentation

Documenting the interview is the process by which the practitioner composes the occupational profile. Taking notes during or immediately after the interview is one method the practitioner will use to document what they learned. In order to preserve the information in the most accurate way, the interviewer must set aside time immediately after the interview to write down everything they remember. If the interviewer plans to take notes during the interview, they should ask the person for permission, especially if the person being interviewed experiences paranoia. It can be helpful to sit in a position that allows the person to view the notes. Being able to review and check the notes for accuracy, as they are being written, can give the person a greater sense of control over the interview outcome.

Just as with interviewing, there is a fair amount of flexibility in how the information is shared with others. The final decisions about how the practitioner will share the profile with other providers will depend largely on the setting. Some settings may encourage a narrative form of documentation, and writing the narrative in the record is one way to construct and share the profile. Another way to construct the profile is through the use of a standardized form. There are several options highlighted in this text. One example is the form used in the Model of Human Occupation Screening Tool (Parkinson, Forsyth, & Kielhofner, 2006). This tool is designed to report both qualitative and quantitative data related to occupational participation, regardless of how it is collected. The practitioner can use this report tool to synthesize and report the occupational profile data and the performance analysis. In addition to the profile, the written treatment plan, including the goals and the treatment strategies, reflects the outcome of the collaborative evaluation process.

Cultural Sensitivity in Interviewing

According to Munoz (2007), culture is inextricably tied to occupational participation. When collecting the data and when interpreting the occupational profile and the analysis of performance, the practitioner must be sensitive to the impact of cultural differences (Munoz, 2007). The phrase *cultural competence* is often used when the role of culture is discussed in the literature related to the helping professions. After many attempts to define the phrase, most experts agree that cultural competence is a complex, multidimensional concept that is difficult to obtain (Lynch & Hanson, 1998; Sue, Arredondo, & McDavis, 1992). A person's culture, once attributed primarily to race and/or ethnicity, is now viewed as forming out of a merging of experiences resulting from variants such as socioeconomic status, age, religion, education, sexual orientation, societal response to disability or illness, and even where and how a person is brought up (Black, 2013). According to Munoz (2007), being a culturally responsible carer is recognizing that not everyone exemplifies what is considered the cultural norm—that, in fact, people are inherently multicultural (Munoz, 2007). Failure to consider the complexity of cultural diversity can result in, at best, ineffective intervention and, at worst, stereotyping based on faulty convictions (Black, 2013).

Although culture is exemplified through a person's profile, interviewers cannot assume they will understand the influence of the person's culture in their daily life simply by interviewing them. Practitioners must establish a basic knowledge of the common cultural experiences for those who seek help in their setting. For example, if the practitioner is working in a community mental health center in an urban area, they would want to learn if the communities around the center are supportive of people with psychiatric disability; if there is a larger concentration of any particular ethnic groups; the cultural influences on health, mental health, and occupation for those particular ethnic groups; and where the communities fall on the socioeconomic ladder. Then, if someone comes into the setting who falls outside the cultural norms in the community, the practitioner will need to do some additional research. Although not everyone embodies the cultural "norm," having knowledge of the person's complex cultural influences helps the interviewer prompt more effectively and gather interview data that are more true to the person's experiences.

Being a culturally responsive carer also means that practitioners must be willing to explore their own cultural identities, including their own prejudices and biases (Munoz, 2007). According to Munoz (2007), practitioners responding in a qualitative study regarding culturally responsive caring stated that they used a constant process of reflective self-awareness as a strategy for checking their assumptions and guarding against bias. A concerted effort to learn about the cultural influences of the people seeking help, along with a willingness to reflect on one's potential for personal bias, can help to ensure that the collaborative evaluation and treatment planning process represents the person's best interest.

The Right of Expression

McDonald and Kidney (2012) argue that it is an ethical responsibility of the interviewer to find a way for people who often lack credibility because of disability or age to exercise their right of expression. Many of the alternative methods for conducting interviews, addressed in the section on interview skills, are valuable tools for ensuring that people with persistent psychiatric disabilities or people with intellectual disabilities are able to exercise that right of expression (Mactavish, Mahon, & Lutfiyya, 2000; Taylor & Bogdan, 1990).

Young children with limited verbal expressive skills are another group of people often perceived as lacking credibility. Practitioners gather information about the occupations of children by talking with the child, parents, teachers, and other significant adults. In most cases, the child has significant input. When a child lacks verbal expressive skills, it is tempting to fall back on the information provided by the parent. Mahoney (2014) suggests that practitioners can gather an occupational profile from the child's perspective by developing a series of simple questions that allow the child to answer by pointing to something, engaging in an activity or demonstrating the answer through actions. "Listening" to the child means paying close attention to the child's interactions with other children and adults, as well as with the physical environment and their toys. The profile that is created through this combination of tasks, questions, and observations will reflect the child's ideas and their desire for participation (Mahoney, 2014).

Another example of people who are often perceived as lacking credibility is people with dementia. Validation therapy techniques, designed to foster communication with an individual with dementia (Feil, 2002), can illicit stories that often result in a rich occupational profile even when their dementia is in the later stages. According to Feil (2002), individuals with dementia experience time in a nonlinear fashion. A picture, a word, or a strong emotion can cause them to relive important moments. When this happens, the person understands the environment and people around them from the perspective of that moment in time. Practitioners who recognize these moments can use them to learn about the person's past occupations. According to Feil (2002), when a practitioner responds with genuine interest by using factual questions that begin with the words when, who, what, and where the person will react by engaging in the interaction. This interaction can reveal important details that can be used to build an occupational profile and engage people in the intervention process. This process also helps the person review important life events and validates their emotional responses. In addition to validation, a practitioner can use memory aids to gather stories. Helen (1998) identifies the Life Story book as a way to help families connect with their family member who has dementia and to help other care providers understand the person as an occupational being. To construct a Life Story book, the individual with dementia works with family members to create the pages of the book. Each page contains a picture or artifact that represents an important life role, achievement, or experience. Through the collection of pictures and artifacts in the book, the reader can begin to develop an image of the person as an active participant in their valued occupations (Helen, 1998). Learning about a person's occupational history though validation or by creating Life Story books often leads to valuable insights regarding the person's actions and behaviors. For example, one gentleman living in a nursing facility was constantly going into other people's rooms and standing over them at night. Using validation, the practitioner discovered that he was once an evening guard at a detention facility for adolescents. Giving him a task to check things around the unit every evening eliminated his previously difficult behavior and gave him a sense of purpose. Validation therapy and Life Story books are tools that help the practitioner complete effective interviews and gather profile data. The occupational profile becomes a story that not only leads to occupation-based interventions for individuals with dementia, but also provides clarity to family and other care providers about the actions of their family member and helps restore important occupations, interpersonal connections, and dignity.

Where to Begin

Interviewing is a skill that develops with time and experience. Practitioners can take several approaches that will develop and hone their interviewing skills more effectively and efficiently. Most practitioners will find it helpful to start with a published, semistructured interview instrument, such as the ones highlighted in this book. These interview instruments provide a ready-made list of questions focused on occupation, as well as clues for building technique. In time, practitioners will identify questions they find most helpful in their settings. In addition to actual instruments, it is valuable to obtain a resource that provides detailed explanations of the basic clinical interviewing skills, such as listening and prompting, as well as other techniques touched on in this chapter. Interview skills can only be developed through the process of actually doing interviews. A therapist can practice by engaging in interviews with friends, strangers at parties, or even with people who call to solicit donations. Because there is no pressure to gather the right information, these small interviews allow the interviewer to focus on building skills for redirecting or prompting. The interviewer can have a colleague observe several interviews and provide constructive feedback. Another option is to record and watch a few interviews. This allows interviewers an opportunity to reflect on their technique, body language, ability to connect with the interviewee, and ability to orchestrate the interview to get the best possible outcome. Lastly, practitioners can ask for feedback from the person they just interviewed. Practitioners gain valuable information about their interview skills when they are open to this feedback.

Summary

The *Framework* (AOTA, 2014) emphasizes the importance of beginning the occupational profile during the initial contact with a person seeking help because the profile guides further decision making related to evaluation and intervention planning. Using an interview methodology is a flexible way for busy practitioners to gather profile information. Interviewing is also an effective way to build rapport and set the stage for a collaborative intervention process. When practitioners develop the skills needed to utilize a variety of interview methods, they are able to obtain the person's perspective regardless of their capacity for expression. Before implementing an interview process in any practice setting, practitioners must make a conscious effort to become more culturally sensitive. Practitioners will benefit from developing a plan to learn and polish their occupation-based interviewing skills. The link to the Occupational Profile published by the AOTA is available at https://www.aota.org/Practice/Manage/Reimb/occupational-profile-document-value-ot.aspx.

References

American Occupational Therapy Association. (2014). Occupational therapy practice framework: Domain and process (3rd ed.). *American Journal of Occupational Therapy, 68*(Suppl. 1), S1-S48.

Asaba, E., & Jackson, J. (2011). Social ideologies embedded in everyday life: A narrative analysis about disability, identities and occupation. *Journal of Occupational Science, 18,* 139-152.

Baron, K., Kielhofner, G., Iyenger, A., Goldhammer, G., & Wolenski, J. (2006). *Occupational Self-Assessment (OSA) Version 2.2.* Chicago, IL: University of Illinois at Chicago, MOHO Clearinghouse.

Black, R. M. (2013). Culture, race and ethnicity and the impact on occupation and occupational performance. In B. A. Boyt Schell, G. Gillen, M. E. Scaffa, & E. S. Cohn (Eds.), *Willard and Spackman's occupational therapy* (12th ed., pp. 173-187). Philadelphia, PA: Lippincott Williams & Wilkins.

Christiansen, C. H. (1999). Defining lives: Occupation as identity: An essay on competence, coherence, and the creation of meaning. *American Journal of Occupational Therapy, 53,* 547-558.

Cohen, A. S., Green, L., & Partnow, S. (2011). *Practicing the art of compassionate listening.* Ashland, OR: The Compassionate Listening Project.

Egan, G. (2009). *The skilled helper: A problem-management and opportunity-development approach to helping.* Belmont, CA: Brooks/Cole, Cengage Learning.

Feil, N. (2002). *The validation breakthrough: Simple techniques for communication with people with Alzheimer's-type dementia* (2nd ed.). Baltimore, MD: Health Professions Press.

Helen, C. R. (1998). *Alzheimer's disease: Activity focused care.* Cambridge, MA: Butterworth-Heinemann.

Keegan, G. (n.d.). *The interview method.* Retrieved from http://www.gerardkeegan.co.uk/resource/interview-meth1.htm

Kielhofner, G., Borell, L., Holzmuller, R., Jonsson, H., Josephsson, S., Keponen, R., … Nygård , L. (2008). Crafting occupational life. In G. Kielhofner (Ed.), *The model of human occupation: Theory and application* (4th ed., pp. 110-125). Philadelphia, PA: Lippincott Williams & Wilkins.

Lynch, E. W., & Hanson, M. J. (Eds.). (1998). *Developing cross-cultural competence: A guide for working with children and their families* (2nd ed.). Baltimore, MD: Paul Brookes Publishing.

Mactavish, J., Mahon, M. J., & Lutfiyya, Z. M. (2000). "I can speak for myself": Involving individuals with intellectual disabilities as research participants. *Mental Retardation, 38,* 216-227.

Mahoney, W. (2014). Practice perk: Developing occupational profiles for younger children. *OT Practice, 25*(15), 18.

Mallinson, T., Kielhofner, G., & Mattingly, C. (1996). Metaphor and meaning in clinical interview. *American Journal of Occupational Therapy, 50,* 338-346. https://doi.org/10.5014/ajot.50.5.338

Mattingly, C., & Lawlor, M. (2000). Learning from stories: Narrative interviewing in cross-cultural research. *Scandinavian Journal of Occupational Therapy, 7*(1), 4-14. https://doi.org/10.1080/110381200443571

McDonald, K. E., & Kidney, C. A. (2012). What is right? Ethics in intellectual disabilities research. *Journal of Policy and Practice in Intellectual Disabilities, 9,* 27-39.

Mindtools. (n.d.). Active listening. Retrieved from https://www.mindtools.com/CommSkll/ActiveListening.htm

Munoz, J. P. (2007). Culturally responsive caring in occupational therapy. *Occupational Therapy International, 14,* 256-280.

Oakley, F., Kielhofner, G., Barris, R., & Reichler, R. K. (1986). The role checklist: Development and empirical assessment of reliability. *Occupational Therapy Journal of Research, 6,* 157-170.

Parkinson, S., Forsyth, K., & Kielhofner, G. (2006). *The Model of Human Occupation Screening Tool (MOHOST), Version 2.0.* Chicago, IL: University of Illinois at Chicago MOHO Clearinghouse.

Remen, R. N. (1996). *Kitchen table wisdom* (9th ed). New York, NY: Riverhead Books.

Roe, D., & Davidson, L. (2005). Self and narrative in schizophrenia: Time to author a new story. *Journal of Medical Ethics: Medical Humanities, 31,* 89-94.

Sommers-Flannagan, J., & Sommers-Flannagan, R. (2009). *Clinical interviewing* (4th ed.). Hoboken, NJ: John Wiley & Sons, Inc.

Story Corps. (n.d.). *Great questions.* Retrieved from http://storycorps.org/great-questions

Sue, D. W., Arredondo, P., & McDavis, R. (1992). Multicultural counseling competencies and standards: A call to the professions. *Journal of Counseling and Development, 70,* 477-486.

Taylor, R. (2008). *The intentional relationship: Occupational therapy and use of self.* Philadelphia, PA: F. A. Davis Company.

Taylor, S. J., & Bogdan, R. C. (1990). Quality of life and the individual's perspective. In R. L. Schalock (Ed.), *Quality of life: Perspectives and issues* (pp. 27-40). Washington, DC: American Association on Mental Retardation.

4

Client-Centered Assessment
The Canadian Occupational Performance Measure

Sue Baptiste, MHSc

*The talent that has to be learned is finding out what someone's passion is and
setting them up to realize that. You don't get the best work from people if
you're guiding them versus them guiding themselves.*
(Cashmore, 2011)

The first iteration of this chapter was completed and published at a time when
the concept and values of client-centered practice were gaining traction across a wide
sweep of health care services, including occupational therapy practice in mental health.
In the course of the growth in use of client-centered practice as a foundational tenet
of much of professional practice and health service delivery (often using the terminology of *person-centered* or *patient-centered*; this requires an independent exploration), the
Canadian Occupational Performance Measure (COPM) itself attracted global interest
and acceptance. Because there exists a much greater understanding of both the concept
and the measure at the time of writing the current version, this chapter will review the
foundational assumptions of client-centeredness as a construct through reflecting on the
literature. The COPM will be explored in some detail, with discussion of the evidence to
support its reliability and validity, as well as its utilization in practice, with specific reference to practice in the areas of mental health and mental illness. Case studies will be provided that illustrate possible applications of the COPM as a gateway step in determining
the patient's perspective upon which to build a therapeutic relationship and process.

Hemphill, B. J., & Urish, C. K. (Eds.). *Assessments in
Occupational Therapy Mental Health: An Integrative Approach,
Fourth Edition* (pp. 53-65). © 2020 Taylor & Francis Group.

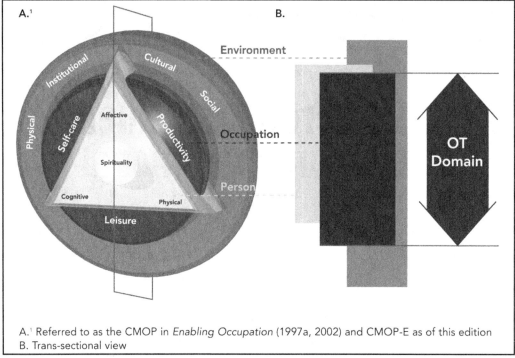

A.[1] Referred to as the CMOP in *Enabling Occupation* (1997a, 2002) and CMOP-E as of this edition
B. Trans-sectional view

Figure 4-1. Canadian Model of Occupational Performance and Engagement. (Reprinted with permission from Polatajko, H. J., Townsend, E. A., & Craik, J. [2007]. Canadian Model of Occupational Performance and Engagement [CMOP-E]. In E. A. Townsend & H. J. Polatajko [Eds.], *Enabling occupation II: Advancing an occupational therapy vision of health, well-being, & justice through occupation* [p. 23]. Ottawa, Ontario, Canada: CAOT Publications ACE.)

Theoretical Basis

History of Development and Previous Versions/ Important Changes to Note in Current Version

The Canadian Model of Occupational Performance (CMOP) was one of the outputs of a consensus process undertaken in the mid-1990s by the Canadian Association of Occupational Therapists (CAOT). The process was another link in the chain that commenced a decade earlier with the development of guidelines for Canadian occupational therapy practice, jointly supported by the CAOT and the Department of Health and Welfare of the federal government of Canada. The book *Enabling Occupation: A Canadian Perspective* (Stanton, Law, & Polatajko, 1997) was the overall outcome of the consensus process within which the CMOP was a central innovation. Since the book's first edition in 1997, the CMOP became one of the core elements of contemporary occupational therapy practice in Canada. With the advent of a second volume of *Enabling Occupation* in 2007 (Townsend & Polatajko, 2013), there was also a second iteration of the original CMOP that is entitled the Canadian Model of Occupational Performance and Engagement (CMOP-E; Figure 4-1). Additionally, there was a new conceptualization of the occupational therapy process that built upon the Occupational Performance Process Model to offer the perspective of the Canadian Practice Process Framework (Figure 4-2). The graphic representations of these new models are introduced, explicated, and illustrated in the second edition of

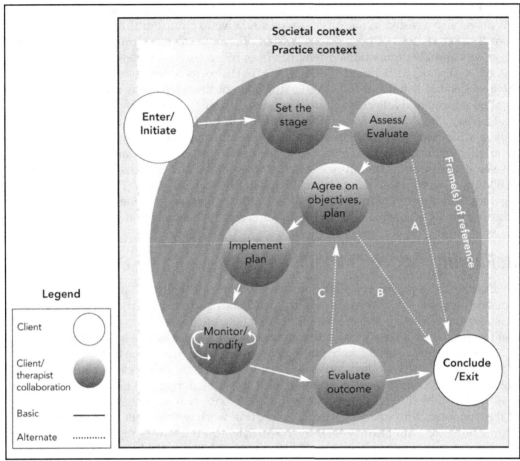

Figure 4-2. Canadian Practice Process Framework. (Reprinted with permission from Polatajko, H. J., Craik, J., Davis, J., & Townsend, E. A. [2007]. Canadian Practice Process Framework. In E. A. Townsend & H. J. Polatajko [Eds.], *Enabling occupation II: Advancing an occupational therapy vision of health, well-being, & justice through occupation* [p. 233]. Ottawa, Ontario, Canada: CAOT Publications ACE.)

Enabling Occupation II (Townsend & Polatajko, 2013). Figures 4-1 and 4-2 are presented here to introduce the reader to the changed images.

Psychometric Properties

The COPM was designed as a client-centered measure that is also occupation focused. The format is that of a semistructured interview with a structured method of scoring that provided measures of occupational performance as perceived by the client across a period of time.

Normative Data

There have been three phases of psychometric evaluation since the launching of the COPM. Phase One included early pilot testing in several Canadian communities ($n = 49$; Law, Baptiste, Carswell, McColl, Polatajko, & Pollock, 1993). This phase was important to the final appearance of the tool in terms of layout, format, and wording. In addition, this phase also assisted in identifying issues relative to clinical utilization and measurement (Law et al., 1993). Phase Two consisted of a more intensive pilot testing involving 256 clients and 219 occupational therapists from 55 practice sites (Law, Polatajko, Pollock, McColl, Carswell, & Baptiste, 1994). These participants were chosen randomly from the membership listings of the CAOT. The value of this phase was inherent within the detailed information collected that pertained to utilization and scoring of the COPM (Law et al., 1994). Phase Three is ongoing since this addresses the validation of the COPM. This is a process that continues throughout the utilization of a tool and is undertaken by many authors and researchers. Different disabilities, countries, and practice settings have emerged from the literature as readily accepting of and responsive to the use of the COPM (McColl, Carswell, Law, Pollock, Baptiste, & Polatajko, 2006). This ensures a growing understanding of the reliability, validity, utility, and responsiveness of a measure—in this case, the COPM. More current information can be obtained from www.thecopm.ca.

Reliability

Ensuring the reliability of an outcome measure speaks to the ability of the tool to replicate the same scores regardless of the conditions surrounding the test situation, such as who completed the assessment and the time taken to do so. The one form of reliability that has relevance to the COPM is that of test-retest (assessment-reassessment).

Seven reliability studies were reviewed in order to determine the test-retest reliability of the COPM. There was clear consensus that the COPM can be repeated and will deliver stable results over differing time periods well above the range that is usually considered reasonable. Many different types of client populations are represented across this section of the literature, with one in particular reporting work with clients with schizophrenia (Pan, Chung, & Hsin-Hwei, 2003). In this article, test-retest was reported as $r = .84-.85$. Specific details regarding the other studies addressed are available in the COPM manual (Law, Baptiste, Carswell, McColl, Polatajko, & Pollock, 2014).

One other element of using the COPM must be mentioned. Although the COPM is ideally a face-to-face interview measure, Kjeken et al. (2005) reported that paper-and-pencil completion of the measure showed reliable results; however, completion of the COPM over the telephone was not as reliable, and therefore not as desirable.

Validity

Many of the different types of validity were tested in relation to the COPM, working with clients from many client groups and in many different practice environments. Those forms of validity illustrated within the literature are the following: concurrent, criterion, convergent, divergent, construct, and content. The studies identified supported the validity of the COPM in the measurement of occupational performance. Sixteen articles were utilized to explore the validity of the COPM. There is a marked range of functional measures, and measures of social and psychological functioning exemplified in the articles appraised for inclusion. Some investigators have taken the approach of stating the degree to which the same occupational performance issues identified by the COPM were identified by other measures. It would appear typical that there is a 50% to 80% congruence; however, the COPM was noted as always identifying more problems. Boyer, Hachey, and Mercier (2000) studied individuals with schizophrenia who received home care services in Canada and reported the following: Work Personality Profile: $r = .53$; Satisfaction With

Performance Scaled Questionnaire: $r = .17-.39$. In the United States, Rochman, Ray, Kulich, Mehta, and Driscoll (2008) reported the following: Pain Disability Index: $r = .75-.79$; visual analog of pain: $r = .42-.39$.

Sensitivity

Sensitivity to change or responsiveness was considered important in determining the ability of a measure to determine changes across time. This can be evaluated in three main ways: by evaluating change while the client is participating in interventions that are known to be effective; by evaluating change across time when improvement or recovery of performance is an expectation; and by comparing change in function rated by the client, family, and therapist. Examples of research reporting responsiveness included two examples relevant to mental health and mental illness within the eight articles. The COPM showed sensitivity to change when used with clients coping with pain in the United Kingdom (Carpenter, Baker, & Tyldesley, 2001), and Australian investigators showed that significant change was detected in both performance and satisfaction in clients with acquired brain injuries.

Assessment Administration

Utility

Utility is an important element of determining the actual use of any measure or tool. If a measure takes a long time to administer when working with a client, chances are that the assessment will not be used accurately because sections may be covered superficially or even omitted. In the case of the COPM, the fundamental principles that are foundational to the measure must be integrated into the manner in which the measure is applied; these are client- and occupation-centered principles. This demands attention to the client telling the story and the therapist interpreting against the scaffolding of the COPM. The assessment necessitates the existence of an emerging partnership between the client and the therapist where goals are shared and respect is mutual.

Many studies ($n = 21$) examined assessment utility. Five key areas were identified that are worthy of note:

1. *Administration time*: 12 to 40 minutes. If the administration takes longer, this is usually because the therapist is guiding the conversation to include details of the illness or injury, back stories that could be included at a later point in the relationship (e.g., spousal circumstances, ethnicity), or content about assessment details and/or ideas for intervention.

2. *Client-centered approach*: When a therapist is comfortable with the client being central to the information exchange, then the COPM flows well. When the therapist tends to be more professionally based and comfortable with the role of expert, then the application of the COPM is less likely to be a smooth process.

3. *Occupation-focused therapy*: The COPM was shown to give a useful structure for establishing a starting place relative to occupational performance problems. Clients reported that they found the COPM easy to understand and that it was helpful in exploring the complexities of understanding their lives at the time of the conversation. The few who did not find it so simple did find the idea of being a partner in their own rehabilitation both interesting and rewarding.

4. *Goal-setting*: There was mention of the COPM being helpful for setting goals and tracking progress. In addition, there was agreement that the role of the COPM as its original purpose, that of an outcome measure, was indeed fulfilled and found to be of particular use.

5. *Ease of communication and documentation:* The COPM definitely helps in defining occupational performance problems. However, in addition and not intentionally, the COPM has become recognized as a way in which the role of occupational therapy and occupational therapists can be readily illustrated to clients, families, and colleagues alike.

Of the 21 articles appraised in relation to utility, 3 had specific relationships to working with clients with mental illness diagnosis and mental health issues (Carpenter et al., 2001; McNulty & Beplat, 2008; Pan et al., 2003).

In these examples from the literature, the findings incorporated the following: the COPM provided a medium for discussing occupational performance issues with clients (Carpenter et al., 2001); time for administration was 23.6 minutes, with difficulty in administration rating at 3.8/7 (Pan et al., 2003); and COPM use led to the naming of more occupational performance problems (McNulty & Beplat, 2008).

Area of Occupation/Performance Skills/ Performance Patterns/Client Factors Assessed

As mentioned within the introduction and detailed description of the COPM, this is an outcome measure for occupational performance. The COPM does not replace the assessment tools used regularly in therapists' work nor does it replace the intervention methods and approaches used in work with clients over time. The COPM is an exoskeleton, populated with the principles and values of client- and occupation-centeredness. The COPM is considered an integrated partner with the CMOP-E and recognized as an essential thread throughout the Canadian Practice Process Framework.

Description of Environment/ Description of Supplies/Materials Required

The COPM can be administered in a regular practice setting as long as the space is comfortable and private with a table for showing the client the COPM measure as it is being explained and applied. The practice setting itself can be institutional, community centered, or home based. The supplies required are copies of the COPM form and a sharp pencil, plus a copy of the COPM manual because the rating scale cards for using with the client are found in the back pocket of the manual. If the therapist is using an online or personal digital assistant version of the COPM, then personal choices need to be made about how the scoring would be best accomplished (e.g., hard copy form for client, hard copy cards for rating). (See more details at www.thecopm.ca.)

Administration

McColl et al. (2005) addressed the particular nature of special applications in using the COPM, including special clinical circumstances. Seven discrete areas were identified and will be addressed here with illustrations from mental health practice.

1. *Legitimacy of the client's point of view*: In many clinical situations, concern was expressed as to whether the client was a reliable source of information about his or her own experience, thus potentially compromising the relevance and quality to the client of the emerging therapeutic plan. It is always difficult to allow the client's priorities to shine through, thus relegating the therapist's goals to the back burner. However, if practicing in a truly client-centered fashion, it is critical to strive for this in every client encounter. This is of particular difficulty when working with clients who are contending with pervasive mental illness and whose form of communication is unfamiliar.

2. *Inclusion of other stakeholders*: Other members or participants in the client's support system are frequently needed as central players in the development and execution of a client-centered treatment plan. While there may be many participants in the process, from the perspective of using the COPM, the core client is the individual or group who seeks to address perceived concerns around occupational performance. In mental health practice, this can include members of the circle of care offering views from their perspectives, but at all times, it is critical that direct input from the identified is sought, however difficult that may be.

3. *Modifications to the approach*: While the COPM has been developed as a semistructured tool, thus implying the use of a standardized approach to the interview and information collection, there are undoubtedly many situations during which adapting the model may be helpful while staying true to the process overall. For example, there may be a need to communicate the message in a way more suited to the cognitive or language skills of the client. In addition, the scoring scheme can appear confusing to some people, and a creative approach to the measurement of performance, importance, and satisfaction can be applied. Examples of this include the use of a happy face to illustrate the number 10 and a sad face to illustrate the number 1.

4. *Use of another person to act as a communication proxy for the client*: Interpreters can be an invaluable resource but should be selected based on their ability to retain an objective position, thus reporting the client's information, opinions, and feelings in an unbiased manner. Another situation where a proxy respondent may be used is when the client is noncommunicative.

   However, being a proxy is not a sound role to assume when trying to elicit the reality of someone's coping and lived experiences with occupational performance. This is a difficult situation for everyone involved and the respondent must be clearly advised **not** to try to represent what is perceived to be the client's viewpoints, but rather should put his or her own interpretations to the side. This should be taken as an opportunity to impart his or her views of how the client appears to cope with life and life tasks; from that should be distilled what the key areas of the client's occupational performance are that impact the other person and may well impact that person's occupational performance as a caretaker of the identified client.

5. *Ability to identify problems*: With many clients, it is necessary to engage in a therapeutic process ahead of the experience of identifying central occupational performance issues. Thus, the timing of the application of the COPM can be critical. Proceeding with the COPM interview too early can suggest that the client is unable to engage, whereas completing the process at a later time can be hampered by decisions and experiences that impact the client's ability to understand his or her own priorities. When working with clients with mental health issues, the key is to have the COPM at hand for that special time when there is clear rapport between therapist and client, with clarity of communication offering that ideal moment to elicit useful information around occupational performance.

6. *Problems with memory and attention*: If clients exhibit problems with concentration or particular signs of tiredness, it is important to consider using the COPM across several occasions rather than trying to complete the whole process at once.

7. *Cultural differences*: In this example, the word *culture* is used broadly and embraces not only ethnic groups but also all other potential cultural filters such as age and stage, socioeconomic status, lifestyle choices, and rural-urban lifestyle expectations. Awareness and respect for cultural diversity are critical components in the application of the COPM and for a client-centered practice approach overall. Considerations of cultural elements include the following: a client's comfort with roles within his or her own life and within the health care system, expectations of experts, understanding of power in a therapeutic relationship, and comfort with standing up for his or her own needs and expressing views and opinions.

Scoring

There are two distinct scores that result from using the COPM—performance and satisfaction—that are rated individually on a scale of 1 to 10. These scores emerge from up to five problems identified by the client as priorities for attention. Five occupational performance problems are suggested as the maximum to address because there can be many that the client perceives as important. Five problems of the occupational therapy assessment and intervention can be addressed at each iteration of the tool; others can then be identified as appropriate, and the process can be undertaken once more. Average scores can be found by adding the problem scores for the individual problems then dividing that total by the number of problems. Change can be identified after a reassessment using the same problems.

Individual scores are unique to each client; therefore, comparing client outcomes is not a useful or appropriate exercise. The truly meaningful scores are those for each client between the different times when the assessment was completed (e.g., Time 1 and Time 2).

The specific manner in which the COPM should be administered and the standard scoring approach make the COPM a standardized measure of occupational performance. However, it is not a norm-referenced measure because this is not congruent with the client-centered approach that is central to the COPM and from the occupational performance model that is one of the foundations. Through a COPM lens, occupation is seen as something individual and subjective.

There are five distinct components of the COPM process, all of which include some elements of the scoring: problem definition, rating performance, selecting problems for scoring, scoring performance and satisfaction, and client reassessment.

1. *Problem definition*: As stated earlier, the COPM is a client-centered instrument, the use of which is unique to each client because the personal nature of the occupational performance issues experienced are anchored in the daily living of each person. With a semistructured process, the therapist-client relationship is established through the client identifying important daily occupations that he or she wishes, needs, or is expected to do but is unable to either undertake or complete. Occupation areas that can be considered include productivity, leisure, and self-care.

2. *Rating performance*: When both partners in the conversation are comfortable with the identification of the occupational performance problems, the therapist then asks the client to rate how important each of these problems are to the client in his or her daily life. This rating is accomplished by considering a scale of 1 to 10. Rating cards are provided with each COPM manual.

3. *Selecting problems for scoring*: In this component, the client chooses a maximum of five problems from the list that he or she rated as important. These five problems will be the foundation of what is addressed during the full assessment and intervention processes. The therapist enters this information into the scoring section of the COPM form so that the importance ratings can form the foundation for intervention planning.

4. *Scoring performance and satisfaction*: Next, the therapist asks the client to use the 10-point scale approach again to determine the level of performance and satisfaction that the client feels for the five priority problems already identified. Once this is accomplished, the therapist calculates the average COPM performance score and the average COPM satisfaction score. These scores regularly range across the full spectrum of possibilities, from 1 to 10. The performance scores and the satisfaction scores are not expected to align. A 1 on the scale indicates poor performance and very low satisfaction, whereas a 10 on the scale represents very good performance and high satisfaction. These ratings are based purely on the client's perceptions of how well he or she does things and how satisfied he or she is with how well he or she is doing them.

5. *Client reassessment*: The final step takes place (1) at a time when an intervention is completed, (2) at a time that was decided on at the time of the first scoring session, or (3) when the client and/or therapist feels that something has changed and that reassessment may be valuable. The same process is followed as occurred the first time, and the therapist then uses these scores to calculate the changes that have taken place between the two assessment events.

Case Studies

In order to help in understanding the potential for applying the COPM within an occupation- and client-centered practice model, the following case studies are offered. Following each patient's story, there are some guiding questions to assist the therapist in considering how the client-centered principles were applied in the case studies and how the COPM assisted in determining the direction for the ongoing therapeutic engagement.

Olivia

Olivia is 16 years old and has a 4-year history of anorexia nervosa. Olivia completed an intensive inpatient eating disorders program where her weight was restored to within 80% of typical weight, participated in group therapy to address the underlying causes of her eating disorder, and learned healthy coping skills to manage challenges. Olivia spent 4 months in the hospital. In order to build on the progress she made in treatment, Olivia was referred to an outpatient eating disorders program at a community hospital close to her home. The occupational therapist at the outpatient program is working with Olivia and her family to help Olivia maintain the medical improvements achieved in the hospital and to continue to address the underlying psychosocial issues related to her eating disorder. The occupational therapist used the COPM in the initial interview, with the main goal to identify occupational performance issues with Olivia and to engage Olivia in the goal-setting process. Olivia responded to the interview well and was active in setting her goals. Olivia stated that she was happy to see the occupational therapist was listening to her goals and not dictating to her what goals she should be working on in therapy. The occupational performance issues (OPIs) identified are summarized in Table 4-1. Olivia

Table 4-1

Canadian Occupational Performance Issues for Olivia

OPI	Interest	Performance (1)	Satisfaction (1)	Performance (2)	Satisfaction (2)
Plan my own meals	10	3	2	8	9
Increase tolerance for walking	7	5	4	9	10
Increase attention span at school in classes	9	2	1	8	8
Feel more confident in social situations outside of classes	10	2	1	7	9

Table 4-2

Guiding Questions to Assist Clinical Reasoning (Olivia)

- Were the principles of client-centered practice realized in this particular case scenario?
  - If so, at which junctures were they most apparent?
- What were the most useful outcomes of using the COPM with this client?
- What elements of your practice are reflected in this scenario?
- Are there components of this process that are familiar?
- Are there components of this process that are new to you?
  - If so, are those components something that you feel have value for your practice?
  - If so, how can you integrate them into your work?

met with the occupational therapist over a 3-month period as progress determined. Session content focused on the skills and resources needed to meet her identified OPIs. Olivia completed a second COPM after 3 months to identify her performance and satisfaction on the original OPIs. Performance and satisfaction ratings at the second COPM are found in Table 4-1. It is apparent that Olivia identified a significant improvement in the performance and satisfaction with each OPI. Olivia remained committed to improving her performance in areas that were important and therefore meaningful for her. Olivia was able to remain out of the hospital and continued to improve with respect to her eating disorder. At the time of discharge from the outpatient program, Olivia was integrated back into her school environment, was becoming more responsible for her meal planning, and was thriving in her social environment (Table 4-2).

Table 4-3

Canadian Occupational Performance Issues for Andrew

OPI	Interest	Performance (1)	Satisfaction (1)	Performance (2)	Satisfaction (2)
Improve sleep and hygiene	8	3	4	7	7
Plan meals that fit my budget and nutritional needs	9	2	2	9	10
Have more energy to attend work	9	3	3	9	9
Participate in recreational ice hockey twice/week	10	1	1	9	9

Andrew

Andrew, a 27-year-old man, was seen by an occupational therapist at a psychiatric day program that focused on weight management through lifestyle changes. This program included educational sessions where Andrew was able to learn more about his illness and began to apply some coping strategies. Andrew was referred to the program by his family physician, who was concerned about Andrew's significant weight gain since he started taking a new (to him) antipsychotic medication. Andrew was diagnosed with schizophrenia at the age of 23 years, after traveling and experiencing a psychotic break that lead to hospitalization. He had completed a community college program in business administration the year before. Andrew started a sedentary job in an office and reported feeling uncomfortable at his current weight, which is 65 pounds above his typical weight. He reported being short of breath and tired all the time. He reported suffering from sleep apnea and had recently started using a continuous positive airway pressure machine. Andrew was once active in recreational sports but did not feel physically able to participate at the time of meeting with the therapist. He was also concerned about an increase in his blood pressure and a family history of diabetes mellitus. Andrew was aware that he needed to continue taking his medications to manage his illness and to continue to function at his job. The occupational therapist met with Andrew at the clinic and together they completed the COPM as part of the initial interview. Andrew stated that he enjoyed participating in the goal-setting process and often referred to the copy of the COPM that he took away from his assessment on that first visit. Andrew also shared the COPM with his family to help them better understand his goals. Table 4-3 summarizes the results of the COPM completed at two points in time. Table 4-4 offers questions to consider relative to providing intervention to the case study for Andrew.

Table 4-4

Guiding Questions to Assist Clinical Reasoning (Andrew)

- Were the principles of client-centered practice realized in this particular case scenario?
  - If so, at which junctures were they most apparent?
- What were the most useful outcomes of using the COPM with this client?
- What elements of your practice are reflected in this scenario?
- Are there components of this process that are familiar?
- Are there components of this process that are new to you?
  - If so, are those components something that you feel have value for your practice?
  - If so, how can you integrate them into your work?

Suggested Further Research

The body of knowledge and understanding related to the COPM grows steadily year by year. When reflecting upon what we know now in comparison with 10 years ago, it is markedly richer. One can only hope then that this progress continues. There is a current body of work ongoing at the time of writing related to the COPM and the relationships between it and the *International Classification of Functioning, Disability and Health* (ICF; World Health Organization, 2001). This work shows some promise in furthering our sense of the importance of linking the foundational principles and intent of the ICF with those of the COPM that are nested within the CMOP-E and the commitment to occupation-focused practice models. With a measure of the nature of the COPM, it cannot be stated too often that there is such a wide range of potential applications for its use. The sense of the work never being done is probably a very true statement here.

Summary

Although the field of mental health practice is one of the historical bases from which occupational therapy grew, and therefore is rich with parallel and similar processes to those experienced in other practice fields, specific challenges remain that are important to identify.

The existence of often very active pathological conditions influence clients' abilities to negotiate and manage their environment in ways that can be very different from those problems and barriers experienced by individuals learning to cope with problems arising from physical conditions. Kusznir, Scott, Cooke, and Young (1996) discuss the results of a research project within which occupational therapists were asked to consider their mental health practice and to reflect on when maintaining a client-centered approach became challenging or impossible. The results of their qualitative analysis revealed five emerging themes:

1. Patient reluctance to become involved in the occupational therapy process
2. Dissonance between opinions or expectations of patients and therapists
3. Difficulty in patients making decisions
4. Lack of fit between the patient decision and skill level
5. Difficulties in modifying the patient environment

Again, these statements in and of themselves may not appear that different from those that could be made by therapists working within other practice settings; however, they do invite a closer examination.

The willingness of a patient to get involved in occupational therapy when coming from the perspective of coping with an episode of mental illness is often clouded by a lack of awareness of how the pathology may be affecting an individual's ability to synthesize and integrate new knowledge and information. In addition, the patient may not be aware of timelines for hospitalization and a potentially quick discharge, which impacts his or her ability to engage in a timely manner. It is at this stage when the role of the therapist as an active partner and as an enabler of change should come to the fore. Being client-centered does not mean that the therapist should wait for the patient to articulate concerns with occupational performance before starting to build the relationship. At times like this, the therapist has the responsibility to be the stronger and more focused one in the partnership by providing suggestions, but listening with care and attention to how those suggestions are received.

References

Boyer, G., Hachey, R., & Mercier, C. (2000). Perceptions of occupational performance and subjective quality of life in person with severe mental illness. *Occupational Therapy in Mental Health, 15*(2), 1-15.

Carpenter, L., Baker, G. A., & Tyldesley, B. (2001). The use of the Canadian Occupational Performance Measure as an outcome of a pain management program. *Canadian Journal of Occupational Therapy, 68*, 16-22.

Cashmore, P. (2011). Mashable's Pete Cashmore on persistence. *Entrepreneur.* Retrieved from https://www.entrepreneur.com/article/219592

Kjeken, I., Dagfinrud, H., Uhlig, T., Mowinckel, P., Kvien, T. K., & Finset, A. (2005). Reliability of the Canadian Occupational Performance Measure in patients with ankylosing spondylitis. *Journal of Rheumatology 32*(8), 1503-1509.

Kusznir, A., Scott, E., Cooke, R., & Young, L. T. (1996). Functional consequences of bipolar affective disorder: An occupational therapy perspective. *Canadian Journal of Occupational Therapy, 63*, 313-322.

Law, M., Baptiste, S., Carswell, A., McColl, M. A., Polatajko, H., & Pollock, N. (1993). *COPM user survey* Unpublished manuscript. McMaster University School of Rehabilitation Science.

Law, M., Baptiste, S., Carswell, A., McColl, M. A., Polatajko, H., & Pollock, N. (2014). *Canadian Occupational Performance Measure manual* (5th ed.). Ottawa, Ontario, Canada: CAOT Publications ACE.

Law, M., Polatajko, H., Pollock, N., McColl, M. A., Carswell, A., & Baptiste, S. (1994). The Canadian Occupational Performance Measure: Results of pilot testing. *Canadian Journal of Occupational Therapy, 61*, 191-197.

McColl, M. A., Carswell, A., Law, M., Pollock, N., Baptiste, S., & Polatajko, H. (2006). *Research on the Canadian Occupational Performance Measure: An annotated resource.* Ottawa, Ontario, Canada: CAOT Publications ACE.

McColl, M. A., Law, M., Baptiste, S., Pollock, N., Carswell, A., & Polatajko, H. (2005). Targeted applications of the Canadian Occupational Performance Measure. *Canadian Journal of Occupational Therapy Abstracts, 72*(5), 298-300.

McNulty, M. C., & Beplat, A. L. (2008). The validity of using the Canadian Occupational Performance Measure with older adults with and without depressive symptoms. *Physical and Occupational Therapy in Geriatrics, 27*(1), 1-15.

Pan, A. W., Chung, L., & Hsin-Hwei, G. (2003). Reliability and validity of the Canadian Occupational Performance Measure for clients with psychiatric disorders in Taiwan. *Occupational Therapy International, 104*, 269-277.

Rochman, D. L., Ray, S. A., Kulich, R. J., Mehta, N. R., & Driscoll, S. (2008). Validity and utility of the Canadian Occupational Performance Measure as an outcome measure in a craniofacial pain center. *OTJR: Occupational, Participation & Health, 28*, 4-11.

Stanton, S., Law, M., & Polatajko, H. (Eds.). (1997). *Enabling occupation: An occupational therapy perspective.* Ottawa, Ontario, Canada: CAOT Publications ACE.

Townsend, E. A., & Polatajko, H. J. (2013). *Enabling occupation II: Advancing an occupational therapy vision of health, well-being, & justice through occupation* (2nd ed.). Ottawa, Ontario, Canada: CAOT Publications ACE.

World Health Organization. (2001). *International classification of functioning, disability and health.* Geneva, Switzerland: Author.

Social Profile
Assessment of Social Participation in Children, Adolescents, and Adults

Mary V. Donohue, PhD, OT/L, FAOTA

*Never doubt that a small group of thoughtful, committed people can change the world.
Indeed, it is the only thing that ever has.*
(Mead, 2017)

The Social Profile is designed to be either an observation tool or a self-scored assessment, depending on the age and cognitive competency of the individual in a group or of a group of individuals (Donohue, 2013). There are two versions of the Social Profile: the Children's version and the Adult/Adolescent version. The assessments are available in the Social Profile manual, which also includes a DVD of the two assessment tools.

The Social Profile is a measure of social participation in activity groups that include the family, classes, schools, clubs, clinics, sports teams, work teams, and community groups. The tool usually measures groups as ranging in interaction across one, two, or three levels of social development (out of five possible levels), thus providing a social profile or continuum of social behaviors while involved in an activity. The developmental level concepts are familiar. They include parallel, associative, basic cooperative, supportive cooperative, and mature levels of participation that manifest during an activity.

Theoretical Basis

Concepts/Construct

In 1932, Mildred Parten performed a study of social participation among 6 preschool children using a repeated measures design by observing each child 60 times, resulting in 360 data points. She observed three levels of participation as the children played. The

Hemphill, B. J., & Urish, C. K. (Eds.). *Assessments in Occupational Therapy Mental Health: An Integrative Approach, Fourth Edition* (pp. 67-75). © 2020 Taylor & Francis Group.

youngest children played parallel to others, side by side. Gradually, they began to have brief associations with children who liked the same activities that they enjoyed. As they became more comfortable playing with others, they began to cooperate with their play-mates, organizing their activity following rules of interaction. Parten (1932) named these levels of social participation as parallel, associative, and cooperative play.

In 1968, Anne C. Mosey, an occupational therapist, added two levels to Parten's (1932) continuum of concepts: an advanced level of cooperative interaction, which can be displayed by adolescents, and a mature level of social interaction, which can be mani-fested by adults. Thus, Mosey (1968) developed a five-level social developmental interac-tion spectrum. For the Social Profile, these concepts are currently labeled supportive, cooperative, and mature social participation (Dildine, 1972). Overall, the construct that underlies the five concepts is cooperation, whether in social groups, at work, in religious groups, or in sports groups.

Another source of the need for emphasis on social participation among healthy indi-viduals can be found in the *International Classification of Functioning, Disability and Health* of the World Health Organization (WHO; 2001). This information can be obtained in Chapters 7 and 9 of the ICF.

History of Development and Previous Versions/ Important Changes to Note in Current Version

In 1999, Donohue defined the theoretical base of the Social Profile to establish the origins of its underlying concepts and the principles of social participation. There was a longer version that clinicians rightfully indicated was not practical as a convenient assess-ment tool. A thorough search of the related literature identified pertinent vocabulary for descriptions of social behaviors in activity groups to compose appropriate items for abstract behaviors, such as social interactions. Ultimately, the adult and adolescent ver-sion of the Social Profile included 39 items. Therapists in pediatric practice requested a children's version of the Social Profile, which now consists of 26 items. Both versions have been used in clinical, classroom, and community settings.

In addition to comprehensive literature searches, 36 groups of children were observed during free play to ascertain what social behaviors naturally emerged at various age lev-els. Adolescents were observed playing in public playgroups. Adult groups in the com-munity were observed to determine whether the behaviors described in Mosey's (1986) theoretical work were typical of current adult social behaviors.

Organization of the items within the Social Profile were divided into three subscales, moving from the most concrete to more abstract items: (1) activity participation, (2) social interaction, and (3) group membership and roles. Activity participation is the most easily observed of the three. Social interaction is also observable, and group membership and roles are more subjective social behaviors.

Psychometric Properties

Normative Data

Observations of 429 children in 36 groups were carried out to determine if Parten's (1932) and Mosey's (1986) age ranges continue to emerge associated with a developmental social behavioral continuum. Children varied in their social development depending on their socioeconomic environment and adult expectations, so although ranges of social abilities were achieved in a standard sequence, individual children and classes of children may vary in their continuum of social growth. The same variation holds true for adolescents depending on the norms of the group in the lunchroom, in extracurricular activities, on the school bus, and in study groups. Maximum capability of social interaction is not always displayed depending on circumstances of adult supervision, school climate, and fatigue levels. Among some adults, mature responsibility is bypassed if an adult wishes to relax and be "retired." A tool such as the Social Profile can provide a graphic picture of how a group's environment fosters maximum social behaviors during an activity (Donohue, 2013).

Reliability

Internal Reliability

Item analysis of the 39 items in the Social Profile was carried out as an initial study of internal reliability, comparing each item with every other item individually to search for overlap and redundancy. The overall alpha reliability coefficient of the Social Profile in the study of 21 groups with 242 children is .7072, a good level of correlation that indicates adequate separateness of the Social Profile items. This result had a Bonferroni correction alpha of .05/4 and a probability level of $p < .001$.

Interrater Reliability

One study was conducted of 15 preschool groups consisting of 187 typically developing children (Donohue, 2005) in age-specific and mixed age groups at free play. The two observers of these groups were psychosocial occupational therapists, and they observed these groups as whole groups using the Social Profile. Subsequently, an intraclass correlation coefficient (ICC; Shrout & Fleiss, 1979; Yaffee, 1998) was used to rate the children who were at parallel, associative, and basic cooperative levels of participation in their activity groups. The two raters' scores correlated highly on parallel and basic cooperative observations (at $p < .05$ or $p < .01$). For parallel behaviors, correlations ranged from $r = .712$ to .902 and for basic cooperative behaviors correlations ranged from $r = .575$ to .798. The observation scores for associative behaviors were not significant. Frequently, associative behaviors are so brief that it is difficult to capture them.

Additional studies of interrater reliability were carried out for psychiatric unit activity groups with general diagnoses, substance abuse, and geriatric groups and for community-based groups of preschool children and senior adults. These studies consisted of 70 observations using the Social Profile (Donohue, 2006, 2013) in 35 groups with 2 occupational therapists and pairs of graduate occupational therapy students. The scores of these observers were examined using an ICC formulation. For the general psychiatric and drug rehabilitation units with 21 group sessions each, the ICC alpha was .8028. For the senior community and preschool groups with 14 group sessions each, the ICC alpha was .8813. Combining these 70 observations together resulted in an ICC alpha of .8359. This total result is moderately high, which is a good score for the agreement of observations of abstract psychosocial behaviors (Table 5-1).

Table 5-1

Interrater Reliability Studies Using the Social Profile

General Psychiatric and Drug Rehabilitation Units Paired occupational therapists and occupational therapy graduate student observers	$n = 21$ group sessions	ICC alpha = .8028
Preschool and Senior Community Groups Paired occupational therapy graduate student observers	$n = 14$ group sessions	ICC alpha = .8813
Combined Data of Group Interrater Observers	$n = 35$ group sessions	ICC alpha = .8359

Validity

Three types of validity evidence were sought for the Social Profile assessment tool: content, construct, and criterion validity.

Content Validity

Donohue (2003) included 11 mental health master clinicians as experts to evaluate the items being proposed for the Social Profile for item clarity and appropriateness related to Parten's (1932) and Mosey's (1968, 1986) theoretical bases. These experts identified the need for specific items in a developmental social schema and evaluated the items for redundancy. These clinicians were asked to identify items as useful, useful but not essential, or not essential. This process reduced the number of items to 39 (Bernard, 2000; Deci & Ryan, 2000).

All of the items were evaluated for authenticity. The author considered the differences between Parten's (1932) and Mosey's (1986) five labels. The concept labels of parallel, associative, basic cooperative, supportive cooperative, and mature groups were clearest in perception of social abilities at these five levels of social development.

In a factor analysis of 21 activity groups of 242 children, Donohue (2003) reported a clear separation of the 3 concepts of parallel level behaviors clustering in the right quadrant, associative level behaviors clustering in the bottom quadrant, and basic cooperative level behaviors clustering in the left quadrant. In these groups of preschool children, the basic cooperative behaviors had the highest loadings of 61%. The associative behavior items had loadings of 11.6%, and the parallel behavior items had loadings of 12.2% (Donohue, 2013).

Construct Validity

The construct selected for the development of construct validity was age groups to be examined in conjunction with the five levels of social participation. In a study of 21 groups of 242 preschool children aged 2 to 5 years involved in free play, Donohue (2003) reported that parallel behaviors occurred most often in 2- to 3-year-olds ($M = 3.2$ years). Associative behaviors were found to be highest in 4- to 5-year-olds ($M = 3.43$ years). Basic cooperative behaviors were seen most frequently in 5-year-olds ($M = 2.72$ years). Five-year-olds also continued to exhibit a high level of associative behaviors ($M = 3.31$ years), as would be expected in a gradual continuum of social growth (Bernard, 2000; Bredekamp & Copple, 2009; Table 5-2).

Table 5-2

Correlation of Four Ages of Preschool Children and Three Levels of the Social Profile

Parallel, Associative, and Cooperative Level Behaviors	Number of Groups	Number of Children	Spearman Correlation	p
Groups aged 2 to 3 years and parallel level	12	131	.8805	.0000
Groups aged 3 to 4 years and associative level	10	134	.7139	.0003
Groups aged 4 to 5 years and basic cooperative level	9	111	.8309	.0000

Table 5-3

Criterion Validity: Correlation of Behaviors and Ages in Parten's (1932) Study With the Social Profile Study[a]

Three Levels of Behaviors	Ages of Children in Both Studies
Highest level of parallel behaviors	2-year-olds
Highest level of associative behaviors	3- and 4-year-olds
Highest level of basic cooperative behaviors	4- and 5-year-olds

[a]Overall Spearman correlation coefficient: .850 ($p < .01$).

Criterion Validity

Parten's (1932) study may be used as a criterion by which to measure the validity of the Social Profile by way of a comparison of their developmental social behavioral scales examining levels of social participation and ages of preschool children. In both studies, Parten (1932) and Mosey (1986), the highest level of parallel behaviors was found among 2-year-olds, the highest level of associative behaviors was seen among 3- and 4-year-olds, and the highest level of basic cooperative behaviors was seen in 4- and 5-year-olds. The correlation of these age levels to the behaviors indicated a Spearman correlation coefficient of .850 ($p < .01$) for 21 groups with 242 children, which is a good correlation of observations of abstract social behaviors (Table 5-3).

Sensitivity

The sensitivity of the Social Profile was studied by Donohue, Hanif, and Wu Berns (2011). The researchers studied psychiatric patients in a typical locked unit activity group. The patients were in the group for 30 days of occupational therapy treatment. Two occupational therapists employed by their units observed 31 patients using the Social Profile upon admission and at discharge to determine if the Social Profile could measure

---

Table 5-4

Sensitivity of the Social Profile to Measure Change in Group Behavior Scores: *t* Test

- Average Social Profile scores in activity group at admission: 62.1666
- Average Social Profile scores in activity group at discharge: 84.333
  - Critical one-tailed *t*-test set at 1.669
  - Observed one-tailed *t*-test set at 4.750
  - $p = .05$
- G-Power test: .835357, with an effect size of 0.5

Adapted from Cohen, Swerdlik, & Phillips, 1995.

---

improvement in activity participation, social interaction, and in-group membership role. Criteria for admission to the study consisted of adequate attendance in the group. A *t* test was employed for this paired sample of data. For this group, the mean for the Social Profile pre-test scores was 62.1666 and the mean post-test scores was 84.333 (Table 5-4). There was a considerable difference between the critical one-tailed test set at 1.669 and the observed one-tailed test set at 4.750 ($p = .05$). A G-Power test revealed a strong difference between the pre-test and post-test of .835357, with an effect size of 0.5, considered a moderate effect size (Dusseldorf University, 2010; see Table 5-4).

Therefore, it is understood that the Social Profile is sensitive enough to measure change in social behaviors after 30 days of treatment on a closed unit. Because other professionals are also treating the patients' behavior on the unit, it is not possible to state that the change was due solely to the intervention of occupational therapy. This could be done in the future if those patients who do not attend the occupational therapy groups are also assessed with the Social Profile.

Assessment Administration

Area of Occupation/Performance Skills/ Performance Patterns/Client Factors Assessed

The Social Profile is designed as an observational tool of psychosocial behaviors of individuals in an activity group and of activity groups as a whole unit. At more advanced levels, the members of the group could self-observe, using the Social Profile as a discussion outline with the therapist or group leader as a moderator. The Social Profile is structured to assess many types of activity groups, including classrooms, therapy groups, gymnasiums, playgrounds, religious groups, family interactions, sporting events, political events, and community meetings.

The performance skills of the Social Profile consist of the Profile's performance patterns or continuum of parallel, associative, basic cooperative, supportive cooperative, and mature levels of participation. A mature group or person in a group should be able to interact at all these levels when appropriate to the activity.

All levels of the Social Profile need to be assessed for all age groups as the activity being observed may be providing a range of parameters limiting the level of participation appropriate for each activity. For example, adults in a movement to music group need to be in parallel participation relative to one another in the activity room.

Description of Environment/ Description of Supplies/Materials Required

The environment for the administration of the Social Profile may be outdoors or indoors in a social situation of any level of participation in a stadium, playground, backyard, dining room, classroom, religious center, team meeting room, board room, locker room, club meeting room, therapy center, or theatre in the round.

Copies of the Social Profile printed from the manual, *Social Profile: Assessment of Social Participation in Children, Adolescents, and Adults* (Donohue, 2013), are needed to conduct the assessment. Within the manual, a flash drive with all the forms necessary for administration is attached to the back cover. This drive includes materials for the Children's and Adult/Adolescent versions of the Social Profile.

Administration

The copies of the Social Profile are usually to be used after leading and/or observing an activity group. The Social Profile may also be used together by an advanced Supportive Cooperative or Mature group to discuss their own interaction for the three areas of activity participation, social interaction, and group membership roles with their leader or moderator present. They could discuss what level they began their interaction and where they have changed levels of participation.

Scoring

The observer using the Social Profile is encouraged to score it as soon as possible after the group meeting. These scores are then carried over to the Social Profile Summary Sheet. If it is meaningful to the group or to the observer, the average of the summaries can be recorded. When reporting these scores to another group leader or professional or team group, the Composite Graph may be used as a summary. The Composite Graph may also be valuable if the observation process is part of a study or research.

Intervention Planning Based on Assessment Results

The assessment results can be examined broadly to determine if the individual or group is performing social behaviors in an age-appropriate manner and in a manner suitable for the environment and group goals. Individual items from the Social Profile may be used to point out goals for modifying behavior of individuals or of the group as a whole. Together, the group leader and the group can create activities that will facilitate participation at the appropriate behavioral level. During times of busyness, holidays, and stress, the group leader can assist the individual or group to maintain their level of group interaction. The leader may also ask the group members how they could modify an activity to make it more appealing. Designing activities together can assist in creating and promoting a healthy social environment. Strategies for sustaining the level of the group's social interactions need to be designed together by the leader and the group members (American Occupational Therapy Association, 2014).

Case Study

An example of a group case includes a planning group for an outing. Group members can be encouraged to identify or create suggestions for where the current group members might like to go, considering the season, the distance, and the hours a community setting is available. The group leader of a basic cooperative level group can establish the ground rule of suggesting three destinations. After the three suggestions are made, the group can discuss how these destinations can help them to become more social members of the community, learning its facilities and healthy settings for becoming comfortable in the community's environment. Then the group can learn how to negotiate for their desirable destination, and a vote can be created. When some group members complain about the selection or decision, they can be encouraged to adapt to the majority choice this week and to be assertive next week about the destination they would desire in the future. Depending on the outcome of the group planning session, the occupational therapist may choose to work on assertive communication skills or further the development of social skills and communication and interaction skills with the group members (Cole & Donohue, 2011). Within the cooperative group, members need to be able to express ideas, respect the rights of others, demonstrate an ability to meet the needs of others, identify and meet goals of the group, and demonstrate motivation to complete an activity. If the occupational therapist discovers during the group planning activity that group members are demonstrating difficulty with these skills, he or she may focus the choice of future intervention on activities that could facilitate skill development in these areas. Examples could include preparing to attend a support group and appropriate level of information sharing, participating in a choir rehearsal, or participating in a community recreational/leisure activity, such as volleyball. The text *Social Participation in Occupational Contexts: In Schools, Clinics, and Communities* (Cole & Donohue, 2011) offers the reader greater insights into the development of social participation interventions across the lifespan.

Suggested Further Research

It is difficult to carry out research about the levels of the Social Profile from week to week in many activity groups where the composition of the participants changes due to other appointments for therapy or with their family or setting. It is proposed to carry out further research on the reliability of the Social Profile for test-retest reliability by using videos that provide stability of material to be viewed.

Summary

The Social Profile has been designed to gauge the current level of a group, and if its performance is suitable for the activity underway. When a group is not up to par for the day, the group leader needs to decide if the activity can be modified to fit the abilities of the group or if the group needs to pull together to create another perspective so it can adapt to a new challenge. The Social Profile facilitates creation of goals together to promote social interactive health for people needing to be a part of their small group and the larger community (WHO, 2001).

References

American Occupational Therapy Association. (2014). Occupational therapy practice framework: Domain and process (3rd ed.). *American Journal of Occupational Therapy, 68*(Suppl. 1), S1-S48.

Bernard, H. R. (2000). *Social research methods: Qualitative and quantitative approaches.* Newbury Park, CA: Sage.

Bredekamp, S., & Copple, C. (Eds.). (2009). *Developmentally appropriate practice in early childhood programs, serving children from birth to age eight.* Washington, DC: National Association for the Education of Young Children.

Cohen, R. J., Swerdlik, M. E., & Phillips, S. M. (1995). *Psychological testing and assessment: An introduction to tests and measurement* (3rd ed.). Mountain View, CA: Mayfield.

Cole, M. B, & Donohue, M. V. (2011). *Social participation in occupational contexts: In schools, clinics, and communities.* Thorofare, NJ: SLACK Incorporated.

Deci, E. L., & Ryan, R. M. (2000). The what and why of goal pursuits. Human needs and self-determination of behavior. *Psychological Inquiry, 11,* 227-268.

Dildine, G. C. (1972). Characteristics of a mature group. In U. Delworth, E. H. Rudow, & J. Taub (Eds.), *Crisis center/hotline: A guidebook to beginning and operating* (pp. 79-81). Springfield, IL: Charles C. Thomas.

Donohue, M. V. (1999). Theoretical bases of Mosey's group interaction skills. *Occupational Therapy International, 6,* 35-51.

Donohue, M. V. (2003). Group profile studies with children: Validity measures and analysis. *Occupational Therapy in Mental Health, 19,* 1-23.

Donohue, M. V. (2005). Social Profile: Assessment of validity and reliability in children's groups. *Canadian Journal of Occupational Therapy, 62,* 164-175.

Donohue, M. V. (2006). Inter-rater reliability of the Social Profile: Assessment of community and psychiatric group participation. *Australian Occupational Therapy Journal, 54,* 49-58.

Donohue, M. V. (2013). *Social Profile: Assessment of social participation in children, adolescents, and adults.* Bethesda, MD: AOTA Press.

Donohue, M. V., Hanif, H., & Wu Berns, L. (2011). An exploratory study of social participation in occupational therapy groups. *Mental Health Special Interest Section Quarterly, 34*(4), 1-4.

Dusseldorf University (2010). G*Power: Users guide—Analysis by design. Web Page of Heinrich-HeineUniversität - Institut für experimentelle Psychologie. Retrieved from http://www.psycho.uniduesseldorf.de/abteilungen/aap/gpower3

Mead, M. (2017). *Quote.* Retrieved from https://en.wikiquote.org/wiki/Margaret_Mead

Mosey, A. C. (1968). Recapitulation of ontogenesis. A theory for practice of occupational therapy. *American Journal of Occupational Therapy, 22,* 426-438.

Mosey, A. C. (1986). *Psychosocial components of occupational therapy.* New York, NY: Raven Press.

Parten, M. B. (1932). Social participation among pre-school children. *Journal of Abnormal and Social Psychology, 27,* 243-269.

Shrout, P. E., & Fleiss, J. L. (1979). Intraclass correlations: Uses in assessing rater reliability. *Psychological Bulletin, 86,* 420-428.

World Health Organization. (2001). *International classification of functioning, disability, and health.* Geneva, Switzerland: Author.

Yaffee, R. A. (1998). *Enhancement of reliability analysis: Application of intraclass correlations with SPSS/Windows v. 8.* New York, NY: New York University.

Activity Card Sort as an Essential Tool to Obtain an Occupational History and Profile in Individuals With Mental Health Challenges

Lisa Tabor Connor, PhD, MSOT, OTR/L
Carolyn M. Baum, PhD, OTR/L, FAOTA

> *Working with my OT and the Activity Card Sort made me realize all the activities that*
> *I used to love doing before my recent struggles. I had the chance to think about how*
> *doing those things again would make me feel like the person I've lost contact with.*
> (Kenny K.)

Occupational therapy holds the professional responsibility to enable people to engage in occupation when health conditions, societal conditions, or disabilities impair or threaten their ability to do that which is important and has meaning for them. People whose occupational performance is limited by mental illness have been the focus of our work since William Tuke opened the York Retreat for the care of the insane in 1796. He pioneered humane methods of treatment for the mentally ill, including providing a pleasant environment and adopting a program involving the therapeutic use of occupational tasks (Whiteley, 2004). The importance of being active in life has been a professional thread since Meyer wrote the theory of occupation (Meyer, 1922) and has been woven into the fabric of our values by leaders like Reilly (1962), Fidler and Fidler (1978), Mosey (1986), and West (1967) and continues today.

The relationship of activity engagement and health is well established. Activity is known to produce positive physical and mental outcomes (Fidler, 1981; Fidler & Bristow, 1992; Jackson, Carlson, Mandel, Zemke, & Clark, 1998; Wilcock, 1999) and protects against cognitive decline and depressive symptoms (Bassuk, Glass, & Berkman, 1999; Hultsch, Hertzog, Small, & Dixon, 1999). Specifically, a randomized clinical trial using an activity intervention had a positive effect on pain, vitality, social functioning, mental health, and life satisfaction (Clark et al., 2012).

Obtaining an occupational history and profile is the starting point of the occupational therapy process (American Occupational Therapy Association, 2014). The occupational profile is the basis for the client and occupational therapist to establish goals, guides how

Hemphill, B. J., & Urish, C. K. (Eds.). *Assessments in Occupational Therapy Mental Health: An Integrative Approach, Fourth Edition* (pp. 77-90). © 2020 Taylor & Francis Group.

the occupational therapist evaluates a client's occupational performance, is the foundation for creating an intervention plan, and guides the selection of appropriate outcome measures to determine if client goals are achieved. Although gathering the occupational profile is fundamental to the entire occupational therapy process, our profession has developed surprisingly few tools to aid in systematically obtaining crucial occupational history and profile information (Kielhofner, Dobria, Forsyth, & Kramer, 2010; Kielhofner et al., 2004; Law, Baptiste, Carswell, McColl, Polatajko, & Pollock, 2005; Matsutsuyu, 1969) and even fewer yet that allow one to quantify participation in occupation. For example, although the Canadian Occupational Performance Measure (Law et al., 2005) is widely used, it does not systematically prompt clients to examine the variety of activities that they perform over a large swath of time. Clinicians usually focus on asking clients to reflect on a typical day, but that may not be an appropriate prompt to help clients imagine resuming some meaningful activities that they performed less frequently or some time ago or to consider engaging in activities that they have not had previous exposure to. For instance, a person who recently experienced homelessness may not have had the opportunity to engage in household maintenance or homemaking activities but may be eager to resume doing them. Another disadvantage of a less structured tool is that a client may have a hard time spontaneously generating a list of previously enjoyed activities without specific prompts about the variety of activities that humans engage in over the course of weeks, months, or even years.

Theoretical Basis

Concepts/Construct

The Activity Card Sort (ACS; Baum & Edwards, 2001, 2008) was born from the need for an objective instrument to evaluate the occupations that individuals engage in beyond self-care and arises from the Person-Environment-Occupation-Performance model (Baum, Christiansen, & Bass, 2015). The ACS evaluates the extent to which people are engaging in a variety of activities in their everyday lives while living in the community, such as maintaining themselves and their loved ones in their homes and engaging in leisure and social activities. Whereas self-care activities, such as feeding, bathing, dressing, and grooming, are generally limited in number and fairly standard across individuals, activities that people do and find personally rewarding and meaningful beyond self-care are varied and personal. For example, although Carolyn enjoys engaging in cooking, hosting friends for dinner, and travel, Lisa enjoys attending live musical performances, engaging in political debates with friends, and attending baseball games. How do you capture individual differences in participation when the number and variety of activities that people engage in are so varied? Further, how do you know if an injury, illness, or a chronic health condition is interfering with participation in occupations if participation levels are disparate among individuals?

The ACS is a tool that allows the clinician to assess the individual's participation in his or her occupations and compare that person's participation to an earlier point in his or her own history. The ACS is a facilitated client-centered interview that uses photographs of 89 activities, allowing the clinician to determine current and previous activities and to see patterns of activity engagement. The ACS is usually performed with the client or with a parent or caregiver proxy respondent if clients have difficulty responding for themselves. The activity cards include 20 instrumental activities (e.g., shopping, household tasks), 35 low-demand leisure activities that do not require a high degree of strength or physical exertion (e.g., watching TV or movies, listening to music), 17 high-demand leisure activities (e.g., walking, sports, yoga), and 17 social activities (e.g., visiting with friends, talking on the phone).

History of Development and Previous Versions/ Important Changes to Note in Current Version

The ACS was initially developed (Baum, 1995; Baum, McGeary, Pankiewicz, Braford, & Edwards, 1996; Baum, Perlmutter, & Edwards, 2000) to assess occupational performance in individuals with cognitive loss due to dementia to assist occupational therapists in helping caregivers engage their loved ones in meaningful activities in order to reduce troublesome behaviors at home. Initially, the ACS was used with caregiver proxies in the case of individuals with cognitive loss. The first version of the ACS included 80 items. Since the first version of the ACS was released as a formal evaluation (Baum & Edwards, 2001), published papers have reported results from community-dwelling healthy older adults (Everard, Lach, Fisher, & Baum, 2000), individuals with stroke (Edwards, Hahn, Baum, & Dromerick, 2006; Hartman-Maeir, Eliad, Kizoni, Nahaloni, Kelberman, & Katz, 2007; Hartman-Maeir, Soroker, Ring, Avni, & Katz, 2007), individuals with Parkinson's disease (Duncan & Earhart, 2011; Foster, Golden, Duncan, & Earhart, 2013; Foster & Hershey, 2011), individuals with schizophrenia (Katz & Keren, 2011), individuals with mental health symptoms such as depression (Adams, Roberts, & Cole, 2011; Bannigan & Laver-Fawcett, 2011; Graven, Brock, Hill, Ames, Cotton, & Joubert, 2011), and many other health conditions (Bailey, Kaskutas, Fox, Baum, & Mackinnon, 2009; Connor, Wolf, Foster, Hildebrand, & Baum, 2014; Foster et al., 2011; Josman, Somer, Reisberg, Weiss, Garcia-Palacios, & Hoffman, 2006; Schreuer, Rimmerman, & Sachs, 2006).

The ACS is used internationally and several cultural derivatives have been created to include culturally relevant activities for individuals around the world. A Hong Kong version (Chan, Chung, & Packer, 2006), an Australian version (Doney & Packer, 2008), an Arab heritage version (Hamed & Holm, 2013), a U.K. version (Laver-Fawcett, Brain, Brodie, Cardy, & Manaton, 2016; Laver-Fawcett & Mallinson, 2013), a Dutch version (Poerbodipoero, Sturkenboom, van Hartingsveldt, Nijhuis-vander Sanden, & Graff, 2015), and a Puerto Rican version (Orellano, Ito, Dorne, Irizarry, & Dávila, 2012) have been published, with several additional versions in development (e.g., Korean version [Lee et al., 2010]), through a consortium of more than 30 international investigators committed to the further development and study of the ACS.

The ACS also was the inspiration for the development of new assessments that use the card sorting methodology to probe participation in children of different ages. The Preschool ACS (Berg & LaVesser, 2006) was designed to obtain an occupational history and profile of preschoolers from their parents. More recently, the Adolescent and Young Adult ACS (AYA-ACS; Berg, McCollum, Cho, & Jason, 2015) was developed to assess participation in emerging adults—individuals in the 17- to 25-year-old transition-to-adulthood period. These assessment tools were constructed through careful research into the common occupations of children and youth of the targeted ages. Like the ACS, the Preschool ACS and the AYA-ACS are psychometrically sound, having good test-retest reliability and validity, and offer clinicians a means to generate client-centered intervention goals.

The current version of the ACS was published in 2008 (Baum & Edwards). The primary modification was changing some of the activities in the assessment. These changes included removing activities that had a low number of responses in a large sample of community-dwelling older adults (e.g., preserving food, hunting), including some specific activities in slightly broader or narrower categories (e.g., mending was included with sewing; travel was replaced with local travel, and an additional card was added for national or international travel), and adding new activities (e.g., going to the doctor, work [paid], playing card games, going to a casino) based on reports from the community sample.

Psychometric Properties

Normative Data

Norms of activity are not published for the ACS. However, as mentioned earlier, the very nature of occupation beyond self-care in adults is extraordinarily varied and personal and is dependent on individual preference, cultural expectations, roles and responsibilities, life circumstances, and societal expectations for people of different ages. The nature of the assessment is that it taps individual preferences and change in activity participation from before illness or injury to afterward and then after intervention. The important information gained is not how a person does relative to his or her peers but rather to him- or herself over a period of time.

During the development of the ACS and particularly in its modification from the first to second editions, interviews and assessments of community-dwelling older adults were conducted to determine which activities ought to be included in the assessment. Prior to the second edition, 317 older adults were interviewed in their homes and given the first edition of the ACS. Participants indicated activities that they did that were not included in the assessment. Furthermore, a few items were found to be extraordinarily low in frequency in this group and were considered for being dropped. In a second sample of 325 individuals 6 months post-stroke, the same group of items was reported as not being done very frequently. Therefore, those items were dropped from the second edition. Likewise, based on these healthy adult evaluations, several items were added to the second edition of the test. As time goes on and cultural norms shift, new activities may need to be added to the ACS to reflect how adults spend their time.

Reliability

The ACS has been found to have both high internal consistency (Carpenter et al., 2007; Chan et al., 2006; Katz, Karpin, Lak, Furman, & Hartman-Maeir, 2003) and high test-retest reliability over a 1-week (Baum & Edwards, 2008) and 2-week period (Carpenter et al., 2007) in healthy older adults. Internal consistency, as measured by Cronbach's alpha coefficients, were found to be 0.71 for Instrumental Activities, 0.71 for Low-Demand Leisure, 0.85 for High-Demand Leisure, and 0.77 for Social Activities, all of which are acceptably high. Test-retest reliability, as measured by intraclass correlations in the Carpenter et al. (2007) study, were all greater than 0.71, with the highest score being for Instrumental Activities (0.89). Other studies have reported even higher test-retest reliability coefficients (Chan et al., 2006; Katz et al., 2003).

Validity

The validity of the ACS is well researched. The ACS was originally developed to examine the relationship between activity participation and caregiver burden. Baum

(1995) and Baum and Edwards (1993) found that in individuals with cognitive loss, the more pre-illness activities that were retained, the fewer disturbing behaviors the person with cognitive loss exhibited. Moreover, the more pre-illness activities retained, the less burdensome caregiving was reported to be.

In a factor analysis conducted by Sachs and Josman (2003) in Israel, a 63-item version of the ACS was found to have a different factor structure in college students ($n = 53$) and in community-dwelling older adults ($n = 131$). Furthermore, the factor structure in the older adult sample was different than the factor structure reported by Baum and Edwards (2001) for healthy older adults in a U.S. sample. In response to differences across cultures, an investigation has since focused on culturally universal vs. culturally specific activities of adulthood around the world (Eriksson et al., 2011). As a result of this work, several cultural-specific derivatives of the ACS have been created (Chan et al., 2006; Doney & Packer, 2008; Hamed & Holm, 2013; Katz & Hartman-Maeir, 2001; Laver-Fawcett & Mallinson, 2013; Laver-Fawcett et al., 2016; Lee et al., 2010; Orellano et al., 2012; Poerbodipoero et al., 2015).

The concurrent validity of the ACS has been demonstrated by examining the relationship of ACS domain scores to subscales from established instruments. In all cases, significant correlations have been obtained with ACS scores and other instruments that purport to tap related constructs. For instance, ACS scores were positively associated with Short Form 12 (SF-12) scores in older adults (Carpenter et al., 2007). ACS-Hong Kong version scores in older adults were correlated with scores on the Comprehensive Quality of Life Scale. In community-dwelling stroke survivors with aphasia (Tucker, Edwards, Mathews, Baum, & Connor, 2012), ACS High-Demand Leisure scores were strongly correlated with SF-36 (Ware & Sherbourne, 1992) Physical Function scores and Stroke Impact Scale (Duncan, Wallace, Lai, Johnson, Embretson, & Laster, 1999) Physical Domain scores; ACS Social Domain scores were significantly correlated with SF-36 Social Function scores; and ACS Total scores were positively correlated with Stroke Impact Scale Participation/Role Function Domain scores.

Sensitivity

The sensitivity of the ACS to detect differences between groups of individuals has been found to be good. For example, Katz et al. (2003) found ACS percent retained and total scores to differ significantly among groups of healthy adults, healthy older adults, caregivers of those with dementia, people with multiple sclerosis, and individuals post-stroke. Edwards et al. (2006) found that individuals with mild stroke who differed in post-stroke activities retained on the ACS also differed in depressive symptoms, SF-12 scores, and Stroke-Adapted Sickness Impact scores.

The sensitivity of the ACS to detect change in individuals over time is uncertain. The instrument relies on self-report, and thus sensitivity to detect change in participation in occupation is dependent on the ability to remember which activities were performed prior to injury or illness and which activities have been done after injury or illness. Likewise, impairments of awareness may have an impact on a person's ability to accurately gauge whether an activity is being done less or has been given up. Generally, clients are excellent reporters of their activity participation, and therefore, their perception of their participation will reflect what is important for the clinician to know to guide the intervention. There is some evidence (Foster et al., 2013) that following a tango intervention in persons with Parkinson's disease their activity participation had improved after 6 months.

Assessment Administration

Area of Occupation/Performance Skills/ Performance Patterns/Client Factors Assessed

The ACS is designed to systematically evaluate occupation from the client's perspective. Information gained from the ACS includes whether the client has ever performed an activity (or performed that activity within a specified time frame) and whether the client continues to do that activity, has given it up, does it less, or has started to do an activity since an injury or illness. The percentage of activities retained in each of four domains (i.e., instrumental, low-demand leisure, high-demand leisure, social activities) is obtained from the instrument. In addition, clients indicate their top five favorite activities. This is an excellent starting point for client- and occupation-centered intervention planning. In the case of clients who have been occupationally deprived, they can indicate five activities that they would like to try, perhaps for the first time. Clients find the ACS engaging, straightforward in its purpose, and understandable from the vantage of its administration. The photographs and the discussions that ensue while the client performs the task build rapport and open a meaningful dialogue about the client's readiness to change how an activity is performed and why a particular activity holds meaning.

Description of Environment/ Description of Supplies/Materials Required

The ACS may be administered in nearly any environment (e.g., in a hospital, clinic, a person's home, school). The ACS requires a small tabletop space to allow the client to group cards into stacks and is best administered where the client and occupational therapy practitioner can converse with little distraction.

The ACS requires that the assessment kit be purchased (Baum & Edwards, 2008). The kit consists of a package of cards (89 photo cards with activity labels and a set of cards with category labels), the ACS test manual, and electronic versions of the record forms that should be printed before administration. The only other item required is a pencil for the examiner to record the client's responses.

Administration

The ACS was designed to be administered for clinical purposes by a registered occupational therapist or certified occupational therapy assistant. The ACS has three separate forms that differ slightly in the categories that a client will sort the cards into. Form A, the Institutional Version, is designed to obtain basic information about the 89 activities. It may be used during an acute hospital or rehabilitation stay before the client has had experience with a new health condition participating in activities in the community. Two labels are placed on the tabletop: Done Prior to Illness/Injury or Admission and Not Done Prior to Illness/Injury or Admission. The client is then asked to sort the cards into the Done or Not Done piles. The occupational therapy practitioner records the client's responses on the printable form that is included in the assessment kit. The form may be entered into the medical record to help occupational therapy practitioners throughout the continuum of care to establish the client's previous level of function and provide occupation-focused treatment targets.

Follow-up with the ACS after discharge would be most appropriately accomplished by administering Form B, the Recovering Version, which is designed to capture change in activity patterns over time. The clinician asks the client to place the cards in the category that best describes his or her involvement with the activity. The client then sorts cards into five stacks with the following labels: Not Done Prior to Current Illness/Injury; Continue to Do During Illness/Injury; Do Less Since Illness/Injury; Given Up Due to Illness/Injury; and New Activity Since Illness/Injury. The occupational therapy practitioner records responses in the appropriate columns for each of the 89 activities. At the end of the sorting activity, the occupational therapy practitioner asks the client to name five activities that are his or her favorite, including ones that may have been given up.

Form C, the Community-Living Version, is designed to be given to older adults living in the community. The category cards are labeled Not Done Since Age 60, Do Now (at the same level as before), Do Less, and Given Up. Participants are asked to sort the 89 photos into the categories that best describe the person's involvement with the activity. The occupational therapy practitioner marks the score sheet in the appropriate column for each activity. The client is asked to choose five favorite activities, including ones that may have been given up.

Although not part of the formal administration of the ACS, the assessment may also be followed by supplemental questions to identify barriers and facilitators the person is experiencing. For example, for the activities placed in the Do Less or Given Up categories, the clinician can explore why the client has given up these activities. A further question may be what it would take for him or her to do it again; such a question may lead to treatment goals and, perhaps, a starting point for environmental modifications to address barriers.

Scoring

Scoring the ACS is based on which form was used to collect the client's occupational history. Form A is designed to give descriptive information about the number and variety of activities that the client engaged in prior to being admitted for the current health event. The number of current activities in each of the domains of instrumental, low-demand leisure, high-demand leisure, and social activities may be noted. However, participation in activities varies widely across individuals.

For Forms B and C, scoring the ACS involves two steps. First, the number of activities in each category in each domain should be tallied based on the score indicated in each column. For Form B, Current Activity is the total of Continue to Do (1 point each), Do Less (0.5 point for each), and New Activity (1 point each). Previous Activity is the total of Continue to Do, Do Less, and Given Up (each activity is given 1 point). Second, the Percent Retained is calculated by dividing Current Activity by Previous Activity scores. Scores should be calculated for each domain separately and for the entire test for a total score for Current, Previous, and Percent Retained.

For Form C, Current Activity is the total of Do Now (1 point each) and Do Less (0.5 point for each) columns. Previous Activity is the total of Do Now (at the same level), Do Less, and Given Up (1 point each). Percent Retained is calculated by dividing Current Activity by Previous Activity scores. Scores should be calculated for each domain separately and for the entire test for a total score for Current, Previous, and Percent Retained. For Forms B and C, the Percent Retained can reflect changes in occupation due to illness or injury and can also reflect change in participation due to intervention to improve occupational performance and participation.

Intervention Planning
Based on Assessment Results

The ACS provides a systematic means to gather critical occupational history and profile information needed to develop an intervention plan. Because of the wide variety of instrumental, leisure, and social activities that it allows the occupational therapy practitioner to assess, clients' priorities are probed systematically and intervention goals are a direct consequence of the evaluation process. Two cases presented below, Nora and Kenny K., illustrate how the ACS facilitates the assessment process and leads directly to intervention planning.

Case Studies

Nora

Nora is an 80-year-old, right-handed woman who experienced a right hemisphere stroke 6 months previously. She has some residual left hemiparesis of her arm and leg, is experiencing left hemianopia, and is having difficulty with complex instrumental activities, such as managing her finances, which is what prompted her referral to occupational therapy for home services. Her 55-year-old daughter is concerned about whether her mother can remain living independently in her own home; her daughter works all day and lives 50 miles away from her mother. The daughter visits every weekend, is currently doing Nora's laundry, and is cooking enough meals for the week, which Nora reheats in the microwave. Nora reports feeling helpless and hopeless in her current situation. She has been referred to occupational therapy for a home safety evaluation and intervention targeted at independent living skills. The occupational therapist administers the ACS, a screening for depression, and a screening for cognitive function.

Based on the results of these assessments, the occupational therapist determines that Nora has a significant number of depressive symptoms, is experiencing cognitive impairment in visual spatial skills and memory, and has retained only 55% of her pre-stroke activities based on the ACS. Nora indicates that she has given up 65% of her instrumental activities and does several other activities less, has given up a significant number of her leisure activities, and has given up all of her social activities except for participating in visits with family. Nora has given up driving and has agreed to sell her car. While completing the ACS, Nora opens up to the occupational therapist about her feelings about her change in activity patterns since her stroke. Nora is satisfied with the help that she receives from her daughter with her laundry and paying her bills, but reports, "I don't want to sound ungrateful, but my daughter is a terrible cook and she prepares food that I would just rather not eat. By the end of the week, I am sick to death of eating the same old thing!" Since her stroke, Nora reports not attending church or the quilting bee. She reports feeling uncertain whether she is able to resume these activities but begins to cry when she tells the therapist, "It just isn't the same just talking on the phone with my friends. I miss them so much." The top five activities that Nora would like to resume doing are cooking, grocery shopping, attending church, needle crafts, and visiting sick friends.

Based on Nora's ACS occupational history and profile, her cognitive and depression screenings, and Nora's self-report, the occupational therapist plans an assessment of Nora's home safety and performance of her desired occupations to determine a treatment plan. After receiving permission from Nora, the occupational therapist notifies Nora's physician regarding her depression screening results. The occupational therapist's initial thoughts, pending further evaluation and determination that Nora can be safe at home with some environmental adaptations and self-management strategies, is that Nora will likely respond positively to some adaptations for cooking, both environmental modifications and simplification of her favorite recipes, some cognitive strategy generation and application to manage her daily tasks, some collaborative problem solving for her transportation issues, and tapping into her social network to enable her to resume some of her desired social activities. The occupational therapist shares these thoughts with Nora and her daughter, and everyone agrees that this is a good plan pending further evaluation at home.

Kenny K.

Kenny K. is a 45-year-old man with schizophrenia who has recently experienced chronic homelessness. He has been living on the street for 6 years since he was laid off from his job as a night-shift custodian at the local community hospital during an episode of acute exacerbation of his psychiatric symptoms. Without a paycheck and no family support, Kenny was unable to pay his bills. His electricity and gas were shut off, and he was evicted from his apartment after 3 months of not paying his rent. Kenny got meals from several local organizations and spent cold winter nights in homeless shelters but reported that "those places are full of liars and thieves. I'm better off on my own where nobody bothers me. I know how to take care of myself."

Several months ago, Kenny was approached by a social worker at a community shelter who helped him secure government assistance and supported housing. The social worker alerted the occupational therapist on staff that Kenny needed assistance with reestablishing his daily routines, particularly maintaining his home and spending his time. The occupational therapist administered the ACS to obtain an occupational history and profile. Kenny agreed that his most immediate goals were reestablishing routines for doing laundry and grocery shopping. What most interested him, however, during the administration of the ACS were the low-demand leisure activities. Kenny's face lit up when he got to the card "Singing in choir/group." He smiled, "Throughout my childhood, I sang in the church choir and even performed a few solos." Kenny then burst into song and revealed his beautiful baritone singing voice. "Singing at church is something I'd really love to do again someday. I just don't know if I can face performing in front of all of those people." Kenny identified spectator sports and reading as other high priority activities that he would like to participate in again. Based on the results of the ACS, the occupational therapist developed a treatment plan to address reestablishing Kenny's routines for grocery shopping, laundry, singing in a group, watching spectator sports, and reading. Her approach would include using monthly, weekly, and daily calendars to help Kenny plan his activities, planning a grocery shopping outing and going to the store to determine supports that Kenny needs, investigating low-stress opportunities to participate in a singing group, finding low-cost options for attending sporting events, and obtaining a library card. While discussing the treatment plan, Kenny declared, "I am looking forward to reconnecting with my old self again. I haven't seen that guy for over 15 years."

Intervention Planning

As illustrated by the two case studies, the ACS is an essential tool for intervention planning and is an ideal entry point into the occupational therapy process because it is designed to obtain an occupational history and profile. The ACS allows the client to systematically review and explore activities that a wide variety of adults report being meaningful occupations to them, so it does not simply rely on the client's report of a typical day or recall of past experiences to develop client goals. The ACS is a tool that can be used flexibly to establish client-centered intervention goals that focus on occupational performance itself, as in Nora's case, or the use of occupation to establish routines, life's rhythms, and engagement and participation in meaningful activity, as in Kenny's case.

The very nature of the ACS allows clients to establish their highest occupational priorities. Therefore, intervention goals directly follow from the assessment process. The ACS does not prescribe the intervention approach that will be necessary to achieve those goals, and the next step in the intervention planning process ought to be performance-based assessment of the client's ability to do the desired occupations and careful consideration of the activity demands and environmental context in which the occupations occur. However, the ACS is an engaging and informationally rich means to both establish rapport with clients and to obtain access to their occupational needs and desires, ensuring a client-centered, collaborative approach to care.

Suggested Further Research

The ACS is both the subject of research and has been an instrument used as an outcome assessment to determine the extent to which individuals are participating in desired activities across the lifespan and after illness or injury. The ACS has been adapted and utilized in many different countries and cultures. In fact, Eriksson et al. (2011) used the ACS and its derivatives to examine both common activities of well older adults in eight places (Israel, Australia, Singapore, Hong Kong, the Netherlands, Korea, Puerto Rico, and the United States) and activities central to Asian culture and activities central to Western culture. Their study revealed that 10 activities were shared across the included countries, whereas there were 16 additional activities that were central to Asian culture but not to Western culture and 18 activities that were central to Western culture but not to Asian culture. The results of this study are important to occupational therapists across the globe to better understand their clients' needed and valued occupations and to help clinicians practice with cultural humility.

In addition to the development and comparison of ACS cultural derivatives, the ACS administration has been adapted so that individuals with aphasia are able to indicate for themselves what their previous and current levels of participation are and what they value in terms of their post stroke participation (Tucker et al., 2012). The Tucker et al. (2012) study demonstrated that people with aphasia were internally consistent in responding to constructs across well-known stroke outcome measures, such as the ACS (Baum & Edwards, 2001), the SF-36 (Ware & Sherbourne, 1992), the Reintegration to Normal Living Scale (Wood-Dauphinée, Opzoomer, Williams, Marchand, & Spitzer, 1988), and the Stroke Impact Scale (Duncan et al., 1999) with minor administration modifications and communication supports. Currently, the ACS is being utilized in a large-scale outcome study examining predictors of stroke recovery in individuals with and without aphasia (e.g., Foley, Nicholas, Baum, & Connor, 2019).

Several studies have used the ACS to examine the participation outcomes of community-dwelling older adults (Carpenter et al., 2007; Everard et al., 2000; Karpin, Hartman-Maeir, & Katz, 2001; Perlmutter, Bhorade, Gordon, Hollingsworth, & Baum, 2010; Sachs & Josman, 2003), as well as in individuals with illness, disease, and injury. For example, Connor et al. (2014) reported decreased participation in community-dwelling individuals with Alzheimer's disease, mild stroke, stroke with aphasia, and Parkinson's disease.

Other investigations have included the ACS as an outcome assessment in individuals with schizophrenia (Katz & Keren, 2011), depression (Leibold, Holm, Raina, Reynolds, & Rogers, 2014), stroke (Edwards et al., 2006; Eriksson, Baum, Wolf, & Connor, 2013; Hartman-Maeir, Soroker, et al., 2007; Spitzer, Tse, Baum, & Carey, 2011; Wolf, Brey, Baum, & Connor, 2012), and congestive heart failure (Foster et al., 2011), as well as those post stem cell transplantation (Lyons, Li, Tosteson, Meehan, & Ahles, 2010). Furthermore, the ACS is now being utilized with success to demonstrate the impact of interventions designed to ameliorate the impact of diseases, such as Parkinson's disease (Duncan & Earhart, 2011; Foster et al., 2013; Katz & Keren, 2011).

Similar to work using the ACS to examine participation outcomes of adults with a wide variety of diseases and disorders, the AYA-ACS was used in research examining participation outcomes of emerging adults. Neurotypical adults in both the United States (Berg et al., 2015) and Taiwan (Wang & Berg, 2013) were studied during the development of the assessment. In addition, the suitability of assessing emerging adults with high-functioning autism with the AYA-ACS was established in both the United States (McCollum, LaVesser, & Berg, 2016) and Taiwanese populations (Wang & Berg, 2014). As the ACS and its age- and cultural-derivatives become more widely utilized as an intervention outcome in future work, we can begin to examine factors that are most important to effect positive change in participation—the ultimate goal of habilitation and rehabilitation interventions.

Summary

Occupational therapy holds the professional responsibility to enable people to engage in occupation when health conditions, societal conditions, or disabilities impair or threaten their ability to do that which is important and has meaning for them. People with mental health challenges whose symptoms interfere with their ability to perform their occupations can benefit from occupational therapy services focused on resuming the things that they need and want to do. Determining the highest priorities for intervention begins with an occupational history and profile and the determination of the client's greatest restrictions in participation. The ACS (Baum & Edwards, 2008) is a psychometrically sound, occupation-focused assessment instrument that is philosophically and empirically aligned with the goals of occupational therapists to understand their clients' highest priorities for intervention. The ACS evaluates the extent to which people are engaging in a variety of activities in their everyday lives while living in the community, such as maintaining themselves and loved ones in their homes and engaging in leisure and social activities. The ACS focuses on activities beyond self-care.

The ACS is comprised of 89 labeled photographs of activities that community-dwelling adults perform in the domains of instrumental, low- and high-demand leisure, and social activities. Clients sort the photographs into categories indicating whether they currently or previously have performed the activities. If a client has an illness or injury, they indicate which activities they have given up or are doing less since that illness or injury. The percentage of activities retained in each of the four domains is then calculated to determine the impact of the illness or injury. In addition, clients choose five of the activities that are most meaningful to them. Therefore, the ACS assists the occupational therapist in creating meaningful, client-centered intervention goals. Because of the utility of the ACS for examining activity participation in both individuals and in groups, the ACS has been the subject of active work to establish reliable and valid derivatives in countries and cultures around the world. In addition, the ACS has been used as an outcome tool to examine the impact that a wide range of health conditions, including mental health conditions such as schizophrenia (Katz & Keren, 2011) and depression (Leibold et al., 2014), have on participation restrictions. Future research using the ACS may help us understand the impact of occupation-based interventions in facilitating the resumption of activities in adults with mental health challenges and improving quality of life.

References

Adams, K. B., Roberts, A. R., & Cole, M. B. (2011). Changes in activity and interest in the third and fourth age: Associations with health, functioning and depressive symptoms. *Occupational Therapy International, 18,* 4-17.

American Occupational Therapy Association. (2014). Occupational therapy practice framework: Domain and process (3rd ed.). *American Journal of Occupational Therapy, 68*(Suppl. 1), S1-S48.

Bailey, R., Kaskutas, V., Fox, I., Baum, C. M., & Mackinnon, S. E. (2009). Effect of upper extremity nerve damage on activity participation, pain, depression, and quality of life. *Journal of Hand Surgery, 34,* 1682-1688.

Bannigan, K., & Laver-Fawcett, A. (2011). Aging, occupation and mental health: The contribution of the Research Centre for Occupation and Mental Health. *World Federation of Occupational Therapists Bulletin, 63,* 55-60.

Bassuk, S. S., Glass, T. A., & Berkman, L. F. (1999). Social disengagement and incident cognitive decline in community-dwelling elderly persons. *Annals of Internal Medicine, 131,* 165-173.

Baum, C. M. (1995). The contribution of occupation to function in person's with Alzheimer's disease. *Journal of Occupation Science Australia, 2,* 59-67.

Baum, C. M., Christiansen, C. H., & Bass, J. D. (2015). The Person-Environment-Occupation-Performance (PEOP) model. In C. H. Christiansen, C. M. Baum, & J. D. Bass (Eds.), *Occupational therapy: Performance, participation, and well-being* (4th ed., pp. 49-55). Thorofare, NJ: SLACK Incorporated.

Baum, C. M., & Edwards, D. F. (1993). Cognitive performance in senile dementia of the Alzheimer's type: The Kitchen Task Assessment. *American Journal of Occupational Therapy, 47*(5), 431-436.

Baum, C. M., & Edwards, D. (2001). *Activity Card Sort.* St. Louis, MO: PenUltima Press.

Baum, C. M., & Edwards, D. (2008). *Activity Card Sort* (2nd ed.). Bethesda, MD: American Occupational Therapy Association.

Baum, C. M., McGeary, T., Pankiewicz, R., Braford, T., & Edwards, D. F. (1996). An activity program for cognitively impaired low-income inner city residents. *Topics in Geriatric Rehabilitation, 12,* 54-62.

Baum, C. M., Perlmutter, M., & Edwards, D. F. (2000). Measuring function in Alzheimer's disease. *Alzheimer's Care Quarterly, 1*(3), 44-61.

Berg, C., & LaVesser, P. (2006). The Preschool Activity Card Sort. *OTJR: Occupation, Participation, and Health, 26,* 143-151.

Berg, C., McCollum, M., Cho, E., & Jason, D. (2015). Development of the Adolescent and Young Adult Activity Card Sort. *OTJR: Occupation, Participation, and Health, 35,* 221-231.

Carpenter, B. D., Edwards, D. F., Pickard, J. G., Palmer, J. L., Morrow-Howell, N., Neufeld, P. S. … Morris, J. C. (2007). Anticipating relocation: Concerns about moving among NORC residents. *Journal of Gerontological Social Work, 49,* 165-184.

Chan, V. W., Chung, J. C., & Packer, T. L. (2006). Validity and reliability of the Activity Card Sort—Hong Kong version. *OTJR: Occupation, Participation and Health, 26,* 152-158.

Clark, F., Jackson, J., Carlson, M., Chou, C.-P., Cherry, B. J., Jordan-Marsh, M., … Azen, S. P. (2012). Effectiveness of a lifestyle intervention in promoting the well-being of independently living older people: Results of the Well Elderly 2 randomized controlled trial. *Journal of Epidemiology & Community Health, 66,* 782-790.

Connor, L. T., Wolf, T. J., Foster, E. R., Hildebrand, M. W., & Baum, C. M. (2014). Participation and engagement in occupation in adults with disabilities. In D. Pierce (Ed.), *Occupational science for occupational therapy* (pp. 107-120). Thorofare, NJ: SLACK Incorporated.

Doney, R. M., & Packer, T. L. (2008). Measuring changes in activity participation of older Australians: Validation of the Activity Card Sort—Australia. *Australasian Journal on Ageing, 27,* 33-37.

Duncan, P. W., Wallace, D., Lai, S. M., Johnson, D., Embretson, S., & Laster, L. J. (1999). The Stroke Impact Scale Version 2.0: Evaluation of reliability, validity, and sensitivity to change. *Stroke, 30,* 2131-2140.

Duncan, R. P., & Earhart, G. M. (2011). Measuring participation in individuals with Parkinson disease: Relationships with disease severity, quality of life, and mobility. *Disability and Rehabilitation, 33,* 1440-1446.

Edwards, D. F., Hahn, M. G., Baum, C. M., & Dromerick, A. W. (2006). The impact of mild stroke on activity participation and life satisfaction. *Journal of Cerebrovascular Disease and Stroke, 15,* 151-157.

Eriksson, G., Baum, M. C., Wolf, T. J., & Connor, L. T. (2013). Perceived participation after stroke: The influence of activity retention, reintegration, and perceived recovery. *American Journal of Occupational Therapy, 67*, e131-e138.

Eriksson, G. M., Chung, J. C., Beng, L. H., Hartman-Maeir, A., Yoo, E., Orellano, E. M., … Baum, C. M. (2011). Occupations of older adults: A cross cultural description. *OTJR: Occupation, Participation and Health, 31*, 182-192.

Everard, K. M., Lach, H. W., Fisher, E. B., & Baum, C. M. (2000). Relationship of activity and social support to the functional health of older adults. *Journal of Gerontology, Psychological Sciences and Social Sciences, 55B*, S208-S212.

Fidler, G. S. (1981). From crafts to competence. *American Journal of Occupational Therapy, 35*, 567-573.

Fidler, G. S., & Bristow, B. (1992). *Recapturing competence: A systems change for geropsychiatric care.* New York, NY: Springer.

Fidler, G. S., & Fidler, J. W. (1978). Doing and becoming: Purposeful action and self-actualization. *American Journal of Occupational Therapy, 32*, 305-310.

Foley, E. L., Nicholas, M. L., Baum, C. M., & Connor, L. T. (2019). Influence of environmental factors on social participation post-stroke. *Behavioural Neurology*, Article ID 2606039.

Foster, E. R., Cunnane, K. B., Edwards, D. F., Morrison, M. T., Ewald, G. A., Geltman, E. M., & Zazulia, A. R. (2011). Executive dysfunction and depressive symptoms associated with reduced participation of people with severe congestive heart failure. *American Journal of Occupational Therapy, 65*, 306.

Foster, E. R., Golden, L., Duncan, R. P., & Earhart, G. M. (2013). Community-based Argentine tango dance program is associated with increased activity participation among individuals with Parkinson disease. *Archives of Physical Medicine and Rehabilitation, 94*, 240-249.

Foster, E. R., & Hershey, T. (2011). Everyday executive function is associated with activity participation in Parkinson disease without dementia. *OTJR: Occupation, Participation and Health, 31*(1), S16-S22.

Graven, C., Brock, K., Hill, K., Ames, D., Cotton, S., & Joubert, L. (2011). From rehabilitation to recovery: Protocol for a randomised controlled trial evaluating a goal-based intervention to reduce depression and facilitate participation post-stroke. *BMC Neurology, 11*, 73.

Hamed, R., & Holm, M. B. (2013). Psychometric properties of the Arab Heritage Activity Card Sort. *Occupational Therapy International, 20*, 23-34.

Hartman-Maeir, A., Eliad, Y., Kizoni, R., Nahaloni, I., Kelberman, H., & Katz, N. (2007). Evaluation of a long-term community based rehabilitation program for adult stroke survivors. *NeuroRehabilitation, 22*, 295-301.

Hartman-Maeir, A., Soroker, N., Ring, H., Avni, N., & Katz, N. (2007). Activities, participation and satisfaction one-year post stroke. *Disability & Rehabilitation, 29*, 559-566.

Hultsch, D. E., Hertzog, C., Small, B. J., & Dixon, R. A. (1999). Use it or lose it: Engaged lifestyle as a buffer of cognitive decline in aging? *Psychology and Aging, 14*, 245-263.

Jackson, J., Carlson, M., Mandel, D., Zemke, R., & Clark, F. (1998). Occupation in lifestyle redesign: The well elderly study occupational therapy program. *American Journal of Occupational Therapy, 52*, 326-336.

Josman, N., Somer, E., Reisberg, A., Weiss, P. L., Garcia-Palacios, A., & Hoffman, H. (2006). BusWorld: Designing a virtual environment for post-traumatic stress disorder in Israel: A protocol. *Cyberpsychology & Behavior, 9*, 241-244.

Karpin, C., Hartman-Maeir, A., & Katz, N. (2001). Leisure and IADL activity characteristics of adult and elderly population in Israel, according to the Activity Card Sort. *Israel Journal of Occupational Therapy, 10*, 3-22.

Katz, N., & Hartman-Maeir, A. (2001). *Activity Card Sort: Israeli version.* Jerusalem, Israel: Hebrew University, Graduate Program in Occupational Therapy.

Katz, N., Karpin, H., Lak, A., Furman, T., & Hartman-Maeir, A. (2003). Participation in occupational performance: Reliability and validity of the Activity Card Sort. *OTJR: Occupation, Participation and Health, 23*, 10-17.

Katz, N., & Keren, N. (2011). Effectiveness of occupational goal intervention for clients with schizophrenia. *American Journal of Occupational Therapy, 65*, 287-296.

Kielhofner, G. Dobria, L., Forsyth, K. & Kramer, J. (2010). The Occupational Self-Assessment: Stability and the ability to detect change over time. *OTJR: Occupation, Participation and Health, 30*, 11-19.

Kielhofner, G., Mallinson, T., Crawford, C., Nowak, M., Rigby, M., Henry, A. & Walens, D. (2004). *Occupational Performance History Interview, version 2.1.* Chicago, IL: University of Illinois.

Laver-Fawcett, A., Brain, L., Brodie, C., Cardy, L., & Manaton, L. (2016). The face validity and clinical utility of the Activity Card Sort—United Kingdom (ACS-UK). *British Journal of Occupational Therapy, 79*, 492-504.

Laver-Fawcett, A. J., & Mallinson, S. H. (2013). Development of the Activity Card Sort—United Kingdom Version (ACS-UK). *OTJR: Occupation, Participation and Health, 33*, 134-145.

Law, M., Baptiste, S., Carswell, A., McColl, M. A., Polatajko, H., & Pollock, N. (2005). *Canadian Occupational Performance Measure.* Ottawa, Ontario, Canada: Canadian Association of Occupational Therapists.

Lee, S. H., Yoo, E. Y., Jung, M. Y., Park, S. H., Lee, J. S., Lee, T. Y. (2010). Development of the Korean Activity Card Sort. *Journal of the Korean Society of Occupational Therapy, 18*(3), 103-117.

Leibold, M. L., Holm, M. B., Raina, K. D., Reynolds, C. F. III, & Rogers, J. C. (2014). Activities and adaptation in late-life depression: A qualitative study. *American Journal of Occupational Therapy, 68*, 570-577.

Lyons, K. D., Li, Z., Tosteson, T. D., Meehan, K., & Ahles, T. A. (2010). Consistency and construct validity of the Activity Card Sort (modified) in measuring activity resumption after stem cell transplantation. *American Journal of Occupational Therapy, 64*, 562-569.

Matsutsuyu, J. S. (1969). The interest check list. *American Journal of Occupational Therapy, 23*, 323-328.

McCollum, M., LaVesser, P., & Berg, C. (2016). Participation in daily activities of young adults with high functioning autism spectrum disorder. *Journal of Autism and Developmental Disorders, 46*(3), 987-997.

Meyer, A. (1922). The philosophy of occupational therapy. *Archives of Occupational Therapy, 1*, 1-10.

Mosey, A. C. (1986). *Psychosocial components of occupational therapy*. Philadelphia, PA: Lippincott Williams & Wilkins.

Orellano, E. M., Ito, M., Dorne, R., Irizarry, D., & Dávila, R. (2012). Occupational participation of older adults: Reliability and validity of the Activity Card Sort—Puerto Rican version. *OTJR: Occupation, Participation and Health, 32*, 266-272.

Perlmutter, M. S., Bhorade, A., Gordon, M., Hollingsworth, H. H., & Baum, M. C. (2010). Cognitive, visual, auditory, and emotional factors that affect participation in older adults. *American Journal of Occupational Therapy, 64*, 570-579.

Poerbodipoero, S. J., Sturkenboom, I. H., van Hartingsveldt, M. J., Nijhuis-vander Sanden, M. W. G., & Graff, M. J. (2015). The construct validity of the Dutch version of the Activity Card Sort. *Disability and Rehabilitation, 38*, 1943-1951.

Reilly, M. (1962). Occupational therapy can be one of the great ideas of 20th century medicine. *American Journal of Occupational Therapy, 16*, 1-9.

Sachs, D., & Josman, N. (2003). The Activity Card Sort: A factor analysis. *OTJR: Occupation, Participation, and Health, 23*, 165-174.

Schreuer, N., Rimmerman, A., & Sachs, D. (2006). Adjustment to severe disability: Constructing and examining a cognitive and occupational performance model. *International Journal of Rehabilitation Research, 29*, 201-207.

Spitzer, J., Tse, T., Baum, C. M., & Carey, L. M. (2011). Mild impairment of cognition impacts on activity participation after stroke in a community-dwelling Australian cohort. *OTJR: Occupation, Participation and Health, 31*(1), S8-S15.

Tucker, F. M., Edwards, D. F., Mathews, L. K., Baum, C. M., & Connor, L. T. (2012). Modifying health outcome measures for people with aphasia. *American Journal of Occupational Therapy, 66*, 42-50.

Wang, H.-Y., & Berg, C. (2013). The development of Adolescent and Young Adult Participation Sort—Taiwanese version. *Occupational Therapy International, 20*, 124-133.

Wang, H.-Y., & Berg, C. (2014). Participation of young adults with high-functioning autism in Taiwan: A pilot study. *OTJR: Occupation, Participation and Health, 34*, 41-51.

Ware, J. E., Jr., & Sherbourne, C. D. (1992). The MOS 36-item Short-Form Health Survey (SF-36): I. Conceptual framework and item selection. *Medical Care, 30*, 473-483.

West, W. L. (1967). The occupational therapist's changing responsibility to the community. *American Journal of Occupational Therapy, 21*, 312-316.

Whiteley, S. (2004). The evolution of the therapeutic community. *Psychiatric Quarterly, 75*, 233-248.

Wilcock, A. A. (1999). Reflections on doing, being and becoming. *Australian Occupational Therapy Journal, 46*, 1-11.

Wolf, T. J., Brey, J. K., Baum, C., & Connor, L. T. (2012). Activity participation differences between younger and older individuals with stroke. *Brain Impairment, 13*, 16-23.

Wood-Dauphinée, S. L., Opzoomer, M. A., Williams, J. I., Marchand, B., & Spitzer, W. O. (1988). Assessment of global function: The Reintegration to Normal Living index. *Archives of Physical Medicine and Rehabilitation, 69*, 583-590.

Part III
Psychological Assessments

Writing as an Assessment Tool in Mental Health

Kristine Haertl, PhD, OTR/L, FAOTA

Writing makes a map,
and there is something about a journey that begs to have its passage marked.
(Baldwin, 1991a, p. 1)

The power of the written word transcends time and space. Historically, cultures have developed written forms and symbols as a means of communication, personal expression, and thought. Writing is powerful; it influences our perceptions, constructs, and worldview. Such forms of written communication may be expressed in the private, public, or personal realm. Personal writing is a unique occupational tool that may be used to enhance personal growth. This chapter presents an innovative approach related to the use of writing in dynamic assessment and intervention within occupational therapy. Given the unique nature of using writing as an assessment tool, the sections of this chapter will differ some from those that cover more traditional means of assessment.

Therapeutic Writing

Therapeutic writing is a form of "client expressive and reflective writing, whether self-generated, or suggested by a therapist/researcher" (Wright & Chung, 2001, p. 278). Writing takes on various forms, which may include the use of written expression, journals, blogs, poetry, unsent letters, and various forms of creative writing and story making. Each form has a unique structure and purpose and may be self-initiated or therapist directed. The following represent examples of commonly used forms of therapeutic writing.

Hemphill, B. J., & Urish, C. K. (Eds.). *Assessments in Occupational Therapy Mental Health: An Integrative Approach, Fourth Edition* (pp. 93-115). © 2020 Taylor & Francis Group.

Journals

The term *journal* refers to a form of personal writing that expresses perceptions, experiences, dreams, and creativity from the perspective of the self. The word comes from the French root word *jour*, meaning "day" (Bender, 2000), and is often used to depict a form of daily writing and reflection. The literature reveals a variety of definitions of journal. Rainer (1978) often used the terms *diary* and *journal* interchangeably, whereas other authors have distinguished a journal from diary writing, identifying the diary as a more formal type of daily writing focused on external events and a journal as writing focused within (Baldwin, 1991b). Murray (1997) asserted, "Journaling is primarily a body/mind/spirit (metaphysical) activity where the journal keeper makes sense of living" (p. 69). The use of journal writing is often instrumental in developing insight and working on personal goals and may be used as a therapeutic tool in rehabilitation.

In personal and rehabilitative writing, the journal may take on a variety of formats, including bound journals, computer-based private journals, and web-based journals. In recent years, the use of electronic forms of journal writing has increased and is now used for both assessment and intervention in mental health settings (Baker & Moore, 2011; Lent, 2009). Such journals lend a new element of choice on private vs. public disclosure, something far more protected in the days of personal paperbound journals. Decisions on the types and formats of journals used are highly personal and based on individual preference, the goals of journaling, and the utility of the journal. Similar to personal journals, the format of the journal within a therapeutic setting will depend on the goals of therapy and a collaborative effort among the client, therapist, and any other identified key persons (e.g., other individuals in a journal writing group). Journal writing has often been used in mental health as a form of intervention, yet within therapy the journal provides a unique tool for ongoing assessment amid the intervention process.

Poetry

Poetry is a form of expressive writing that may be included within a journal or written on its own. Poetry therapy utilizes both existing poems and the creation of poetry to facilitate therapeutic connections and personal healing (Chavis, 2011; Haertl, 2014; Mazza, 2003). Clark (2007), a mental health consumer with schizoaffective disorder, provided a fascinating account of personal poetry analysis from preadmission to several hospitalizations through his recovery process. The author used his poetry to increase understanding of his healing journey. The use of poetry in the therapeutic process may be done individually or within a group and includes the use of various forms and techniques, including, but not exclusive to, prescriptive poetry, poetry stems, and narratives (Chavis, 2011; Mazza, 2003). The National Association of Poetry Therapy (www.poetrytherapy.org) provides a variety of resources, conferences, and credentialing for interested therapists.

Letter Writing

Letter writing has been long used as a therapeutic tool in mental health intervention (Green & Lambert, 2013; Steinberg, 2000). It may take on the form of a means of communication between the therapist and client or may be used as a technique (e.g., unsent letters) for a client to explore communication with someone or something he or she has a personal conflict or dilemma with. Such techniques allow for personal reflection, insight, and feedback from the therapist. Therapeutic letter writing may also be used in order for a client to work on emotional regulation and to process difficult emotions (Prasko, Diveky, Mozny, & Sigmundova, 2009). Decisions regarding whether and with whom to share the letter writing is a partnership agreement between the therapist and client, as are the nature and use of the techniques throughout therapy.

Additional Forms of Therapeutic Writing

Though an exhaustive discussion of therapeutic writing is beyond the scope of this chapter, many additional forms of writing are used in mental health. Perhaps the most well-known techniques are those of James Pennebaker (Pennebaker, 1997; Pennebaker & Beall, 1986; Pennebaker & Seagal, 1999; Ramirez-Esparza & Pennebaker, 2006). In controlled studies conducted on expressive writing, people who expressed their deepest thoughts in writing for 15 to 20 minutes on at least 3 occasions demonstrated a number of physiological health benefits, including fewer medical-related health visits, improved immune function, and reduced stress (Pennebaker, 1997; Ramirez-Esparza & Pennebaker, 2006). Additional techniques involving expressive writing, which may or may not be directed by the therapist, as well as more formal therapeutic writing activities, have been used with a variety of cognitive behavioral and psychodynamic approaches to evaluation and intervention. The following sections will present a brief history, research, theoretical approaches, and uses of writing in the occupational therapy evaluation and intervention process.

Writing and Mental Health

Historical Roots

Writing has long been recognized for its therapeutic properties in its various forms. Historically, therapeutic writing was mainly used within the context of self-help approaches implementing cognitive and behavioral techniques (Wright & Chung, 2001). Prior to the more recent emphasis on expressive writing, Progoff (1975, 1992) developed an intensive journal process that emphasized a variety of written forms to facilitate self-awareness and personal expression. Progoff spent decades developing his techniques, utilizing theoretical principles from depth psychology. Progoff's (1975, 1992) Intensive Journal process involves the use of multiple sections within the journal designed to look at the self from different perspectives. Progoff emphasized the importance of daily logs, meditations, life dimensions, spirituality, dreams, and personal reflection in order to facilitate personal growth through both the process and product of journal writing. The author's journal writing techniques continue to be used in various forms throughout the world.

Following Progoff's work and the onset of this widespread interest in expressive writing, Pennebaker (Pennebaker, 1997; Pennebaker & Beall, 1986; Pennebaker & Seagal, 1999; Ramirez-Esparza & Pennebaker, 2006) developed a specific writing technique involving 15 to 20 minutes of in-depth writing on emotionally relevant materials. Progroff's techniques have been heavily expanded upon and researched. In recent years, additional writing applications have focused on psychoanalytic Freudian and cognitive Adlerian approaches (Schneider & Stone, 1998), emphasizing the relationship between writing and psychological adjustment, as well as the use of electronic versions of expressive writing, journals, and blogs (Baker & Moore, 2011; Haberstroh, Trepal, & Parr, 2005; Lent, 2009). Although writing has long been used in mental health, the past 2 decades have marked an insurgence of evidence-based support for the use of writing in therapy.

Current Applications and Research

Prior to 2000, literature and research on therapeutic applications of writing were largely focused within psychology and counseling in adult populations (Hall & Hawley, 2004; Jordan & L'Abate, 1995; L'Abate, 1991, 1999; Ulrich & Lutgendorf, 2002) and based on the use of various writing techniques in both individual and group therapy. In recent years, populations studied extend to people with addiction (Grasing, Mathur, & Desouza, 2010; Knoetz, 2013), youth (Walker & Kelly, 2011), post-traumatic stress disorder (Stockton, Joseph, & Hunt, 2014), cancer (Horowitz, 2008), the general population (Haertl, 2014), and several other clinical populations throughout the lifespan. Applications of reflective and journal writing strategies have also been extensively used in the academic realm in order to facilitate critical-thinking skills in students within the classroom and fieldwork settings (Griffith & Frieden, 2000; Ritchie, 2003; Ruthman, Jackson, Cluskey, Flannigan, Folse, & Bunten, 2004; Spalding & Wilson, 2002). Writing strategies used within clinical and academic settings often focus on developing personal insight on the part of the client or student. Insight may be gained by personal reflection and analysis, by cooperative dialogue and feedback with the therapist or teacher, or through use of peer feedback from other clients or students. Within such settings, individual, environmental, and therapeutic factors lead to the development of the purpose of the assigned writing and ultimately to the selection of the format of writing, reflection, and feedback.

Research on the use of therapeutic writing has suggested promising results in a variety of areas, yet continued research is needed, particularly in the rehabilitative fields. One of the most well-known studies on the use of writing within psychotherapeutic approaches is that of Pennebaker (Pennebaker, 1997; Pennebaker & Beall, 1986; Pennebaker & Seagal, 1999; Ramirez-Esparza & Pennebaker, 2006) in studies of undergraduate students who participated in a regimented program of writing on stressful/traumatic events. These studies demonstrated statistically significant improvement in physiological measures (e.g., blood pressure, skin conductance) in students who wrote about personal traumatic events. A subsequent meta-analysis by Smyth (1998) suggested that the effect sizes of studies on personal writing about stressful events seem to imply that expressive writing may lead to improved psychological health and well-being.

Additional research on therapeutic writing techniques has demonstrated a variety of benefits. Brady and Sky (2003) found in a qualitative study of 15 older learners (average age: 69.2 years) that journal writing facilitated improved personal coping skills with daily life and contributed to self-expression and the ability to reflect on and integrate meaning in life. Hall and Hawley (2004) conducted a study on the use of interactive process notes, which involved peer sharing of personal writing within a group setting. The study suggested that the use of interactive process notes might facilitate increased client insight, yet drawbacks include questions of confidentiality among the client, peers, and the group facilitator. Haertl (2014) found that writing connected individuals to the spiritual realm, was integral to identity formation, and facilitated perspective taking and personal growth.

Wright (2002) reviewed research on therapeutic outcomes of writing and cited a number of studies suggesting benefits of therapeutic writing to include (1) greater client control within the therapeutic relationship, (2) the provision for an outlet of emotional expression, and (3) increased client participation in the healing process. Additional applications of therapeutic writing include use of poetry therapy, bibliotherapy, expressive forms of writing, and structured workbooks (McArdle & Byrt, 2001). In recent years, there has been increased research on the efficacy of the therapeutic effects of writing, including a number of meta-analyses that have led authors to assert use of writing as evidence-based practice (Frattaroli, 2006; Frisina, Borod, & Lepore, 2004; Horowitz, 2008; Lee & Cohn, 2009).

Despite the fact more than 90 studies have focused on the therapeutic use of writing (Lee & Cohn, 2009), a paucity of research in rehabilitation exists; thus, future research should consider how to best incorporate therapeutic writing into rehabilitation.

Application to Occupational Therapy

The intrinsically personal nature of writing is well-suited to reflective client-centered practice and may be used in academic and clinical realms. Although expressive writing techniques and journaling may be included in the use of meaningful occupations within the context of the therapeutic relationship, little is written on the use of writing in occupational therapy settings. Writing may be incorporated in mental health occupational therapy both within evaluation and intervention, particularly in expressive, psychodynamic approaches, as well as use of cognitive behavioral techniques (Haertl, 2019; Haertl & Christiansen, 2011). Specific uses of this modality within these frames of reference will be described further.

Denshire (2002) wrote about the power of personal reflective writing and its influence on the role as a therapist. The author asserted the importance of personal reflection in developing subjective ways of knowing and valuing the personal self within the therapy context (Denshire, 2002). Similarly, client-centered, occupation-based frames of reference, such as the Person-Environment-Occupational Performance Model (Baum, Christiansen, & Bass, 2015; Christiansen & Baum, 1997), the Ecology of Human Performance Process Model (Fearing, Law, & Clark, 1997), and the Model of Human Occupation (Kielhofner, 2002, 2008), all stress the importance of meaningful occupational engagement within the therapeutic context involving client choice, perspective, and meaning. Through use of expressive writing, the client is afforded opportunities to express personal thoughts, feelings, and ideas in a context that may feel safer than direct self-report. The client has a unique opportunity to develop a relationship with the journal and personal writing itself, a relationship that is sustainable over time (Thompson, 2004).

Haiman, Lambert, and Rodrigues (2005) wrote of the benefits of using various expressive techniques, such as poetry and journal writing, in adolescent mental health occupational therapy and suggested that writing techniques encourage emotional expression and personal exploration. Such techniques may be applied in the rehabilitation setting to a variety of populations across the lifespan (Brady & Sky, 2003; Levitt, 2005; Murray, 1997; Stone, 1998).

Journal Writing in the Occupational Therapy Evaluation-Intervention Continuum

The *Occupational Therapy Practice Framework: Domain and Practice, Third Edition,* identifies the occupational therapy process as including the evaluation (i.e., development of occupational profile and analysis of occupational performance), intervention, and outcomes assessment phases (American Occupational Therapy Association [AOTA], 2014). The evaluation process refers to the entire spectrum of information gathering through use of historical information, interviews, observations, and formal assessments, whereas assessments denote use of a particular tool or technique. Assessments are often a measure of client function in a particular context and time. Assessment results may be fairly static when the client is at baseline and function remains stable, yet often mental health clients are in a perpetual state of fluctuation in daily function; such variability lends itself well to means of assessment that measure change over time. Within the occupational therapy process in mental health, clients with insight may help develop the occupational profile, not only through interviews and history taking, but also through expressive writing techniques used to portray their past, present, and future. Such an approach affords the therapist the opportunity to listen to the client perspective and may be repeated through the course of therapy.

Christiansen, Haertl, and Rogers (2011) wrote of the dynamic interactive state of evaluation when used repeatedly throughout the therapy process. The use of repeated evaluations assists the therapist and client in measuring change as related to personal therapeutic goals. Given the fact that the nature of therapeutic writing implies an ongoing practice, the literature most often presents it in the context of intervention, yet the fluidity of writing provides opportunities for use throughout the evaluation-intervention continuum.

Within occupation-based practice, therapists seek to engage clients in meaningful activities throughout the therapeutic process. Client interest and follow-through with writing assignments will vary based on personal preference, experience with writing, and the context in which it is presented. Given the highly personalized, ongoing nature of therapeutic writing, it may be used both as a dynamic means of assessment within the evaluative process and as a unique intervention tool applicable to a variety of theoretical perspectives.

L'Abate (1991) presented four types of writing assignments often used in therapy: open-ended writing, focused writing, guided writing, and programmed writing. Open-ended writing techniques are more free flowing and client generated, such as the techniques used from psychodynamic perspectives. Focused and guided techniques provide the client with direction in relation to the writing content (e.g., write about how you feel when you are depressed, answer the following questions), yet allow the individual freedom within the guided writing. Programmed writing techniques often include prescriptive worksheets or a series of homework assignments designed for a specific purpose. The therapist must consider client factors along with theoretical perspectives in determining the type, format, and duration of journal writing that will take place.

Frame of Reference and Theoretical Perspectives

In order to use therapeutic writing within the evaluation and intervention continuum, the occupational therapist should have an understanding of techniques and applications, as well as ethical and client considerations, and should have a theoretical basis for which the writing process will be used. Information and resources related to journal writing are presented in Appendix A. Key questions the therapist should ask prior to use of journal writing are presented in Table 7-1.

The following presents a brief summary of possible applications for use of therapeutic writing within the evaluation-intervention continuum. The techniques are only a sample of those available, and although they are presented within a specific frame of reference, many techniques are applicable across several therapeutic approaches.

Table 7-1

Key Questions a Therapist Should Ask Prior to the Use of Therapeutic Writing

- What is my knowledge and use of writing as an assessment and intervention tool?
- What are the therapeutic needs of the client, and how will use of therapeutic writing meet these needs?
- What form of writing techniques will be used and how often (e.g., computer-based/internet or hardbound journals, homework-based, letter writing, poetry, structured assignments)?
- Who will the writing be shared with (e.g., client, therapist, peers, others)?
- What level of confidentiality will be maintained?
- Do the client's occupational profile and other factors lend themselves to use of therapeutic writing (e.g., client's writing skills, capacity for insight, motivation)?
- Is the client interested in the use of writing, and is follow-through likely?
- What is the underlying theoretical background/frame of reference used?
- Will the techniques extend beyond therapy (e.g., will the client engage in writing outside of therapy and/or will the client continue this modality upon discharge)?
- How will the outcomes be monitored?

Object Relations/Psychodynamic Techniques

The application of psychodynamic principles to occupational therapy practice assumes that psychological constructs contribute to an individual's occupational and social behaviors (Bruce & Borg, 2002). The use of expressive and projective writing techniques within this approach may bring up thoughts and emotions that are within the unconscious or subconscious (Adams, 1990; Bruce & Borg, 2002; Haertl & Christiansen, 2011; Progoff, 1992). The therapist serves as a guide within this approach, not an analyst. Through the use of therapeutic writing within this frame of reference, the therapist seeks to achieve a collaborative relationship with the client in order to "mutually assume responsibility for assessment, identification of intervention goals, and development of an intervention plan, and to work together cooperatively during the intervention process" (Bruce & Borg, 2002, p. 91).

Stream of Consciousness

Stream of consciousness writing stems from the psychodynamic principles of Freud (Adams, 1990; Senn, 2001) and includes techniques such as flow writing, expressive free writing, and dream analysis. Within stream of consciousness writing, writers utilize tactile, auditory, associative, and subliminal impressions to influence writing. A related form of expression often used within journals, map of consciousness, not only includes the use of words but also encourages creative spontaneous expression, including use of drawings, diagrams, and symbols in conjunction with the use of words (Rainer, 1978). In both stream of consciousness and map of consciousness, clients are encouraged to explore areas of the unconscious through free-form writing, often initiated with a particular word or topic. Once the idea is introduced, the client is encouraged to write or draw whatever comes to mind. One of the most common types of stream of consciousness writing is flow writing, or free writing.

Flow Writing and Free Writing

Flow writing and *free writing* are terms used to denote writing techniques that encourage the free expression of thought over a period of time. The client may be given a specific topic to write about, but generally there is a fair amount of freedom allowed within this type of journal entry. The client is encouraged to write whatever comes to mind. Clients may be offered a set amount of time to write (Baldwin, 1991a) or encouraged to write as long as they would like to do so. Gute and Gute (2008) asserted that, within the use of flow writing, individuals may become so consumed they lose sense of time and self. This technique may also be helpful when the client/writer experiences writer's block within the journal (Rainer, 1978) and may facilitate new insights or a sense of catharsis (Hilsdon, 2004). Benefits of flow writing include the opportunity for free expression of thoughts and feelings and the ability to access the unconscious (Adams, 1998; Rainer, 1978). Hilsdon (2004) recommended the following options for flow/free writing:

- Consider whether to use a time limit for the free write.
- Clients may be guided with a trigger word or phrase.
- Encourage writing without judgment or censorship.
- Refrain from returning to the entry to edit or change.
- Work with the client to determine insights gained from the writing.

Within mental health settings, the client and therapist may wish to revisit the entry immediately after it is written or may choose to wait for a period of time because it allows the client time between the writing and review in order to explore the entry for potential themes, meanings, and insights.

Expressive Writing

Expressive writing has been shown to have positive effects on physiological factors, mood (Grasing et al., 2010), and personal growth (Stockton et al., 2014). Forms of expressive and creative writing may be used through a variety of techniques, including the writing of stories, poetry, and narratives. Art therapist Dr. Lucia Capacchione has written several books on creativity and journal writing and introduced a creative journal approach (1989) designed for feelings exploration through use of writing and drawing exercises. Of most notable interest in her technique is the encouragement of use of the nondominant hand, forcing expanded use of the creative means within the brain. According to Campbell (2000), the use of the nondominant hand encourages recruitment of the nondominant side of the brain. Such expression may be more difficult for the writer but may tap into some unconscious/creative areas that are not often used. Additional techniques within the journal should explore personal expression regarding topics of meaning, areas of difficulty, and plans for future goals. Horowitz (2008) suggested the following when utilizing Pennebaker's prescriptive writing, which involves a minimum of 15 minutes writing about highly emotional events:

- Utilize a place where the writer will not be disturbed.
- Have the client write about topics he or she has been worrying about or that have had a negative effect on health.
- Decide whether to write about the same or different topics each time.
- Consider reviewing the writing either with the self or therapist.
- Decide whether you will eventually keep or destroy the writing.

Additional expressive writing styles may be incorporated throughout the evaluation and intervention process.

Dream Exploration

Dream exploration may be used as an access to the unconscious, bridging the dream life to our waking hours (Adams, 1990; Progoff, 1975, 1992; Rainer, 1978). Dreams offer a way to make sense of the world through intersubjective and relational means (Kirtsoglu, 2010). The use of dream exploration and dream analysis comes out of the psychoanalytic applications of psychology and is best used by trained therapists. Occupational therapists generally are not trained in dream analysis; however, the client may wish to explore dreams within the journal. Through the recording of dreams, clients may gain insights into themes of importance in their lives. Adams (1990) suggested the following techniques for improving dream recall:

- Keep a notebook and pen by the bed
- Record the dream immediately upon awakening, even if in the middle of the night
- Go to sleep with the intention of remembering your dreams
- Visualize writing down the dreams upon awaking
- Write whatever comes to you upon wakening (do not censor)
- Be good-natured in the process of dream recall

Dreams may often be frightening or confusing. Progoff (1992) emphasized the importance of recording the dreams without initial judgment or analysis and asserted "… to do that would, in the first place, have the effect of rationalizing the symbolic material and thus violating the fact that its nature is inherently non-rational" (p. 203). The author stressed the importance of recording dream materials in an unbiased manner and revisiting the material later, recording any insights without overanalysis. In addition to dream logs, the use of meditation or twilight imagery may be used to invite thoughts, images, and dreams in a state between the sleep/wake cycle (Progoff, 1975, 1992; Rainer, 1978). *Twilight imagery* is a term used to denote a state between levels of consciousness (Progoff, 1992). The journal writer enters the state through a process of meditation and imagery, which may bring about images that are later reviewed for correlation with life events and themes of meaning.

Special Considerations in Applying Psychodynamic Applications to Assessment

Within the psychodynamic framework, therapists uphold the importance of developing client insight; therefore, client capacity for realistic thinking and self-reflection should be considered (Bruce & Borg, 2002). The content of expressive writing must be considered in the context of the environment, client factors, and personal meaning. The therapist and client work together in a collaborative relationship, identifying themes that may be of importance with relationship to life history, current experience, and therapeutic goals. Questions for consideration in expressive writing are considered in Table 7-2.

If expressive writing techniques are used in the evaluation process, the client and therapist must maintain a collaborative relationship throughout the planning, writing, and discussion of the content. Therapists should ensure that the writing does not bring up issues or questions that compromise the client's ability to cope; therefore, ethical considerations must be adhered to. Written expression and use of follow-up dialogue provide rich sources of information regarding client perception, sources of meaning, cognitive status, dynamic changes within the client's psyche, and potential areas for goal and intervention planning. In using therapeutic writing as an assessment tool, dialogue and teamwork must be maintained at all times among the client, therapist, and intervention team.

Table 7-2
Questions to Consider When Using Expressive Writing
• What was the experience of the client during the writing process? Was it therapeutic?   • What are the client's thoughts, feelings, and experiences with relation to the process and product of the writing?   • What does this writing content say about client events, experiences, thoughts, feelings, and ego functions?   • Are there themes that relate to other examples of the client's writing, therapy, and/or past or current experience?   • What does the writing say about client meaning, and how does this apply to identified strengths, needs, and goals?   • What insights can be gained from the writing? How can these insights be utilized in the therapeutic process and in pursuit of improved occupational performance?   • Where will the therapeutic writing process go from here?

Cognitive Behavioral Techniques

Cognitive behavioral interventions stem from social learning theory and the work of theorists such as Bandura, Ellis, and Beck, theorists who emphasized the dynamic interplay between thought and behavior (Haertl & Christiansen, 2011). The cognitive behavioral frame of reference assumes that (1) thinking influences behavior, (2) thinking can be self regulated, and (3) desired behavioral change may occur through structured learning and acquired skills (Stein & Cutler, 2002). This frame of reference often involves skill building through the use of structured homework assignments, daily personal tracking sheets, and the teaching of coping skills, such as relaxation training and exercise. Use of therapeutic writing and journal techniques may involve structured assignments followed by self-reflection, group interaction, or feedback and dialogue between the client and therapist. A key focus within this frame of reference is the development of personal insight and skills in order to maximize function and quality of life through the development of coping skills and meaningful healthy occupational patterns.

Homework/Structured Writing

According to L'Abate (1991), the use of writing assignments is advantageous in the provision for structure in therapy, yet it is important such assignments do not overcontrol the assessment and intervention process. In order to remain dynamic and client-centered, occupational therapists must select and adapt writing assignments based on the context and client needs and desires.

Several resources are available to guide structured writing (Adams, 1998; Bender, 2000; Hering, 2013; Jacobs, 2004). Therapists may choose to utilize prescriptive writing or may wish to adapt homework assignments based on the goals of the evaluation and intervention process. Typically, clients engage in writing homework as part of an ongoing assessment and intervention process within individual or group therapy. If used as a part of a group, decisions should be made as to how confidentiality will be maintained and how much of the personal writing will be shared with the therapist and peers. Through the use of homework, clients are often asked to complete a structured writing assignment with the intention of later revisiting the assignment for personal analysis or feedback from peers or the therapist. Assignments may be used to gauge and track progress on personal goals or may be used in order to further the assessment and intervention process through the development of new goals and practice of skill building. Appendix A provides suggested resources to assist with the facilitation of structured journal writing.

Lists

The use of lists in conjunction with therapeutic writing provides a means to organize thoughts around a particular topic. Lists are powerful tools due to their simplistic, informative, and efficient properties (Campbell, 2000). Lists may be used for a variety of purposes, including self-expression, such as in the instance of exploring anxiety (e.g., 10 things that I am stressed about right now), for problem solving (e.g., 5 things I can do to cope with my stress), or for the development of insight (e.g., 5 key events in my life). The structuring of lists may include lists of short words, phrases, or sentences (e.g., list of friends) or more detailed lists (e.g., 10 favorite memories from college).

Progoff (1975, 1992) introduced a type of list he termed *stepping stones*. Within this technique, the writer is encouraged to list significant events that have occurred in the client's life. The list of stepping stones is akin to looking at personal marker events in one's own life, a practice that fits well not only into the cognitive behavioral frame of reference, but also into developmental theories and frames of reference. Following the list of stepping stones, the journal writer and therapist review the journal entry for themes of importance throughout the life span and identify areas for further exploration in the assessment-intervention continuum.

Adams (1990) asserted the utility of using longer lists within journal writing and introduced an additional listing technique titled *Lists of 100*. Examples of lists she identified include lists of fears, lists of stressors, and lists of things never grieved. Adams (1990) suggested that use of extensive lists often provides greater depth and unfolds into three parts: (1) things held in the conscious mind (generally the first third of the list), (2) repetition and themes that arise in the list, and (3) things that arise from the subconscious. Extensive lists may be used to assess for themes and insights and to facilitate goal planning.

Clustering

Similar to lists, clustering is a writing technique that may be used to organize thoughts and feelings around a particular topic. Clustering is the use of cognitive mapping strategies and involves the connection of words and topics to similar words and topics (Adams, 1990; Campbell, 2000). The use of clustering is not isolated to journal writing; it is often used in academic settings to facilitate student learning of a topic. Campbell (2000) suggested the use of clustering as a means of undercutting tension or anxiety often caused by writing. Perhaps one of the most basic techniques is the mapping of words where one word is placed in a box and lines are drawn to additional boxes with associated words. Although clustering is a useful tool, it should not be overused because it is highly structured and limits free expression of thought. However, it is a useful tool for organizing thoughts and beginning exploration of a particular topic.

Dialogue

Progoff (1975, 1992) introduced the writing technique of using dialogue to explore relationships with other individuals, with the self, or with inanimate objects. Generally, when selecting a source for dialogue, a person or object is chosen with which there is unfinished business, a significant event occurred, or there is some area that needs more

Table 7-3

Questions Following Dialogue

- Is there anything more to be written?
- What thoughts and emotions were experienced during the writing, following the writing, and now?
- What perceptions and insights does the dialogue present?
- Is there unfinished business to attend to?
- What do you hope to gain from the dialogue?
- What strategies can be used for personal growth following the dialogue process?

insight. Progoff (1975, 1992) discussed the use of dialogue with individuals (relationships), works (significant activities in life), the body, society, and events. Green and Lambert (2013) asserted that the use of dialogue may be incorporated into other writing techniques, such as letter writing. Adams (1990) suggested additional areas for dialogue, including emotions, objects, subpersonalities/symbols, and areas of resistance. In order to engage in the dialogue, Adams (1990) suggested the importance of taking time to enter into a state in which the writer is cognitively and emotionally prepared to write the dialogue. The use of imagery and meditation may be helpful, and it is important for the writer to be gentle on the self when engaged in the process. Following the written product, the writer (and possibly therapist) should revisit the dialogue and consider questions presented in Table 7-3.

The following presents an example of a short journal dialogue between a 36-year-old depressed mother (Jane) and her deceased 18-year-old son (Mark), who died in an accident while under the influence of alcohol (excerpt from Jane's journal):

Me: Daily my stomach curls, I sob, and I don't think there is a reason to go on. I can't deny that I am angry you are dead; I question why you always drank, and some days I want to scream "I told you so!!" but it cuts me apart to know you will never hear my voice again.

Mark: You're one to talk you hypocrite!! I never drank that much, and you were always so hard on me, I know you never cared as much for me as you did for your job!! It seemed that you were always working, never home, and you know that you GUZZLED TOO!!!

Me (crying!): I'm sorry! I did my best! Why will no one forgive me? Why can't I cope? Why is my life full of eating, sleeping, and drinking? I can't go on!!!

Following an extended version of this excerpt, Jane and the therapist identified key areas for intervention planning and goal setting, including her chemical dependency issues, stress management, and finding meaningful occupational activities within a daily schedule in order to improve her quality of life. In addition to the occupational therapy approach, the entire team made a collective plan as to how to address her issues of grief/loss, self-esteem, depression, and chemical dependency. The use of a small journal excerpt provided a wealth of information within the assessment process.

Unsent Letters

As briefly discussed earlier, a technique similar to dialogue is the use of unsent letters. The client is encouraged to write a letter designed for one-way communication to someone/something of significance. The letter may be written about a past hurt, about a time of meaning, or about continued questions in life. According to Adams (1990), "unsent letters are marvelous tools for the three C's—catharsis, completion, and clarity" (p. 172). Such letters can help bring closure to issues of difficulty or may be used to bring new insights to something or some relationship that has caused hurt, anxiety, stress, or some other psychological need that should be expressed. Unsent letters are meant for the individual writer and are generally not intended to actually be sent to the person of correspondence; however, the journal or therapy session may also be used to write a practice letter to someone with whom correspondence, confrontation, or communication is anticipated to be difficult. The use of unsent letters can provide a venue for clients to self-evaluate with the therapist the patterns of communication and to consider healthy means of expression. Letter writing may also be used in addictions, as the individual writes to those he or she has hurt; discussions occur with the therapist as to whether they should actually be sent or should remain unsent (Hagerdorn, 2011). Rainer (1978) stressed that therapists and clients should caution against overuse of unsent letters because they may encourage a preoccupation with the written product and avoidance of actual feelings expressed to the individuals with whom communication is intended. Therapists using the unsent letters technique should explore with the client the significance of the letter as related to occupational themes, social relationships, life satisfaction, and areas for future work.

Reflective Writing

There are many types of reflection often used in academia (Samrajya, 2014) and in therapeutic settings for personal growth (Wright, 2005). While some reflective writing techniques are done as homework for students or clients, often it is an integral part of journal writing. Progoff (1975, 1992) spoke of the importance of revisiting the journal in order to develop new insights and add new entries based on reflections of previous writing. Therapists may work with clients to structure reflective writing entries in order to have space for writing future insights upon revisiting the writing. One such technique, the double entry, utilizes half a page for the actual writing and leaves half the page blank for future reflections and insights. Reflections may be retroactive based on a particular journal entry or may be single entries designed to reflect on any area of life, therapy, or personal significance. Following a review of the reflections, the client and therapist work together to assess progress toward goals, personal growth, and areas for future development.

Use of Writing in Dialectical Behavioral Therapy

Dialectical behavioral therapy (DBT) is a broad cognitive behavioral strategy originally designed to treat clients with borderline personality disorder, but it since has been applied to a number of populations, including those with depression, substance abuse, and eating disorders. Linehan (1993) developed the method based on the premise that individuals who have lived in invalidating environments often develop maladaptive skills for coping and emotional regulation. Use of the DBT program generally involves a structured weekly psychotherapy session as well as an intensive group session designed to teach adaptive coping skills, such as emotional regulation, interpersonal effectiveness, and assertiveness training. Occupational therapists are often involved as facilitators of the skill training component of DBT. Within the group, clients use a diary card to track incidents, events, and reactions, and in retrospect often evaluate their performance in the situation. Diary cards are useful not only for intervention purposes, but also in assessment and ongoing tracking of personal progress (Haertl & Christiansen, 2011). DBT groups also involve a series of homework sheets and may incorporate the use of therapeutic writing or a journal to facilitate insight related to the skills taught. A key consideration when facilitating DBT groups is the impact of skills training on occupational performance and the maintenance of open communication with the client's psychologist and other team members. Consistency of approach is important when facilitating skills training and therapeutic writing applications.

Additional Considerations Within the Cognitive Behavioral Frame of Reference

Within the cognitive behavioral frame of reference, a key focus is the development of insight to influence growth and change. The writing and homework assignments are often incorporated in stages designed to bring about awareness, practice adaptive skills, and develop an internal locus of control designed to follow through with the skills throughout life. In order for the achievement of such goals to be met, the therapist continually works with the client to assess progress through review and discussion of the homework and journal assignments. Progress will depend on client motivation, capacity for insight, the therapeutic relationship, and contextual factors. Academic literature identifies various factors necessary for individual capacity and willingness to reflect including the following (Paterson, 1995):

- Developmental level
- Perceived trustworthiness of the teacher (therapist)
- The clarity of expectations
- The quality of the feedback process

When utilizing reflective practice within occupational therapy, therapists should consider the client's capacity for insight, willingness to write, and amount of structure needed to meet the needs of the client, context, and therapeutic process.

Spirituality

Often, mental health clients have to deal with grief, loss, and bereavement related to their illness, personal trauma, and/or a chasm between their goals for the self, conceptualizations of perceived self, and current life events contributing to the actual self. The use of therapeutic writing is a powerful place to work through bereavement and loss, find a place of meaning, and explore personal spirituality and belief systems.

The AOTA's (2014) *Framework* acknowledges the spiritual dimensions of our lives as an important client factor that conveys personal meaning and purpose in life. Spirituality affects the development of the self and influences occupational patterns. Writing is a powerful tool for exploration of spirituality and matters of personal meaning. Baldwin (1991a) wrote of the power of the journal and personal writing to facilitate exploration of meaning within and beyond ourselves. The author asserted, "Spiritual writing expands the interior conversation of consciousness to include your relationship with the sacred ... You are in conversation with something you perceive as beyond, or deep within, yourself. It is this inclusion of the sacred that spiritualizes the writing" (Baldwin, 1991a, p. 23). Through the use of spiritual questions, reflections, and expressive writing, clients may work with the therapist to gain insight into areas of meaning with relation to personal existence. Occupational therapists are not formal spiritual leaders, yet issues of spirituality, value, and meaning should be addressed because they are intrinsic to occupational performance and quality of life. As themes of meaning unfold within the writing, the therapist and client work together to develop goals and interventions surrounding lifestyle, meaningful activities, and occupations that contribute to personal quality of life, wellness, and the ability to cope with loss, work through grief, and explore spiritual matters as they relate to individual occupational performance.

Applying Therapeutic Writing to Occupational Therapy Assessment

The use of writing techniques in mental health assessment is a dynamic process and should flow from assessment to intervention. Prior to utilizing therapeutic writing for assessment, therapists must determine how writing will fit into the evaluation-intervention continuum. Decisions must be made on the writing styles and format (e.g., which techniques to use, whether to use electronic media, with whom it will be shared), theoretical approach, client readiness, and utility to achieve desired outcomes. By definition, therapeutic writing is a fluid, ongoing process; therefore, structure must be built into therapy in order to align writing techniques used with opportunities for assessment, goal planning, and intervention. Assessment of the writing should be a collaborative process between the therapist and client and, if applicable, peers (e.g., if in a shared writing or journal group). Some individuals choose to use therapeutic writing within a group format; therefore, decisions must be made as to how much is shared with peers and who is involved in the feedback process. Generally, the assessment process is ongoing and involves looking at original entries, collaborating with the client to develop a goal plan, and periodically revisiting future entries to track progress. Clients may also be asked to engage in formal self-assessments; therefore, structured questions or goals may be written, such as within a journal or use of tracking sheets for client self-evaluation.

Schneider and Stone (1998) suggested that various writing techniques work best within three separate stages of therapeutic change:

1. Reflection stage
2. Cognitive reconstruction stage
3. Creative construction stage

Within the reflection stage, clients engage in expressive techniques designed to look at perceptions, views, and experiences. This first stage may be used as a means of assessment by which the client's current view of oneself, key life issues, strengths, and needs are addressed. Through the writing process and the revisiting of entries, the client and therapist develop new insights and are challenged to recognize, interpret, and assimilate the insights into their view on life. During the cognitive reconstruction stage, clients use the insights gained and develop new insights, outlooks, and goals for themselves. During the creative construction stage, the therapist and client work together to help the client develop an internal locus of control (empowerment of the client from within) in order to utilize personal skills in meaningful occupational patterns. Throughout this process, the client is encouraged to practice skills, including positive coping, healthy decision making, and meaningful occupational engagement. Thus, therapeutic writing provides unique opportunities for expression, insight, and personal growth.

Format

The use of therapeutic writing may take a variety of forms, including computer-based journals, web-based journals and blogs, hard copy journals or writing activities, and structured workbooks. In addition to the format, therapists must consider the structure for assessment and intervention, including the therapeutic approach, theoretical application, and whether the writing process will be done individually or within a group. If writing is introduced in a group, it is often easiest to have all clients use the same techniques, yet Stone (1998) asserted the importance of individualizing the writing approach in order to maximize follow-through during and after therapy. As a result, the use of groups should have some consistency in approach yet also have enough freedom for client expression and individuality. Decisions must also be made as to whether groups will involve face-to-face interactions or the use of a computer-based journal or blog approach. The use of online journal sites or specialized software often allows clients to determine which entries are public and which are private. Such flexibility may be useful in both individual and group journal approaches and offers the client freedom for personal expression and privacy, an area integral to personal journal writing (Baldwin, 1991b). The danger of using an web-based journal in a group format is that the group facilitator has less control over the group exchange, particularly in asynchronous formats; therefore, the therapist must use caution when setting up web-based journal groups in order to adequately facilitate and structure the process for entry submissions, as well as facilitate ongoing interchange. If journal groups are used, particularly web-based groups, careful selection must take place regarding the clients' ability for insight, capacity for empathy in social interaction, and client skill related to conflict management and assertiveness. With careful set up, structure, and client selection, groups can be an excellent way to develop client insight and promote empowerment within a peer-support model. The use of other techniques, such as mindfulness, may be used to augment the writing group and enhance personal reflection and insight (Poon & Danoff-Burg, 2011).

Self-Assessment

Throughout the writing process, clients should be encouraged to partake in self-assessment, particularly when used as part of the occupational therapy evaluation. The addition of reflective questions is often used in academia and has utility in therapeutic writing as well. An example of self-reflection may include the use of a series of prescribed writing activities in the coping group in order to reflect on insights from the writing content over time. Examples of reflective questions can be found in Table 7-4.

The use of self-assessment techniques may later be shared with the group, therapist, or both so that the client can be held accountable for personal goals. The group may also be structured for open discussion and feedback regarding the client's self-assessment and may be used to consider current progress and future goals. The use of didactic processes and periodic feedback may facilitate self-understanding, as well as opportunities to practice healthy social interactions.

Additional means of self-assessment may include the use of a journal with reflective entries, tracking sheets, checklists, and ongoing discussions with the therapist. When utilizing writing activities for insight and self-assessment, it is important for the therapist to provide clear expectations and feedback regarding the purpose of the writing activities, the means by which they will be used, the expectations, and the depth of reflection expected (Srimavin & Darasawang, 2004). Providing clear expectations and

Table 7-4
Reflective Questions
• What did I learn from my writing and this group regarding my current coping patterns and how they influence my daily life?   • What coping skills have been most successful for me to avoid maladaptive behaviors?   • What progress have I made on my goal to (list goal)?   • Have I completed or do I need to revise or change my goals?   • What is my plan in order to address these goals for the next week?   • What type of writing reflections could help me gain insight on goal attainment?

use of a collaborative approach is imperative to maximize meaningful use of therapeutic writing. Therapists may encourage clients to incorporate outside writing or journals that may extend beyond therapy and provide an ongoing therapeutic outlet once the therapy sessions are finished.

Additional Considerations

Occupational Therapy Approach

In current psychosocial occupational therapy practice, there is often a blending of roles and intervention approaches in the mental health service team. The use of therapeutic writing is not unique to occupational therapy, and much of the writing on its use is within the fields of clinical and counseling psychology. Writing has many therapeutic properties (Haertl, 2014; Haertl & Christiansen, 2011) and is well suited to occupational therapy, particularly when considered as a means of meaningful occupational engagement, as well as a conduit toward the provision of improved occupational performance. The use of writing within the assessment-intervention continuum should have meaning to the client, consider the process and product of the journal within the *Framework* (AOTA, 2014), and be linked to the evaluation and intervention goals aimed at improving occupational performance, life satisfaction, and quality of life. As the client engages in the writing process, a plan should be in place to consider the future utility of personal writing as an ongoing part of the individual's daily life post discharge.

Ethical Considerations

In deciding whether to use writing as a part of therapy, occupational therapists must take into account ethical considerations, such as the expertise of the therapist, the appropriateness of writing for the context and the client, and the means by which it will be used. L'Abate (1999) identified the importance of the client's willingness and interest in the use of writing as a means of therapy. In utilizing a client-centered approach, the decision to use writing and the format that will be used should involve client input. Discussions should be centered on expectations, the format, and the degree of confidentiality that will be maintained. Therapists must caution against promising confidentiality if the client's safety or the safety of others is put at risk; therefore, clear guidelines, expectations, confidentiality, and boundaries must be established prior to the onset of therapy. If writing is used within a group, additional considerations include the establishment of trust and

---

Table 7-5

Key Questions for
Occupational Therapists Using Therapeutic Writing

- What is the therapist's expertise in this area?
- Is the use of therapeutic writing well suited to this population?
- How will the therapeutic approach be unique to occupational therapy?
- How will this modality be assimilated into other areas of the client's treatment and other modalities used by the team?
- What is the therapeutic approach and rationale for using writing in this context?
- Does the therapist have the skills to educate the client, team members, and public regarding the use of therapeutic writing?

---

confidentiality codes within the group, the freedom for clients to determine how much will be personally shared, and the provision for a structured group process, conversation, and conflict management if an uncomfortable topic emerges within the group. For trust to be developed, the therapist must also facilitate and educate clients on the importance of nonjudgmental attitudes within the group process. Clients should have some capacity for insight and empathy when assigned to groups utilizing shared writing strategies.

Additional confidentiality concerns include client privacy regarding the accessibility of the journal or writing activities to others. If clients are in a facility with shared bedrooms, concerns may arise regarding privacy. The therapist and client should establish a plan for how the writing will be kept safe from others, what portions of the journal or writing activities may be completely private (i.e., client access only), and what sections will be accessible to the therapists or to others (if in a group setting). Sometimes within a group setting, the actual writing itself may not be fully shared, but clients have the freedom to openly discuss particular insights that are meaningful to the group.

Therapist Expertise

Within the therapeutic process, the occupational therapist must utilize clinical reasoning and a therapeutic approach to determine means to facilitate desired change (Bruce & Borg, 2002). Although there is evidence to support the benefits of therapeutic writing (Brady & Sky, 2003; Miller, 2014; Walker & Kelly, 2011), little is written on conceptualizations of the use of therapeutic writing in occupational therapy. Occupational therapists are uniquely trained in the study of occupation in conjunction with the person, environment, and context; therefore, they have a unique set of skills that are used to determine meaning, useful engagement, and the utility of writing within the therapeutic process. However, when utilizing any means of assessment and intervention, therapists must consider their own expertise. Table 7-5 offers the occupational therapist questions to consider prior to the use of therapeutic writing.

It is imperative the occupational therapist possess a rationale and theoretical basis for the use of writing within therapy and the ability to articulate the evidence to support its use. Several workshops, organizations, books, and resources exist to provide support and education in the use of therapeutic writing (see Appendix A).

Case Study

Marcy is a 19-year-old woman recently admitted to New Start Day Program due to depression, suicidal ideation, and anorexia nervosa. Marcy recently graduated from high school with high honors and numerous athletic awards in gymnastics. In addition to athletics, she was the editor of the school newsletter and a participant in the poetry club. She originally planned to attend a local major university, but due to increasing depression and medical concerns secondary to a significant drop in her weight (5′6″, 95 pounds), her primary physician convinced her to take a semester off.

Marcy grew up in a single-parent household with one younger sister. Her father left when she was 5 years old, and she has not seen him since. Marcy has been on medication for her diagnosis of depression for about 1 year but has never experienced a psychiatric hospitalization, nor has she ever attended day treatment. She did briefly see a counselor at school, and the question of her eating patterns came up, but at the time she was not referred for medical intervention. During the summer following graduation, she reported increased feelings of stress and depression related to a fear of failure and recent separation from her best friend, who has moved away to college. Her general practitioner referred her to the New Start program due to the multidisciplinary approach and comprehensive services provided by the program, including its psychiatric, residential, vocational, and recreational programs. As part of the day program, Marcy was referred for occupational therapy assessment and intervention.

In the initial occupational therapy interview, Marcy admitted to being depressed but experienced difficulty verbalizing her feelings and the events surrounding the depression and eating disorder. She indicated interests in writing, poetry, literature, and exercise, yet admitted that she did not feel like participating in any leisure activities. Given her writing interests, Marcy agreed to participate in writing and journal activities as part of her ongoing assessment and intervention. As part of an assessment battery during the second week of therapy, Marcy completed an unsent letter journal entry to her father. The following is a short excerpt:

Dear Dad,

They say I'm sick but I feel fine, just a little depressed, that's all. I shouldn't be here anyways; I should be in class working on a degree in education. Why is it that no matter how much I try, I always screw things up? Anyways, you wouldn't care, you never call and mom never mentions your name anyways. I wanted to go to college, and now I've screwed that up too; it seems the world hates me, that's all. My life is crap. I sleep, get up, watch TV, and listen to tunes. Janna [her friend] is gone and there's nothing to do. I never write anymore and have no energy. So what's the big deal? They say I don't eat; I eat fine. They say I'm not ready for school; they say, they say, they say!! Why doesn't anybody ever listen to me?!!

Following her writing, Marcy was asked to write a follow-up reflection indicating any insights she had from her letter. Due to her depression, the occupational therapist decided she would need a structured format for reflection; therefore, she was asked to consider the following questions:

- What feelings and memories came to you as you were writing?
- What feelings do you have now?
- What does this entry say about what is important to you?
- Is your lifestyle how you would like it to be?

- What could you change?
- What are your goals?
- How can we work toward the goals in occupational therapy?
- Was the process of writing helpful? If so, how?

Marcy identified that she was angry, frustrated, and depressed as she wrote her entry. Although she initially identified magnified feelings of depression during the writing process, she stated that writing helped her sort through some things that were bothering her, including the lack of communication with her father, the feeling of helplessness and failure to achieve her goals, the loss of control, and the lack of pleasure in her life. From the initial assessment entry, the occupational therapist developed an occupational profile as presented in the *Framework* (AOTA, 2014) that identified occupational barriers, including her depression, eating disorders, self-concept, and family issues, all of which posed difficulties in successfully achieving her goals to attend school and create a meaningful life. Strengths and interests identified included Marcy's athleticism, intelligence, interest in writing and poetry, and willingness to engage in therapy. It was determined the role of the family would further need to be explored. The therapist collaborated with Marcy and identified initial goal areas including the development of coping skills, increased meaningful engagement in activities of interest, and development of a plan for return to school. In addition, Marcy was to work on her eating disorder concerns in therapy and in collaboration with the entire treatment team. A plan was developed for Marcy to attend DBT treatment, to engage in ongoing journal writing, and to work individually with the therapist to examine lifestyle patterns and means to enhance her quality of life through meaningful activities.

Summary

Writing provides a unique tool within the occupational therapy evaluation-intervention continuum. As therapists' use of writing within occupational therapy continues, research is needed regarding the unique role, efficacy, and clinical utility of the various writing approaches in practice. Writing is highly individualized and fits well into client-centered practice, yet should be used in conjunction with other, more formal means of assessment. Through the use of therapeutic writing, clients can gain insight, work on personal goals, and have an ongoing venue for reflection and personal growth that can be carried throughout life.

References

Adams, K. (1990). *Journal to the self: Twenty-two paths to personal growth.* New York, NY: Warner Books.

Adams, K. (1998). *The way of the journal: A journal therapy workbook for healing* (2nd ed.). Baltimore, MD: Sidran Institute Press.

American Occupational Therapy Association. (2014). Occupational therapy practice framework: Domain and process (3rd ed.). *American Journal of Occupational Therapy, 68*(Suppl. 1), S1-S48.

Baker, J. R., & Moore, S. M. (2011). Creation and validation of the personal blogging style scale. *Cyberpsychology, Behavior and Social Networking, 14*, 379-385.

Baldwin, C. (1991a). *Life's companion: Journal writing as a spiritual quest.* New York, NY: Bantam Books.

Baldwin, C. (1991b). *One to one: A new and updated edition of the classic self-understanding through journal writing.* New York, NY: M. Evans and Company.

Baum, C. M., Christiansen, C. H., & Bass, J. D. (2015). The Person-Environment-Occupation-Performance model. In C. Christiansen, C. Baum, & J. Bass (Eds.), *Occupational therapy: Performance, participation and well-being* (pp. 49-55). Thorofare, NJ: SLACK Incorporated.

Bender, S. (2000). *A year in the life: Journaling for self-discovery.* Cincinnati, OH: Walking Stick Press.

Brady, E. M., & Sky, H. Z. (2003). Journal writing among older learners. *Educational Gerontology, 29,* 151-163.

Bruce, M. A., & Borg, B. (2002). *Psychosocial frames of reference: Core for occupation based practice.* Thorofare, NJ: SLACK Incorporated.

Campbell, A. (2000). *Your corner of the universe: A guide to self-therapy through journal writing.* Lincoln, NE: ASJA Press.

Capacchione, L. (1989). *The creative journal: The art of finding yourself* (2nd ed.). Tarzana, CA: Newcastle Publications.

Chavis, G. G. (2011). *Poetry and story therapy: The healing power of creative expression.* Philadelphia, PA: Jessica Kingsley Publishers.

Christiansen, C., & Baum, C. (1997). Person-environment occupational performance: A conceptual model for practice. In C. Christiansen & C. Baum (Eds.), *Occupational therapy: Enabling function and well-being* (2nd ed., pp. 47-70). Thorofare, NJ: SLACK Incorporated.

Christiansen, C., Haertl, K. L., & Rogers, S. (2011). Evaluation to plan intervention. In C. Christiansen, & K. Matuska (Eds.), *Ways of living: Intervention strategies to enable participation* (4th ed., pp. 45-88). Bethesda, MD: AOTA Press.

Clark, T. (2007). Poetry and self recovery. *The Royal Australian and New Zealand College of Psychiatrists, 15,* S1-S3.

Denshire, S. (2002). Reflections on the confluence of personal and professional. *Australian Journal of Occupational Therapy, 49,* 212-216.

Fearing, V. G., Law, M., & Clark, J. (1997). An occupational performance process model: Fostering client and therapist alliances. *Canadian Journal of Occupational Therapy, 67,* 7-15.

Frattaroli, J. (2006). Experimental disclosure and its moderators. *Psychological Bulletin, 6,* 823-865.

Frisina, P. G., Borod, J. C., & Lepore, S. L. (2004). A meta-analysis of the effects of written emotional disclosure on the health outcomes of clinical populations. *Journal of Nervous and Mental Disease, 192,* 629-634.

Grasing, K., Mathur, D., & Desouza, C. (2010). Written emotional expression during recovery from cocaine dependence: Group and individual differences craving intensity. *Substance Use and Misuse, 45,* 1201-1215.

Green, A., & Lambert, N. (2013). Revisit the forgotten art of letter writing. *Mental Health Practice, 16,* 30-34.

Griffith, B. A., & Frieden, G. (2000). Facilitating reflective thinking in counselor education. *Counselor Education and Supervision, 40,* 82-93.

Gute, D., & Gute, G. (2008). Flow writing in the liberal arts core and across the disciplines: A vehicle for confronting and transforming academic disengagement. *Journal of General Education, 57,* 191-222.

Haberstroh, S., Trepal, S., & Parr, G. (2005). The confluence of technology, and narrative approaches in group work: Techniques and suggestions for using interactive e-journals. *Journal of Creativity in Mental Health, 1,* 29-44.

Haertl, K. (2014). Writing and the development of the self-heuristic inquiry: A unique way of exploring the power of the written word. *Journal of Poetry Therapy, 27,* 1-14.

Haertl, K. (2019). Coping and resilience. In C. Brown, V. Stoffel, & J. Munoz (Eds.), *Occupational therapy in mental health: A vision for participation* (2nd ed.). Philadelphia, PA: F. A. Davis.

Haertl, K., & Christiansen, C. (2011). Coping skills. In C. Brown & V. Stoffel (Eds.), *Occupational therapy in mental health: A vision for participation* (pp. 313-329). Philadelphia, PA: F. A. Davis.

Hagerdorn, B. (2011). Using therapeutic letters to navigate resistance and ambivalence: Experiential implications for group counselling. *Journal of Addictions and Offender Counseling, 31,* 108-126.

Haiman, S., Lambert, W. L., & Rodrigues, B. J. (2005). Mental health of adolescents. In E. Cara & A. MacRae (Eds.), *Psychosocial occupational therapy: A clinical practice* (2nd ed., pp. 298-325). Clifton Park, NY: Delmar Publishers.

Hall, J., & Hawley, L. (2004). Interactive process notes: An innovative tool in counseling groups. *Journal for Specialists in Group Work, 29,* 193-205.

Hering, K. (2013). *Writing to wake the soul: Opening the sacred conversation within.* New York, NY: Atria Books.

Hildsdon, J. (2004). After the session: Free writing in response. In G. Bolton, S. Howlett, C. Lago, & J. K. Wright (Eds.), *Writing cures: An introductory handbook of writing in counselling and therapy* (pp. 212-220). New York, NY: Brunner-Routledge.

Horowitz, S. (2008). Evidenced based health outcomes of expressive writing. *Alternative and Complementary Therapies, 14,* 194-198.

Jacobs, B. (2004). *Writing for emotional balance.* Oakland, CA: New Harbinger Publications.

Jordan, K. B., & L'Abate, L. (1995). Programmed writing and therapy with symbiotically enmeshed clients. *American Journal of Psychotherapy, 49,* 225-236.

Kielhofner, G. (2002). *Model of Human Occupation: Theory and application* (3rd ed.). Baltimore, MD: Lippincott Williams & Wilkins.

Kielhofner, G. (2008). *Model of Human Occupation: Theory and application* (4th ed.). Baltimore, MD: Lippincott Williams & Wilkins.

Kirtsoglu, E. (2010). Dreaming the self: A unified approach towards dreams, subjectivity and radical imagination. *History and Anthropology, 21,* 321-335.

Knoetz, J. (2013). Sandworlds, storymaking and letter writing: Therapeutic sandstory method. *South African Journal of Psychology, 43,* 459-469.

L'Abate, L. (1991). The use of writing in psychotherapy. *American Journal of Psychotherapy, 45,* 87-98.

L'Abate, L. (1999). Taking the bull by the horns: Beyond talk in psychological interventions. *Family Journal, 7,* 206-220.

Lee, H. S., & Cohn, L. D. (2009). Assessing coping strategies by analyzing expressive writing samples. *Stress and Health, 26,* 250-260.

Lent, J. (2009). Journaling enters the 21st century: The use of therapeutic blogs in counseling. *Journal of Creativity in Mental Health, 4,* 68-73.

Levitt, V. B. (2005). Anxiety disorders. In E. Cara & A. MacRae (Eds.), *Psychosocial occupational therapy: A clinical practice* (2nd ed., pp. 1193-1234). Clifton Park, NY: Delmar Publishers.

Linehan, M. M. (1993). *Skills training manual for treating borderline personality disorder.* New York, NY: The Guilford Press.

Mazza, N. (2003). *Poetry therapy: Theory and practice.* New York, NY: Brunner-Routledge.

McArdle, S., & Byrt, R. (2001). Fiction, poetry, and mental health: Expressive and therapeutic uses of literature. *Journal of Psychiatric Mental Health Nursing, 8,* 517-524.

Miller, W. R. (2014). Interactive journaling as a clinical tool. *Journal of Mental Health Counseling, 36,* 31-42.

Murray, S. (1997). The benefits of journaling: "Stories are medicine" "art is medicine." *Parks & Recreation, 32,* 68-75.

Paterson, B. L. (1995). Developing and maintaining reflection in clinical journals. *Nurse Education Today, 15,* 211-220.

Pennebaker, J. W. (1997). Writing about emotional experiences as a therapeutic process. *Psychological Science, 8,* 162-166.

Pennebaker, J. W., & Beall, S. (1986). Confronting a traumatic event: Toward an understanding of inhibition and disease. *Journal of Abnormal Psychology, 95,* 274-281.

Pennebaker, J. W., & Seagal, J. D. (1999). Forming a story: The health benefits of narrative. *Journal of Clinical Psychology, 55,* 1243-1254.

Poon, A., & Danoff-Burg, S. (2011). Mindfulness as a moderator in expressive writing. *Journal of Clinical Psychology, 67,* 881-895.

Prasko, J., Diveky, T., Mozny, P., & Sigmundova, Z. (2009). Therapeutic letters: Changing the emotional schemas using writing letters to significant caregivers. *Activitas Nervosa Superior Rediviva, 51,* 163-167.

Progoff, I. (1975). *At a journal workshop: The basic text and guide for using the intensive journal.* New York, NY: Dialogue House.

Progoff, I. (1992). *At a journal workshop: Writing to access the power of the unconscious and evoke creative ability.* New York, NY: Penguin Putnam Books.

Rainer, T. (1978). *The new diary: How to use a journal for self-guidance and expanded creativity.* Los Angeles, CA: Penguin Putnam.

Ramirez-Esparza, N., & Pennebaker, J. W. (2006). Do good stories produce good health? *Narrative Inquiry, 16,* 211-219.

Ritchie, M. A. (2003). Faculty and student dialogue through journal writing. *Journal for Specialists in Pediatric Nursing, 8,* 5-12.

Ruthman, J., Jackson, J., Cluskey, M., Flannigan, P., Folse, V. N., & Bunten, J. (2004). Using clinical journaling to capture critical thinking across the curriculum. *Nurse Education Perspectives, 25,* 120-123.

Samrajya, L. B. (2014). Reflective practice through journal writing and peer observation: A case study. *Turkish Online Journal of Distance Education, 15,* 189-204.

Schneider, M. F., & Stone, M. (1998). Processes and techniques of journal writing in Alderian therapy. *Journal of Individual Psychology, 54,* 511-531.

Senn, L. C. (2001). *The many faces of journaling: Topics and techniques for personal journal writing.* St. Louis, MO: Penn Central Press.

Smyth, J. M. (1998). Written emotional expression: Effect sizes, outcome types, and moderating variables. *Journal of Consulting Clinical Psychology, 66,* 174-184.

Spalding, E., & Wilson, A. (2002). Demystifying reflection: A study of pedagogical strategies that encourage reflective journal writing. *Teachers College Record, 104,* 1393-1421.

Srimavin, W., & Darasawang, P. (2004). Developing self-assessment through journal writing. Published Proceedings of the 2003 Independent Learning Conference. Retrieved from https://www.researchgate.net/publication/228609049_Developing_self-assessment_through_journal_writing

Stein, F., & Cutler, S. K. (2002). *Psychosocial occupational therapy: A holistic approach* (2nd ed.). Albany, NY: Delmar Publishers.

Steinberg, D. (2000). *Letters from the clinic: Letter writing in clinical practice for mental health professionals*. London, United Kingdom: Routledge.

Stockton, H., Joseph, S., & Hunt, N. (2014). Expressive writing and post-traumatic growth: An Internet based study. *Traumatology, 20,* 75-83.

Stone, M. (1998). Journaling with clients. *Journal of Individual Psychology, 54,* 535-545.

Thompson, K. (2004). Journal writing as a therapeutic tool. In G. Bolton, S. Howlett, C. Lagon, & J. Wright (Eds.), *Writing cures: An introductory handbook of writing in counseling and therapy* (pp. 72-84). New York, NY: Brunner-Routledge.

Ulrich, P. M., & Lutgendorf, S. K. (2002). Journaling about stressful events: Effects of cognitive processing and emotional expression. *Annals of Behavioral Medicine, 24,* 244-250.

Walker, S., & Kelly, M. (2011). The introduction of an early warning signs journal in an adolescent inpatient unit. *Journal of Psychiatric and Mental Health Nursing, 18,* 563-568.

Wright, J. (2002). Online counseling: Learning from writing therapy. *British Journal of Guidance Counseling, 30,* 285-298.

Wright, J. K. (2005). Writing therapy in brief workplace counselling. *Counselling and Psychotherapy Research, 5,* 111-119.

Wright, J., & Chung, M. C. (2001). Therapeutic writing: A review of the literature. *British Journal of Guidance Counseling, 29,* 277-291.

Creative Participation Assessment

Jane Ryan, MBA/CHM, LOTR, CLT;
Daleen Casteleijn, B OccTher, M OccTher, PhD;
and Wendy Sherwood, DipCOT, MSc, PhD

To achieve the greatest success, the occupational therapist must be capable of meeting each patient with
original responsibility, with reality, with initiative and in fact with himself/herself.
(du Toit, n.d.)

What is creativity? What does creativity have to do with occupational therapy? Are we treating only those skilled with visual/movement arts? Is the ballerina, interior designer, painter, or potter the only one who can receive occupational therapy services for physical disabilities, as well as cognitive disabilities and mental health issues? What about the average person? Creativity reaches far more areas of living than you can imagine and is not exclusive to the dancer, interior designer, painter, or sculptor. Creativity in everyday life is how each person exerts maximum effort in his or her daily life to successfully problem solve issues as they arise (Coffey, Lamport, & Hersch, 2015). Therefore, what is creative ability and why is occupational therapy such an important part of it? To answer these questions, this chapter will discuss the Vona du Toit Model of Creative Ability (VdTMoCA) and the Creative Participation Assessment (CPA).

History

Vona du Toit, a South African occupational therapist, believed that clients have the ability to behave with creativity, which influences the effect of their engagement in treatment, their ability to resolve their problems, and their ability to adjust to their specific disability (du Toit, 1962). The work of Buber, Rogers, and Piaget and the belief that the quality of participation in purposeful activities influences the meaning of human life led to the development of the theory of creative ability (Joubert, 2019), the beginnings

Hemphill, B. J., & Urish, C. K. (Eds.). *Assessments in*
Occupational Therapy Mental Health: An Integrative Approach,
Fourth Edition (pp. 117-136). © 2020 Taylor & Francis Group.

of which is evident in du Toit's (1962) dissertation *Initiative in Occupational Therapy*. Her untimely death in 1974 inspired her South African occupational therapy colleagues to debate, observe, and research her legacy to bring it to the rightful place in occupational therapy service delivery, encompassing the holistic occupational therapy philosophy held worldwide. The VdTMoCA is a model of occupational therapy in South Africa and has been used widely for more than 50 years. In addition to being widely used in South Africa, the model is used in the United Kingdom and Japan (Sherwood & Wilson, 2019; Walters, Sherwood, & Mason, 2014). Research has been conducted on aspects of the model, spearheaded by Casteleijn (2014), Casteleijn and Smit (2002), De Witt (2003), and Sherwood (2016). The VdTMoCA is focused on recovery and strengths and can be used with a variety of clients, from children diagnosed with neurological conditions or sensory problems to adults with learning disabilities/intellectual impairment (Sherwood, 2017), psychiatric diagnoses and/or physical disabilities such as acquired head injury and stroke, and older adults with dementia (Sherwood, 2021). It is applicable across any occupational therapy practice setting. Although widely utilized in other countries, occupational therapists trained in the United Kingdom and South Africa who are employed in the United States are working to educate occupational therapists in the United States on this occupation-based model.

The CPA was developed by Dain van der Reyden (van der Reyden, Casteleijn, Sherwood, & De Witt, 2019) for occupational therapists to clinically observe behaviors and identify the level of creative ability in an individual. Sound knowledge of the VdTMoCA is needed by the occupational therapy practitioner to merge information gained from interviews, collateral, and observing client behavior, particularly during activities and occupational performance tasks in a range of situations. Upon completion of this process, the practitioner refers to items and descriptors of ability across levels of creative ability to rate the client on the CPA. Careful analysis of the findings leads to establishing the client's level of creative ability (De Witt & Sherwood, 2019). The brevity of the descriptors on the CPA assumes that the user has sufficient understanding of the components and levels of creative ability, therefore the descriptors are cues only. Competent use of the CPA requires being fully conversant with the VdTMoCA, especially the components, levels, and phases of creative ability (De Witt & Sherwood, 2019).

Upon completion of the CPA, occupational therapists can utilize their clinical reasoning abilities to determine how the components of creative ability are impacting the client's performance to facilitate effective occupational therapy intervention (De Witt & Sherwood, 2019).

Concepts/Constructs

Vona du Toit (2015) viewed creative ability in two parts. First, in the context of the person ("man") with uniqueness—an indivisible psyche, soma, and spirit—as being an indivisible part of the world and having the need for purposeful activity, which includes working and contributing to the world through interaction, being an integral part of humanity, and having a need for environmental stimulation. Developed on a continuum of identification, it is the development of individual needs within a widening environment that culminates into responsibility to one's fellow man. Each person must have the desire for participation in purposeful activity or occupation, and this desire leads to recovery, growth, and development in physical, mental, and psychosocial needs (du Toit, 1974). Decisions must originate from the client's own self (I) to enhance the relationship with his or her world—one's fellow man (Thou), materials and objects (It) as per the work of Buber. This occurs through acting on the world (activity participation), through which one defines and redefines oneself during life. The individual must assume responsibility for one's own acts, which ultimately determine one's becoming (du Toit, 1962). The ultimate goal is to have the client reach a relationship with people/objects/situations. Where oneness/identification absorbs with moment/person/activity. This is also called the *You-Me (I-Thou) moment* (Buber, 1971).

Second, du Toit (2015) viewed creative ability in the context of occupational therapy. Occupational therapists use purposeful activity as a treatment medium to impact illness and disability. Therefore, human occupation can and will influence well-being and health in all individuals with physical and psychiatric disabilities. The spiritual component of human occupation has to be acknowledged and is the catalyst to optimum holistic functioning in the human (du Toit, 1962, 1974). Therefore, occupational therapy treatment is focused on increasing total participation in life. This inspires total participation of the client receiving occupational therapy services (du Toit, 1974). Thus, treatment focus is graded from attention to occupational performance such as basic self-care activities to full participation in life, including preparedness in participation in work/productive activities. As one of the four treatment principles, the occupational therapist utilizes therapeutic use of self to engage with the client with a significant sense of vitality, energy, sensitivity, responsiveness, and initiative. Therapeutic use of self is essential because the occupational therapist must demonstrate skill and knowledge in all interventions and is used with the other treatment principles to grade and facilitate purposeful activity by adapting variables such as the environment, activity, cognitive components, physical movement, and handling of the person to encourage the maximum purposeful participation of the client. The occupational therapy treatment plan must be unique to each client and encompasses the following components:

- Application technique within the selected activity to stimulate volition, motivation, and active participation
- Activity must be purposeful and meaningful
- Client "must do with" not be "done to"

Therefore, the VdTMoCA is seen as inseparable from occupational service delivery as the model embraces the fundamental philosophy of occupational therapy (du Toit, 2015).

Creative Ability Defined

Creative ability is defined as "the manifestation of one's motivation in action resulting in a tangible or intangible product, which is directed by volition—the will to be and to direct one's own life" (van der Reyden & Sherwood, 2019, p. 64). Creative ability develops within the context of the client's creative capacity—the maximal creative potential a client has that will most likely develop under optimal circumstances. This varies from client to client and is influenced by factors such as intelligence, personality, mental health, environmental opportunities, and physical/emotional security. An assumption of the VdTMoCA is that every individual has potential for growth, hence therapists aim to enable fulfilment of creative potential.

Maximum effort is needed for growth (van der Reyden & Sherwood, 2019). The client must exert effort at the boundaries of his or her own creative ability in order to master challenges and create something new, thus extending his or her creative ability. Effort

Figure 8-1. Concepts of creative ability.

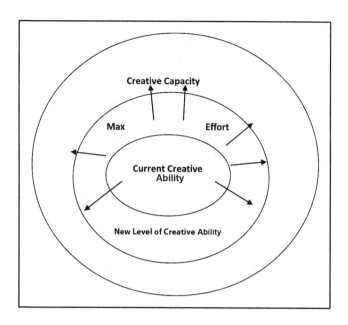

is central to what are termed the growth factors, that is, (1) the creative response (preparedness to exert effort), (2) creative participation (activity participation with effort), and (3) the creative act (tangible and/or intangible products as the result of (1) and (2). *Creative response* is defined as the positive attitude/response the client displays toward any opportunity.

Creative response precedes creative participation. This reflects preparedness to use all resources (effort) to participate, anticipate pleasure, and gain or acknowledge the presence of anxiety regarding individual capabilities and outcomes (du Toit, 1970). *Creative participation* is "active engagement in activity with effort, through which there is the potential to bring about something new in one's self and/or the external world" (van der Reyden & Sherwood, 2019, p. 70). The client needs to take action rather than be a passive participant in all areas of occupation and needs to engage in daily areas of occupation in such a way that abilities and resources are challenged. A *creative act* is defined as the final result of creative response and creative participation, in terms of producing an end product, tangible or intangible, that has meaning and purpose to the client (du Toit, 1970).

Creative ability is depicted in Figure 8-1. The largest circle represents the whole creative capacity of each individual. The smallest circle depicts the client's current creative ability. The goal of this model is to enable the client's exertion of maximum effort to expand his or her creative capacity beyond the current boundaries (middle circle). Occupational therapy intervention is well suited to assist the client in expanding his or her creative ability. Once the occupational therapist has identified the client's level of creative ability, interventions can be chosen and the client can be engaged in intervention to facilitate growth in creative ability, or if more relevant, maintain and/or prevent decline in creative ability.

A fundamental concept of creative ability is volition. Both the occupational therapist and the client need to work together to achieve the occupational growth needed to facilitate positive changes in the individual. Volition is "the act of being willing to resolve something by making a decision or choice; the power or faculty of willing; will power" (van der Reyden & Sherwood, 2019, p. 68). Hence, volition has two components that drive growth: choice and will (du Toit, 1970), translating the choice or intention to act into action (action is the expression of volition and motivation; van der Reyden & Sherwood, 2019). Hence, motivation influences volition and action—"motivation is the want, need or desire to do something" and volition "is the will to be and to direct one's own life, evident in directedness and commitment to action" (van der Reyden & Sherwood, 2019, p. 69). Motivation within the client is not static and has different foci at different stages of occupational performance development, decline, or recovery. Vona du Toit's identification of the relation between motivation, volition, and action lead to the establishment of the levels of creative ability. There are nine different and sequential levels of creative ability, each possessing specific qualities, which during the course of development are directed at developing life tasks for each individual. Each level describes changes in the quality of the person's ability to form relational contact with others, situations, materials, and objects in the environment and characteristics of occupational behavior, engagement in occupations and an individual's ability to live, work, and play within the community. The establishment of the levels were informed by Vona du Toit's observations of children diagnosed with cerebral palsy and autism and adults with mental health disorders and spinal cord injuries (du Toit, 2015). These observations led to the development of levels of creative ability that described activity participation in a sequential order.

The levels of creative ability are shown in Table 8-1.

The occupational therapy practitioner's role is to identify the volition and motivation of each client and determine how to establish treatment interventions to elicit appropriate action to facilitate occupational engagement of the client.

Therapist-Client Interaction Within the Vona du Toit Model of Creative Ability

Within each of the nine levels of creative ability, there are three phases. The client move through these phases dependent upon the occupational performance behaviors demonstrated at each phase within the level. The first phase is defined as the *therapist-directed phase*, because the occupational therapist directs most of the participation. The occupational therapist is instrumental in controlling the environment and stimuli as much as possible, which creates an environment for the client to experience success during occupational performance within the activity. The occupational therapist must work to address and lessen anxiety to ensure success by providing the "just-right" challenge (Figure 8-2).

The second phase is the *patient-directed phase* (client/service user-directed). Within this phase, the client directs participation, demonstrates increased anxiety control, and performs consistently within identified occupational roles according to the level. The client experiences a sense of accomplishment (Figure 8-3).

The third phase is the *transitional phase*. The client shows characteristics of the current level in addition to characteristics of the level above. The occupational therapist is challenged to stimulate the client to accept more challenges in occupational performance in his or her daily life, while assisting to keep anxiety levels at the "just-right" level to spark participation in new situations successfully at the next higher level of creative ability (Figure 8-4).

Table 8-1

Levels of Creative Ability: Volition and Action Ability

Level	Volition	Action
9	Competitive contribution	Society-centered action
8	Contribution	Situation-centered action
7	Competitive participation	Competitive-centered action
6	Active participation	Norm transcendence, individualistic and inventive action
5	Imitative participation	Imitative norm-compliant action
4	Passive participation	Norm awareness, experimental action
3	Self-presentation	Constructive explorative action
2	Self-differentiation	Destructive action
		Incidental constructive action
1	Tone	Purposeless and unplanned action

Adapted from van der Reyden et al., 2019.

Figure 8-2. Diagram of the therapist-directed phase within any level of creative ability.

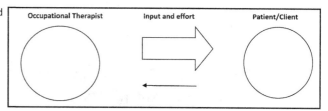

Figure 8-3. Diagram of the client-directed phase within any level of creative ability.

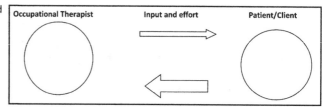

The characteristics of each phase will be discussed during the description of the characteristics of each level of creative ability. Du Toit (1970) stated that the development of creative ability happens within the boundaries of a person's creative potential, which develops under maximum circumstances.

The CPA was developed by Dain van der Reyden, a South African occupational therapist (De Witt & Sherwood, 2019; van der Reyden, 1998). The CPA is not an assessment per se; rather it is a method for recording and analyzing client behavior considering the level of creative ability demonstrated.

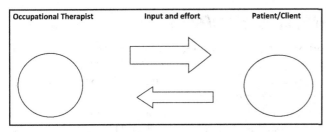

Occupational Therapist	Input and effort	Patient/Client

Figure 8-4. Diagram of the transition phase within any level of creative ability.

A full occupational therapy evaluation of a client's creative participation (addressing all areas of occupation; reviewing the client's past medical and occupational history and physical and mental disabilities; interviewing and performing observations within active occupational performance tasks including social situations) should be completed to establish the person's level of creative ability. The evaluation process assists the occupational therapist in combining all knowledge, clinical reasoning, and clinical observations of the client's creative ability (De Witt & Sherwood, 2019). Initially, practitioners gain a sense of the individual's level of creative ability from these data, which leads to gaining greater clarity through observation of an individual's creative participation in unfamiliar activities. These are particularly useful for assessing each component of creative ability, as unfamiliar activities place greater demand on executive functioning, initiative, emotional control, and effort—in fact all of the components, which can enable a person's level of creative ability to become more evident than when doing familiar activities (De Witt & Sherwood, 2019). In choosing an activity that is unfamiliar to the client, it is graded so that it is doable for the person on the assumed level of creative ability, but with a challenge that will require exertion of effort considering the following: objects and their properties, space demands, social demands, sequencing and timing, required actions and performance skills, required body functions and structures. The occupational therapy practitioner must be extremely familiar with the activity due to the potential need to grade the activity up or down. Usually, an activity that takes 45 minutes to complete is adequate, but the time is likely to be reduced for clients on the levels of Tone and Self-Differentiation. When considering activity choice, the physical and social environment, as well as cultural, personal, temporal, and virtual contexts, must be considered (American Occupational Therapy Association, 2020).

Clinical reasoning and skilled observations are essential for the occupational therapy practitioner. The occupational therapist must observe the client's attitude and his or her ability to relate to materials, objects, people, and situations within the environment, both internally and externally. Further, the occupational therapist should observe the client's ability to initiate, and sustain effort within the chosen activity, as well as his or her ability to continue the same level of performance if the activity is repetitive in nature (De Witt, 2014). The occupational therapist observes the client's quality of performance and examines the standards the client establishes relative to execution, engagement, and completion of the activity. The occupational therapist considers the level of supervision required for the activity, the amount of environmental structure necessary for the client's successful participation, and the ability to handle the tools/materials required by the task, as well as the ability to meet socially acceptable norms. The occupational therapist observes the client's level of anxiety and ability to cope with anxious feelings when presented with a new activity, as well as the client's response to active participation. The client's decision making and problem solving with the task are also observed.

Psychometric Properties

The CPA has been extensively studied by Casteleijn and Smit (2002) and Casteleijn (2014) and has been determined to be a reliable and valid instrument. The Volitional Questionnaire was utilized to study the criterion validity, while construct validity and internal consistency of the CPA were established on a population of persons with schizophrenia (Casteleijn & Smit, 2002). The results indicated the CPA was a valid and reliable assessment of motivation in clients diagnosed with schizophrenia (Casteleijn & Smit, 2002). The assessment was studied as a measure to confirm the levels of creative ability as described by the VdTMoCA through the use of Rasch analysis. Results indicated the levels present in the CPA measured increasing amounts of the construct of creative ability (Casteleijn, 2014). When analyzed with the Functional Levels Outcome Measure (FLOM) and the Activity Participation Outcome Measure (APOM), the APOM was the only instrument that integrated the phases within the model (i.e., therapist directed, patient directed, transitional) within the scoring of the assessment. The research indicates that the levels of creative ability were accurate, valid, and resemble measurement that is linear (Casteleijn, 2014). The limitation presented within the study was that each of these instruments (i.e., CPA, FLOM, APOM) utilized differing levels of creative ability for scoring. Additionally, each measurement utilized different terminology. This could be concerning, but Casteleijn (2014) posits that differing terminology may be present due to different interpretations of the assumptions of the VdTMoCA. A benefit of this flexibility of interpretation of the model did not appear to negatively impact scoring as it was reported to be accurate across measures (Casteleijn, 2014).

Assessment Administration

The CPA (van der Reyden et al., 2019) addresses six of the nine levels of creative ability as described by Casteleijn and Holsten (2019) in considering the following observed behaviors as the 12 items to rate on the form:

1. Action
2. Volition
3. Make relational contact with tools/objects
4. Materials
5. People and situations
6. Task concept and concept formation
7. Product
8. Assistance/supervision required
9. Behavior
10. Norm awareness
11. Anxiety and emotional responses
12. Initiative and effort (De Witt & Sherwood, 2019)

The occupational therapist gains as much information as possible on the individual's creative ability for familiar and unfamiliar activities including in social situations, across four occupational performance areas (Personal Management, Social Ability, Work Ability, Constructive Use of Free Time) and records the client's behaviors and responses on the one-page assessment form, marking an X or highlighting each box within the table to select the most accurate description of each component of creative ability, as evidenced in action for the majority of the time.

The occupational therapist adds the number of Xs placed in each column at the bottom. The highest number indicates the overall level of creative ability the client is functioning at. For example, if the occupational therapist observes the client to demonstrate 10 behaviors within the Self-Differentiation column and two behaviors in the Self-Presentation column, the client would be identified to be functioning at the Self-Differentiation level. Any Xs in the level above the overall level such as in Self-Presentation in the aforementioned example, these indicate strengths the occupational therapist can utilize within treatment to work to develop areas that are lower and require intervention.

If there are components identified with Xs in the level below the overall level, these inform intervention to improve client engagement in occupation and his or her creative ability. The CPA (van der Reyden et al., 2019) is presented in Table 8-2 and Appendix B.

Creative Participation Assessment

To accompany the CPA, the occupational therapist should document the tasks/situations/activities that were used for assessment purposes and that the CPA scorings are informed by. It is advised that occupational therapists complete the CPA; however, occupational therapy assistants and other professionals can be sought out by the occupational therapist to provide information regarding the client's creative ability (De Witt & Sherwood, 2019). The occupational therapist must be well versed in the VdTMoCA and the CPA in order to use the CPA competently. Occupational therapists are directed to the VdTMoCA Foundation (UK) for information on resources and training opportunities regarding the model and the assessment.

Occupational Therapy Practice Framework and Creative Participation Assessment

The CPA relates directly to numerous areas of the *Occupational Therapy Practice Framework: Domain and Process, Fourth Edition* (AOTA, 2020). All areas of occupation can be addressed when conducting the CPA, with the exception of rest and sleep, based upon the choice of activities and situations the occupational therapist utilizes. Through engagement in a task/activity necessary to complete the CPA, the occupational therapist can observe performance skills such as motor, process, and social interaction skills. All contexts and environments are of significant concern to the occupational therapist in the choice of activities, tasks and situations utilized to complete the CPA. The *Framework* (AOTA, 2020) addresses occupation and activity demands, and these are closely aligned with the CPA, specifically focusing on objects and their properties, social demands, required actions and performance skills, relevance and importance to the client, sequence and timing, and space demands (AOTA, 2020).

Table 8-2

Creative Participation Assessment

Levels of Creative Ability

	Tone	Self-Differentiation	Self-Presentation	Passive Participation	Imitative Participation	Active Participation
Action	Undirected and unplanned; purposeless	Incidentally constructive or destructive (1- to 2-step task)	Constructive explorative (3- to 4-step task)	Fairly product centered; norm awareness experimental (5- to 7-step task)	Product centered; follows the norm (7- to 10-step task)	With originality; transcends norm/expectations
Volition	Egocentric; to maintain existence	Egocentric; to differentiate self from others	Seems willing to try to present self; unsure	Robust; directed to attainment of skill	Directed to produce a good product; acceptable behavior	Directed to improvement of product, procedures, or systems
Handle Tools and Materials	Not evident; unaware	Only simple everyday tools (e.g., spoon); poor handling	Basic tools for activity participation; poor handling	Appropriate; limited skill	Appropriate, good use and care	With initiative, skill evident
Relate to People	No awareness	Fleeting awareness	Selective identification; responds and tries to communicate, superficial interpersonal relations	Communicates, initiates contact, conversation; spectator role	Communicates/interacts; open to others' views; may be assertive	Close interpersonal relations; intimacy evident; can assist others

(continued)

Table 8-2 (continued)

Creative Participation Assessment

Levels of Creative Ability

	Tone	Self-Differentiation	Self-Presentation	Passive Participation	Imitative Participation	Active Participation
Handle Situations	No awareness of different situations	No or fleeting awareness; no ability shown to cope; inappropriate	Partial awareness, stereotypical handling; makes effort, but unsure or timid	Follower/spectator; manages fairly in a variety of situations; participates in passive way	Comprehends and manages variety of situations; appropriate behavior.	Can interpret, evaluate, adapt, and adjust, according to need or plan
Task Concept	No task concept; basic concepts	No task concept; basic and elementary concepts	Partial task concept (developing); compound concepts	Full task concept; extended compound concepts (abstract element)	Consolidated task concept; integrated abstract concepts	Abstract reasoning; organization, planning, individualization
Product	None	No product	Simple, familiar activities or part thereof; process oriented; poor quality product	Product fair quality; aware of expectations/norms; needs direction	Product good quality; norms internalized; with norm compliance; meets expectations	Open labor market quality; can adapt, modify, evaluate
Assistance/ Supervision Needed	Total assistance including physical assistance; supervision, assistance, needs (24-hour) nursing care constant supervision	Physical assistance and constant supervision; requires full-time care	Constant supervision needed for task completion	Regular supervision	Guidance needed; regular supervision for new activities and tasks; occasional supervision for known activities	Occasional guidance needed in training for new skills; takes full responsibility and helps to supervise others

(continued)

Table 8-2 (continued)

Creative Participation Assessment

Levels of Creative Ability

	Tone	Self-Differentiation	Self-Presentation	Passive Participation	Imitative Participation	Active Participation
Behavior	Haphazard, disorientation and bizarre behavior	Little or inappropriate reaction, disorientation and bizarre behavior	At times inappropriate or strange behavior; hesitant, unsure but willing to try out	Follower, participates passively, occasionally inappropriate or hesitant behavior	Socially acceptable behavior; symptoms generally controlled	Socially acceptable behavior; shows originality; may decide to act contrary to norm with appropriate and original behavior
Norm Awareness	None noted	None noted	Starts to be aware of norms for appearance and behavior, but not for task or product norms	Norm awareness for appearance, behavior, task, and product	Norm compliance; does as expected, meets required standard for product, procedure, and social behavior	Norm transcendence (does better or more, adapts); transcend norms in activities as well as situations
Emotional Responses and Anxiety	Limited responses; positive/negative	Limited, uncontrolled basic emotions displayed (positive or negative); shows fleeting comfort and discomfort, satisfaction or dissatisfaction	Broader range of emotions, intensity, frequency, and duration not always appropriate; low self-esteem and anxiety present	Refined nuances of emotions evident; prone to immobilizing effects of anxiety; low self-esteem; intensity, frequency, and duration better controlled in known situations	Full range of emotions, mostly controlled and makes effort to control emotions; maybe immobilized by anxiety	Shows compassion, picks up subtle differences in emotions; ↑ self-awareness; anxiety used positively

(continued)

Table 8-2 (continued)

Creative Participation Assessment

Levels of Creative Ability

	Tone	Self-Differentiation	Self-Presentation	Passive Participation	Imitative Participation	Active Participation
Initiative and Effort	None noted	No initiative; fleeting, minimal; effort not sustained	Initiative usually inappropriate; effort inconsistent, not sustained; low frustration tolerance	Hesitant to use initiative and put own ideas forward; courage to exert effort but needs guidance or assistance when problems are encountered	Initiative seldom used, prefer to follow the norm; sustained effort in known task, able to handle occasional failures	Initiative is original and frequently used; exert maximum effort over extended period of time
Total per Level						

Level of creative ability:

Phase within level:	Therapist directed
	Patient directed
	Transitional

Reprinted with permission from van der Reyden, D. (2018). *Creative participation assessment*. Unpublished assessment.

Case Study

Rebekah, a divorced 56-year-old woman who is estranged from her family of origin, was referred for home health occupational therapy services. Two adult children were aware of their mother's health conditions but were disinterested in a relationship with her. The medical record provided a social history that was conducted by the social worker. This reported the client's self-esteem was quite low and her behavior was child-like in nature. The client sustained a cerebrovascular accident secondary to a history of cocaine use and alcohol abuse for the past 10 years. Upon review of her medical record, the occupational therapist noted the client presented with a flaccid right upper extremity due to the cerebrovascular accident, was right-hand dominant prior to the cerebrovascular accident, and had experienced seizures that were controlled with prescribed medication. The client lived in a one-bedroom apartment in an independent living apartment complex.

When the occupational therapist arrived for the initial visit with the client, she observed dirty laundry throughout the apartment and a strong smell of urine. Initially, Rebekah stated she did not need occupational therapy services, as she had "someone" to assist her in completing self-care and home maintenance tasks. Upon further discussion, Rebekah identified that possibly she could benefit from "some" services. As such, the client and the occupational therapist identified the need to improve the client's skills in bathing, dressing, toileting, and simple grooming. During the initial assessment, the client reported she often drinks alcohol in the evening, sometimes to the point of intoxication, and then would experience difficulty getting to the toilet to void. As a result, the client would leak urine onto the bedroom carpet and bathroom floor before reaching the toilet. This behavior placed the client at greater risk of falling. The occupational therapist inquired about falls, and initially the client denied falling; however, the client later admitted to numerous falls, which most often occurred during the night as a result of slipping on her own urine. Initially, the client was resistant to using a bedside commode; however, after significant discussion about the negative consequences that could occur as a result of continued falls, the client agreed to obtain and use a bedside commode. Further, dignity issues were discussed relative to safety and toileting. The client shared that she had been in recovery in the past but had returned to alcohol use due to the limitations she was experiencing functionally, as well as frustration of not being able to leave her home and feeling socially isolated. The occupational therapist discussed the importance of using medical equipment to ensure safety and listened to the client's concerns relative to increasing substance use and isolation. The client reported she was embarrassed to have others to her home and to go out in public due to her inability to effectively control her bladder, as well as to clean herself to not smell of urine.

A tub transfer bench was used during bathing, and the client was independent in the use of this piece of medical equipment. However, during bathing the client demonstrated difficulty manipulating the soap and reaching her back to wash due to the flaccid right upper extremity. The occupational therapist provided a long-handled sponge and a bath glove that enabled the client to complete bathing independently. The client reported to the occupational therapist at a later time feeling an increased sense of accomplishment and motivation to engage in self-care tasks due to increasing independence in the completion of these tasks. Rebekah was independent in grooming with the use of compensatory hand grip to open and close toothpaste, shampoo and conditioner bottles, and lotion.

A quad cane was used for safe ambulation, and a friend of the client attached a small basket to it to hold her cell phone, keys, and wallet. Rebekah needed maximum assistance in cleaning, mopping the bathroom and kitchen floors, and making her bed. The client was independent in folding her clothes but relied on someone else to complete the task of washing and drying her laundry. Meals consisted of mostly TV dinners, crackers/cheese, and potato chips/dip. The client was independent in the use of the microwave. The client had an electric can opener that she was independent in using. In the evening, she would frequently begin drinking and at times would not eat an evening meal. Sometimes, the client would go without eating breakfast or lunch and just drink beer in the evening to the point of intoxication. Although prior to her stroke she enjoyed an active social life, due to her functional limitations she began to isolate herself. She had a boyfriend with whom she was intimate; however, she recently experienced fewer visits from him. Rebekah's CPA identified her at the self-presentation level, with some areas emerging into the passive participation level with norm awareness action.

Occupational therapy intervention was used to improve her level of creative ability and to get the client to be a major part of the goal setting for each visit; a total of 30 visits that were 1 hour in length were completed over two certification periods. Initially, the activities of daily living tasks of bathing and toileting were addressed. The client was educated on the safe use of the bedside commode for nighttime use and trained on its emptying and cleaning; in addition, pelvic rotator cuff exercises were provided to improve bladder and bowel functioning.

The client was motivated to address being able to make her bed using a one-handed technique, especially managing the fitted sheet. The occupational therapist demonstrated the technique to her, from folding the sheets to applying the sheets onto the bed. Bed making and manipulation of the sheets were addressed over several sessions for the client to demonstrate competence. The occupational therapist worked with Rebekah to learn how to use a foam cleaner on her mattress, couch, chair, and carpet using a long-handled scrub brush. Once the cleaner was dry, the client was instructed on how to use the vacuum cleaner and the appropriate attachments to ensure all surfaces were clean.

Mopping the kitchen and bathroom floors was a task the client was encouraged to problem solve on how to safely complete. Previously when the client leaked urine, she would try to clean it at the time with a rag or bath towel, and as a result had sustained several falls. After addressing the safety concerns and when the bathroom and kitchen floors should be cleaned, the client chose the bathroom and kitchen sink rather than a mop bucket as the tile floors were confined to about 10 square feet in each room. Rebekah was able to squeeze the mop using her left hand, pressing the mop head against the sink to be wet/damp enough to clean the floors, and a second dry mop was used to dry the floors to prevent slipping.

At the end on the intervention period, the client had improved from Self-Presentation with explorative constructive action to the Passive Participation level with norm awareness experimental action, patient-directed phase. Because of her increased independence in self-care at home, the client invited friends she had met in recovery to her home and began working to not drink alcohol to cope with negative feelings. After obtaining a sponsor, she could attend an Alcoholics Anonymous meeting. The client reported that she knew alcohol was a detriment to her health and had discontinued alcohol use. Rebekah began attending a Bible study group weekly with individuals who resided in her apartment complex. As she was no longer embarrassed to have individuals enter her home, she invited neighbors over and everyone would bring something to share for dinner. This social activity was occurring at least once per month.

Use of the Vona du Toit Model of Creative Ability in Intervention

Following the aims and treatment principles for each level of creative ability (van der Reyden et al., 2019), treatment is always directed at what the person can do, and with activity participation that has a satisfying process and end products. Presenting the client with activities from all areas of occupational performance needs to be selected and graded according to each client's motivation and needs as per his or her level of creative ability in order to make each treatment session count (van der Reyden et al., 2019). Some of the most important tools the occupational therapist has are clinical reasoning, observation, and adaptability of lessening or upgrading the demands of the activity used during treatment.

The occupational therapist must be familiar with the nuances of the activity presented to the client. This ensures that a just-right challenge is provided and appropriate adjustments are made during active occupational performance. This enables the client to experience success and improve motivation to return and continue using occupational skills acquired during intervention.

The treatment planning worksheet can be utilized to assist the occupational therapist in analyzing occupational performance tasks and planning interventions. This sample worksheet is completed based on Rebekah's case study (Table 8-3). This worksheet assists the occupational therapist to accurately document the treatment session and progress achieved within the session.

Summary

Casteleijn (2014) stated that, although more research is needed with assessments of creative ability, the levels is a valid measure of the amount of creative ability in a person. However, all occupational therapy practitioners who apply the VdTMoCA should have completed training in all aspects of the model. The VdTMoCA provides promise to the profession of occupational therapy and demonstrates specific distinct value to the clients who receive occupational therapy services throughout the world (Birkhead, 2021; Carpenter et al., 2021; Jeffries, 2021; Murphy, 2021). An occupational therapist, Vona du Toit (2015) developed the model; another occupational therapist, Dain van der Reyden (van der Reyden et al., 2019), developed the CPA. Gillen (2013, as cited in Padilla & Griffiths, 2017) suggested that occupational therapy practitioners need to utilize occupation and performance-based assessments and stop using non–occupation-based assessments. The VdTMoCA and the CPA meet Gillen's directive. Occupational therapists and students are encouraged to engage in research focused upon the VdTMoCA and the CPA. Additional assessment research and training opportunities on the APOM grounded in the VdTMoCA (Casteleijn, 2017) exist. The occupational therapy practitioner must have thorough knowledge of the VdTMoCA before the using the CPA or APOM. The VdTMoCA and the CPA support the profession of occupational therapy through addressing all areas of domain and practice within the profession.

Table 8-3

Sample Treatment Planning Worksheet

Client: Rebekah   Level of creative participation: Self-Presentation
Date: August 15, 2019   Activity: Mopping the kitchen and bathroom floors

Occupational Performance Areas	Description of Level	Planning Activity	Outcomes
Action	5- to 7-step task, preparing water, mop.	Available tools are presented to client: mops, cleaning solution. Task is 5 to 7 steps.	Client prepared for session. Tools were ready for session, discussed technique and problem solved for safe completion of task.
Volition	Client motivated to engage in task to improve living environment.	Client prepared with all tools.	Client was excited to be able to clean her environment and showed willingness to engage in the activity.
Tools/materials	Client followed verbal cues on holding mop with left hand and technique to ring mop one-handed.	Client obtained cleaning solution, 2 mops prior to session.	Client was familiar with mop but not the bucket, her habit was to rinse the mop in the kitchen sink.
Relating to people	Client followed verbal instructions provided by occupational therapist very well.	Occupational therapist is competent in compensatory technique to be utilized with client; ready to demonstrate when needed/provide verbal cues.	Client related easily to the occupational therapist.
Situational handling skills	Client manages variety of problems within the environment and participates in the situation as a follower.	Demonstration, verbal cues on technique and problems that could arise within the situation.	Client follows and masters simple techniques to facilitate engagement in mopping task with supervision.
Task concept/sequence	Manages abstract and concrete concepts well considering potential problems that could arise within the situation.	Number of verbal cues after initial instruction to be kept at a minimum. Encourage client to problem solve.	After instructions from therapist, client initiated the task independently, executed the steps with good quality, and decided independently when she was done with the mopping. She needed prompting from the therapist to complete the task (rinsing the mop and restore it). She showed task satisfaction at the end of the activity.

(continued)

Table 8-3 (continued)

Sample Treatment Planning Worksheet

Occupational Performance Areas	Description of Level	Planning Activity	Outcomes
Product—tangible/ intangible	Client is aware of expectations of the end product to be achieved (floors mopped— tangible, satisfaction at task completed— intangible).	Clear instructions provided, allow client to fail and problem solve small, safe, issues.	Mopping was done well. She used her own strategy to wring mop with one, nondominant hand, independently.
Assistance/ supervision required	Regular supervision.	Independent mastery of one-handed technique observed at end of session.	Needed prompting to end activity (rinsing and restoring tools).
Behaviors expected/ exhibited	Follower. Participated passively, at times, bizarre behaviors can be demonstrated.	Keep client focused on task and praise as needed.	No bizarre behaviors. Client expressed satisfaction and pride in her task she completed.
Norm awareness	Client is aware of the norms of the task and expectations.	Clear instructions on expectations provided during task instruction the client is to complete.	Client exhibited good understanding of the norms of mopping (habituated task) but not restoring tools afterward.
Anxiety and emotional responses	Anxiety can be poorly controlled.	Occupational therapist to be well prepared on all problems that might arise with this task.	Client experienced a sense of satisfaction with the end product (clean floor) of the task well done. No anxiety as therapist guided her through the task.
Initiative and effort	Effort made. More correct actions.	Willing to put more effort into task.	Signs of initiative in using non-dominant hand to assist in wringing the mop.
Specialized techniques needed	One-handed technique to mop. Use side of sink to squeeze out mop head.	Demonstrate parts of technique to client to initiate problem solving.	Client mastered technique well.
Environmental adjustments/ adaptation	Use of sink.	None.	Client chose to use sink not a bucket.

Acknowledgments

Jane Ryan wishes to acknowledge the following individuals: Ms. Dain van der Reyden for her insight in developing the CPA, Ms. Patricia De Witt for her research and contributions to the VdTMoCA, Dr. Daleen Casteleijn for her research on the CPA and outcome measurement, Dr. Wendy Sherwood for her research on effort as a component of creative ability, supporting practitioners through supervision and provision of training, and the VdTMoCA Foundation UK for encouraging research. Lastly, Ms. Ryan expresses significant and sincere gratitude to Dr. Christine Urish for her encouragement, assistance, and guidance in the writing and editing of the chapter.

References

American Occupational Therapy Association. (2020). Occupational therapy practice framework: Domain and process (4th ed.). *American Journal of Occupational Therapy, 74*(Suppl. 2).

Birkhead, S. (2021). Making sense of dementia—A multi-sensory approach based on the first four levels of the Vona du Toit Model of Creative Ability. In W. Sherwood (Ed.), *Perspectives on the Vona du Toit Model of Creative Ability: Practice, theory and philosophy.* Watford, England: International Creative Ability Network.

Buber, M. (1971). *Between man and man.* London, United Kingdom: Routledge.

Carpenter, C., Jordan, S., Lawrence, J., London, A., Reilly, J., Southon, M., & Summers, L. (2021). Application of the VdTMoCA to occupational therapy within a High Secure Mental Health Hospital. In W. Sherwood (Ed.), *Perspectives on the Vona du Toit Model of Creative Ability: Practice, theory and philosophy.* Watford, England: International Creative Ability Network.

Casteleijn, D. (2014). Using measurement principles to confirm the levels of creative ability as described in the Vona du Toit Model of Creative Ability. *South African Journal of Occupational Therapy, 44,* 14-19.

Casteleijn, D. (2017). *Activity Participation Outcomes Measure training manual.* Unpublished document.

Casteleijn, D., & Holsten, E. (2019). Creative ability – its emergence and manifestation. In D. Van der Reyden, D. Casteleijn, W. Sherwood, & P. De Witt. (Eds.). *The Vona du Toit Model of Creative Ability: Origins, constructs, principles and application in occupational therapy* (pp. 106-146). Vona & Marie du Toit Foundation.

Casteleijn, D., & Smit, C. (2002). The psychometric properties of the Creative Participation Assessment. *South African Journal of Occupational Therapy, 32,* 6-11.

Coffey, M. S., Lamport, N. K., & Hersch, G. I. (2015). *Creative engagement in occupation: Building professional skills.* Thorofare, NJ: SLACK Incorporated.

De Witt, P. A. (2003). Investigation into the criteria and behaviours used to assess task concept. *South African Journal of Occupational Therapy, 33*(1).

De Witt, P., & Sherwood, W. (2019). Assessment of creative ability. In D. van der Reyden, D. Casteleijn, W. Sherwood, & P. De Witt (Eds.), *The Vona du Toit Model of Creative Ability: Origins, constructs, principles and application in occupational therapy* (pp. 148-199). Pretoria, South Africa: Vona & Marie du Toit Foundation.

du Toit, V. (1962). Initiative in occupational therapy. In V. du Toit (Ed.), *Patient volition and action in occupational therapy* (5th ed.). Pretoria, South Africa: Vona and Marie du Toit Foundation.

du Toit, V. (1970). Creative ability. In V. du Toit (Ed.), *Patient volition and action in occupational therapy* (5th ed.). Pretoria, South Africa: Vona and Marie du Toit Foundation.

du Toit, V. (1974). The background theory related to creative ability which leads to work capacity within the context of occupational therapy for the cerebral palsied. In V. du Toit (Ed.), *Patient volition and action in occupational therapy* (5th ed.). Pretoria, South Africa: Vona and Marie du Toit Foundation.

du Toit, V. (2015). *Patient volition and action in occupational therapy* (5th ed.). Pretoria, South Africa: Vona and Marie du Toit Foundation.

Jeffries, L. (2021). Seclusion: The end of the road for occupational therapy or a new route with the Vona du Toit Model of Creative Ability? In W. Sherwood (Ed.), *Perspectives on the Vona du Toit Model of Creative Ability: Practice, theory and philosophy.* Watford, England: International Creative Ability Network.

Joubert, R. (2019). Theoretical paradigms and influences underpinning the development of the Vona du Toit Model of Creative Ability. In D. van der Reyden, D. Casteleijn, W. Sherwood, & P. De Witt (Eds.), *The Vona du Toit Model of Creative Ability: Origins, constructs, principles and application in occupational therapy* (pp. 44-57). Pretoria, South Africa: Vona & Marie du Toit Foundation.

Murphy, L. (2021). Implementing the VdTMoCA on an inpatient mental health rehabilitation ward for clients with complex needs. In W. Sherwood (Ed.), *Perspectives on the Vona du Toit Model of Creative Ability: Practice, theory and philosophy.* Watford, England: International Creative Ability Network.

Padilla, R., & Griffiths, Y. (Eds.). (2017). *The Eleanor Clarke Slagle lectures in occupational therapy 1955-2016: A professional legacy centennial edition.* Bethesda, MD: AOTA Press.

Sherwood, W. (2016). An investigation into the theoretical construction of effort and maximum effort as a contribution to the Theory of Creative Ability. PhD Thesis. University of the Witwatersrand, Johannesburg. Retrieved from http://wiredspace.wits.ac.za/handle/10539/21261

Sherwood, W. (Ed.). (2017). *The Vona du Toit Model of Creative Ability: A practical guide to occupational therapy for people with learning disabilities.* Northampton: Vona du Toit Model of Creative Ability Foundation (UK).

Sherwood, W. (Ed.). (2021). *Perspectives on the Vona du Toit Model of Creative Ability: practice, theory and philosophy.* International Creative Ability Network.

Sherwood, W., & Wilson, S. (2019). International perspectives: An illustration of the VdTMoCA beyond South Africa. In D. van der Reyden, D. Casteleijn, W. Sherwood, & P. De Witt (Eds.), *The Vona du Toit Model of Creative Ability: Origins, constructs, principles and application in occupational therapy* (pp. 246-264). Pretoria, South Africa: Vona & Marie du Toit Foundation.

Van der Reyden, D. (1998). The South African Model of Creative Participation. In V. du Toit. (2015). *Patient volition and action in occupational therapy* (5th ed.). Vona and Marie du Toit Foundation.

Van der Reyden, D., Casteleijn, D., Sherwood, W., & De Witt, P. (Eds.). (2019). *The Vona du Toit Model of Creative Ability: Origins, constructs, principles and application in occupational therapy.* Pretoria, South Africa: Vona & Marie du Toit Foundation.

Van der Reyden, D., & Sherwood, W. (2019). The Vona du Toit Model of Creative Ability core constructs and concepts. In D. Van der Reyden, D. Casteleijn, W. Sherwood, & P. De Witt. (Eds.), *The Vona du Toit Model of Creative Ability: Origins, constructs, principles and application in occupational therapy* (pp. 58-105). Vona & Marie du Toit Foundation.

Walters, J. H., Sherwood, W., & Mason, H. (2014). Creative activities. In W. Brandt, J. Fieldhouse, & K. Bannigan (Eds.), *Creek's occupational therapy and mental health* (5th ed., pp. 260-276). Edinburgh, Scotland: Churchill Livingstone.

The Kawa (River) Model
Culturally Relevant Assessment in Occupational Therapy Mental Health Practice

Brock Cook, BA, OT
Michael K. Iwama, PhD, MSc, BSc, BScOT

Life is like the river,
sometimes it sweeps you gently along and sometimes the rapids come out of nowhere.
(Smith, n.d.)

Occupational therapy has experienced rapid global expansion over the past 2 decades as more countries, communities, and health care institutions have embraced and recognized its restorative, enabling, and empowering qualities. However, this growing appreciation for occupational therapy has raised several important challenges for the profession as it strives to be relevant and meaningful in meeting the needs of culturally diverse people and communities (Iwama, Thompson, & Macdonald, 2009).

Similar challenges face occupational therapists as they strive to meet the needs of their diverse clients in mental health practice contexts. As industrialized societies progress from the modernist era into the postmodern era, our familiar understanding of people's health states and conditions are also expanding from focusing on embodied pathologies (i.e., those located in the body, including the brain) toward an understanding of health and well-being that increasingly brings into account the physical and social environment or context.

In mental health, this progress can be seen in new movements, such as Recovery (Anthony, 1993), that shift traditional emphases from embodied pathology and professional prescriptive care to social context and person-centered and directed care. The aims are not necessarily to cure disease or enhance one's ability to act and perform according to some external set standard of "normal." Rather, the aim is to support and help the person through a process of change through which he or she may improve his or her health and wellness, live a self-directed life, and strive to achieve his or her full potential (Anthony, 1993). In this manner, the person is supported to recover a way of

Hemphill, B. J., & Urish, C. K. (Eds.). *Assessments in Occupational Therapy Mental Health: An Integrative Approach, Fourth Edition* (pp. 137-152). © 2020 Taylor & Francis Group.

living a satisfying, hopeful, and contributing life, even with limitations caused by the illness. Recovery involves the development of new meaning and purpose in one's life as one grows beyond the catastrophic effects of mental illness (Anthony, 1993).

In addition to the familiar traditional practice of helping individuals who have been diagnosed with a particular health condition achieve or return to some universally acceptable standard or norm, occupational therapists practicing in current and emerging mental health contexts are becoming increasingly interested in helping their clients move toward performance targets that are realistic and meaningful for the client to recover or attain. In order to practice in such a manner, occupational therapists require theoretical frameworks and assessment paradigms that support and enable comprehension and appreciation of how daily life experience and challenges look from the client's perspective (Iwama, 2003). The client's unique narrative of his or her everyday life becomes a central framework of focus—a reference point or narrative from which treatment plans are derived, appreciated, and considered.

In this chapter, a relatively new model of occupational therapy practice is introduced. The Kawa (Japanese for "river") Model (Iwama, 2006) is the newest, substantial model of occupational therapy. Recognized as a versatile framework that can function as an assessment treatment modality as well as a theoretical guiding framework, its utility as an assessment is explained in this chapter. Although at the time of this writing the Kawa Model is still relatively unknown in the North American occupational therapy discourse, the Kawa Model's emergence, as evidenced in the growing body of professional publications worldwide, attests to its potential to support current and future occupational therapy practice. The Kawa Model is the first substantial model of occupational therapy practice to emerge outside of the English-speaking, Western world and is the first practice framework to emerge from clinical practice through a process of qualitative research. A model based on the use of a familiar metaphor of nature to depict a person's life journey, the Kawa Model is purported to be easily understood and used by both occupational therapy clients and therapists alike.

Deductive and Inductive Assessment

Each person's experience and interpretation of day-to-day life is uniquely constructed. Each client's experience and interpretation of daily life is appreciated as being particular and unique. No two people with the diagnosis of schizophrenia will have the exact same experience of everyday life, nor will their interpretations of their daily life experiences be identical. They may share common features or markers of distinction, such as a similar pattern of symptoms associated with a psychiatric diagnosis such as schizophrenia, but the individual experience and comprehension of daily life experience will differ. What may be considered to be a problem to one person may not necessarily be considered as much of a problem to another person given the same diagnosis. In order to identify/illuminate issues that occur uniquely in an individual's daily life experiences, and therefore consider an occupational therapy response that is relevant and effective in meeting the unique daily life needs of the client, an inductive approach to assessment may be considered.

In deductive assessment, the categories and criteria for measurement are familiarly standardized and set (Anthony, 1993). Each assessment or test has a set of specific concepts and criteria to which the client's responses or observed performances are measured and compared against. All individuals are measured and assessed universally, and performance outcomes are then evaluated according to preestablished normative data.

Conversely, in inductive assessment approaches, there are no predetermined categories and criteria to guide the processes of inquiry. Concepts of importance and of particular meaning to the person *emerge*. Such emergent concepts and related principles can form new postulates or theories that become the subject of further study and validation. In this process of further study and validation, deductive inquiry methods involving the use of established tests and assessments yielding reliable information are often indicated.

Inductive assessment and inquiry can often yield unique narratives or stories of the client's experience of the world, told in the person's own words and on his or her own terms. These narratives often go beyond the immediate boundaries of the person's identified pathology or diagnosis and can provide a more comprehensive appreciation of the person in the rich context of his or her surrounding environment and circumstances, set in a historical continuum.

River Metaphor:
A Powerful Tool for Inductive Reasoning

If a metaphor could be selected to explain this interconnected dynamic of person in context of an environment and circumstances, we might say that the client's experience of everyday life is like a river. The flow qualities of the client's river are shaped by a constellation of factors, including the river walls, rocks, and driftwood that appear in the channel to either enhance or impede life flow. The occupational therapist's role, in following this metaphor of the river to depict the client's life journey, would be to enhance and enable better life flow. The occupational therapist, from the perspective of the river metaphor, could be described as a *life-flow enabler*.

In this chapter, the river metaphor is introduced as an assessment framework that guides the occupational therapist in drawing out the client's narrative or perspective of everyday life. *Kawa* metaphorically forms the basis on which the client's unique narrative can be used as a common vehicle of understanding between client and occupational therapist.

The Kawa Model

Origins

In the late 1990s, a group of Japanese occupational therapy practitioners set about creating a new model of occupational therapy practice that was simple and useful and that would exemplify the purpose, aims, and processes of their profession. Most importantly, they wanted the new model to be understandable for clients and professionals to readily use. In order to achieve these requirements, the creators of the model chose to base the emergent framework on a metaphor of nature, a river to depict a person's life journey and experience of everyday living. Most of the established models of occupational therapy in that era favored metaphors of machines, of systems and mechanical logic.

During the early stages of development of the Kawa Model, it had been assumed that the model would only be relevant for practice in Japanese contexts. However, they would discover that the metaphor of the river to depict people's life journeys would resonate with people of many different cultures around the world—even in Western countries. The Kawa Model is now taught in more than 500 occupational therapy education programs around the world and is used in occupational therapy practices across 6 continents.

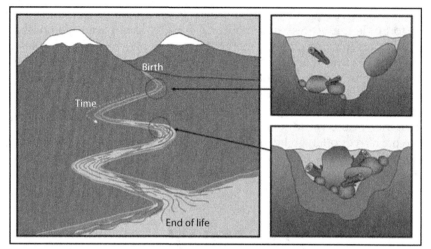

Figure 9-1. A river is a metaphor for a person's life journey. A cross-sectional view of the river at points along its length reveal different and unique configurations of the river's components.

Figure 9-2. Four basic components of the river combine to determine the river's boundaries, shape, and flow.

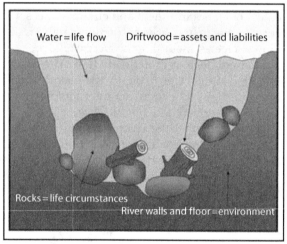

Structure and Components

The complex dynamic that characterizes an Eastern perspective of harmony in life between self and environment might be best explained through a familiar metaphor (Lakoff & Johnson, 1980) of nature. Life is a complex, profound journey that flows through time and space, like a river (Figure 9-1). An optimal state of well-being in one's life, or river, can be metaphorically portrayed by an image of strong, deep, unimpeded water flow. Aspects of the environment and the dynamic phenomena that occur within it, like the integrated dynamics that occur among the various components that comprise a river, can influence and affect that flow. Rocks (life circumstances), walls and floor (environment), and driftwood (assets and liabilities) are all inseparable parts of a river that determine its boundaries, shape, and flow (Figure 9-2). Occupational therapy's purpose in this metaphorical representation of a human being, then, is to enable and enhance life flow.

Water

Water metaphorically represents the person's life energy or life flow. Fluid, pure, spirit, filling, cleansing, and renewing are some of the meanings and qualities commonly associated with this natural element. Just as people's lives are bounded and shaped by their surroundings, people, and circumstances, the water flowing as a river touches the rocks, banks, and all other elements that form its context. Water envelopes, defines, and affects these other elements in a similar way to how the same elements affect the water's volume, shape, and flow rate. When life energy or flow weakens, the occupational therapy client, whether individually or collectively, can be described as unwell or in a state of disharmony. When it stops flowing altogether, as when the river releases into a vast ocean, end of life is met.

In the Western world, with so much of our consciousness focused on the independent, agent self, there may be a tendency to overlook or underestimate the importance that place and context play in determining the forms, functions, and meanings of human occupation. Imagining how certain aspects of one's surrounding context can limit or enable one's state of being can be challenging if we have spent a lifetime learning context, environment, and circumstances as aspects of one's existence that require conquering and subjugating.

Through the vantage of the Kawa Model, a person's state of well-being coincides with life flow. Occupational therapy's overall purpose in this context is to enhance life flow, regardless of whether it is interpreted at the level of the individual, institution, organization, community, or society. Just as there are constellations of interrelated factors/structures in a river that affect its flow, a rich combination of internal and external circumstances and structures in a client's life context combine to determine his or her life flow.

With regard to assessment, the Kawa Model affords a holistic, comprehensive, and integrated perspective of the client in the context of his or her environment and circumstances.

River Banks and Floor

The river's banks and floor are the structures/concepts from the river metaphor that stand for the person's social and physical environment. The physical environment is just that, the physical structures and features of the location in which a person exists and carries out his or her activities of daily living. This can be a person's house, apartment, a temporary shelter, or workplace. The river banks and floor can also represent the person's social context—mainly those who share a direct relationship with the person. Depending on which social frame is perceived to be the most important to a person in a given instance and place, the social environs can represent family members, workmates, friends in a recreational club, or classmates.

Aspects of the surrounding social frame on the person can affect the overall flow (volume and rate) of the Kawa. Harmonious relationships can enable and complement life flow. Increased flow can have an agent effect upon difficult circumstances and problems as the force of water displaces rocks in the channel and even create new courses through which to flow. Conversely, a decrease in flow volume can exert a compounding, negative effect on the other elements that take up space in the channel (Figure 9-3). If there are obstructions (rocks and driftwood) in the watercourse when river walls and floor are thick and constricting, the flow of the river is especially compromised. As can be imagined, the rocks in this river can directly butt up against the river walls and floor, compounding and creating larger impediments to the river's usual flow.

Figure 9-3. All components of the river are interrelated and are in dynamic change.

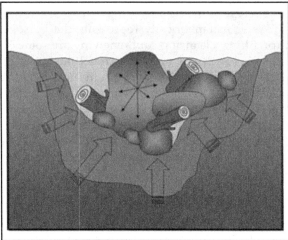

Like all other elements of the river, these concepts are always interpreted in relation to the whole, taking into consideration all other elements of the person's context and his or her interrelations/interdependencies.

Rocks

In the Kawa Model, rocks represent discrete circumstances that are considered impediments to one's life flow. They are life circumstances perceived by the client to be problematic and difficult to remove. Most rivers, like people's lives, have such rocks or impediments, of varying size, shape, and number. Large rocks, by themselves or in combination with other rocks, jammed directly or indirectly against the river walls and banks (environment) can profoundly impede and obstruct flow. The client's rocks may have been there since the beginning, such as with congenital conditions; they may appear instantaneously, as with a sudden illness or injury; or they may even be transient.

The impeding effect of rocks can compound when situated against the river's walls and floor (environment). For example, a person's level of coping with auditory hallucinations can become challenging when moving into a particularly noisy and crowded environment. In another example, functional difficulties associated with a neurological condition can change according to the environmental context. A (physically) barrier-free environment can decrease one's disability, as can social and/or political/organizational environments that are accepting of people with disabling conditions. Once the client's perceived rocks are known (including their relative size and situation), the therapist can help to identify potential areas of intervention and strategies to enable better life flow. The broader contextual definition of disabling circumstances necessarily brings into play the client's surrounding environment. Therefore, occupational therapy intervention can include treatment strategies that expand beyond the traditional patient to his or her social network and even to policies and social structures that ultimately play a part in setting the disabling context.

The concepts and the contextual application of the Kawa Model are by natural design flexible and adaptable. Each client's unique river takes its important concepts and configuration from the situation of the person in a given time and place. The definition of problems and circumstances are broad—as broad and diverse as our clients' worlds of meanings. In turn, this particular conceptualization of people and their circumstances foreshadows the broad outlook and scope of occupational therapy interventions, when set in particular cultural contexts.

The person, be it an individual or a collective, ideally determines the specific rocks and their number, magnitude, form, and situation in the river. As with all other elements of the model, if the client is unable to express his or her own river, family members or a community of people connected with the issue at hand may lend assistance.

Driftwood

Driftwood represent the person's personal attributes and resources, such as his or her values (e.g., honesty, thrift), character (e.g., optimism, stubbornness), personality (e.g., reserved, outgoing), special skills (e.g., carpentry, public speaking), and immaterial (e.g., friends, siblings) and material (e.g., wealth, special equipment) assets that can positively or negatively affect the person's circumstance and life flow.

Like driftwood, they are transient in nature and carry a certain quality of fate or serendipity. They can appear to be inconsequential in some instances and significantly obstructive in others, particularly when they settle in among rocks and the river walls and floor. On the other hand, they can collide with the same structures to nudge obstructions out of the way. A client's religious faith and sense of determination can be positive factors in persevering to erode or move rocks out of the way. Receiving a grant to acquire specialized assistive equipment can be the piece of driftwood that collides against existing flow impediments and opens a greater channel for one's life to flow more strongly.

Driftwood are a part of everyone's river and are often like intangible components possessed by each unique client of occupational therapy. Effective therapists pay particular attention to these components of a client's or community's assets and circumstances and consider their real or potential effect on the client's situation and daily life experiences.

Spaces (Between Obstructions): The Promise of Occupational Therapy

In the Kawa Model, spaces are the points through which the client's life energy (water) flows, and these spaces represent occupation, in the way that Western occupational therapists have discussed it. When the metaphor of a river depicting the client's life flow becomes clearer, attention turns to the spaces between the rocks, driftwood, and river walls and floor. These spaces are as important to comprehend in the client as are the other elements of the river when determining how to apply and direct occupational therapy. For example, a space between a functional impairment such as depression (a rock) and a social group or person (in the river walls and floor) may represent a certain social role, such as parent, company worker, or friend.

Water naturally coursing through these spaces can work to erode the rocks, river walls, and floor and over time can transform them into larger conduits or channels for life flow (Figure 9-4). This effect reflects the latent healing potential that each person naturally holds within him- or herself and in the inseparable context. Thus, occupational therapy in this perspective retains its hallmark of working with the client's abilities and assets. It also directs occupational therapy intervention toward all elements (in this case, a medically defined problem, various aspects and levels of environment) in the context (see inner image, Figure 9-4).

Spaces, then, represent important targets for occupational therapy. They occur throughout the context of the self and environs, between the rocks, walls and floor, and

Figure 9-4. Spaces are potential channels for greater flow and are defined by the components that combine to form their qualities and boundaries.

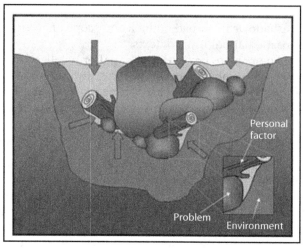

driftwood. Spaces are potential channels for the client's flow, allowing the client and therapist to determine multiple points and levels of intervention (see Figure 9-4). In this way, each problem or enabling opportunity is bounded by and appreciated in a broader context.

Rather than attempting to reduce a person's problems (i.e., focusing only on rocks) to discrete issues that are isolated out of their particular contexts (similar to the rational processes in which client problems are identified and discretely named/diagnosed in conventional Western health practice), the Kawa Model framework compels the occupational therapist to view and treat issues within a holistic framework, seeking to appreciate the clients' identified issues within his or her integrated, inseparable contexts. Occupation is therefore regarded in wholes—to include the meaning of the activity to self and community to which the individual inseparably belongs and not just in terms of psychological or biomechanical components, nor as individual pathology and function.

Phenomena and life circumstances rarely occur in isolation. By changing one aspect of the client's world, all other aspects of his or her river change. The river's spaces represent opportunities to problem solve and focus intervention on positive opportunities, which may have little direct relation to the person's medically defined condition.

By using this model, occupational therapists in partnership with their clients are directed to stem further obstruction of life energy/flow and look for every opportunity in the broader context to enhance it (Figure 9-5).

Harmony: The Essence of Human Occupation

What has been illustrated throughout the descriptions of the Kawa Model's components is the underlying ontology of the Kawa framework: Everything is interconnected. The Kawa Model's central point of reference is not the individual but rather harmony—a state of individual or collective being in which the person, be it the self or community, is in balance with the context that it is a part of. Here, the essence of such harmony is conceptualized as life energy or life flow. Occupational therapy's purpose is to help the client enhance and balance this flow. In this balance, there is coexistence, a synergy between elements that affirm interdependence. How can one come to terms with one's circumstances? How can harmony between the elements, of which one is merely one part, be realized? How and in what way can occupational therapy assist this construction of well-being?

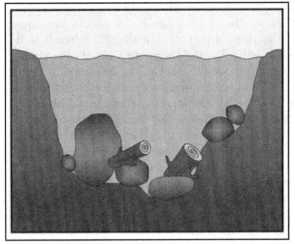

Figure 9-5. Using the Kawa Model, the aim of occupational therapy is to enhance life flow.

How Can the Kawa (River) Metaphor and Its Concepts Be Employed in the Client Assessment Processes in Mental Health Care Contexts?

Through the perspective of the river metaphor, based on an ontology in which self and context are inseparably interconnected, the occupational therapist aspires to comprehend as much as possible the client's real world of meanings in his or her experience of the flow or state of well-being, with the ultimate objective of enabling and supporting a better life flow. The Kawa Model and its interrelated concepts are used as a framework to draw out the client's narrative of his or her experience of daily life.

If we were to assume that every person's narrative of his or her experience of daily life was unique and different from another person's, then we might then assume that no single universal assessment or set of concepts created in a particular (cultural) place and time could accurately capture and explain the client's experience and interpretation of daily life reality. It would then be fair to ask whether a framework/assessment like the Kawa Model, with certain defined concepts (e.g., water, rocks), could abet the same erroneous pattern of applying a set of concepts universally to all clients regardless of diversity. Therapists using the Kawa Model attempt to avoid this problematic pitfall by reversing the power dynamic inherent in the assessment process. Rather than taking the concepts and principles of the Kawa Model and applying them through a standard protocol to all clients in a consistent manner, the therapist encourages the client to use the river metaphor to give an authentic account of how his or her daily life is flowing. Through this process, the client is empowered to tell his or her story through a metaphor of nature that both the client and therapist can relate to. The client constructs and names the concepts and can explain the principles that tie the concepts together. In essence, the client becomes a theorist who builds a model or narrative to explain his or her day-to-day life circumstances to the occupational therapist in a way that both parties can mutually understand.

Consistent with the client-centered and culturally relevant qualities often associated with the Kawa Model (Iwama, 2006), assessment protocols can vary according to context and location. The most common format of the Kawa Model's application appears to be in its drawing form, in which an image of a river to depict the client's life journey is constructed. It has been the authors' experience to see the Kawa Model presented as an exercise in which the client is asked to draw a picture of a river. This tends to be prevalent in English-speaking societies, such as the United Kingdom, Canada, the United States, Australia, and New Zealand. In Spain, as well as in various locations in South America, the assumption is almost always that the client and occupational therapist construct the client's river drawing together. In societies like Japan's, where social hierarchy is celebrated according to Confucian ethic, almost always the therapist constructs the drawing, followed by requests for the client to clarify and validate the resulting narratives. Some occupational therapists working in facilities that are predominantly medical-model oriented have reported that they rarely ever refer to a river drawing or image. In such cases, the five concepts of the Kawa Model are organized as assessment categories in tabular form. A table with five column headings—Life Flow (Water), Difficulties (Rocks), Environment (River Walls), Personal Factors (Driftwood), and Areas of Potential Improvement (Spaces)—is constructed and then filled with pertinent client information, specific instruments/tests, and outcomes to further assess the client's status and progress, time lines, and goals. As can be readily imagined, the Kawa Model can be repeated at appropriate times along the client's treatment continuum.

Case Studies

Two brief cases that describe the use of the Kawa Model in occupational therapy mental health care settings are presented to give the reader a sense of how the Kawa Model and its concepts are used in actual practice. The Kawa Model's use in assessment application is highlighted, although the model is versatile and often employed as a guide for occupational therapy processes and as a treatment modality in itself.

A growing list of resources spanning various media relating to the Kawa Model is available online through popular social media outlets. Written publications, video and slide presentations, blog entries, and live discussion forums pertaining to the model can be accessed through popular search engines.

Anjali S.

Community Mental Health Care/Case Management Care
The following brief summary was provided by the referring agency:
- 38-year-old woman of South Sea Islander/Asian background
- Diagnosis of paranoid schizophrenia
- Deaf since age 6 years due to degenerative health condition
- Poor English
- IQ tested as 70
- Family lives 700 miles away
- Noncompliant with medication
- 17 admissions to an acute unit in the past 12 months
- Very difficult to engage with due to limited communication

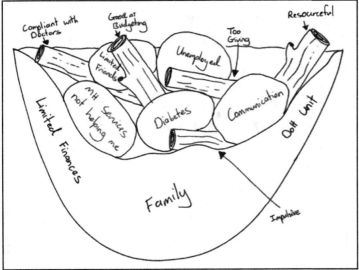

Figure 9-6. Anjali's Kawa drawing (in cross-section view).

The agency reported that the person had been described by previous caregivers as being difficult to work with and that she often threw unpredictable tantrums. They also reported that Anjali frequently displayed impulsive and disinhibited behaviors.

The occupational therapist decided to try the Kawa Model based on its visual-spatial characteristics. The therapist was aware of potential communication difficulties as English was not the client's first language. The concepts of the Kawa Model were explained via written communication and through a visual example of the occupational therapist's own Kawa drawing.

Anjali was asked by her therapist to draw at least two diagrams of her river: a longitudinal view to show some of those experiences she has had through her life that she deemed to be important and a cross-sectional view to show her view of life at this very moment. The client explained that the model itself was easy to understand. The therapist also found that the model was easy to explain, even with very basic levels of communication (Figure 9-6).

The person identified that many of the largest difficulties she faced were based around communication difficulties with others. Note that there is no mention in the resultant Kawa drawing of any of the symptoms of schizophrenia that she experienced, and no mention of her medications, which had been the two main focus points in previous treatment plans.

From this initial assessment approach using the Kawa Model, the occupational therapist and client collaboratively agreed upon a treatment plan based on engagement in meaningful activities. The first prioritized area of intervention focused on the identified communication difficulties. The person was empowered to teach basic sign language to the occupational therapist. They started with the most important signs required for basic health conversations: doctor, nurse, medication, food, money, family, happy, and sad, as well as those for numbers and dates. Sessions became about the person empowering the therapist, and this sense of purpose became something that Anjali looked forward to and eagerly engaged in.

Anjali was engaged with a deaf services charity in her community that supported her in finding work in a local café. This increased her circle of friends, improved her finances, and eliminated her status of being unemployed. Together, Anjali and the occupational therapist

Figure 9-7. Anjali's second Kawa drawing (in cross-section view).

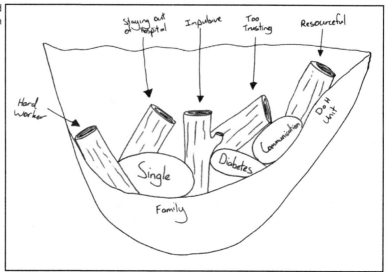

explored alternative communication methods for keeping in touch with her family. Anjali worked on writing regular letters, which helped satisfy her need for connection with her family. As the change in her circumstance indicates, her original Kawa drawing no longer stood as an accurate representation of her present situation, so the process of constructing an up-to-date Kawa drawing was repeated (Figure 9-7). This process of producing Kawa drawings was repeated multiple times throughout the process and used to guide and mediate the therapeutic work that Anjali and the therapist performed together. This method of treatment-informed care enabled Anjali to control the direction and focus of treatment throughout the therapy process. The Kawa Model played an integral part in this process not only as an assessment but also as an outcome measure and self-reflection tool.

Jason B.

Acute Mental Health Inpatient Unit Occupational Therapy
The following brief summary was derived from the patient's chart:
- 80-year-old man of North American background
- Working diagnosis of depression
- No contact with family other than with partner
- Attempted suicide by hanging
- First presentation to mental health services
- Isolated and not interacting with staff

On the psychiatry acute care ward, Jason would keep to himself, isolating himself to his room. He would not interact with any of the other patients or staff. He was often observed to be crying quietly in his room and while moving about the ward. Other staff had attempted to engage with him, but he would not respond to them at all. Jason seemed so saddened, he could barely form a conversation for more than a minute at a time. At this stage, the occupational therapist decided to try using the Kawa Model with Jason. It was thought that the Kawa Model could be used as a visual medium to enable the client to process his thoughts and then convey them to the occupational therapist in an understandable way.

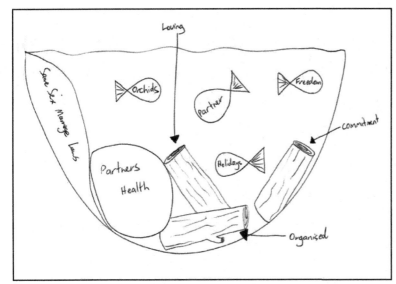

Figure 9-8. Jason's Kawa drawing (in cross-section view) of his life flow prior to depression.

The concept of the Kawa Model was explained to Jason, and then assessment using the Kawa Model was completed over several 15-minute sessions. During the first session, Jason found something about his current situation greatly distressing. He was unable to contain his emotions, and he could not complete the Kawa Model assessment activity. While being aware of his current state of distress, Jason was able to recall feeling okay 6 months previously, before the depression had started (Figure 9-8). He reported that they had a "great life back then." The discussion focused on exploring his life flow.

Another component was added to his Kawa Model: Fish. Fish were added in order to represent the things in his life that he felt had contributed to his feeling of flow. He identified that his partner was a large proponent of his flow. Jason explained that over the past 5 decades, he and his partner never spent more than a weekend apart from each other. His life's work and love of orchid farming was also a large source of value for him. He also identified that he and his partner would travel often and that this sense of freedom had always fulfilled him. Using the Kawa Model to assess historical engagement in activities allowed Jason to feel more comfortable in discussing the events of his life and to share possible factors that may have been affecting his current mental state.

When Jason and his occupational therapist traced his Kawa drawings back to the present day, Jason revealed that he had given away all of his orchids 4 months previously. He reported that he just "lost all interest in gardening." He then revealed that 2 months prior to giving away his orchids, his partner of 50 years had been moved into a nursing facility due to deteriorating health. By the time of his admission to the psychiatry acute care ward, he stated that he had not seen his partner in 3 weeks and did not even "know if he was okay" (Figure 9-9).

Guilt was identified as a negative personal factor in his Kawa Model, which he had attributed to the fact that he "loved his partner very much" and "couldn't look after him anymore" on his own.

The geographical barrier that was keeping him from his partner on a daily basis was explored and community access support workers were engaged to support him to visit his partner daily. He was able to reengage in his carer role by assisting his partner around meal times and by helping him access books and magazines to entertain him. Jason understood that his being available to support his partner had a positive benefit on his

Figure 9-9. Jason's second Kawa drawing (in cross-sectional view) of his current life flow.

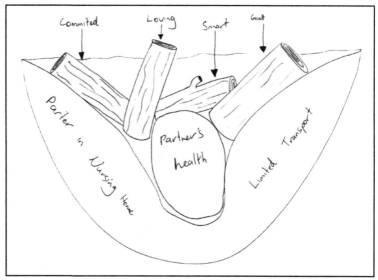

partner's health. His aim was to use the identified personal attributes of being committed and loving to chip away at the stone identified as his partner's health in order to reduce its impact on their combined flow.

Jason gradually rediscovered his joy of gardening and would often take new plants to put in his partner's room, where they would discuss them as they always had. As his engagement in these activities increased, he reported that the feelings of depression and guilt gradually subsided.

The Kawa Model applied as an assessment in Jason's case appeared to be effective and useful on a number of levels. The Kawa Model facilitated the establishment and building of rapport between the client and occupational therapist. The ensuing narrative allowed Jason to identify and make sense of his current situation. The Kawa Model helped to create a chronological and visual representation of Jason's daily life experience that was then used as the basis for the occupational therapy treatment plan.

Additional Considerations

Over the past decade, case studies of the model's application have emerged across the spectrum—from neonatal to end of life, from individuals to organizations and communities, and across the medical categories of rehabilitation and mental health. A search of Kawa Model case studies conducted through the internet (particularly social media) will quickly yield a growing body of information spread across six continents.

Perhaps the Kawa Model's most special feature is in its potential utility in mediating a more client-centered approach to understanding the client and his or her daily living needs. Rather than the health professional dictating the terms and means of care for the client based solely on the professional's perspective and expertise, the Kawa Model achieves the opposite by becoming a vehicle of mutual understanding between client and therapist. The Kawa Model can be used effectively to bring forth the client's narrative, or model, in which the concepts and the principles that connect the concepts are manufactured and explained by the client in his or her own words.

A Client-Centered Perspective and Practice

To be truly client centered, the client's views of his or her realities and circumstances should not be forced to comply with someone else's manufactured framework of culturally bound concepts and principles. The therapist using the Kawa Model first recognizes the uniqueness of each person's situation/context and then follows this with an inquiry into the person's experience and perspective of everyday life. The structure and meanings of the river metaphor takes shape according to the person's views of his or her circumstances in appropriate cultural context.

The Kawa Model can be used to derive what concepts, meaningful and germane to the client's perspective of life, need to be appreciated and explored further. Once those unique and meaningful concepts are determined, the therapist can proceed to select tools/instruments and methods that will effectively gather pertinent information. These chosen instruments should also be culturally safe and nonexploitative. Equipped with the Kawa framework, occupational therapists do not become dependent on a particular measurement tool or procedure to inform them of what their interventions should be. Rather, therapists are challenged and guided toward understanding the client's occupational issues in proper context and have a clearer sense of what needs to be measured and studied further and why. The instruments are chosen judiciously according to the requirements of the client's case, in proper context, and set in harmony with occupational therapy's mandate.

Summary

Occupational therapy proceeds when the client privileges the occupational therapist to develop an interest in his or her day-to-day circumstances and world of meanings. To appreciate the complex dynamic between people's day-to-day realities and their contexts and to deliver meaningful interventions that support a better state of harmony in people's lives, occupational therapists require approaches that are guided and informed by theory and instruments that are culturally relevant and safe for their clients (Iwama, 2006). The Kawa Model represents one example of the kind of theoretical material that occupational therapy may need to develop if it is to retain its relevance and effectiveness as it transcends cultural borders (Iwama, 2003).

Assessment is widely regarded as a necessary, pivotal element of health care processes and typically forms the common starting point for professional care intervention. The outcomes of assessment processes define a baseline, a starting point in the continuum of care that follows. Assessments determine the benchmarks to which care plans and strategies are aimed. They inform the factors along which occupational therapy is directed, structured, and evaluated and define the endpoints worth aiming for.

Assessments can also help to define and validate the person's state of being with respect to identifying key issues and matters requiring attention and intervention. They can assist in deriving a standard baseline of performance that can be compared with established normative data. The resulting data can help to define what aspects of the client's state of being and performance compare with others in similar states or circumstances.

In traditional medical model–oriented settings, the problems and issues that form the centers of concern for attending care professionals are often assumed to reside in the person's body. Embodied pathology includes not only the musculoskeletal systems, but also the neurological and endocrine systems. The location and quality of the experience associated with embodied pathologies subsequently direct treatment (including invasive and noninvasive). As approaches to treatment in mental health continue to move toward the environment, and particularly the social, intervention and treatment are moving progressively out of the person's body into the environment, particularly the social environment and context.

By taking a broad view of the person embedded in the rich context of their day-to-day circumstances, the Kawa Model, when employed in mental health assessment, can help both the therapist and client to appreciate the client's experience of day-to-day life. By being able to gain greater access to how day-to-day experiences look and feel from the perspective of the client, through their words, explanations, and images, the resulting occupational therapy interventions gain greater potential to be more tangible, meaningful, and intimately relevant to those who matter most.

References

Anthony, W. A. (1993). Recovery from mental illness: The guiding vision of the mental health service system in the 1990's. *Psychosocial Rehabilitation Journal, 16*(4), 11-23.

Iwama, M. (2003). Toward culturally relevant epistemologies in occupational therapy. *American Journal of Occupational Therapy, 57*, 582-588.

Iwama, M. (2006). *The Kawa Model: Culturally relevant occupational therapy.* London, United Kingdom: Churchill Livingstone.

Iwama, M. K., Thompson, N. A., & Macdonald, R. M. (2009). The Kawa Model: The power of culturally responsive occupational therapy. *Disability Rehabilitation, 31*(14), 1125-1135. https://doi.org/10.1080/09638280902773711

Lakoff, G., & Johnson. M. (1980). *Metaphors we live by.* Chicago, IL: University of Chicago Press.

Smith, E. (n.d.). Emma Smith quotes. Retrieved from https://www.goodreads.com/quotes/300539-life-is-like-the-river-sometimes-it-sweeps-you-gently

Part IV
Cognitive Assessments

10

Performance-Based Assessments and Neuropsychological Assessments
A Comparison

Glen Gillen, EdD, OTR, FAOTA
Emily Raphael-Greenfield, EdD, OTR/L, FAOTA

Occupation is as necessary as food and drink.
(Knowles, 1995)

The aims of this chapter are to promote the use of performance/occupation as the primary assessments for use by occupational therapy practitioners and to compare and contrast performance-based assessments to traditional neuropsychological assessments. The chapter will provide detailed examples of three performance-based assessments and briefly familiarize readers with assessments that may be used by our colleagues in other disciplines.

Comparing and Contrasting Performance-Based Assessments and Neuropsychological Assessments

There are different schools of thought in regard to the potential assessment methods and tools that can be used with our clients. For the purpose of this chapter, the authors will be discussing, comparing, and contrasting what can be described as performance/occupation assessments that use real-world tasks in natural contexts as the means to evaluate everyday living skills and the factors/skills that support or limit performance with neuropsychological (i.e., pen-and-paper, table-top) assessments. The reader is referred to Table 10-1 for a summary.

Hemphill, B. J., & Urish, C. K. (Eds.). *Assessments in Occupational Therapy Mental Health: An Integrative Approach,* Fourth Edition (pp. 155-178). © 2020 Taylor & Francis Group.

Table 10-1

A Comparison of Performance-/Occupation-Based Assessments and Neuropsychological Assessments

Performance-/Occupation-Based Assessments	Neuropsychological (Pen-and-Paper or Table-Top) Assessments
Use real-world tasks as the means of assessing everyday function and factors/skills that support or limit performance	Use novel and isolated cognitive manipulations to document the presence or absence of impairments
Examples of included items are cooking, shopping, money management, self-care, and homemaking	Examples of included items are trail making, clock drawing, naming animals, drawing pentagons, citing number strings, and spelling backward
Examples of tools include AMPS, EFPT, ESI, MET, and TOGSS	Examples of tools include MMSE, MoCA, SLUMS, WCST, and Trails A and B
Performed in natural contexts such as kitchens, bathrooms, and malls	Performed in office settings to control for distractions
Requires multitasking	Requires single or dual tasking
Ecologically valid	Low ecological validity
Identifies abilities or difficulties in performing real-world tasks	Low to moderate associations with measures of everyday living
Consistent with occupational therapy's philosophy	Primarily developed for philosophies that guide our colleagues in other disciplines

Abbreviations: AMPS = Assessment of Motor and Process Skills; EFPT = Executive Function Performance Test; ESI = Evaluation of Social Interaction; MET = Multiple Errands Test; MMSE = Mini Mental State Examination; MoCA = Montreal Cognitive Assessment; SLUMS = Saint Louis Mental Status Examination; TOGSS = Test of Grocery Shopping Skills; WCST = Wisconsin Card Sorting Test.

Performance-based assessments that involve actual doing of everyday occupations are promoted as the methods, materials, and settings of the assessments because they approximate the real world that is being examined and therefore are ecologically valid. Ecological validity is a critical concept for occupational therapy practitioners to consider. This concept refers to whether one can generalize from observed behavior in testing to natural behaviors in the real world (Chaytor & Schmitter-Edgecombe, 2003) and is the foundation of occupational therapy assessment.

The choice of assessment will influence whether testing is considered ecologically valid. For example, if the occupational therapy practitioner is concerned that executive dysfunction is a limiting factor related to occupational performance, he or she has several choices of assessments to consider. The Wisconsin Card Sorting Test (WCST; Berg, 1948) is measure of neuropsychological functioning, assessing abstract thinking, cognitive flexibility, and executive function and impairment. Developed by our colleagues from psychology, it uses a variety of novel card sorting tasks (low ecological validity) as the means of assessment. The middle-ground of ecological validity can be described as simulation tasks. An example of this type of assessment is the Behavioural Assessment of the Dysexecutive Syndrome (Wilson, Evans, Emslie, Alderman, & Burgess, 1998). Developed by colleagues in psychology and neuropsychology, the Behavioural Assessment of the Dysexecutive Syndrome uses simulation tasks, such as planning how to remove a cork from a test tube and planning a trip to the zoo. Finally, one may consider using everyday tasks in natural contexts to document the executive functions that support or limit everyday performance (the highest level of ecological validity). The Executive Function Performance Test (EFPT; Baum, Connor, Morrison, Hahn, Dromerick, & Edwards, 2008; see Chapter 15), developed by occupational therapists, uses the real-world tasks of cooking, medication management, bill paying, and telephone use as the means of assessment. It is imperative that occupational therapy practitioners use performance-/occupation-based assessments that, by definition, are ecologically valid as their primary means of assessment.

Assessment of Motor and Process Skills
Theoretical Basis

Concepts/Construct

The Assessment of Motor and Process Skills (AMPS) is a test of a person's ability to perform personal activities of daily living (ADL) tasks and instrumental activities of daily living (IADL) tasks. The motor and process performance skills included in the AMPS are referred to as ADL skills. Performance skills are the "smallest observable actions or units of occupational performance that we can observe as a person carries out his or her daily life tasks" (Fisher & Griswold, 2014b, p. 249). One can also consider performance skills as "the goal-directed actions a person carries out one-by-one during naturalistic and relevant daily life task performances" (Fisher & Griswold, 2014b, p. 251). Performance skills should not be confused with body functions. Body functions (e.g., praxis, strength, memory, visual processing, coordination) describe what the person's body systems do, whereas performance skills describe what the person does in relation to task objects while engaging in meaningful occupations (Fisher & Griswold, 2014b).

History of Development and Previous Versions/ Important Changes to Note in Current Version

The AMPS has been in development since 1985 and is currently in its eighth edition. Since its inception, the AMPS has been based on three assertions (Fisher & Jones, 2014a): (1) occupational therapy services must be client centered, (2) evaluations and interventions must be occupation-focused and occupation-based, and (3) the occupational therapy process is most effective when organized in a top-down manner. The original research version of the AMPS included 12 tasks, and the original standardization sample included 64 participants. There are presently over 100 tasks (representing both personal ADLs and IADLs) included on the AMPS. The standardization sample is now greater than 140,000 participants, and there are more than 13,000 calibrated raters worldwide.

Psychometric Properties

Normative Data

The current AMPS standardization sample is based on 148,158 people. The ages range from 3 to 103 years. The standardization sample can be divided into the following diagnostic groups: well, frail old, mild disabilities, those with developmental disorders, cerebrovascular accident, other neurological disorders, those with intellectual disabilities, musculoskeletal disorders, medical/sensory disorders, those with schizophrenia or thought disorders, other psychiatric disorders/autism, dementia, other memory disorders, and multiple/unknown disorders. This sample includes people from across the globe, including the United States, Ireland, Asia, South America, the Middle East, United Kingdom, and New Zealand. The ADL motor ability ranged from 3.95 to -3.00 logits and the ADL process ability ranged from 3.00 to -2.00 logits. Positive values indicate more ADL ability (Fisher & Jones, 2014a).

Reliability

Studies that have examined test-retest reliability of the AMPS reveal high test-retest reliability, indicating the AMPS measures remain consistent from one test session to the next. Data from a small sample of older adults revealed test-retest reliabilities of $r = .91$ for the AMPS motor skill scale and $r = .90$ for the AMPS process skill scale. In a larger study, Rockwood, Doble, Fisk, MacPherson, and Lewis (1996) reported test-retest coefficients of $r = .90$ for the motor skill scale and $r = .87$ for the process skill scale.

Kirkley and Fisher (1999) examined parallel forms (alternate forms) of reliability and obtained reliability coefficients of $r = .91$ for the motor skill scale and $r = .85$ for the process skill scale. Fisher, Liu, Velozo, and Pan (1992) reported a high intrarater reliability coefficient of $r = .93$ in a sample of Taiwanese participants without disability.

Fisher and Jones (2014a) reported that when the data for the current standardization sample was analyzed, the many-faceted Rasch equivalent of Cronbach's alpha was $r = .92$ for the ADL motor measures and $r = .91$ for the process measures. This further supports the very high reliability of the AMPS measures.

Validity

The AMPS validity has been addressed in multiple studies. Specifically, studies have determined that the AMPS can be validly used with both men and women, across various ages, and from people from various worldwide regions and cultures (i.e., North America, United Kingdom, Republic of Ireland, Nordic countries, other European countries, Australia, New Zealand, and Asian countries; Fisher & Jones, 2014a). There is a substantial body of evidence that the AMPS can be used validly for a variety of diagnostic groups, including cerebrovascular accident, dementia, multiple sclerosis, those with mental retardation, and those with psychiatric disorders (Fisher & Jones, 2014a). For example, Moore, Merritt, and Doble (2010) aimed to determine whether there are significant differences in ADL ability and ADL skill profiles between samples of individuals with bipolar disorder depression ($n = 158$), bipolar disorder mania ($n = 200$), and schizophrenia ($n = 200$) using the AMPS. The authors found that no clinically significant differences were found in mean ADL ability. The ADL process skill item *attends* was more difficult for those with bipolar disorder mania than for those with bipolar disorder depression. This difference did not disrupt the measurement model. The authors concluded that the findings also provide solid evidence that valid measures of ADL ability are generated when individuals with bipolar disorder and schizophrenia complete the AMPS (Moore et al., 2010). Readers are directed to the Center for Innovative OT Solutions (http://www.innovativeotsolutions.com/tools/amps) for detailed references related to the validity of the AMPS.

Sensitivity

Although standard error of measurement (SE) is considered a reliability index, it also reflects the sensitivity of the measure in evaluating change. The mean SE for the people in the current standardization sample was 0.25 logit on the ADL motor scale and 0.20 logit on the ADL process scale. If two individual measures differ by at least 2 SE, there is a significant difference between measures. Ceiling effects have not been noted within the AMPS due to the wide range of tasks that are included. In addition, the problem of limited sensitivity is minimized when using the AMPS because the therapist observes the smallest observable units of ADL task performance; therefore, very small changes in the quality of ADL performance can be observed (Fisher & Jones, 2014a).

Assessment Administration

Area of Occupation/Performance Skills Assessed

The AMPS evaluates the following areas of occupation: personal ADLs and IADLs. Examples of personal ADLs included in the AMPS are eating a meal, dressing, showering, using an electric razor, and hair care. Examples of multiple IADLs include preparing beverages and food (e.g., eggs, French toast, sandwiches, snacks, salads), housecleaning, bed-making, laundry, table setting, plant care, outdoor maintenance tasks, shopping, and pet care (Fisher & Jones, 2014b).

The AMPS also measures the quality of 16 ADL motor and 20 ADL process performance skills. Motor skills are defined as occupational performance skills (e.g., ADL motor skills) observed as the person interacts with and moves task objects, and moves oneself around the task environment (Fisher & Jones, 2014a). The specific motor skills evaluated on the AMPS include the following: stabilizes, aligns, positions, reaches, bends, grips, manipulates, coordinates, moves, lifts, walks, transports, calibrates, flows, endures, and paces.

Process skills are defined as occupational performance skills (e.g., ADL process skills) observed as a person (1) selects, interacts with, and uses task tools and materials; (2) carries out individual actions and steps; and (3) modifies performance when problems are encountered (Fisher & Jones, 2014a). The specific process skills evaluated on the AMPS include the following: paces, attends, heeds, chooses, uses, handles, inquires, initiates, continues, sequences, terminates, searches/locates, gathers, organizes, restores, navigates, notices/responds, adjusts, accommodates, and benefits.

Description of Environment/ Description of Supplies/Materials Required

The AMPS can be administered in either a clinic or home setting. The environment should be a natural, task-relevant environment. A clinic setting is defined as any environment that is not the client's home environment or where the client is living. Therefore, hospital or clinical settings, classrooms, and day treatment centers are considered clinic settings (Fisher & Jones, 2014a). Home settings are defined as any setting, other than a hospital, where a client is currently living and are considered a home environment. Examples include houses, apartments, assisted living, group homes, and nursing homes (Fisher & Jones, 2014a).

Each AMPS task is described in the AMPS user manual (Fisher & Jones, 2014b). Each description includes a heading of required tools and materials. All of the tools and materials are natural, everyday objects found in natural environments. Two examples follow:

1. Task C-1: Cold cereal and beverage for one person. Required tools and materials include: dry cereals (e.g., bran flakes, muesli, granola), milk or cream, prepared beverages (e.g., juice, milk, tea, iced tea), and kitchen.

2. Task L-3: Loading and starting a washing machine. Required tools and materials include: washing machine, a load of dirty laundry (no large items such as sheets or bed coverings), soap/detergent (liquid or powder), and a laundry basket.

Administration

The authors of the AMPS describe the administration as occurring in nine phases. These phases and their abbreviated descriptions include (Fisher & Jones, 2014a):

1. Preparing to test a person: Initiating the process of establishing the client-centered performance context, establish rapport and collaborative relationships, prepare for the occupational therapy interview

2. Interviewing the client: Identify priorities, introduce AMPS, establish task contract

3. Observing and implementing a standardized performance analysis: Summarize contract, initiate task observation, observe at least two AMPS tasks, take notes

4. Score the AMPS observation: Record on the score form, rate the quality of occupational performance for each task, rate the functional level, and score each AMPS task observation

5. Enter the raw scores into the computer-scoring software and generate AMPS reports

6. Interpret and document the person's AMPS results: Interpret the ability measures relative to a criterion of competence as using a norms-based perspective, interpret need for assistance, define and group actions that the person does not perform effectively, and document the results

7. Define and interpret reasons for the person's ineffective ADL performance: Determine resources and limitations that contribute to the ineffective task performance

8. Plan and implement occupation-based intervention: May include adaptive occupation, occupational skills training, person factor or body functions training, and/or occupation-based education programs

9. Reevaluate for enhanced ADL task performance

Scoring

Following each AMPS observation, the person's overall quality of performance on the task regarding increased effort, decreased efficiency, decreased safety, and assistance is provided. The person's overall ability to live in the community is then rated as independently, with minimal assistance or supervision, or moderate to maximal assistance. Each of the 16 motor and 20 process skills are then scored as the following: competent performance that supports the action progression and yields good outcomes (4 points); questionable performance that yields uncertain outcomes (3 points); ineffective performance that disrupts or interferes with the actual progression and yields undesirable outcomes (2 points); or severely deficient performance that impedes the action progression and yields unacceptable outcomes (1 point; Fisher & Jones, 2014a).

The raw scores for each task observation are entered into the AMPS computer-scoring software to generate AMPS reports. The software considers the challenge of the various tasks, items of various difficulties, and the rater's severity. The AMPS measurement model, which incorporates the use of Rasch analysis, is able to account for these different facets to generate equal-interval, linear measures of the quality of individuals' ADL performance. When the data are subjected to Rasch analysis, the raw ordinal scores are converted into linear units of measurement called logits (i.e., log odds ratios). The software then generates the following AMPS reports:

- AMPS Performance Skill Summary
- AMPS Raw Score Report, AMPS Graphic Report (on which each client's ADL motor and ADL process ability measures are plotted along a continuum of more to less ability)
- Results and Interpretation Report
- Progress Report

Scores are then interpreted relative to a criterion of competence and via using a norm-based perspective (Fisher & Jones, 2014a). When ADL motor and ADL process ability measures are below the criterion-referenced cutoffs, it indicates that the person demonstrated at least some degree of clumsiness or increased physical effort (i.e., below the ADL motor cutoff at 2 logits) and/or some degree of inefficiency (time-space disorganization; i.e., below the ADL process cutoff at 1 logit).

Intervention Planning Based on Assessment Results

Interventions from the results of the AMPS may be guided by the American Occupational Therapy Association's (AOTA, 2014) *Occupational Therapy Practice Framework: Domain and Process, Third Edition*, as well as the Occupational Therapy Intervention Process Model (OTIPM; Fisher, 2009). Use of the OTIPM in conjunction with the *Framework* ensures that occupational therapy services are client centered, the evaluation occurs in a top-down manner, the evaluation and intervention methods used are occupation based and/or occupation focused, and the documentation is occupation focused (Fisher, 2009). Based on the results of the AMPS, the following intervention models may be utilized from the OTIPM (Fisher, 2009, 2013):

- Compensatory models: The planning and implementation of adaptive occupations that involve practicing and learning to perform daily life tasks using adaptive equipment, assistive technology, compensatory strategies, modifications to the physical environment, and/or modifications to the social environment.
- Educational models: The planning and implementation of educational programs for groups of clients that maintain a focus on learning about aspects of performance of daily life tasks.
- Acquisitional models: The planning and implementation of acquisitional occupations in the form of occupational skills training focused on the client reacquiring, developing, or maintaining occupational skill in the context of performing targeted daily life tasks.
- Restorative models: The planning and implementation of restorative occupations focused on the client restoring, developing, or maintaining person factors or underlying body functions in the context of performing relevant daily life tasks.

Consistent with the AOTA's (2014) *Framework*, the client-centered approach embraced by the AMPS helps to ensure that all goals and outcomes remain client centered throughout the occupational therapy process.

Case Study

Cliff is a 25-year-old man who is living with schizophrenia. He was first diagnosed in college, where he was in a pre-med program while working part time at a local deli. While his first 2 years in college were uneventful, he became increasingly disheveled, was paranoid that his roommate was stealing from him, began missing work and classes, and eventually developed psychotic features (i.e., hallucinations, thought disorders, delusions). He has been living with his parents since his diagnosis, has held multiple jobs for short periods, and spends most of his days in the basement watching television and playing video games. There has been increasing tension between Cliff and his parents as to his lack of family role and "not doing anything." Cliff is consistently fighting with his parents, stating that he would like to move out and that he would like to be on his own despite the lack of a plan. Cliff's parents spoke to the occupational therapist (Jeff) at the day program that Cliff inconsistently visits about this issue, reporting they could help him out financially but were concerned for his safety if he moved out.

Jeff decided to administer the AMPS as an objective way to measure whether Cliff would be safe on his own in the community. Cliff chose two AMPS tasks in conjunction with Jeff that he would be observed performing (Task R-1: shopping and Task I-23: packing a lunch). These tasks are considered being of average difficulty and harder than average, respectively.

In terms of rating quality of performance on the tasks, Jeff rated Cliff in the category "minimal" in regard to increased effort, decreased efficiency, decreased safety, and assistance provided. Jeff rated Cliff's overall ability to live in the community as with minimal assistance or supervision. In terms of specific performance skill items, several items were scored as questionable or ineffective performance. Examples of problematic specific items were the following: paces, attends, initiates, continues, adjusts, accommodates, calibrates, flow, and searches/locates. Cliff's raw scores were entered into the software and the AMPS Graphic Report was generated. Cliff was above the ADL motor cutoff but below the ADL process cutoff at 1 logit. ADL process ability measures that are below the cutoffs may indicate that the client demonstrated unsafe performance and/or needed assistance during the task performance. This confirmed Jeff's assessment that Cliff would need assistance to live in the community. After reviewing the findings with Cliff, Jeff shared the AMPS results with Cliff's parents after Cliff gave permission. Using the AMPS findings, Cliff and Jeff collaborated on an intervention plan that focused on compensatory strategies related to independent living skills (e.g., meal preparation, budgeting), as well as occupational skills training focused on the client reacquiring and developing independent living skills (e.g., community mobility, work tasks, housekeeping).

Evaluation of Social Interaction
Theoretical Basis

Concepts/Construct

The Evaluation of Social Interaction (ESI) is a standardized assessment of the quality of a person's social interaction that is directly observed and criterion referenced (Fisher & Griswold, 2014a). The purpose of the ESI is to establish an occupation-focused measurement of the quality of a person's social interaction as it is observed in a natural ecological context in order to provide a baseline performance, plan occupational therapy interventions, and assess change over time and/or the effectiveness of occupational therapy services. The ESI allows social interactions to be evaluated according to cultural expectations; it is both culture specific and not subject to cultural bias.

Key constructs that underlie the ESI include the following: Social interaction is the exchange of nonverbal and verbal communications and social behaviors between two or more people within the context of everyday activities. Social exchange is a specific social interaction event that serves a specific purpose. Social interaction skills, a type of performance skill, are the small, observable units of social behavior that can be viewed as more or less a social interaction skill or a performance error that reflects decreased social effectiveness or appropriateness (Fisher & Griswold, 2014a). The intended purpose of a social interaction is the desired goal of the person participating in the social exchange. Overall quality of social interaction is the entire evaluation of the person's competence while interacting with a social partner in a particular social exchange. The ESI quality of social interaction measure (ESI Measure) is a statistically computed number that represents a person's place on the continuum of social interaction quality. It is estimated using Rasch analysis and is based on 54 raw ESI item scores (27 for each social exchange). Weighting of the ESI items is based on their relative difficulties, the relative challenge of each type of social exchange (social exchange challenge), the relative severity of the individual rater, and each person's quality of social interaction (person ESI Measure).

Fisher's (2013) OTIPM explains how the ESI fits into occupational therapy practice. The key concepts of this model include the client-centered performance context, direct observation of the client's task performance, implementation of performance analysis of selected tasks, a true top-down clinical reasoning process that distinguishes between the client's observed and perceived problems, setting of client-centered and occupation-focused goals, planning and implementing occupation-based and/or occupation-focused interventions, and conclusion with a reevaluation stage (Fisher & Griswold, 2014a).

History of Development and Previous Versions/ Important Changes to Note in Current Version

The rationale for developing the ESI was the recognition of the importance of the quality of social interaction to participation in everyday activities. Social interaction is necessary for, and observable during, engagement in all occupations, including ADLs, IADLs, work, education, leisure, rest, and social participation and is an important determinant of a person's quality of life (Fisher & Griswold, 2014a). People with mental health issues often break social convention rules, which leads to their diagnosis and stigmatization. Other professionals have tried to measure social interaction by using rater checklists, questionnaires, role play, and videotaped scenarios. These have significant limitations, including being based on someone else's report or the client's self-report, which may not be reliable; emphasis placed on isolated parts of social interaction or underlying body functions rather than viewing a person's social interaction gestalt; do not reflect a person's real social interaction within a natural context; and do not evaluate both the sending and receiving of social messages (Fisher & Griswold, 2014a). Unlike other professionals, occupational therapists have the know-how to use and interpret an occupation-based assessment of social interaction within the context of occupational performance (Fisher & Griswold, 2014a).

The beginnings of the ESI are traced to the 1992 occupational therapy Doble and Magill-Evans taxonomy of social interaction. Englund, Bernspang, and Fisher (1995) expanded this model and created the Assessment of Social Interaction (ASI), which included 25 social interaction skills with operational definitions; it was also based on the Model of Human Occupation's Assessment of Communication and Interaction Skills. In 1995, Fisher and Kielhofner published Englund's taxonomy of social interaction skills, along with the taxonomies of motor and process skills, categorizing all of them as performance skills, which were distinguished from underlying physical, cognitive, or emotional body functions. The same methodology utilized by the AMPS and the School AMPS was adopted for the ASI, including the four-category rating scale and the format of defining each skill with scoring examples. From 2002 to 2006, Fisher further refined the social interaction skill definitions and related them to the World Health Organization's *International Classification of Functioning, Disability and Health* constructs (Fisher & Griswold, 2014a).

Fisher published the first research edition of the ESI in 2006, which entailed major revisions of operational definitions, scoring examples, and intended purposes of social interaction. In 2014, Fisher and Griswold (2014a) published the second research edition of the ESI, adding additional social interaction skills and further clarifying the intended purposes categories.

The first edition of the ESI was published by Fisher and Griswold in 2006, which measured 27 social interaction skills, included ratings of environmental and social partner characteristics, as well as used 6 intended purposes; the first edition was based on scores for 468 participants performed by 28 raters. The second edition of the ESI was published by Fisher and Griswold in 2010, which was based on 1140 participants with 98 raters and both criterion-based and norm-based interpretations became possible, including normative data for global age groups (9 to 15, 16 to 50, and 51 to 90 years). The third edition of the ESI, published in 2014 (Fisher & Griswold, 2014a), utilized 27 social interaction skills, 7 intended purposes, and 38 specific social interaction codes and was based on 6514 participants and 512 raters. This edition was accompanied by the release of the Occupational Therapy Assessment Package (OTAP), a software program that generates an ESI Results Report, an ESI Raw Scores Report, and an ESI Progress Report, which allow a person's quality of social interaction to be evaluated according to criterion- and norm-referenced standards (Fisher & Griswold, 2014a).

Psychometric Properties

Normative Data

The current edition of the ESI utilized a sample of 6552 participants for standardization purposes; approximately two thirds of the sample was composed of healthy individuals aged 2 to 92 years (Fisher & Griswold, 2014a). The sample was divided into the following six global groups: well persons; children at risk or persons with mild disabilities;

individuals with psychiatric disorders; individuals with developmental disabilities; individuals with neurological disorders; and individuals with medical conditions, dementia, and multiple and/or unknown disorders. Approximately half of the sample was men (43%). Approximately 30% of the sample were tested in Scandinavia, approximately 25% were Asian, approximately 20% were from the United Kingdom and Ireland, 11% were from Australia, 8% were from North America, and the remainder were from Europe (Fisher & Griswold, 2014a).

The mean ESI Quality of Social Interaction Measures (ESI Measures) are expressed as logits, which refer to log-odds probability units. In the ESI, logits refer to the linearized increments of quality of social interaction along the social interaction measurement scale. An analysis of variance test confirmed that there is a significant relationship between ESI Measures and age, with ESI Measures gradually increasing until age 18 years, plateauing in adulthood; however, from ages 30 to 39 years, there is a significantly higher mean ESI Measure and a gradual decline begins starting at age 70 years (Fisher & Griswold, 2014a). The ESI Measures or logits for the 4099 typically developing individuals in the standardization sample range from -1.3 logits for individuals aged 2 years to 0.8 logits for individuals aged 80 years and older (Fisher & Griswold, 2014a).

Reliability

Inter- and intrarater reliability have both been established for the ESI. The approach used to determine these two types of reliability for the ESI was to demonstrate that all individual raters scored each person in a consistent manner and each individual rater scored all of the persons he or she rated consistently using goodness of fit statistics with the Rasch model. According to Fisher and Griswold (2014a), in the ESI standardization sample of 6552 individuals, there were 511 raters; 96.5% of these raters demonstrated acceptable goodness of fit for both inter- and intrarater reliability, which supports high overall rater reliability for the ESI.

The ESI Measures have been found to be reliable when testing is repeated with a single individual or a group of individuals. When the ESI is administered, the person is usually observed in two separate social exchanges that differ in some way (i.e., intended purpose of the social exchange; familiarity, age, and quality of social interaction of the social partner; environment; time of day). Comparison of these two social exchange ratings are considered as separate but parallel and form a conservative estimate of reliability of the ESI Measure due to the potential sources of error that can occur. The ESI Measures for the sample of 6507 individuals comparison between the first and second social exchanges were the same for 59.8% of the raters, which revealed a high reliability coefficient of $r = .92$ (Fisher & Griswold, 2014a). The tradeoff between the stability of the ESI Measures and its concurrent ability to detect change or its sensitivity was also examined. A low standard error for ESI Measures combined with high reliability coefficients means that the ESI results between two sets of data adequately detected change while retaining its stability (Fisher & Griswold, 2014a).

Validity

Earlier versions of the ESI, including the ASI and research editions of the ESI, demonstrated that the instrument has a number of different types of validity because of its use of the Rasch analysis. Internal scale validity is defined as the inclusion of test items that are unidimensional (test only one concept). One way to determine internal scale validity is to make certain that at least 95% of the test items exhibit statistical goodness of fit with the Rasch model (Englund et al., 1995). Bond and Fox (2007) concluded that 21 of 25 items displayed acceptable goodness of fit with the Rasch model. The most recent study of internal scale validity of the ESI conducted by Asplund and Forsberg (2006) demonstrated that all but one item exhibited acceptable goodness of fit with the Rasch model.

Person response validity, defined as score patterns matching expectations of the model, is determined in a similar manner, and Englund et al. (1995) concluded that 14 of 16 participants demonstrated acceptable goodness of fit. High person response validity was seen in Simmons, Griswold, and Berg's (2010) more recent study of 128 individuals, aged 4 to 73 years, who were well adults and children, adults with neurological and psychiatric disabilities, and children with developmental disorders. Ninety-six percent of the participants demonstrated acceptable goodness of fit (Simmons et al., 2010).

Another important measure of the validity of an instrument is to determine if the normative values for the ESI are valid with both gender groups. A number of recent research studies indicate that the ESI is free of bias with regards to gender. For example, Søndergaard and Fisher (2012) did not find significant gender effects (F $[1,90] = 1.43$, $p = .24$) in a sample of gender-matched well adults ($n = 16$) or who had neurological/psychiatric disorders ($n = 16$).

Determining if an instrument is cross-culturally valid for testing people from different countries and world regions is accomplished by verifying that results apply in a similar way to people from different cultural backgrounds. Although it is believed that there are important cultural differences in social interaction skills and cultural norms of what is satisfactory social interaction, the ESI was designed to take into account the cultural expectations for good-mannered, considerate, and appropriately timed social interaction in the cultural context where the person is living. Fisher, Berg, and Saito (2012) looked at ESI results for 4075 participants from 8 countries/world regions, with 62% identified as well individuals and 38% with a disability. They did not find that any of the 48 intended purpose calibration comparisons among countries/world regions (8 countries/regions x 6 intended purposes) differed significantly. When Fisher and Griswold (2014a) investigated the most recent ESI standardization sample (5623 participants), they found that none of the 48 intended purpose calibration comparisons differed significantly by country/world region. They also compared item difficulty calibrations and found that less than 2% were significantly different among countries/regions. They concluded that the ESI items, as well as the intended purposes, were free of cross-cultural bias between global world regions (e.g., Asia and Scandinavia) and within world regions (e.g., Korea and Japan; Fisher et al., 2012).

Sensitivity

The ability of an instrument to differentiate among different groups and to detect change is referred to as its *sensitivity* and is another way to measure its validity. The ESI is able to detect differences within the well adult population who have differing levels of quality of social interaction. The ESI is also capable of distinguishing differences in quality of social interaction between well adults and adults with diagnosed stroke, schizophrenia, traumatic brain injury, and intellectual disabilities. The ESI was sensitive enough to detect differences between children who are typically developing and those with mild or at-risk disabilities. According to ESI results, children with identified disabilities have a significantly lower quality of social interaction than typically developing children (Fisher & Griswold, 2014a). The limitations of the ESI include that it cannot be used to evaluate children younger than age 2 years and people who do not attempt to communicate or cannot produce either spoken or signed speech (Fisher & Griswold, 2014a).

Assessment Administration

Area of Occupation/Performance Skills Assessed

All areas of occupation included in the *Framework* can involve social interaction skills (AOTA, 2014). These include ADLs, IADLs, rest and sleep, education, work, leisure and social participation (AOTA, 2014). Social participation involves the use of activities to support engagement in family and community, as well as involvement in a subgroup of activities that involve social exchanges. Many areas of occupation are usually carried out alone, such as bathing, showering, toileting, dressing, personal hygiene, and grooming, but if a person develops a problem in functioning independently, an aide or assistant may be necessary to help carry out these activities and necessitates the use of social interaction skills. When social skills are required for an occupation, they can be assessed with the ESI.

According to the *Framework*, performance skills are observable components of action that exemplify an implicit functional purpose and underlie people's ability to engage in activities and occupations (AOTA, 2014). Performance skills are subdivided into motor, process, and social interaction skills. The 27 social interaction skills listed in the *Framework* (AOTA, 2014) were derived from Fisher's body of work with the ESI and her OTIPM. The ESI assesses a person's quality of carrying out each of these 27 skills (Fisher & Griswold, 2014a).

Description of Environment/ Description of Supplies/Materials Required

After the initial referral for an occupational therapy evaluation of social interaction skills and the interview with the client to determine the types of social interaction that are of importance and of concern to the client, and the client has agreed to being observed, the time and place for two performances of social exchanges must be scheduled. Fisher and Griswold (2014a) refer to these environmental characteristics of the ESI as ecologically relevant settings with typical social partners. The ESI is best done in a real setting where the problematic social interaction typically takes place with the client's actual social partners. If it is not possible to observe the client in his or her typical physical and social environment, an alternative setting needs to be chosen, which is ideally selected and any obstacles are negotiated with the client and therapist. The alternative setting must contain similar contextual characteristics to the actual setting in terms of the types of social interaction allowed, usual noise level, number of people, and a matching primary social partner. The setting and primary social partners in the two observed social exchanges should be different (Fisher & Griswold, 2014a).

Materials required for the ESI include a pencil and paper for the therapist to take observational notes that capture the progression of the social exchange, as well as the timing of the social interaction. The therapist must record what was said as well as the nonverbal messages and behaviors, including each speaker's tone of voice and gestures. Several note-taking strategies are suggested for the ESI, including dividing the paper into columns for Words Heard, Notes Taken, and Interpretations of Observations. Therapists must try to record the types of messages sent, as well as the types of response given in reply, categorizing it as a Comment (C), Question (Q), Suggestion (S), or Opinion (O).

Administration

The ESI begins with an interview to identify social interaction concerns with the client or the client's constellation (i.e., the people the client lives or works with and who experience problems interacting with the client). The most important purpose of the interview is to determine if an ESI observation would be helpful and what are the social interactions that concern the client. While developing therapeutic rapport with the client, the therapist gathers information about contextual external and internal factors, contextual resources and limitations, and client-reported strengths and limitations of task performance related to social interaction. The therapist decides if the ESI should be administered and identifies the types of social situations that the client desires to change.

The occupational therapist observes the client in at least 2 social exchanges with a client-selected purpose and scores the occupational performances on 27 social interaction skills (ESI items) within ecologically relevant contexts and with social partners who are part of, or similar to, real members of the client constellation. The ESI allows the therapist to observe limitless social exchanges that meet one of seven global purposes (i.e., gathering information from others; sharing information with others; problem solving or decision making; collaborating and producing; acquiring goods and services; providing or serving goods and services; conversing socially or engaging in small talk). The intended purposes of the two social exchanges that are observed should be different.

The 27 ESI items are organized into 7 categories that describe the universal performance skills that are a part of all social exchanges: (1) initiating and terminating social interaction; (2) producing social interaction; (3) physically supporting social interaction; (4) shaping content of social interaction; (5) maintaining flow of social interaction; (6) verbally supporting social interaction; and (7) adapting social interaction.

There are a number of practical considerations that the therapist must attend to during the observation: (1) diminishing the impact of the therapist on the social exchange under observation; (2) determining the beginning and ending of a social interaction; (3) deciding when it is suitable to observe two or more consecutive social exchanges; (4) deciding if an observed social exchange was too easy; (5) handling unexpected and disruptive social interactions; and (6) defining who is the primary social partner.

Scoring

Each of the two social exchange observations are scored on the ESI Score Form using the following recording steps: (1) demographic information; (2) characteristics of each observed social exchange; (3) the number of social partners and identification of the primary social partner; (4) characteristics of the primary social partner; (5) overall comfort level; (6) person's overall quality of social interaction; (7) primary social partner's overall quality of social interaction; and (8) score for each of the 27 ESI items (Fisher & Griswold, 2014a). The ESI raw scores are recorded one by one for both social exchanges using a standardized procedure to ensure valid and reliable results. The best way to do this is to use the ESI item definitions and scoring examples that are contained in Appendix G of the ESI manual. The therapist must match up the observed client's social behavior and level of skill with the criteria for each score.

A general principle for scoring the ESI items is that they are criterion referenced, not norm referenced, and that the criterion that is utilized is competence, which means social appropriateness, social maturity, and the absence of any disruption of social interaction. Each ESI item is rated on a four-category rating scale: 4 = competent performance,

3 = questionable performance, 2 = ineffective performance, and 1 = severely limited performance. Explicit rules for scoring include the following:

- Each skill is considered separately.
- When in doubt between two scores, the lower score is given.
- Competent skill is displayed by socially appropriate interaction.
- The therapists do not base any of their scores on what they think the person should, could, or might have done, but only on what messages were heard, behaviors were observed, and responses were given.

The final step of scoring involves entering the scores into the computer's OTAP software, which performs a multifaceted Rasch analysis that simultaneously adjusts for three factors: (1) the amount of challenge of the social exchange's intended purpose; (2) the difficulties of each ESI item; and (3) the rater calibration severity of the rater. The OTAP converts the ESI raw score into a single, linear quality of social interaction measure (the ESI Measure), which is reported in all documentation (Fisher & Griswold, 2014a). The preliminary report contains a Summary of Main Findings, including Criterion-Referenced and Norm-Referenced Findings and Specific Findings, which itemize the person's most competent social interaction skills and the specific social interaction skills that diminish the quality of the person's social interaction.

Intervention Planning Based on Assessment Results: Utilizing *Occupational Therapy Practice Framework* Language

The therapist uses the ESI report to interpret and document the results of the ESI, as well as to create and document the client's goals. The ESI utilizes language from the *Framework* (AOTA, 2014) to evaluate the performance skills pertaining to social interaction skills. After categorizing social interaction skills into strengths and limitations, the therapist creates clusters of interrelated behaviors for both strong and limiting social interaction skills using terminology and observable examples of behavior from the *Framework* (AOTA, 2014). Based on the clusters, baseline statements are developed. After interpreting the person's ESI Measure compared to the competence criterion, the therapist can compare the person's ESI Measure to the social interaction measures of well individuals of the same age using a norm-based perspective. The therapist then collaborates with the client to decide upon client-centered, occupation-focused goals, which will target particular areas of occupational performance involving social interaction skills that are important to the client. The therapist has the option of entering the person's skill item clusters, baseline statements, and occupation-focused goals into the OTAP software to generate a Final ESI Results Report (Fisher & Griswold, 2014a).

Using the ESI item difficulty hierarchy, the therapist establishes priorities for intervention. Clients obtain greater success when they begin working on easier rather than more challenging skills, as well as skills they acknowledge being a problem. In order to plan an effective intervention, the therapist analyzes what resources and barriers within the client's performance context are impacting the person's clusters of limited social skills. A model for intervention is selected from one of the following: adapting the occupation, including its methods, equipment, and environment; designing educational programs, such as seminars and workshops that promote discussion of occupational performance; focusing on occupational skills training that promotes the attainment of skills within the natural environment of doing the occupation; or concentrating on training of body functions, which are underlying physical, cognitive, and emotional capacities (Fisher & Griswold, 2014a).

Case Study

Bruce was referred for an occupational therapy evaluation due to his perceived difficulties on the job. The occupational therapist, Elyse, gathered information in an interview with Bruce about the external and internal contextual factors that were impacting his occupational performance. After interviewing Bruce's boss, the occupational therapist learned that there had been customer and coworker complaints about Bruce's work enough so that the boss was considering letting him go, even though the boss would like to be supportive. Bruce works in an office as a navigator for the state health care plan. He spends a lot of time on the phone, but on some projects, he is required to work with other staff members. The occupational therapist then focused on the specific types of social interactions required for his job, the ones that were easier and those that were more challenging for him. Bruce told the occupational therapist that he liked making small talk during breaks with his coworkers (Conversing Socially/Small Talk), but he was very irritated by having to listen to customers that "go on and on and do not get to the point" (Gathering Information) and collaborating with his coworkers on a planning project where he said he becomes confused and overwhelmed (Problem Solving or Decision Making). The occupational therapist asked Bruce if she could observe him while he was talking to a customer and while working on a project with coworkers. Although Bruce was not okay with allowing the occupational therapist to listen during a privileged phone conversation, he said he would not mind being observed at work with his coworkers if his boss did not object. They made arrangements with Bruce's boss for the occupational therapist to observe him at work. Bruce was comfortable telling his coworkers that Elyse was observing him to help him improve his work skills.

Once Elyse arrived at the worksite, she no longer interacted with Bruce and became an observer. She observed him in two social exchanges with his coworkers. The first was in the lounge with one coworker where Bruce was able to make coffee and appropriately share that he had watched four basketball games over the weekend. He also inquired about his coworker's plans for the upcoming weekend. The second social exchange was with his team of two other staff members and the team leader. The team leader presented a work plan that required the division of labor among all present. Bruce immediately became defensive, stating that he always worked harder than everyone else in the office. He did not make eye contact and turned away in his seat from the three others at the table. The team leader tried to reassure Bruce that everyone was working harder because of increased enrollment in the health plan. Bruce became argumentative, stating that he had a harder time because he had to deal with so many "whiny, long-winded customers." The team leader acknowledged that there were many problems with the computer system and individual clients could be "really challenging!" After arguing, Bruce stood up and left the room.

Elyse took notes during each social exchange. She organized her notes. She scored both social exchanges on two ESI Score Forms, using the ESI item definitions and scoring examples that are contained in Appendix G of the ESI manual to rate each ESI item. She entered 4s (readily and consistently) for Approaches/Starts and Concludes/Disengages for the first social exchange that involved Conversing Socially/Small Talk. She scored 1s (severely limited) for Turns Toward, Looks, Regulates, Expresses Emotions, and Disagrees for the second social exchange that involved Problem Solving or Decision Making. She entered all of his raw scores into the *Framework* (AOTA, 2014) and received an ESI Measure of 0.5 for Bruce, which revealed that he was mildly to moderately ineffective and/or immature at social interaction. She established goals collaboratively with Bruce that would enable him to address his clustered limitations in social interaction skills, including the following: Looks, Turns Toward (Bruce will make eye contact with coworkers at least 25% of the time), Disagrees, and Expresses Emotions (Bruce will express disagreement with coworkers in a socially appropriate manner, using a respectful volume and tone; Fisher & Griswold, 2014a).

The collaboratively developed intervention plan followed the educational model. Bruce became upset when interacting with demanding customers. He lacked assertiveness and listening skills and carried this anger inappropriately into his team meeting. He did not realize that his coworkers also found some customers challenging. The team leader began a series of classes that focused on developing strategies to deal with problematic customers. Using the ESI enabled Bruce to feel better understood by his team leader and coworkers and helped to improve his ESI scores when the occupational therapist reevaluated him 3 months later after the conclusion of the educational classes, and he was able to keep his job.

Multiple Errands Test
Theoretical Basis

Concepts/Construct

The Multiple Errands Test (MET) is an assessment of the impact of executive function impairments on the performance of a shopping task within a real-world context. Its purpose is to predict the ability of clients with mild cognitive impairments whose difficulties are not detected by traditional neuropsychological tests to carry out everyday tasks in naturalistic surroundings.

Keys constructs that underlie the MET include the following: the meaning of executive function; traditional tests of executive function; the difference between real-world assessments of executive function and performance-based tests of executive function; and the need for site-specific tests and lack of a standardized scoring system for the many versions of the MET. *Executive function* refers to a combination of high-level cognitive skills that includes initiating, planning, hypothesizing, thinking flexibly, making decisions, monitoring of the self, incorporating feedback, and making judgments (Dawson et al., 2009). It is most noticeably manifested when a person is challenged by novel, nonroutine experiences that are endemic to daily life. Traditional office-based, pencil-and-paper neuropsychological tests of executive function, such as the Stroop Test and the WCST, were not created to measure deficits that are most apparent in the management of the unpredictable complexity of everyday functioning, but rather were developed to measure significant problems at the impairment level. The MET, originally developed by psychologists Shallice and Burgess (1991), requires site-specific adaptations and local maps and has resulted in the creation of several different versions. Occupational therapists Morrison et al. (2013) remedied the MET's lack of a standardized and objective rating scale, as well as norms that distinguish scores for healthy participants and those with mild executive function deficits.

History of Development and Previous Versions/ Important Changes to Note in Current Version

Shallice and Burgess created the original MET in 1991 and discovered significant differences between inpatients and healthy controls in organization, rule breaks, and efficiency in the following tasks: clients had to shop in several stores for a list of items with a limited amount of money, check in with the evaluator 15 minutes into the test, and gather four specific types of information. Newer versions include the following: Knight, Alderman, and Burgess (2002) created a simpler version (MET-HV) for hospitalized patients in a hospital gift shop; Alderman, Burgess, Knight, and Henman (2003) designed one for a community shopping center or outpatient setting (MET-SV); and Rand, Basha-Abu Rukan, Weiss, and Katz (2009) designed a virtual MET (V-MET). Dawson et al. (2009) created the Baycrest version of the MET, which compared the performance of 27 outpatients with traumatic brain injury or stroke with healthy controls and further established the MET-HV's interrater reliability and ecological validity. Morrison et al. (2013) based the newest version (MET-R) on the earlier hospital versions but created an administration manual and an observation form, defined efficiency in terms of rule breaks, and developed a simple scoring system with operationally defined measures of total time, the number of locations visited, the number of tasks completed, the total rule breaks, and performance efficiency. The purpose of the MET-R is to increase its usefulness within the clinic, as well as its user-friendliness for the examiner.

Psychometric Properties

Normative Data

The normative sample for the original version of the MET consisted of three healthy controls (Shallice & Burgess, 1991). The normative sample for the Baycrest version was 25 healthy matched controls (Dawson et al., 2009). The normative sample for the MET-R was 21 matched control participants. According to Asher (2014), there are cutoff scores for numbers of errors for different MET versions when comparing clients to healthy participants; 7 total errors on the MET-HV indicates impaired functioning, whereas 12 total errors on the MET-SV is an indicator of impairment. In addition to the total rule breaks, the MET-R created a new score, performance efficiency, which is the ratio of the total number of tasks ($n = 17$) divided by the total number of locations needed to complete all the tasks ($n = 5$); the perfect performance efficiency for the MET-R (3.4) was normalized to a score of 1.0 (Morrison et al., 2013).

Reliability

With the MET-SV, Alderman et al. (2003) found interrater reliability that ranged from (0.81) on the score of interpretation failures and (1.00) on rule breaks with an internal consistency measured with Cronbach's alpha score of 0.77 (Asher, 2014). With the Baycrest version of the MET, the interclass correlation coefficients were high (0.71 to 0.88; Dawson et al., 2009). With the MET-R, interrater reliability for all test sections was extremely high, with interclass correlation coefficients of 1.00 (Asher, 2014).

Validity

Many types of validity have been established for the MET-SV, MET-HV, V-MET, and MET-R, including ecological, face, and construct. *Ecological validity*, defined as the degree to which a deficient score on the test relates to problems with daily functioning, has been established with significant correlations between scores on the MET-R and Baycrest version and other standardized measures of executive function and IADL performance (Dawson et al., 2009). For example, the MET-R discriminated between participants with and without mild cerebrovascular accident ($p = .002$) on the following assessments: the National Institutes of Health Stroke Scale, which measures stroke-related neurological impairment; the Functional Independence Measure; the Stroke Impact Scale; and the EFPT (Morrison et al., 2013). The Baycrest version revealed good to strong correlations ($p > .50$) between the MET-SV and other standardized measures of IADL and everyday function, including the Dysexecutive Questionnaire, the Mayo-Portland Adaptability Inventory, the Sickness Impact Profile, and the AMPS (Dawson et al., 2009). Due to the fact that all task performance is directly observed, all versions of the MET have good face validity (Asher, 2014). Concurrent validity was established for the MET-R by correlating scores with EFPT results, a valid measure of executive function in people who are post stroke. A moderate correlation of $r = -.55$ was found, which was expected due to differences in task demands, the support of the examiner, and the amount of structure in the testing environment (Morrison et al., 2013).

Sensitivity

The ability of an instrument to differentiate among different groups and to detect change is referred to as its *sensitivity* and is another way to measure its validity. All of the MET versions have distinguished between people with brain lesions, including traumatic brain injury and stroke, and matched healthy controls. For example, performance on the Baycrest version significantly discriminated between people with acquired brain injury and healthy controls ($p < .05$; Dawson et al., 2009). Published reports of the use of the MET with different groups of psychiatric patients include La Paglia et al.'s (2013) study of the V-MET with groups with obsessive-compulsive disorder and schizophrenia disorders and Caletti et al.'s (2013) study of the MET-HV with patients with bipolar and schizophrenia disorders; both research studies included healthy controls. Both clinical populations made more inefficiency errors than healthy controls on the V-MET, including not using the map, not making reference to the task instruction list during the test, and not demonstrating the ability to recognize their own errors and self-correct, even though on standard neuropsychological tests, such as the Mini Mental State Examination, the patients with obsessive-compulsive disorder had results more similar to the healthy controls than the patients with schizophrenia (La Paglia et al., 2013). Both patient groups in Caletti et al.'s (2013) research completed significantly fewer tasks and made more task errors than the healthy controls on the MET-HV. Gillen and Raphael-Greenfield have unpublished data from the evaluation of clients with extensive histories of substance use using the Baycrest version of the MET that documented rule breaks, incomplete tasks, inefficiency, and extended use of time.

Assessment Administration

Area of Occupation/Performance Skills/ Performance Patterns/Client Factors Assessed

The areas of occupation evaluated by the MET are IADLs, with specific attention to shopping and community mobility. The performance skills assessed within the MET are primarily the process skills, including the following: paces, attends, heeds, chooses, inquires, initiates, continues, sequences, terminates, searches/locates, gathers, navigates, notices/responds, and adjusts. The client factors addressed within the MET include the higher-level cognitive and executive function.

Description of Environment/ Description of Supplies/Materials Required

The environments of the MET have varied with each real-world version of a different shopping place, including hospital gift shops (Dawson et al., 2009; Knight et al., 2002; Morrison et al., 2013), a shopping mall (Alderman et al., 2003), and two virtual reality versions (Rand et al., 2009; Raspelli et al., 2010). Some versions have necessitated access to postal drops and house phones, but modification of the local maps published with each of the different versions is expected and encouraged.

The main supplies and materials usually required include a clipboard, a task list that contains the purchase of small food/candy/drink items, a rule list, a map of the shopping area and hospital lobby, money, a blank greeting card and envelope, access to a watch or clock, a backpack, and a pen or pencil.

Administration

All of the versions involve the examiner observing the participant with the proviso that the participant cannot speak to the examiner unless it is one of the tasks. All of the versions determine in some way that the participant has read and understood all of the instructions and rules before self-initiating the test. All versions provide the participants with a task and rule list, as well as a map of the shopping area, and require the participants to perform 12 to 17 tasks, which must be completed within the constraints of 9 rules. All versions time the test, and some tests terminate the test after 45 minutes even if the participant has not completed all of the tasks (Morrison et al., 2013). During the test administration, the examiner follows the participant from an observable distance and documents performance on a site-specific scoring form (Dawson et al., 2009; Morrison et al., 2013).

Scoring

All participants rate themselves on expected and real performance using a Likert scale before beginning any of the versions of the test by checking off statements ranging from hopeless to excellent. Scoring of all versions is based on the number of errors made by the participant, including inefficiencies, rule breaks, failures of interpretation, task failure, and incorrectly asking the examiner for help (Morrison et al., 2013). The MET-R records total scores (including time), locations visited, tasks, passes (times participant visits any location), and rule breaks (Asher, 2014). The MET-R has created a reliable, more objective scoring system that can be used with the local versions of the test.

Intervention Planning Based on Assessment Results

The MET is especially useful for the clinical identification of people who appear to be unimpaired and do not present with memory, attention, or motor skill problems but who exhibit executive function difficulties in their daily lives in complex, naturalistic environments. Several features of the MET make it more relevant to clinical practice because of the ways it increases executive function challenge by increasing task novelty, using multiple overlapping task demands, and the adoption of novel rules while carrying out familiar tasks and routines. All of these features may increase the sensitivity of the MET to elusive executive function difficulties (Morrison et al., 2013). Clients with these types of problems are usually discharged without follow-up care because their deficits are not detected by routine rehabilitation tests. At home, they often self-impose their own restrictions on their daily functioning, avoiding complex and demanding environments, such as busy stores and other community sites, and not returning to overstimulating work environments. With younger, better-educated people experiencing more subtle executive function impairments due to increased incidence of mild cerebrovascular accidents, a test such as the MET will have important clinical utility in the future. Morrison et al. (2013) have suggested the importance of using the MET-R with acute inpatients who do not have insight into the nature of their problems with daily functioning before they are discharged to increase their awareness. In addition, the MET requires interactions with strangers, which could present additional challenges for people with executive function, self-confidence, and social cognition problems.

Case Study

Ann was referred for an occupational therapy evaluation of her readiness to be discharged from a psychiatric inpatient unit where she has been stabilized on medications and participated consistently in all individual and group treatment sessions on the unit for 4 weeks. She was diagnosed with schizophrenia, and this was her first hospitalization. She is in her mid-20s and lives with her husband. She will attend a partial hospitalization program, as well as a psychosocial club for 2 months and then plans to return to work. She states that she is eager to be discharged. When asked what problems she anticipates she will have post discharge she states, "None!" With the occupational therapist she takes the elevator down to the hospital's busy lobby where she states that the crowds are making "me feel real nervous." The therapist walks with her to a quiet corner where they can talk quietly, carry out some deep breathing, and review the test materials together. After Ann feels calmer, she completes the Likert scale check-off form rating her expected performance, listens to the therapist's reading of the task and rule lists, makes a mark on the map indicating her current location in the lobby, and repeats both the task and rule lists aloud to the therapist.

Although Ann has completed all of the preliminary steps and is deemed ready to begin the test, she dawdles and requires further encouragement to begin. She begins by buying a Pepsi and a birthday card rather than the indicated Coca-Cola and get well card; it takes her 8 minutes to choose the card and 10 minutes to decide on a bag of chips and a candy bar. She does not buy any stamps at the gift shop nor does she mail the addressed envelope to her doctor. From a distance, the therapist notes that Ann is not using the map to help her complete the test nor is she using her watch to keep track of time. After 10 minutes, she does not meet the therapist at the main information desk as instructed nor does she make the telephone call to the occupational therapy office. Ann is able to obtain the opening and closing times of the gift shop and the price of a candy bar, but she leaves blank the number of entrances/exits on the first floor of the hospital lobby. After 45 minutes, the therapist tells Ann that the test is over.

On the way back to the unit, Ann states that she is "relieved" that she has finished the test and expresses new concerns about her readiness for discharge. The therapist scores Ann's results and found 10 total errors, which indicates impaired performance when compared with healthy samples. The results of the MET are shared with Ann and her husband in the next family meeting. It is decided that her discharge will be delayed by 1 week, and her husband has agreed to take time off from his job to accompany his wife to her partial hospitalization program and psychosocial club until she feels acclimated to these new contexts. The results of the MET will be shared with the occupational therapist in the partial hospitalization program who will continue to address executive function skills in real-life situations with Ann.

An Overview of Neuropsychological Assessments

As it is common for occupational therapy practitioners to work on interprofessional teams, it is important to have some understanding of the assessments used by our colleagues in other disciplines (e.g., psychology, neuropsychology, neurology, psychiatry). Three common examples of valid and reliable tools are the Montreal Cognitive Assessment (MoCA; Nasreddine et al., 2005), the Saint Louis Mental Status Examination (Tariq, Tumosa, Chibnall, Perry, & Morley, 2006), and the Mini Mental State Examination (Folstein, Folstein, & McHugh, 1975). As summarized in Table 10-1, these tools aim to document the presence or absence of various cognitive impairments. The findings from these tools may help the occupational therapist corroborate his or her findings, help clarify findings when there are discrepancies in the observations of everyday tasks, or help the occupational therapist focus his or her observations if he or she has the findings prior to the occupational therapy evaluation. For example, the MoCA evaluates attention deficits via repeating a list of digits forward and backward, serial subtraction by 7 starting at 100, and indicating every time the letter "A" is heard when a list of letters is read. As the occupational therapist prepares for an observation of meal preparation, he or she may keep these findings in mind to help organize observations of potential errors that may be made due to attention deficits during the meal preparation observation. Examples may include the following:

- Background noise distracts the client, leading to task interruption and "off-task" behaviors (poor selective attention/distraction)
- Not being able to monitor two burners at the same time (poor dividing of attention)

- Requiring cues to continue the cooking tasks (decreased sustained attention/vigilance)
- And/or not able to attend back to the task of cooking after a brief social conversation with the therapist (poor attentional switching)

Summary

Clients with major mental illness and substance use disorders often obtain normal results on office-based psychological and neuropsychological tests given in quiet, distraction-free environments that are under the complete control of the evaluator. They proceed to have difficulty functioning in their communities, which is often confirmed by behavioral observation, self-report, and reports by significant others. The AMPS, the ESI, and the MET provide valid and reliable measures of easily overlooked problems of executive and social functioning for people with mental health issues in everyday living in stressful and cognitively and socially complex occupational environments. Occupational therapists have a professional obligation to link their assessments and interventions with the everyday lives and functioning of their clients and the expertise to utilize performance-based assessments with proven ecological validity as their primary mode of evaluation.

References

Alderman, N., Burgess, P. W., Knight, C., & Henman, C. (2003). Ecological validity of a simplified version of the Multiple Errands Shopping Test. *Journal of the International Neuropsychological Society, 9*, 31-44.

American Occupational Therapy Association. (2014). Occupational therapy practice framework: Domain and process (3rd ed.). *American Journal of Occupational Therapy, 68*(Suppl. 1), S1-S48.

Asher, I. E. (2014). *Asher's assessment tools: An annotated index for occupational therapy* (4th ed.). Bethesda, MD: AOTA Press.

Asplund, M., & Forsberg, E. (2006). *Evaluation of social interaction skills of persons with good overall social ability: One step towards establishing the usability of the ESI version 2.* Unpublished bachelor thesis, Department of Occupational Therapy, Umea University, Umea, Sweden.

Baum, C. M., Connor, L. T., Morrison, T., Hahn, M., Dromerick, A. W., & Edwards, D. F. (2008). Reliability, validity, and clinical utility of the Executive Function Performance Test: A measure of executive function in a sample of people with stroke. *American Journal of Occupational Therapy, 62*, 446-455.

Berg, E. A. (1948). A simple objective technique for measuring flexibility in thinking. *Journal of General Psychology, 39*, 15-22.

Bond, T. G., & Fox, C. M. (2007). *Applying the Rasch model: Fundamental measurement in the human sciences* (2nd ed.). Mahwah, NJ: Lawrence Erlbaum.

Caletti, E., Paoli, R. A., Fiorentini, A., Cigliobianco, M., Zugno, E., Serati, M., ... Altamura, A. C. (2013). Neuropsychology, social cognition and global functioning among bipolar, schizophrenic patients and healthy controls: Preliminary data. *Frontiers in Human Neuroscience, 7*(661), 1-14.

Chaytor, N., & Schmitter-Edgecombe, M. (2003). The ecological validity of neuropsychological tests: A review of the literature on everyday cognitive skills. *Neuropsychology Review, 13*, 181-197.

Dawson, D. R., Anderson, N. D., Burgess, P., Cooper, E., Krpan, K. M., & Stuss, D. T. (2009). Further development of the Multiple Errands Test: Standardized scoring, reliability, and ecological validity for the Baycrest version. *Archives of Physical Medicine and Rehabilitation, 90*(11 Suppl.), S41-S51.

Englund, B., Bernspang, B., & Fisher, A. G. (1995). Development of an instrument for assessment of social interaction skills in occupational therapy. *Scandinavian Journal of Occupational Therapy, 2*, 17-23.

Fisher, A. G. (2009). *Occupational therapy intervention process model: A model for planning and implementing top-down, client-centered, and occupation-based interventions.* Ft. Collins, CO: Three Star Press.

Fisher, A. G. (2013). Occupation-centered, occupation-based, occupation-focused: Same, same or different? *Scandinavian Journal of Occupational Therapy, 20*, 162-173.

Fisher, A. G., Berg, B., & Saito, S. (2012). *Is it possible to develop a cross-cultural test of social interaction?* Paper presented at the International Symposium on Implementing Occupation-Focused and Occupation-Based Services, Copenhagen, Denmark.

Fisher, A. G., & Griswold, L. A. (2006). *Evaluation of social interaction.* Fort Collins, CO: Three Star Press.

Fisher, A. G., & Griswold, L. A. (2010). *Evaluation of social interaction* (2nd ed.). Fort Collins, CO: Three Star Press.

Fisher, A. G., & Griswold, L. A. (2014a). *Evaluation of social interaction* (3rd ed.). Fort Collins, CO: Three Star Press.

Fisher, A. G., & Griswold, L. A. (2014b). Performance skills: Implementing performance analyses to evaluate quality of occupational performance. In B. A. B. Schell, G. Gillen, M. E. Scaffa, & E. S. Cohn (Eds.), *Willard & Spackman's occupational therapy* (12th ed., pp. 249-264). Philadelphia, PA: Wolters Kluwer.

Fisher, A. G., & Jones, K. B. (2014a). *Assessment of motor and process skills. Vol. 1: Development, standardization, and administration manual* (7th ed.). Fort Collins, CO: Three Star Press.

Fisher, A. G., & Jones, K. B. (2014b). *Assessment of motor and process skills. Vol. 2: User manual* (8th ed.). Fort Collins, CO: Three Star Press.

Fisher, A. G., & Kielhofner, G. (1995). Skill in occupational performance. In G. Kielhofner, *A model of human occupation: Theory and application* (2nd ed.). Baltimore, MD: Williams & Williams.

Fisher, A. G., Liu, Y., Velozo, C., & Pan, A. W. (1992). Cross-cultural assessment of process skills. *American Journal of Occupational Therapy, 46,* 876-885.

Folstein, M. F., Folstein, S. E., & McHugh, P. R. (1975). "Mini-mental state." A practical method for grading the cognitive state of patients for the clinician. *Journal of Psychiatric Research, 12,* 189-198.

Kirkley, K. N., & Fisher, A. G. (1999). Alternate forms reliability of the Assessment of Motor and Process Skills. *Journal of Outcome Measurement, 3,* 53-70.

Knight, C., Alderman, N., & Burgess, P. W. (2002). Development of a simplified version of the Multiple Errands Test for use in hospital settings. *Neuropsychological Rehabilitation, 12,* 231-255.

Knowles, F. E. III. (1995). Memories of Dr. Dunton. *Maryland Psychiatrist Newsletter.* Retrieved from http://www.dunton.org/archive/biographies/William_Rush_Dunton_Jr.htm

La Paglia, F., La Cascia, C., Cipresso, P., Rizzo, R., Francomano, A., Riva, G., & La Barbera, D. (2013). Psychometric assessment using classic neuropsychological and virtual reality based test: A study in obsessive-compulsive disorder (OCD) and schizophrenic patients. Lecture Notes of the Institute for Computer Sciences, Social-Informatics and Telecommunications Engineering, LNICST 05/2014. In *4th International Symposium on Pervasive Computing Paradigms for Mental Health, MindCare 2014.*

Moore, K., Merritt, B. K., & Doble, S. E. (2010). ADL skill profiles across three psychiatric diagnoses. *Scandinavian Journal of Occupational Therapy, 17,* 77-85.

Morrison, M. T., Giles, G. M., Ryan, J. D., Baum, C. M., Dromerick, A. W., Polatajko, H. J., & Edwards, D. F. (2013). Multiple Errands Test—Revised (MET-R): A performance-based measure of executive function in people with mild cerebrovascular accident. *American Journal of Occupational Therapy, 67,* 460-468.

Nasreddine, Z. S., Phillips, N. A., Bédirian, V., Charbonneau, S., Whitehead, V., Collin, I., … Chertkow, H. (2005). The Montreal Cognitive Assessment (MoCA): A brief screening tool for mild cognitive impairment. *Journal of the American Geriatrics Society, 53,* 695-699.

Rand, D., Basha-Abu Rukan, S., Weiss, P. L., & Katz, N. (2009). Validation of the Virtual MET as an assessment tool for executive functions. *Neuropsychological Rehabilitation, 19,* 583-602.

Raspelli, S., Carelli, L., Morganti, F., Poletti, B., Corra, B., Silani, V., & Riva, G. (2010). Implementation of the multiple errands test in a NeuroVR-supermarket: A possible approach. *Studies in Health Technology and Informatics, 154,* 115-119.

Rockwood, K., Doble, S. E., Fisk, J. D., MacPherson, K. M., & Lewis, N. (1996). *Measuring functional change in elderly adults with Alzheimer's disease.* Final report to Alzheimer Society of Canada. Halifax, Nova Scotia, Canada: Dalhousie University.

Shallice, T., & Burgess, P. W. (1991). Deficits in strategy application following frontal lobe damage in man. *Brain, 114,* 727-741.

Simmons, C. D., Griswold, L. A., & Berg, B. (2010). Evaluation of social interaction during occupational engagement. *American Journal of Occupational Therapy, 64,* 10-17.

Søndergaard, M., & Fisher, A. G. (2012). Sensitivity of the Evaluation of Social Interaction Measures Among people with and without neurologic or psychiatric disorders. *American Journal of Occupational Therapy, 66*(3), 356-362. http://dx.doi.org/10.5014/ajot.2012.003582

Tariq, S. H., Tumosa, N., Chibnall, J. T., Perry, M. H. III, & Morley, J. E. (2006). Comparison of the Saint Louis University Mental Status Examination and the Mini-Mental State Examination for detecting dementia and mild neurocognitive disorder—A pilot study. *American Journal Geriatric Psychiatry, 14,* 900-910.

Wilson, B. A., Evans, J. J., Emslie, H., Alderman, N., & Burgess, P. (1998). The development of an ecologically valid test for assessing patients with a dysexecutive syndrome. *Neuropsychological Rehabilitation, 8,* 213-228.

Cognitive Disabilities Model
Allen Cognitive Level Screen–5 and Allen Diagnostic Module (2nd Edition) Assessments

Catherine A. Earhart, BA, OT Cert, OTR/L
Deane B McCraith, MS, OT/L, LMFT

Self-fulfillment is a combination of what the person can do (cognitively realistic), will do (psychologically relevant), and may do (contextually and environmentally possible). Self-fulfillment is experienced while doing significant activities that use one's full capacity to function. … Occupational therapy … reaffirm(s) the right of each individual, no matter how disabled, to engage in self-fulfilling activities.
(Allen, 1994)

The Cognitive Disabilities Model (CDM) is an intervention model designed to guide occupational therapy practice with individuals who have temporary or permanent cognitive disabilities or impairments that affect safe participation in valued daily activities (Allen, 1982, 1985; Allen & Blue, 1998; Allen, Earhart, & Blue, 1992; McCraith & Earhart, 2018). This chapter features two standardized, theory-, performance-, observation-, and evidence-based assessments associated with the CDM:

1. Three forms of the Allen Cognitive Level Screen, version 5: Allen Cognitive Level Screen–5 (ACLS-5) and Large Allen Cognitive Level Screen–5 (LACLS-5; Allen, Austin, David, Earhart, McCraith, & Riska-Williams, 2007) and Disposable Large Allen Cognitive Level Screen–5 (LACLS-5[D]; Allen Cognitive Group/ACLS and LACLS Committee, 2016).

2. Allen Diagnostic Module (2nd Edition [ADM-2]; Earhart, 2006).

A third assessment associated with the CDM, the Routine Task Inventory–Expanded (RTI-E; Katz, 2006), is featured in Chapter 12.

These assessments are measures of functional cognition for individuals with existing or suspected changes in cognitive capacities that impact their functional performance. Occupational therapy practitioners use scores from these assessments, criterion referenced to the Allen Cognitive Scale of Levels and Modes of Performance (Allen Cognitive Scale), along with other evaluation findings, to plan interventions that compensate for the impact of cognitive disabilities or impairments (limitations) on occupational performance and optimize the use of available functional cognitive abilities (strengths) for safe

Hemphill, B. J., & Urish, C. K. (Eds.). *Assessments in Occupational Therapy Mental Health: An Integrative Approach, Fourth Edition* (pp. 179-210). © 2020 Taylor & Francis Group.

participation in valued everyday activities. This is accomplished by creating a fit between a person's available functional cognitive abilities and the cognitive complexity of activity demands of the activities a person wants and needs to do. The expected outcome of this intervention approach is safe, successful, satisfying engagement and participation in valued activities in supportive environments.

In the context of the evaluation and intervention process described in the *Occupational Therapy Practice Framework: Domain and Process, Third Edition* (American Occupational Therapy Association [AOTA], 2014), these assessments are top-down, occupation- and performance-based assessments that yield information that contributes to analysis of occupational performance by identifying and describing:

- Disabilities or impairments in functional cognitive capacities and available functional cognitive abilities (mental functions, a client factor) that impact occupational performance and are inferred from observations of what a client pays attention to and performance skills as the client engages in activities
- Activity demands, activity patterns, and environmental supports that appear to fit with the client's available functional cognitive abilities

Interventions focus on enabling engagement in meaningful activities by:

- Modifying and adapting activities and environments (physical and social)
- Establishing and restoring attentional and performance skills within the client's available functional cognitive abilities
- Maintenance of and prevention of decline in functional cognitive abilities

Initially, the CDM and associated assessments were developed for patients in mental health settings with psychiatric disorders (e.g., Allen, 1985, pp. 79, 267-362; Cairns, Hill, Dark, McPhail, & Gray, 2013; Chapleau, Seroczynski, Meyers, Lamb, & Buchino, 2012; David & Riley, 1990; Helfrich, Chan, & Sabol, 2011; Henry, Moore, Quinlivan, & Triggs, 1998; Katz & Perelman, 1993; McAnanama, Rogosin-Rose, Scott, Joffe, & Kelner, 1999; Penny, Mueser & North, 1995; Raweh & Katz, 1999; Scanlan & Still, 2013; Schubmehl, Barkin, & Cort, 2018; Shapiro 1992; Su, Tsai, Su, Tang, & Tsai, 2011; White, Meade, & Hadar, 2007). Over time, they have been studied and used with adolescent, adult, and older populations with varied clinical conditions and diagnoses, including neurologic and developmental disorders, and in a variety of practice settings (Allen, 1985, pp. 79, 267-362; Allen et al., 1992, pp. v-vi, 241-280, 328-338; McCraith & Earhart, 2018, pp. 470-472).

First, this chapter presents the major CDM theories and concepts that are the foundation for the featured theory-based assessments. Next, each assessment is described and the development, psychometric properties, administration, scoring, and score interpretation are discussed. Then, intervention planning and implementation with a summary of intervention outcome evidence based on use of scores from the two featured assessments are described. Finally, a case study illustrates use of the assessments in the evaluation and intervention process guided by the CDM and the *Framework* (AOTA, 2014).

This chapter is an overview. Use of the CDM and the two assessments require more in-depth knowledge and supervision to become skilled in administration, scoring, and interpretation of scores for use in intervention planning and implementation. For a thorough articulation of the CDM, see *Occupational Therapy Treatment Goals for the Physically and Cognitively Disabled* (Allen et al., 1992), *Understanding the Modes of Performance* (Allen, Blue, & Earhart, 1995), and the chapter "Cognitive Disabilities Model: Creating Fit Between Functional Cognitive Abilities and Cognitive Activity Demands" (McCraith & Earhart, 2018). In addition, refer to the *Manual for the Allen Cognitive Level Screen–5 (ACLS-5) and the Large Allen Cognitive Level Screen–5 (LACLS-5), First Edition* (Manual-1; Allen et al., 2007) and the *Allen Diagnostic Module: Manual (2nd Edition)* (Earhart, 2006). A second edition of the manual for the ACLS-5, LACLS-5, and the LACLS-5[D] is planned for publication in Fall 2020 (Allen Cognitive Group/ACLS and LACLS Committee [ACG/ACLS Committee]). Readers are also referred to www.allencognitive.org for videos and other resources related to applications of the CDM and the two assessments discussed in this chapter.

Cognitive Disabilities Model
Theories and Concepts

The key theories and concepts that form the foundation of the CDM and inform use of the two assessments discussed in this chapter are:

1. Functional Cognition
2. Information Processing Model
3. Allen Cognitive Scale of Levels and Modes of Performance
4. Hierarchy of Cognitive Complexity of Activity Demands
5. Task/Activity Analysis and Equivalence
6. Whole Person Perspective and the Biopsychosocial Model

Functional Cognition

The complex, multifaceted relationship between function and cognition has been central to the theoretical foundation of the CDM since it was first introduced (Allen, 1985, pp. 3, 31). The two assessments discussed in this chapter are standardized, performance-based, observational assessments designed to estimate *functional information processing capacities* (Allen, 1985, 1999; Allen & Blue, 1998) or *functional cognition* (Allen et al., 2007; Austin, 2009; Earhart, 2006; McCraith, Austin, & Earhart, 2011; McCraith & Earhart, 2018; Pollard & Olin, 2005; Wesson, Clemson, Brodaty, & Reppermund, 2016; Wesson & Giles, 2019). In the CDM, functional cognition is defined as "the integrated functioning of the brain's cognitive processes that guide performance of everyday activities in varied environments" (McCraith & Earhart, 2018). The focus is on *global* or integrated functioning of the brain's cognitive processes, an approach that differs from approaches that focus on the brain's domain-specific, distinct cognitive functions and processes such as memory, visual perception, or language.

Information Processing Model

In the CDM, the complex, dynamic relationship between cognition and function is further understood in the context of the information processing (IP) model (Allen, 1985, p. 40, 1999; Allen & Blue, 1998; McCraith & Earhart, 2018). As conceptualized in the CDM, the IP model consists of a closed loop of four dynamically interrelated phases.

1. The *input phase* triggers the processing of information. Sensory cues in the environment capture a person's attention and are passed to the next phase to be processed as a precursor to performance.

2. In the *throughput phase*, basic cognitive functions and processes (e.g., encoding, filtering, retrieving, and storing information), as well as higher level executive functions and processes (e.g., problem solving, decision making, and learning) work together to transform the information for use in guiding and managing performance.

3. In the *output phase*, this transformed information guides use of performance skills (e.g., involuntary, voluntary, and imitated motor actions; process skills; and verbal and social behaviors), which enable engagement and participation in basic and complex activities.

4. The *feedback phase* completes the IP loop by ensuring that evaluative information available to the person during or after performance becomes new sensory cues for input and processing. This supports the ongoing, successful maintenance, modulation, and modification of occupational performance.

Mental energy or processing speed influences all four phases of the IP model. In addition, the processing of information through each phase may be unconscious, conscious, or a combination of both.

Practitioners use observations of function, specifically what individuals pay attention to during the input phase and their use of performance skills while engaged in activities in the output phase, as the basis for identifying *patterns of performance* from which to infer the available cognitive capacities or strengths that are not observable in the throughput phase. Practitioners may ask clients to talk out loud about what they are sensing, thinking, feeling, experiencing, or doing to better understand what they are consciously aware of as part of inferring clients' functional cognitive capacities. Refer to McCraith and Earhart (2018, pp. 472-474) and Levy (2018, pp. 105-127) for a more detailed discussion of the IP model and the role of memory in the context of the CDM.

In summary, functional cognition encompasses the phases of the IP model and also describes the construct measured by the two assessments featured in this chapter.

Allen Cognitive Scale of Levels and Modes of Performance

The Allen Cognitive Scale is a hierarchical, cumulative, ordinal 27-point scale that describes functional cognitive abilities and provides the criteria for scoring the two assessments featured in this chapter. The scale is comprised of six levels numbered 1-6. Within each level, there are five hierarchical modes, which are labeled .0, .2, .4, .6, and .8. It is important to stress that this sequential use of numbers reflects a nominal (descriptive) and ordinal labeling system; it should not be confused with an interval system in which the distance between numbers is equal and can be averaged arithmetically. In a validity study of three ADM-2 assessments, Austin (2009; McCraith et al., 2011) found significant support for the use of the modes as distinct gradations of capacity within Levels 3 and 4 on the Allen Cognitive Scale based on the Rasch method of analysis. Austin was also some support for Level 5, but the sample size for this level was insufficient to support a definitive finding.

Table 11-1 illustrates the sequence of the 6 cognitive levels and 27 modes. The titles reflect a prominent, observable, voluntary motor action associated with each level and mode. Within each cognitive level, the modes appear to progress in a predictable pattern of relative stability with the .4 modes being the most stable and consistent with the overall characteristics of each level. The fewest and simplest available functional cognitive capacities are described by Level 1. Successive levels describe additional capacities of increasing variety and complexity that are *cumulative* up the scale, with the most complex capacities associated with the fully developed, typical adult brain described by Level 6. The same

Table 11-1

Allen Cognitive Scale: Titles of 6 Cognitive Levels and 26 Modes of Performance

Titles of Levels[a]	Titles of Modes[b]				
	.0	.2	.4	.6	.8
(Preconscious state prior to Level 1)	Coma				
Level 1: Automatic Actions	1.0 Withdrawing from noxious stimuli	1.2 Responding to stimuli with one sensory system	1.4 Locating stimuli	1.6 Rolling in bed	1.8 Raising body part
Level 2: Postural Actions	2.0 Overcoming gravity and sitting	2.2 Righting reactions and standing	2.4 Aimless walking	2.6 Directed walking	2.8 Using grab bars
Level 3: Manual Actions	3.0 Grasping objects	3.2 Distinguishing objects	3.4 Sustaining actions on objects	3.6 Noting effects on objects	3.8 Using all objects
Level 4: Goal-Directed Actions	4.0 Sequencing familiar actions	4.2 Differentiating features of objects	4.4 Completing a goal	4.6 Personalizing features of objects	4.8 Learning by rote memorization
Level 5: Exploratory Actions	5.0 Comparing and changing variations in actions and objects	5.2 Discriminating among sets of actions and objects	5.4 Self-directed learning	5.6 Considering social standards	5.8 Consulting with others
Level 6: Planned Actions	Typically functioning adult brain and functional cognitive capacities				

[a]Titles of the levels are a prominent, observable, voluntary motor action associated with the level.

[b]Titles of the modes are an observable functional cognitive behavior characteristic of mode.

Developed by C. A. Earhart and D. McCraith (2015) and revised (2020) for educational use. © 2020 C. A. Earhart, Pasadena, CA, and ACLS and LACLS Committee, Camarillo, CA. Reprinted with permission.

point on the scale identifies both the severity of cognitive disability and available functional cognitive abilities. Thus, practitioners assume that individuals have all of the functional cognitive abilities at and below their specified level/mode on the scale. Functional cognitive abilities above that point on the scale are typically considered unavailable for use (Allen & Blue, 1998; Allen et al., 1992, 1995; McCraith & Earhart, 2018).

Drawing on the IP model and *Framework* (AOTA, 2014) terminology, each cognitive level and mode is characterized by its associated attributes, including:

1. Observable attributes:
   ◦ Sensory cues that capture and sustain attention
   ◦ Performance skills, including motor (e.g., grasping, manipulating, reaching), process (e.g., pacing, choosing, sequencing), and social interaction (e.g., sharing, questioning, initiating, engaging others)
   ◦ Typical verbalizations or verbal content expressed
2. Other qualitative and quantitative attributes that may be observed or inferred:
   ◦ Characteristics of occupational performance such as purpose, attention span, processing speed, learning, and problem solving
   ◦ Descriptions of apparent conscious awareness of self and personal, temporal, physical, and social contexts and environments
3. Inferred underlying cognitive processes such as executive functions

In addition, the descriptions of each level and mode include the typical patterns of performance that might be expected when engaging in activities, such as activities of daily living (ADLs) and instrumental activities of daily living (IADLs), along with important safety considerations and suggestions for modifying or adapting the cognitive complexity of activity demands to enable optimal use of available functional cognitive abilities at a given level and mode (Allen et al., 1995).

Table 11-2 summarizes the sensory cues attended to, spontaneous and imitated motor actions observed, inferred purpose, and attention span that characterize each of the six cognitive levels (Allen, 1985; Allen et al., 1992, 1995). The general types of activities that match these available functional cognitive abilities, as well as typical expectations for supervision and assistance to ensure safety and success in performance of everyday activities, are summarized.

Hierarchy of Cognitive Complexity of Activity Demands

The Allen Cognitive Scale serves a dual purpose. It provides an analysis of the cognitive complexity of both the functional cognitive capacities of individuals and the activity demands of activities (Allen, 1985; McCraith & Earhart, 2018). Therefore, Austin (2009; McCraith et al., 2011) described the scale as having two hierarchies: the hierarchy of functional cognition and the hierarchy of activity demands. Austin observed that this dual use of the Allen Cognitive Scale is similar to identifying both the cognitive complexity of functional cognitive reading abilities of a *third-grade child* and the cognitive complexity of activity demands of a book that the child reads as a *third-grade level book*.

Skilled practitioners who use the CDM apply knowledge of both hierarchies along with activity analysis skills in the evaluation process to introduce activity demands with known cognitive complexity as a means for verifying available functional cognitive abilities. In the intervention process, practitioners analyze the cognitive complexity of activity demands as part of creating a fit between clients' available functional cognitive abilities and the activities they need and want to do. Refer to the PDF download titled *Analysis*

Table 11-2

Summary of Functional Cognitive Abilities for the Allen Cognitive Scale's 6 Cognitive Levels With Intervention Guidelines

Cognitive Level	1 Automatic Actions	2 Postural Actions	3 Manual Actions	4 Goal-Directed Actions	5 Exploratory Actions	6 Planned Actions
Functional Cognitive Abilities						
Sensory cues attended to	Subliminal cues	Proprioceptive cues	Tactile cues	Visible cues	Related cues	Symbolic cues
Motor actions: Spontaneous	Automatic	Postural	Manual Manipulations	Goal-directed	Exploratory	Planned
Imitated	None	Approximate	Manipulations	Replications	Novelty	Unnecessary
Purpose/intent	Arousal	Comfort	Interest	Compliance	Self-control	Reflection
Attention span	Seconds	Minutes	Half hours	Hours	Weeks	Past/future
Intervention Guidelines						
Occupational therapy activities	Sensory stimulation	Gross motor exercise	Tasks with repeated actions	Tasks with several steps	Concrete tasks	Conceptual tasks
ADL assistance	Initiate and complete tasks	Initiate and complete tasks	Initiate, set up, and prompt actions	Provide materials in familiar locations	Identify hazards	Provide resources
Safety	Ensure intake, skin integrity	Prevent wandering	Remove hazardous objects	Solve new problems	Issue warnings	Provide resources
Supervision	24 hour	24 hour	Frequent checks	Live alone with daily checks	Live alone with weekly checks	None

Developed by C. A. Earhart (2015a) for educational use. © 2015 C. A. Earhart, Pasadena, CA and ACLS and LACLS Committee, Camarillo, CA. Reprinted with permission.

of Modes of Performance for the Allen Cognitive Scale's Hierarchies of Functional Cognition and Activity Demands for a detailed analysis of both hierarchies with examples (available from www.allencognitive.org).

Task/Activity Analysis and Equivalence

Practitioners also use the Allen Cognitive Scale's hierarchies of functional cognition and activity demands to analyze and identify activities that appear to have activity demands of equivalent cognitive complexity. This process is referred to as estimating *activity equivalence*. Practitioners rely on the processes of activity analysis and equivalence to identify activities and environments that are both meaningful to individuals and most likely to be safe, realistic choices based on individuals' available functional cognitive capacities.

Whole Person Perspective and the Biopsychosocial Model

The CDM embraces the biopsychosocial model's emphasis on the whole person and the view that biological, psychological, and social factors all play a significant role in understanding human functioning (Allen & Blue, 1998, p. 237). Allen (1994) simplified these components of function into "what the person CAN DO, WILL DO, and MAY DO." Can Do refers to what is biologically realistic for safe participation in everyday activities, including functional cognitive capacities, as well as other medical, physical, and developmental capacities that may impact function. Will Do refers to what is psychologically relevant to the person, such as motivation, values, and interests. May Do refers to what is socially and environmentally possible, such as available family and caregiver supports, financial resources, transportation, accessibility, legal factors, and cultural or religious beliefs and expectations.

In the CDM, when there is a fit among Can Do (realistic functional cognitive and other biologic capacities), Will Do (meaningful activities), and May Do (social/environmental supports), *best ability to function* is achieved. When there is a misfit among Can Do, Will Do, and May Do, the whole person's best ability to function is impacted and dysfunction occurs.

Evaluation Process in the Cognitive Disabilities Model

As part of the overall evaluation process in the CDM, information related to Will Do and May Do is obtained by interviewing clients and their family members and others who are involved in their care. In many mental health settings, as well as other practice settings, this is also part of developing the person's occupational profile. The two standardized assessments featured in this chapter focus on assessing functional cognition or what a person Can Do.

The evaluation process also stresses the importance of considering all client factors and performance skills that might impact occupational performance, such as physical capacities (e.g., low vision, hand tremors, physical disabilities, low energy) or other mental functions (e.g., hallucinations or focal deficits in perception or memory, verbal skills). For this purpose, a variety of other approaches and assessments designed to address these concerns may be used to complete the overall evaluation process before proceeding to intervention. Initial evaluation data, including occupational profile and occupational performance analyses, may also be used as part of the ongoing evaluation and intervention process to detect changes over time in functional cognitive capacities and the resulting impact on occupational performance and engagement in meaningful activities.

Before describing the two assessments featured in this chapter, it is useful to describe several CDM-based evaluation principles that the assessments have in common. First, it is important that individuals demonstrate their highest level of functional cognitive capacity or best ability to function. Several recommendations address this principle:

- Assistive devices typically used by the individual, such as glasses, hearing aids, or splints, should be used. Qualified translators may also be helpful when a language barrier is identified.

- Assessment activities need to be relevant and meaningful to individuals to foster motivation to perform at their best and to use their highest level of functional cognitive capacity. When use of standardized assessments is not feasible or meaningful to the individual, practitioners may select a nonstandardized activity based on an analysis of the cognitive complexity of its activity demands.

- When the cognitive complexity of activity demands for desired activities match or fit individuals' highest level of functional cognitive capacity, individuals are more likely to demonstrate optimal performance using these capacities (Allen et al., 1992).

- Activities are likely to be ignored if the cognitive complexity of their activity demands is greater than an individual's functional cognitive abilities.

Another evaluation principle addresses safety in unexpected or new situations, a central concern in the CDM. Novel or unfamiliar activities are more likely to require processing and learning new information for responding safely and appropriately in these situations. Observations of performance in ADLs containing a preponderance of familiar elements are more likely to overestimate available functional cognitive abilities because they often draw on habitual or procedural memories. For this reason, standardized ADM-2 assessments, addressed later in this chapter, utilize craft projects that are less familiar in order to present more opportunities for new learning and problem solving with novel information. This approach is useful when it is necessary to make predictions about how a person will safely function outside the controlled environment of the treatment facility (Allen & Blue, 1998, p. 228).

A third principle focuses on the importance of discovering "what types of cues capture an individual's attention, how a person best learns new information, what strategies the person uses to solve problems, and how the person responds to unfamiliar situations" (McCraith et al., 2011, p. 394; see also McCraith & Earhart, 2018, pp. 481-482). Therefore, in addition to requiring that practitioners have skilled expertise for observation, activity analysis, and selection of assessment activities, the administration process for both assessments requires use of a dynamic interactive process of probing and grading the cognitive complexity of activity demands. These options are incorporated into the administration process for the two assessments featured in this chapter.

Figure 11-1. ACLS-5 with three stitching tasks set up for administration. (© 2018 ACLS and LACLS Committee, Camarillo, CA. Reprinted with permission.)

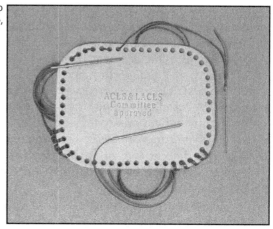

Allen Cognitive Level Screen–5, Large Allen Cognitive Level Screen–5, and Disposable Large Allen Cognitive Level Screen–5
Description

The ACLS-5, LACLS-5 and LACLS-5[D] are three forms of a standardized screen of functional cognition designed to provide a *quick estimate* of functional cognitive capacities within Allen Cognitive Levels/Modes 3.0 to 5.8. The standard form, the ACLS-5, is intended for general use. The larger form, the LACLS-5, is intended for use with clients who have vision or hand impairments. The disposable form, the LACLS-5[D], is intended for single or serial use with individuals for whom infection control is required. All three forms provide opportunities to observe current functional cognitive capacities related to the sensory cues the person pays attention to, new learning and problem-solving abilities, and the use of performance skills as they are applied within three standardized and carefully designed stitching tasks with activity demands that increase in cognitive complexity. As screens, these assessments may be used to detect unknown or suspected problems in functional cognition or to identify potential functional cognitive abilities or strengths. They are understood to provide an estimate of available functional cognitive abilities at a given point in time.

The assessment consists of learning to make three increasingly complex stitches through holes on a piece of leather (or chipboard for the LACLS-5[D]) by using information from sample stitches, directions and cues provided by the administrator, and motor and sensory feedback from the materials and process of completing the stitching tasks. Figure 11-1 shows the three stitches set up for administration of the ACLS-5.

Successful performance of each stitching task implies that the individual has the set of functional cognitive capacities that match the cognitive complexity of activity demands associated with that task; that is, they demonstrate understanding and use of the sensory cues from the materials, the administrator's demonstrated and verbal directions, and the feedback from their own performance actions while making the stitches.

Table 11-3 presents an activity analysis of selected task elements in the running, whip, and single cordovan stitching tasks and illustrates their correspondence to the cognitive complexity described in the Allen Cognitive Scale's hierarchy of activity demands ranging from level/mode 3.0 to 5.8.

Table 11-3

Analysis of Cognitive Complexity of Activity Demands for ACLS Version 5 Stitching Tasks

Task Elements	Activity Demands for ACLS-5 Stitching Tasks		
	Running Stitch Task	Whipstitch Task	Single Cordovan Stitch Task
Demonstrated steps	One step	Short sequence	Long sequence
Purpose	Repeat familiar actions	Make three stitches that match sample	Discover how to make three stitches that match sample
Motor actions	Hold objects Grasp/release needle Push needle through hole Pull lace tight Move in a line L → R	Grasp/release lace Turn/rotate lace	Fine motor manipulation of lace to tighten stitch
Visual and spatial cues	Immediate visible effects of actions on objects Shape of stitch	Striking, visible features: color/texture of lace Front/back, number	Details of complex cue: tension, angle, relative position, direction of lace
Verbal cues	Nouns, verbs specifying an action	Adjectives describing the features of objects	Adverbs describing relationships between objects
Learning	Imitate familiar action	Imitate short sequence of steps	Imitate long sequence OR Self-directed trial and error
Problem solving	None OR Stops actions	Match striking visual cues Reverse actions	Match complex visual cues Alter action sequence
ACLS Scores/ Allen Cognitive Scale	3.0 3.2 3.4 3.6 3.8	4.0 4.2 4.4 4.6 4.8	5.0 5.2 5.4 5.6 5.8
Complexity	Less complex ————————————————————▶ More complex		

Developed by C. A. Earhart (2020) for educational use. © 2020 C. A. Earhart. Reprinted with permission.

History of Assessment Development

Five standardized versions of the ACLS and LACLS have been described, although others have been developed for limited use in research (Allen et al., 2007). For a detailed discussion of the psychometric evidence for versions 1 through 4, see Allen and Blue (1998).

Allen Cognitive Level Screen, Versions 1 Through 5

The nonstandardized, original version of the ACLS assessment, known as the *Cognitive Levels Test*, was developed in the early 1970s. The first standardized version, the Allen Cognitive Level–Original (ACL-O), was published by Moore (1978). The materials used in this version have remained largely unchanged in subsequent versions, including the standard ACLS-5. Similarly, most administration processes have remained the same for all three forms of version 5 of the ACLS assessment.

Version 2, the Allen Cognitive Level–Expanded (ACL-E; Allen et al., 1992), added scoring options and increased the number of required stitches for each of the three stitching tasks from two to three to decrease the probability that individuals might complete stitches correctly by chance (Earhart & Allen, 1988).

A larger version, the Large Allen Cognitive Screen (LACLS), originally based on the ACLS-E, was introduced by Kehrberg, Kuskowski, Mortimer, and Shoberg (1992) for use with individuals with decreased visual acuity and impaired hand function.

Version 3, the Allen Cognitive Level Screen–1990 (ACLS-90; Allen et al., 1992), adopted a change in administration proposed by Josman and Katz's (1991) research version, the Allen Cognitive Level–Problem Solving (ACL-PS). The ACL-PS introduced the single cordovan stitch without a demonstration in order to observe exploratory learning associated with Allen Cognitive Level 5. The ACLS-90 has the most extensive and substantive body of psychometric evidence to support reliability and validity of the ACLS assessment.

Version 4, the ACLS–2000 (Allen & Earhart, 2000), simplified the scoring criteria by eliminating the odd-numbered scores and combining theoretically compatible scores into even-numbered scores (.0, .2, .4, .6, .8) consistent with the even-numbered modes described in the Allen Cognitive Scale.

Version 5, introduced in the *Manual for the Allen Cognitive Level Screen–5 (ACLS-5) and the Large Allen Cognitive Level Screen–5 (LACLS-5)* (Allen et al., 2007), was developed in response to feedback from clinicians, educators, and researchers who believed that a more professionalized, informative assessment manual was needed to meet the clinical and scholarly expectations of the professional community. This version instructs the administrator to continue to the next stitching task whether or not the person has completed three correct stitches. This replaces the previous instruction to end the assessment when the person failed to make a stitch after two demonstrations. This change was introduced to reduce a possible ceiling effect by ending the assessment too soon. The enhancements and additions to the manual for version 5 were guided by the *Standards for Educational and Psychological Testing* (American Educational Research Association [AERA], 1999). The disposable form of the LACLS-5, the LACLS-5[D], was introduced by the ACG/ACLS Committee (2016) for single or serial use with one client for whom infection control is required.

Psychometric Properties

This summary of psychometric evidence focuses on studies using the ACLS-5 and LACLS-5 as described in Manual-1, the LACLS-5[D], and version 3, the ACLS-90 (Allen et al., 1992), which has the most extensive and substantive published psychometric evidence for the ACLS assessment. For a more detailed description and reviews of these studies, as well as studies using other versions of the ACLS, refer to Allen and Blue (1998); Allen, Earhart, and Blue (1992); Allen, Austin, and colleagues (2007); McCraith, Austin, and Earhart (2011); and McCraith and Earhart (2018). In addition, a report on the psychometric properties of the three forms of version 5 of the ACLS is periodically updated and available from www.allencognitive.org.

Reliability

The interrater reliability evidence across all versions and forms of the ACLS that were developed between 1978 and 2007 has been high, with reported correlations ranging from $r = .91$ to .99. In eight studies investigating the consistency of scores between different raters, researchers found ratings at the high end of this range in studies using the ACLS-90 (Henry et al., 1998; Keller & Hayes, 1998; Lee, Gargiullo, Brayman, Kinsey, Jones, & Shotwell, 2003; McCraith & Henry, 2003; Penny et al., 1995; Raweh & Katz, 1999; Velligan, Bow-Thomas, Mahurin, Miller, Dassori, & Erdely, 1998; Velligan, True, Lefton, Moore, & Flores, 1995). An additional study using a Chinese translation of the ACLS-90 (Su et al., 2011) also reported a high correlation for interrater reliability of $r = .98$.

In a pilot study of the LACLS-5, interrater agreement was 100% after margin of error was accounted for among a convenience sample of five therapists with varied exposure to any version of the ACLS (Helfrich & McCraith, 2015).

The ACG/ACLS Committee recently completed an interrater reliability analysis as part of a form equivalence study for the three forms of version 5 of the ACLS assessment. The interclass correlation coefficient with a 95% confidence level, a measure of interrater reliability, was selected for the analysis because it provides a probabilistic estimate of the generalization of findings to larger populations. In addition, an absolute agreement analysis was used because it assesses how closely different therapists assign a screen score to the same client, a very important consideration for use of scores in clinical practice. The interclass correlation coefficient findings were as follows: 0.80 for the ACLS-5, 0.93 for the LACLS-5, and 0.91 LACLS-5[D]. While the results for all three forms were good to excellent, the 0.80 for the ACLS-5 was puzzling given the excellent findings previously reported for this version and earlier versions of the ACLS assessment. Review of feedback from practitioner-raters who participated in this study strongly suggests that the clients' performance while completing the ACLS-5 on the five videos used for this study were difficult for practitioner-raters to score because the administrator's hand or the client's hand tended to obscure the client's performance on the ACLS-5, the standard form of version 5. This problem was not reported by practitioner-raters for the other two larger forms, the LACLS-5 and LACLS-5[D]. For a prepublication copy of the methodology and data analysis for this study, email contact@allencognitive.com.

Equivalence across the three forms of version 5 of the ACLS assessment, measured by the interclass correlation coefficient, was found to be 0.99 with a 95% confidence level, an excellent level of reliability (Koo & Li, 2016). This demonstrates that the three forms are highly equivalent. In other words, they are parallel forms of the same cognitive assessment. A client is likely to receive the same score regardless of which form they are administered. This finding supports an earlier finding by Kehrberg et al. (1992) that found the ACL-E, version 2 (Earhart & Allen, 1988), to be significantly correlated with the LACL-E in 49 participants with Alzheimer's disease ($r = .95$, $p < .0001$).

Validity

As with reliability evidence, there is a strong body of research supporting validity across various earlier versions and forms of the ACLS developed between 1978 and 2007.

Seven published studies of persons with psychiatric disorders described significant correlations between various top-down measures of ADLs and IADLs and the ACLS-90 (Keller & Hayes, 1998; McAnanama et al., 1999; Secrest, Wood, & Tapp, 2000; Velligan et al., 1995, 1998; Wilson, Allen, McCormack & Burton, 1989) and the LACLS-90 (Ziv, Roitman, & Katz, 1999). Significant correlations between the ACLS-2000 (Earhart & Allen, 2000) and scores from a self-report measure, the Practical Skills Test (Chang, Helfrich,

& Coster, 2013), were found for a homeless population. For individuals with psychiatric conditions, researchers found significant correlations between the ACLS-90 scores and living situation (Henry et al., 1998; McAnanama et al., 1999) and social competence (Penny et al., 1995).

More recently, two validity studies with persons in mental health settings reported moderate but significant associations between the LACLS-5 and level of independence (Scanlan & Still, 2013) measured with a functional independence rating by Collister and Alexander (1991) and medication adherence (Cairns et al., 2013) measured with the Medication Adherence Rating Scale by Thompson, Kulkami, and Serge (2000).

Several validity studies have focused on the relationship between the ACLS-90 or the LACLS-5 and the Assessment of Motor and Process Skills (AMPS), a top-down measure of functional cognition based on performance of various ADLs and IADLs. Wesson et al. (2017) reported a moderately significant relationship between the LACLS-5 and the AMPS Process score for community-living older adults with mild cognitive impairment and mild dementia. For persons at home after their first stroke, Marom, Jarus, and Josman (2011) also reported moderately significant correlations between the LACLS-90 and the AMPS Process score. These findings support the ecological validity of the assessment.

A significant relationship has been demonstrated between global cognition measured by the Mini-Mental State Examination (Folstein, Folstein, & McHugh, 1975) and the ACLS-90 (Su et al., 2011) and the ACLS-5 (Okamura, Takeshita, Teramoto, Aida, & Kino, 2010) and the LACLS-5 (Wesson et al., 2017). Additional evidence of significant associations between various cognitive domains (e.g., attention, concentration, executive functions, memory, language, visuo-constructional skills, etc.) and the ACLS-90 (David & Riley, 1990; McCraith & Henry, 2003; Secrest et al., 2000; Velligan et al., 1998) and the ACLS-5 (Rojo-Mota, Pedrero-Perez, Huertas-Hoyas, Merritt, & MacKenzie, 2016; Schubmehl et al., 2018) have been reported for persons with addictions and psychiatric disorders.

Researchers have established that mean ACLS and LACLS scores may be used to differentiate between distinct populations. For example, in two studies using the ACLS-90, one focused on adolescents with and without mental illness (Lee et al., 2003), and the other focused on older adults with and without dementia (Ziv et al., 1999). A more recent study found that the LACLS-5 discriminated between normal adults and adults with mild dementia and between normal adults and adults with mild cognitive impairment, but not between adults with mild cognitive impairment and normal adults (Wesson et al., 2017).

A review of seven studies by researchers in the United States, Canada, and Israel that addressed the relationship between ACLS and LACLS scores and ethnicity, level of acculturation, and gender have consistently shown that these variables do not impact ACLS scores (McCraith et al., 2011). Results related to the relationship between level of education and ACLS scores have been more mixed (Roitman & Katz, 1996; Velligan et al., 1995).

As a criterion-referenced assessment, evidence verifying the validity of the Allen Cognitive Scale is also important. Austin's (2009; McCraith et al., 2011) Rasch-based study provided evidence to support the presence of distinct modes of performance in the scale with individuals who had mental illness, particularly for the modes in Allen Cognitive Levels 3 and 4. There was also evidence of support for the modes in Level 5, but the sample size for this level was insufficient to be conclusive. For individuals with schizophrenia, Su et al. (2011) found evidence to support significant differences between Allen Cognitive Levels/Modes 4 and 5. The Level 5 group had higher mean scores for measures of processing speed, verbal memory, and working memory. More recently, a study by Regier, Hodgson, and Gitlin (2017) lends support to the hierarchies of functional cognition and activity demands for Allen Cognitive Levels 3 and 4.

There are a growing number of intervention outcome studies that provide validity evidence for several versions of the ACLS and LACLS by demonstrating that use of scores from these assessments contributes to practitioners' ability to provide effective interventions. These studies are described in the Intervention and Outcomes sections in this chapter.

Finally, many experts and other stakeholders reviewed and contributed to the content of Manual-1 (Allen et al., 2007). This extensive, collaborative process provides another important source of validity evidence for version 5 of the ACLS assessment.

Assessment Administration

Area of Occupation/Performance Skills/
Performance Patterns/Client Factors Assessed

The ACLS-5, LACLS-5, and LACLS-5[D] provide an estimate of functional cognition (available cognitive mental functions) for engaging safely in valued everyday activities. This estimate is inferred from (a) observations of what individuals pay attention to in their external and internal or personal environments and their performance skills as they engage in activities and (b) from analysis of the cognitive complexity of activity demands, activity patterns, and contextual and environmental supports that appear to fit with the person's cognitive mental functions and desired activities and occupations they need and want to do.

Description of Environment/
Description of Supplies/Materials Required

The ACLS-5, LACLS-5, and LACLS-5[D] are supported by a comprehensive manual, Manual-1 (Allen et al., 2007), designed to inform and guide administrators in the set up of the assessment and the environment for administration. Even though the LACLS-5[D] is not included in Manual-1, with minor exceptions, this manual is currently used for the set up, administration, and scoring of LACLS-5[D]. The LACLS-5[D] will be included in the second edition of the manual due to be published in Fall 2020.

Although they are standardized and similar, the materials for version 5 vary depending on the form of the assessment. The ACLS-5, shown in Figure 11-1, is considered the standard form. It consists of a 4- x 5-inch tan leather rectangle with rounded corners. The back side of the rectangle is rough in texture, and the front side is smooth and bears the imprint "ACLS & LACLS Committee approved." Fifty-six 1/8-inch-diameter prepunched holes around the perimeter of the leather are used to make the three stitching tasks. A large-eyed, blunt needle with waxed linen thread is used to make the running stitch. A brass, threaded, locking needle with 1/8-inch-wide leather lace is used to make the whipstitch and the single cordovan stitch.

The LACLS-5, shown in Figure 11-2, uses the same materials as the standard ACLS-5, except that it has larger cues. The leather rectangle is 6 x 7 inches with 53 1/4-inch-diameter prepunched holes around the perimeter. In addition, the waxed thread and needle are replaced with a textured shoelace with a plastic tip to make the running stitch. A 3/16-inch-wide leather lace is used to make the other two stitches.

The LACLS-5[D], shown in Figure 11-3, uses the same materials as the LACLS-5, except the leather rectangle is replaced with a sturdy, grayish chipboard rectangle with the front side distinguished from the back side by the "ACLS & LACLS Committee approved" imprint. If administrators use brass needles to make the whipstitch and single cordovan stitches, the needles must be sanitized between use with different people by

Figure 11-2. LACLS-5 with three stitching tasks set up for administration. (© 2018 ACLS and LACLS Committee, Camarillo, CA. Reprinted with permission.)

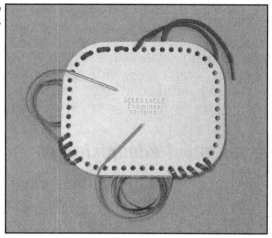

Figure 11-3. LACLS-5[D] with three stitching tasks set up for administration. (© 2016 ACLS and LACLS Committee, Camarillo, CA. Reprinted with permission.)

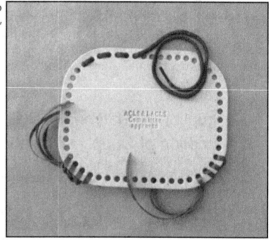

following established facility procedures. If administrators elect not to use needles with the leather laces, one end is cut at an angle to form a pointed tip. This disposable form, intended for persons who have infection control needs, is to be disposed of after single or serial use with one client by following the established procedures of the facility.

Latex is present in the leather lace used in all three forms. Administrators are advised to take precautions for persons allergic to latex and to follow the established latex safety policies in their facility.

Set up of the assessment and the environment and positioning of the administrator and client in preparation for administration are the same for all three forms of version 5 of the ACLS. Before beginning administration, each form should be set up with three correct sample stitches in place for each of the three stitching tasks as described in the manual. Figures 11-1, 11-2, and 11-3 illustrate this set up.

When possible, the environment should have minimal distractions and good lighting. The administrator sits next to the person being assessed, at an angle to facilitate observation of the person's facial expressions and other behavioral responses during the assessment and close enough to facilitate holding the assessment, set up for administration, in front of the person while demonstrating stitches and observing the person's actions.

Administrators may sit to the right or left of the person. The assessment also may be administered at bedside or while standing.

Administration

Administrators should have experience working with individuals who have temporary or permanent cognitive disabilities or impairments, and should have been trained or mentored in the use of the CDM and in the use of standardized assessments. If formal training in the CDM and administration of the ACLS is not available, new administrators should work with an experienced administrator or mentor.

The administrator uses the standardized verbal statements and demonstrations prescribed in the manual to introduce the three stitching tasks starting with the least complex running stitch, then the whipstitch, and ending with the most complex single cordovan stitch. The administrator introduces the next stitching task to the person on successful completion of three correct stitches or after the client fails to complete three correct stitches following two demonstrations of the stitch. There is no time limit for the assessment. Unlike previous versions, version 5 does not end the assessment when the person is unable to complete a stitch as directed. Instead, in version 5, the administrator continues to the next stitch to avoid a ceiling effect. The administrator ends the assessment when the person completes all three stitching tasks correctly or incorrectly; fails to correct errors in the most complex task, the single cordovan stitch, after two demonstrations; refuses to watch the demonstration of any stitch; requests to end the assessment; refuses to continue the assessment; or expresses or is observed to demonstrate significant anxiety or distress verbally or nonverbally, despite supportive cues from the administrator.

For some individuals, this screening assessment may not meet the criteria for being a meaningful activity. Therefore, when introducing it to a person, it is important to explain the relevance of the assessment to the person's situation in addition to the standardized explanation of the screening assessment's purpose contained in the manual. This potential limitation of the screening assessment reinforces the importance of verifying ACLS scores with standardized or nonstandardized skilled observations of performance in activities meaningful to the person.

Assigning and Interpreting Scores

Scores are assigned and interpreted within the context of the CDM. Three scoring tables, one for each stitching task, provide 16 possible scores ranging from less than 3.0 to 5.8. Using clinical reasoning, the administrator compares observations of the person's pattern of performance to the scoring table in the manual for the most complex stitching task completed and assigns the score that most closely matches his or her observations. Although scores are criterion referenced to the Allen Cognitive Scale, they need to be interpreted in light of what is appropriate for screening assessments. The score is an indicator, or estimate, of available functional cognitive abilities at a moment in time. Before establishing the person's cognitive level/mode on the Allen Cognitive Scale, screen scores should be verified with further skilled observations of performance in other meaningful activities or with other standardized assessments, such as the ADM-2 assessments (Earhart, 2006) or the RTI-E (Katz, 2006) associated with the CDM or other functional cognitive assessments. In determining the validity of the score, administrators also consider other client factors, such as physical impairments, as well as the person's motivation (Will Do), and environmental/contextual factors, such as distractions or possible familiarity with the assessment (May Do).

Figure 11-4. Examples of ADM-2 assessments (Earhart, 2015b). (© 2015 C. A. Earhart. Reprinted with permission.)

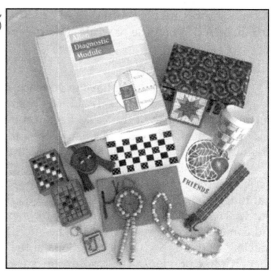

Allen Diagnostic Module (2nd Edition)
Manual and Assessments
Description

ADM-2 assessments (Earhart, 2006) are a collection of 27 currently available standardized, craft-based activities that offer individuals opportunities to use available functional cognitive abilities for learning and solving predictable problems while making a functional object such as greeting card, visor, or placemat. Figure 11-4 illustrates examples of ADM-2 assessments. Each ADM-2 assessment is designed to introduce activity demands with an identified range of cognitive complexity within levels 3.0 and 6.0 on the Allen Cognitive Scale. The variety of content and processes used in the assessments allows administrators to collaborate with individuals in selecting an assessment activity that is meaningful (Will Do) and within the individuals' expected functional cognitive capacities (Can Do). The ADM-2 assessments employ a dynamic, interactive process that includes offering the individual choices within parameters represented by a completed sample and the active collaboration of the administrator who may adjust the cognitive complexity of activity demands to facilitate performance. This dynamic process allows practitioners to identify the conditions, including supervision and other contextual factors, that support safe and successful performance for the individual.

The ADM-2 assessments may be used to verify estimates of functional cognitive ability based on the ACLS score with observations of patterns of performance that emerge as the individual engages in problem solving and new learning required by the activity over an extended period of time. Serial observations of performance in ADM-2 assessments can help practitioners monitor changing patterns of performance that may reflect changing functional cognitive capacities, especially in acute or declining conditions. The preponderance of unfamiliar elements in these craft-based assessments makes them particularly suitable for examining problem solving in novel conditions that may suggest an individual's capacity to engage in adaptive behaviors to ensure his or her safety in changing conditions or novel environments.

History of Development

The original Allen Diagnostic Module (ADM-1; Earhart, Allen, & Blue, 1993) assessments were developed in response to requests by practitioners for efficient, cost-effective, and reliable assessments to verify ACLS scores and to meet growing demands for productivity and accountability in practice. Extensive pilot testing by skilled practitioners with adult and adolescent psychiatric patients identified reliable rating criteria, referenced to the Allen Cognitive Scale, for 24 crafts projects designed to be successful at multiple levels of ability. The administration manual and standardized assessment kits were produced by S&S Worldwide (www.ssww.com), a large arts and crafts supply company. Over time, several ADM assessments were discontinued and additional assessments targeting special populations were developed, including a safety series for prevocational assessment and activities that may be completed with one hand.

The ADM-2 (Earhart, 2006) includes 27 currently available assessments (of the 33 originally in this edition) and a substantially expanded administration manual revised according to the *Standards for Educational and Psychological Testing* (AERA, 1999.)

Table 11-4 lists 27 currently available ADM-2 assessments in order of the cognitive complexity of their activity demands, as reflected in a range of potential scores for each assessment. Lower scores are associated with less cognitively complex activity demands, whereas higher scores indicate more cognitively complex activity demands. All ADM-2 assessments offer opportunities for successful engagement at the multiple levels of functional cognitive abilities suggested by the scores criterion-referenced to the corresponding level/mode on the Allen Cognitive Scale. Administration protocols for ADM-2 assessments with asterisks are available as downloads at www.allencognitive.org and include specifications for self-manufacturing assessment kits.

Psychometric Properties

The following summary of psychometric evidence is not exhaustive, but it is representative of the body of evidence supporting use of the ADM-2 assessments.

Interrater Reliability

Interrater reliability has been moderately high to high, as reported for 11 ADM-1 assessments (Roitman & Katz, 1996). High interrater reliability ($r = .99$) was found for the Recessed Tile Box, an ADM-2 assessment (Henry, McCraith, & St. Germain, 2000). In a study of the ADM-2 Placemat and Leather Key Fob assessments using Rasch analysis, Austin (2009; McCraith et al., 2011) found minimal variation in the severity with which eight occupational therapy practitioners applied the rating criteria. Results also suggested that the majority of 41 rating criteria on the ADM-2 assessments appear to support a one-dimensional functional cognition construct, although a small number of criteria appear to vary based on person factors, such as low vision, mania, and English-language fluency.

Validity

In Austin's (2009; McCraith et al., 2011) Rasch-based study, 89.9% of the 161 individuals demonstrated responses to specific rating criteria that were expected based on their other responses during the assessment. Of the 10.1% of individuals whose responses were unexpected on the basis of their other responses, many of these responses were related to behaviors that were affected by the individual's lack of fluency in English, low vision, mania, and/or florid psychosis.

Table 11-4

Range of Scores Based on Cognitive Complexity of Activity Demands for Allen Diagnostic Module (2nd Edition) Assessments

ADM-2 Assessments	Allen Diagnostic Module Scores/Cognitive Levels/Modes														
	3.0	3.2	3.4	3.6	3.8	4.0	4.2	4.4	4.6	4.8	5.0	5.2	5.4	5.6	5.8
Mug	■	■	■	■	■										
Placemat	■	■	■	■	■										
Visor*	■	■	■	■	■										
Frog note holder	■	■	■	■	■										
Whale note holder	■	■	■	■	■										
Felt turtle	■	■	■	■	■	■									
Bargello bookmark*	■	■	■	■	■	■	■	■	■						
Bead kit I	■	■	■	■	■	■									
Recessed tile box	■	■	■	■	■	■	■	■	■	■	■	■	■	■	■
Tile trivet	■	■	■	■	■										
Storage box			■	■	■	■	■	■	■	■	■	■			
Button bookmark				■	■	■	■								
Button frame				■	■	■	■	■	■						
Fabric notebook															
Ribbon card*						■	■	■	■						
Leather key fob															
Turtle key ring								■	■						
Jute purse															
Jute tote bag							■	■	■	■	■	■	■	■	■
Bead kit II															
Fabric-covered box								■	■	■	■	■	■		
Heart key ring															
Secretary box w/stencil										■	■	■	■	■	■
Stenciled greeting card*										■	■	■	■	■	■
Initial key ring*										■	■	■	■	■	■
Needlepoint flag magnet															
Needlepoint coaster													■	■	■

*Directions and video available online at www.allencognitive.com.

Updated by Earhart (2015c) based on Earhart (2006). © 2015 C. A. Earhart. Reprinted with permission.

Two studies addressed the relationship among ADM-2 scores, ACLS-5/LACLS-5 scores, and other measures of cognition. Moderate correlation between ADM-1 scores and LACLS scores for earlier versions was reported by Roitman and Katz (1996). A strong correlation ($r = .72$, $p < .001$) was found between the scores from ACLS-90 and scores for the Recessed Tile Box, an ADM-2 assessment. A modest association was found between the Recessed Tile Box, ACLS-90, and several subtests of the Wechsler Memory Scale–Revised and the Wisconsin Card Sorting Test (McCraith & Henry, 2003).

Assessment Administration

Area of Occupation/Performance Skills/
Performance Patterns/Client Factors Assessed

The ADM-2 assesses functional cognition. This includes identifying impairments and abilities in mental functions that impact occupational performance. This is inferred from observations of what a person pays attention to and performance skills as the individual engages in activities and from analysis of the cognitive complexity of activity demands, activity patterns, and contextual and environmental supports that appear to fit with the individual's mental functions and desired activities.

Description of Environment/
Description of Supplies/Materials Required

Environmental considerations are specified in the administration protocol for each assessment in the ADM-2 manual (Earhart, 2006) and include features such as sinks, cupboards, and trash cans that allow opportunities to observe problem solving related to clean-up or self-directed exploration. Most ADM-2 assessments require a flat working surface, such as a table top or tray table, but some may be accomplished while sitting in bed (e.g., Ribbon Card) or standing (e.g., Bargello Bookmark). The environment should be well lit and distraction free, with adequate space for administrators to observe performance while engaging in the dynamic administration process.

Required supplies include the ADM-2 manual (Earhart, 2006), which includes guidelines for use and administration protocols for all assessments; standardized kits for the selected assessments; and additional supplies and tools such as scissors, brushes, and glue sticks specified in the administration protocol. Manufactured assessment kits are available through S&S Worldwide at www.ssww.com, and some assessment kits may be self-manufactured according to specifications in protocols available as downloads from www.allencognitive.org. Administrators are encouraged not to alter materials or tools specified in the protocol (e.g., using liquid glue in place of a glue stick) because this may affect validity of scores. One or more completed samples of the finished project must be completed prior to administration. Samples represent the standard end-product used to guide the individual's problem-solving process. Making the sample acquaints administrators with the particular properties of materials and processes, as well as the predictable problems that need to be solved within the activity.

Administration

In selecting which ADM-2 assessment to use, administrators consider assessments containing activity demands whose cognitive complexity as indicated by the range of scores matches or exceeds the person's current functional cognitive abilities, typically

Figure 11-5. Observing performance in ADM-2 Ribbon Card assessment (Earhart, 2015d). (© 2015 C. A. Earhart. Reprinted with permission.)

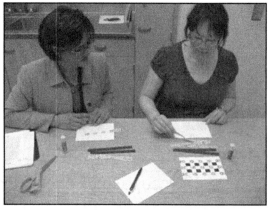

estimated by ACLS scores or other skilled observations of performance. Occupational profile data (i.e., client factors such as physical limitations, cultural beliefs, personal preferences, or familiarity with the activity) collected prior to administration should be considered as well. To promote engagement in the outcome, practitioners offer individuals a choice between two or more ADM-2 assessments whenever possible and encourage them to keep the object they produce.

Practitioners who use ADM-2 assessments generally utilize several assessments that match the range of functional cognitive abilities typically encountered in their practice setting rather than using all 27 currently available assessments. The ADM-2 assessments are not timed and may be completed in more than one session; however, administrators need to consider the possible impact of this practice when interpreting scores.

The administration protocol specifies the set up of the assessment materials including positioning the materials and the sample(s) for individual and group assessments. Figure 11-5 illustrates set up and positioning of the administrator, person being assessed, and materials for individual assessment with the ADM-2 Ribbon Card assessment.

During the assessment administration, instructions provided to the person are selected by the administrator to support differing levels of ability; for example, in assessments with activity demands of Level 3 cognitive complexity, familiar actions may be demonstrated one action at a time. In assessments with activity demands of Level 4 cognitive complexity, a short sequence of actions in a new procedure may be demonstrated, accompanied by simple verbal statements. Small groups of up to four individuals who are engaged in the same ADM-2 assessment in proximity may be monitored simultaneously by skilled administrators.

An overview of the dynamic administration process used for all ADM-2 assessments is detailed in the "Guidelines for Use" section in the ADM-2 manual (Earhart, 2006). Although the person controls and directs performance within the activity, administrators may influence performance by introducing information of known complexity in the form of questions, prompts, or cues to clarify abilities or to adjust the cognitive complexity of activity demands to observed abilities to ensure a successful activity experience. To assist administrators, suggested prompts and cues are provided in the assessment protocol. Recognizing typical patterns may be helpful at points where errors may be attributed to either Can Do limitations or Will Do decisions based on personal preferences.

Assigning and Interpreting Scores

Assigning and interpreting scores of ADM-2 assessments requires clinical reasoning as the administrator reflects on all the data observed throughout the activity, compares all observed behaviors to the sets of behaviors in the rating criteria that constitute a score, and assigns the score that most closely matches the pattern of performance observed. A single score may be assigned when the preponderance of behaviors matches behaviors at one score; atypical patterns of performance are further investigated or explained by considering additional data collected during the intervention process or from the occupational profile. When it is not possible to identify causative factors, it may not be appropriate to report a single score. As with ACLS scores, determining the validity of ADM scores requires administrators to consider other factors that might have impacted the individual's performance, including familiarity of the activity or particular elements within the activity, additional cognitive or physical impairments, symptoms such as pain or perceptual disturbances, interest and motivation, lack of adaptive equipment, distractions in the social or physical environment, and time of day. The dynamic administration process allows administrators to intervene to identify such factors during the assessment by asking the person to verify suspected complications (e.g., Can you see clearly? Are you in pain right now? Does this activity interest you? Are you trying your best?). ADM assessments with equivalent cognitive complexity that involve use of different materials and processes may be offered serially to confirm an observed pattern of performance and to avoid identified confounding variables such as familiarity.

Intervention and Outcomes in the Cognitive Disabilities Model

All intervention approaches in the CDM are designed to *create a fit* between the cognitive complexity of activity demands of valued activities and what is cognitively realistic (Can Do), psychologically relevant (Will Do), and socially and environmentally possible (May Do) for the person (McCraith & Earhart, 2018). This process of creating a fit assumes the involvement of individuals and caregivers to identify Will Do and May Do. It also requires practitioners to analyze the cognitive complexity of activity and environmental demands of valued activities to ensure that the cognitive complexity of activity demands fit individuals' available functional cognitive capacities or to identify other realistic and equivalent activity options that are most apt to be performed safely and successfully.

Intervention Approaches

Within the intervention focus and process of the CDM, the selection of an intervention approach is not only based on evaluation results including Can Do, Will Do, and May Do but also targeted outcomes. In addition, the selection may be influenced by the stability of a person's mental or physical health (e.g., improving, stable, declining). For example, in acute care settings, persons frequently have cognitive limitations that will likely *improve* over time with medications, a supportive milieu, and other interventions. In community, long-term care, and home care settings for individuals with persistent mental illness or other more permanent physical and cognitive disabilities, their conditions are more likely to be *stable* for periods of time or to *decline* over time. Practitioners may use serial assessments to monitor improvement, stabilization, and decline in functional cognitive abilities in order to make recommendations that support ongoing best ability to function.

Several types of intervention approaches described in the *Framework* (AOTA, 2014) are appropriate for use by practitioners within the context of the CDM. These approaches frequently complement each other as part of an overall intervention.

Modifying Activities and Environments

As discussed previously, within the CDM the primary intervention approach focuses on compensating for functional cognitive disabilities or limitations and enhancing functional cognitive abilities by modifying environments and activities rather than by changing an individual's available cognitive capacities through remediation. For example, a dressing routine may be modified by bundling a complete set of clothing items in the order they are to be donned to support independence in dressing for an individual functioning in Allen Cognitive Level/Mode 3.8. For modification of environments, human and nonhuman, food preparation might be modified by posting steps for food preparation for an individual functioning in Allen Cognitive Level/Mode 4.8; educating caregivers to provide assistance that matches current capacities, such as setting up familiar objects of self-care in visible locations for an individual functioning in Allen Cognitive Level/Mode 4.0; or starting actions for an individual functioning in Allen Cognitive Level/Mode 3.4.

Establish and/or Restore

In the context of the CDM, performance skills and activity patterns, such as routines, may be learned or resumed if they are within the person's functional cognitive capacities as described by the Allen Cognitive Scale. Scores from CDM-based assessments may provide information about the type of assistance and number of repetitions that will facilitate new learning or the restoration of skills and patterns of performance. For example, individuals functioning in Allen Cognitive Level/Mode 4.4 would typically be able to learn how to deposit a disability check, learn a bus route, or how to best bag groceries with demonstrations of each step and repeated practice, assuming that the demands of the task did not change. The case study in this chapter illustrates a combination of this approach and modify/adapt for a person with permanent cognitive disability, but stable, available functional cognitive abilities and overall health.

It should be noted that, although the CDM focuses primarily on compensatory interventions, it does not exclude the possibility that when an optimal fit is achieved between individuals' best ability to function and their engagement and participation in valued activities, this may offer the optimal conditions for restoration of functional cognitive capacities.

Maintenance and Prevention

Maintenance and prevention are closely aligned in the CDM approach to intervention, regardless of the stability of a person's condition. Maintaining a person's best ability to function may create optimal conditions for preventing or slowing decline in functional cognition or for creating the optimal conditions for improvement in functional cognitive abilities. In addition, preventing or minimizing risks and hazards is central to promoting safety, a significant intervention outcome of the CDM. This may involve recommending environments that are an optimal fit with a person's functional cognitive abilities or providing caregiver training about how to modify activities and environments to maintain and support a person's available functional cognitive abilities or to prevent or slow decline in functional cognitive abilities. In addition, maintaining a person's best ability to function requires training caregivers to recognize a change in function that may indicate the need for reevaluation by skilled practitioners.

Resources for Intervention

For a more in-depth discussion of intervention approaches within the context of the CDM, refer to Allen and Blue (1998); Allen, Blue, and Earhart (1995); Allen, Earhart, and Blue (1992); and McCraith and Earhart (2018). For specific guidelines based on an in-depth analysis of the cognitive complexity of functional cognitive capacities and activity demands with suggestions for possible activities and safety precautions for each level and mode of performance, refer to Allen, Blue, and Earhart (1992); Allen, Earhart, and Blue (1995); and Pollard and Olin (2005). Program descriptions that incorporate the principles of the CDM also offer useful resources, for example, Bieber and Keller (2005); Earhart and Riska-Williams (2014); Gitlin et al. (2009, 2010); Helfrich, Chan, and Sabol (2011); Ngoh, Lewis, and Connolly (2005); and Warchol (2004).

Intervention Outcomes and Evidence

The primary outcome of interventions in the CDM is safe, successful, and satisfying engagement and participation in valued activities in supportive environments and contexts that fit the person's available functional cognitive capacities. In the CDM, this outcome is also referred to as achievement of the person's best ability to function (Allen & Blue, 1998; McCraith & Earhart, 2018).

A growing number of published outcome studies, including several large randomized controlled trials, with interventions based on the CDM and assessments described in this chapter, demonstrate that use of scores from these assessments contributes to practitioners' ability to provide effective interventions. Several studies for adults and older adults with mental illness, including those with acute conditions and others with serious conditions at risk for homelessness, have demonstrated the usefulness of the CDM model and the ACLS-90 to guide effective interventions (Chapleau et al., 2012; Raweh & Katz, 1999).

Two outcome studies with hospitalized older adults have demonstrated the feasibility of using the CDM and the ACLS-90 to guide effective interventions (Holm et al., 1999; Ngoh et al., 2005). Four other studies used scores from the ACLS-5, LACLS-5, and ADM-2 to guide an occupational therapy intervention as part of the Tailored Activity Program (Gitlin et al., 2009), one with hospitalized older adults described by Kvedar and Alonzi (2014) and published by Gitlin et al. (2016). The other three studied community-dwelling older adults with dementia and their caregivers, two by Gitlin et al. (2009, 2010) and the third described by Howell (2014) and published by Gitlin, Mann, Vogel, and Arthur (2013). Wesson et al. (2013) demonstrated the feasibility of using the CDM and the LACLS-5 to guide interventions in a falls prevention program with older adults living in the community.

Case Study

The following case illustrates a community-based mental health evaluation, intervention, and outcome by an occupational therapy practitioner using the CDM and the ACLS-5 and the ADM-2 assessments (Earhart, 2011).

Occupational Profile

Data were collected in interviews with Chris and his parents. Chris is a 21-year-old single man who was diagnosed with autism at 3 years of age. He lived with his parents and two siblings after graduation from high school, but recently moved into a mobile home in a safe, residential neighborhood. The mobile home was purchased by his parents so that he could be more independent. Chris follows a familiar daily routine to complete his immediate self-care (i.e., bathes; grooms; takes medication; prepares a few simple meals of microwavable dinners, canned soups, and sandwiches). He has been trained to ride the bus to familiar locations, do his laundry at home, make a simple purchase, and write out a rent check to his mother. His parents assist him to budget his disability check, shop for food and other items, travel to new locations, and plan new activities. Chris rides his bike for some of these activities when the route is familiar and deemed safe by his parents. They check on him daily in person or by phone. Chris has no other medical problems and has never engaged in substance abuse. Chris works 4 hours each day at a restaurant wrapping silverware in napkins, a job arranged by his mental health case manager. Chris's parents report that Chris is typically compliant and very proud of his ability to follow rules and learned routines.

Request for Service

Chris's parents were no longer able to provide him with a ride to the bus station to get to work each morning. Chris wanted to get to the bus by himself but did not know how to accomplish this. His parents supported his desire to be independent but were concerned about his safety. This resulted in the client and caregiver goal that Chris will be able to get to the bus station safely by himself every weekday to catch the bus to work.

Occupational Performance Assessment

The ACLS-5 was selected to screen for possible functional cognitive disability that might impact Chris's ability to safely get to the bus station by himself. Chris completed three correct running and whipstitches but was unable to complete any correct single cordovan stitches after two demonstrations, for a score of 4.4. To verify this screen score, Chris was given a choice between two ADM-2 assessments, the Ribbon Card and the Leather Key Fob, both of which contain activity demands with cognitive complexity of 4.0 to 5.0 on the Allen Cognitive Scale. Chris selected the Leather Key Fob (Will Do). Chris completed this activity with assistance, which included demonstration of all new action sequences, orientation to errors that were not strikingly apparent, and demonstration of solutions to errors that he made but could not correct. Chris imitated new action sequences but recalled them imperfectly at times. He recognized a striking mismatch of visual cues as an error and would typically ask for help. These observations best matched the set of behaviors described in the score of 4.4 on the rating criteria, which are criterion referenced to Mode 4.4 on the Allen Cognitive Scale. When asked to evaluate which part of this activity was hardest for him, he replied, "All of it." However, he remarked earlier that some steps were "easy." Chris also stated that he enjoyed the activity and was pleased that he could use the key fob to hold his house keys.

Other skilled observations during Chris's performance included the observations that Chris answered questions with short, concrete responses without elaboration and that he requested help readily and accepted it because, as he stated, "I have autism, and I need help with things." Important contextual and environmental considerations were that

Chris lived in a safe, residential neighborhood about 1.5 miles from the bus station and his parents were willing to assist with recommended interventions.

Interpreting Occupational Profile and Performance Data

Scores of 4.4 on both standardized ACLS-5 and ADM-2 assessments, observations of Chris's verbal behaviors, self-awareness, and reported need for daily supervision and assistance to plan complex IADLs appeared consistent with the typical pattern of performance described by Allen Cognitive Level/Mode 4.4. Since Chris had no other identified medical problems and did not engage in substance abuse or other behaviors that are known to jeopardize functional cognitive abilities, the practitioner judged that Chris appeared to be currently displaying stable Allen Cognitive Level/Mode 4.4 functional cognitive abilities.

Analyzing Activity Demands and Contextual and Environmental Supports to Determine Realistic Targeted Outcomes

Two potential realistic (Can Do) options to achieve Chris's valued goal were identified: walking to the bus station or riding his bike (a familiar skill). By analyzing the cognitive complexity of activity demands of walking and riding to the bus station and comparing them to Chris's current assessed capacity, the practitioner identified the following relevant considerations:

- Determining a safe route to the bus stop required Allen Cognitive Level/Mode 6.0 functional cognitive abilities.
- Chris would require assistance to determine a safe route and repeated demonstration to learn the identified route based on current Allen Cognitive Level/Mode 4.4 abilities (Can Do).
- While walking on the sidewalk, which requires Allen Cognitive Level/Mode 2.6 functional cognitive abilities, was safer than biking, which requires Allen Cognitive Level/Mode 4.4 abilities, if familiar, it would take three times longer and would significantly impact Chris's morning routine.
- Biking would better fit into Chris's existing schedule but would expose Chris to the hazards of sharing the road with other vehicles.
- Chris was not likely to scan for other vehicles, a skill requiring Allen Cognitive Level/Mode 4.6 abilities; therefore, he would be at greater risk for a collision.
- Teaching Chris to scan was not realistic, but exposure to this hazard might be reduced by instructing Chris to ride his bike on the sidewalk. Chris was likely to comply as he understood and was reportedly proud of his ability to follow rules.

When presented with both options, Chris chose riding his bike to the bus station (Will Do). Chris's parents supported this choice and were willing to provide assistance to meet safety needs and to teach Chris this new routine (May Do).

Targeted Outcome

Chris will be able to independently travel to his weekday job by following specified safety precautions for riding his bike from his home to the bus stop 1.5 miles away using residential sidewalks along a route determined by his Dad.

Intervention Plan

In consultation with Chris and his parents, the following activity modifications and assistance for establishing a safe new routine that fit with Chris's Allen Cognitive Level/Mode 4.4 functional cognitive abilities were established to ensure a safe and successful outcome:

- Dad assembled and checked Chris's bike for safety and identified a safe route on residential street sidewalks.
- Chris agreed to wear a helmet, carry his cell phone, and follow the route identified at all times.
- Dad accompanied Chris on repeated trial runs, pointing out striking visual landmarks along the route, until Chris appeared to learn the route.
- To ensure his safety, Chris practiced calling Dad using a preset number on his cell phone if he encountered a problem or emergency. Chris took this responsibility seriously.

Outcome of Intervention

On his first unsupervised bike ride, Chris used the wrong crosswalk at the only major intersection and could not proceed across the highway because there was no painted crosswalk on that side of the street. Perplexed, he phoned his dad, stating, "I don't know what to do. The cars will not stop for me." Dad deduced that Chris had crossed the street in the wrong direction, and instructed him to go back across the street and use the other painted crosswalk. Chris followed his Dad's directions and, after this incident, biked to the bus by himself successfully each morning. It is important to note that in addition to establishing a new skill for Chris by modifying/adapting the cognitive complexity of activity demands in his valued activity, this intervention both maintained his best ability to function and prevented a possible decline in function.

Suggested Further Research

The psychometric evidence for both CDM-based assessments featured in this chapter, as well as the growing body of intervention outcome evidence for the CDM, has been summarized in this chapter. More peer-reviewed, published psychometric studies are needed for the current versions of these two assessments to ensure that they continue to meet the evidence-based criteria for best practice in occupational therapy. Additional research examining the relationship between the three forms of the ACLS-5 and between these forms and the ADM-2 assessments would strengthen the validity of these assessments as measures of functional cognition and their relationship to the Allen Cognitive Scale. In addition, although some of the ADM-2 assessment activities have been studied, it would be useful to have psychometric data on each of them and their relationship to each other.

While there is a growing body of evidence supporting use of scores from the two featured assessments in this chapter to guide CDM-based interventions, determining the degree to which use of these assessments influences intervention outcomes is another rich area for research. Because occupational therapy practitioners use the CDM to guide their practice with a wide range of populations in varied settings, researchers also need to examine the effectiveness of a wider range of intervention applications based on the CDM and scores from CDM-based assessments with varied populations.

Summary

Although the CDM's core theoretical concepts, principles for evaluation and intervention, and the associated assessments have remained similar over the past 45 years, they have also evolved as a result of extensive clinical experience and expertise and research evidence to meet the changes in occupational therapy and health care practice and to ensure current best practice (Allen, 1985; Allen & Blue, 1998; Allen et al., 1992; McCraith et al., 2011; McCraith & Earhart, 2018). Use of the *Framework* (AOTA, 2014) is an important aspect of best practice in occupational therapy. Therefore, this chapter has described the three forms of version 5 of the ACLS assessment and the ADM-2 in the context of the *Framework* (AOTA, 2014) and current CDM theoretical concepts and principles. These two functional cognitive assessments yield information for understanding functional cognitive capacities that impact occupational performance for individuals with temporary or permanent functional cognitive disabilities. This information is inferred from observations of what a person pays attention to and performance skills as the person engages in activities and from analysis of the cognitive complexity of activity demands, activity patterns, and environmental supports that appear to fit with the person's functional cognitive abilities. These evaluation findings, along with other evaluation data, are used to plan and implement compensatory interventions that optimize use of available functional cognitive abilities by creating a fit between a person's functional cognitive abilities and the cognitive complexity of activity demands of the person's desired activities, contexts, and environments. The expected outcome of this occupational therapy intervention approach is safe, successful, satisfying engagement and participation in valued activities and occupations in supportive contexts and environments. In the words of Claudia K. Allen, for the person with a cognitive limitation or disability "self-fulfillment is experienced while doing significant activities that use one's full capacity to function … [Thus, occupational therapy] reaffirm[s] the right of each individual, no matter how disabled, to engage in self-fulfilling activities" (Allen, 1994).

References

Allen, C. K. (1982). Independence through activity: The practice of occupational therapy (psychiatry). *American Journal of Occupational Therapy, 36*, 731-739.

Allen, C. K. (1985). *Occupational therapy for psychiatric diseases: Measurement and management of cognitive disabilities*. Boston, MA: Little, Brown and Company.

Allen, C. K. (1994). The disabled human mind. Unpublished manuscript.

Allen, C. K. (1999). *Structures of the cognitive performance modes*. Ormond Beach, FL: Allen Conferences, Inc.

Allen, C. K., Austin, S. L., David, S. K., Earhart, C. A., McCraith, D. B., & Riska-Williams, L. (2007). *Manual for the Allen Cognitive Level Screen–5 (ACLS-5) and Large Allen Cognitive Level Screen–5 (LACLS-5)*. Camarillo, CA: ACLS and LACLS Committee.

Allen, C. K., & Blue, T. (1998). Cognitive disabilities model: How to make clinical judgments. In N. Katz (Ed.), *Cognition and occupation in rehabilitation: Cognitive models for intervention in occupational therapy* (pp. 225-280). Bethesda, MD: American Occupational Therapy Association.

Allen, C. K., Blue, T., & Earhart, C. A. (1995). *Understanding the modes of performance*. Ormond Beach, CA: Allen Conferences, Inc. Available at www.ssww.com.

Allen, C. K., & Earhart, C. A. (2000). *Allen Cognitive Level Screen (ACLS) 2000: Test manual*. Colchester, CT: S&S Worldwide.

Allen, C. K., Earhart, C. A., & Blue, T. (1992). *Occupational therapy treatment goals for the physically and cognitively disabled*. Bethesda, MD: American Occupational Therapy Association.

Allen Cognitive Group/ACLS and LACLS Committee. (2016). *Disposable Large Allen Cognitive Level Screen (LACLS[D]) with three stitching tasks set up for administration)*. Camarillo, CA: Author.

Allen Cognitive Group/ACLS and LACLS Committee. (2018a). *ACLS-5 with three stitching tasks set up for administration*. Camarillo, CA: Author.

Allen Cognitive Group/ACLS and LACLS Committee. (2018b). *LACLS-5 with three stitching tasks set up for administration*. Camarillo, CA: Author.

American Educational Research Association. (1999). *Standards for educational and psychological testing*. Washington, DC: Author.

American Occupational Therapy Association. (2014). Occupational therapy practice framework: Domain and process (3rd ed.). *American Journal of Occupational Therapy, 68*(Suppl. 1), S1-S48. 10.5014/ajot.2014.682006.

Austin, S. A. (2009). Hierarchies of abilities and activity demands in the Allen Diagnostic Module (2nd ed.): A validity study. Unpublished doctoral dissertation, University of Illinois, Chicago, IL.

Bieber, D. C., & Keller, B. (2005). Falls and the client with dementia: Using the occupational profile and Allen cognitive level to direct care. *Gerontology: Special Interest Section Quarterly, 28*(2), 1-3.

Cairns, A., Hill, C., Dark, F., McPhail, S., & Gray, M. (2013). The Large Allen Cognitive Level Screen as an indicator for medication adherence among adults accessing community mental health services. *British Journal of Occupational Therapy, 76*, 137-143.

Chang, F. H., Helfrich, C. A., & Coster, W. J. (2013). Psychometric properties of the Practical Skills Test (PST). *American Journal of Occupational Therapy, 67*, 246-253.

Chapleau, A., Seroczynski, A. D., Meyers, S., Lamb, K., & Buchino, S. (2012). The effectiveness of a consultation model in community mental health. *Occupational Therapy in Mental Health, 28*, 379-395.

Collister, L., & Alexander, K. (1991). *The Occupational Therapy Domestic and Community Skills Assessment, research edition*. Melbourne, Victoria, Australia: La Trobe University.

David, S. K., & Riley, W. T. (1990). The relationship of the Allen Cognitive Level Test to cognitive abilities and psychopathology. *American Journal of Occupational Therapy, 44*, 493-497.

Earhart, C. A. (2006). *Allen Diagnostic Module: Manual* (2nd ed.). Colchester, CT: S&S Worldwide.

Earhart, C. A. (2011). Case example: Chris [Teaching Case]. In C. A. Earhart (2011, October). Using the Cognitive Disabilities Model to Guide Interventions. Presented at the 35th Annual Occupational Therapy Association of California Conference. Sacramento, CA.

Earhart, C. A. (2015a). *Summary of functional cognitive abilities for the six cognitive levels with intervention guidelines*. Camarillo, CA: ACLS and LACLS Committee.

Earhart, C. A. (2015b). *Examples of Allen Diagnostic Module (2nd ed.) assessments*. Pasadena, CA: Author.

Earhart, C. A. (2015c). Range of scores based on complexity of activity demands for Allen Diagnostic Module (2nd ed.) assessments. In C. A. Earhart, *Allen Diagnostic Module: Manual* (2nd ed.). Colchester, CT: S&S Worldwide.

Earhart, C. A. (2015d). *Observing performance in Allen Diagnostic Module, 2nd Edition: Ribbon Card assessment*. Pasadena, CA: Author.

Earhart, C. A. (2020). *Analysis of complexity of activity demands for ACLS version 5 stitching tasks*. Pasadena, CA: Author.

Earhart, C. A., & Allen, C. K. (1988). *Cognitive disabilities: Expanded activity analysis: Analysis of craft processes and cognitive stimulation and response*. Los Angeles, CA: University of Southern California.

Earhart, C. A., Allen, C. K., & Blue, T. (1993). *Allen Diagnostic Module: Instruction manual* (1st ed.). Colchester, CT: S&S Worldwide.

Earhart, C. A., & McCraith, D. (2020). *Titles of six cognitive levels and 26 modes of performance*. Camarillo, CA: ACLS and LACLS Committee.

Earhart, C. A., & Riska-Williams, L. (2014). The perfect fit: Creating sustainable communities of participation for elderly persons with dementia. Retrieved from https://www.allencognitive.com/pdf-downloads/

Folstein, M. F., Folstein, S. E., & McHugh, P. R. (1975). Mini-mental state: A practical method for grading the cognitive state of patients for the clinician. *Journal of Psychiatric Research, 12*, 189-198.

Gitlin, L. N., Mann, W. C., Vogel, W. B., & Arthur, P. B. (2013). A non-pharmacologic approach to address challenging behaviors of Veterans with dementia: Description of the tailored activity program-VA randomized trial. *BMC Geriatrics, 13*(96). https://doi.org/10.1186/1471-2318-13-96

Gitlin, L. N., Marx, K. A., Alonzi, D., Kvedar, T., Moody, J., Trahan, M., & Van Haitsma, K. (2016). Feasibility of the Tailored Activity Program for hospitalized (TAP-H) patients with behavioral symptoms. *Gerontologist, 57*, 575-584.

Gitlin, L. N., Winter, L., Dennis, M. P., Hodgson, N., & Hauck, W. W. (2010). A biobehavioral home-based intervention and the well-being of patients with dementia and their caregivers: The COPE randomized trial. *Journal of the American Medical Association, 304*, 983-991.

Gitlin, L. N., Winter, L., Vause-Earland, T., Herge, A. E., Chernett, N. L., Piersol, C. V., & Burke, J. P. (2009). The Tailored Activity Program to reduce behavioral symptoms in individuals with dementia: Feasibility, acceptability, and replication potential. *Gerontologist, 49*, 428-439.

Helfrich, C. A., Chan, V. C., & Sabol, P. (2011). Cognitive predictors of the life skill intervention outcomes of adults with mental illness at risk for homelessness. *American Journal of Occupational Therapy, 65,* 277-286.

Helfrich, C. A., & McCraith, D. (2015). *A pilot study of the inter-rater reliability of the ACLS-5 and LACLS-5.* Camarillo, CA: Allen Cognitive Group/ACLS and LACLS Committee.

Henry, A., McCraith, D., & St. Germain, T. (2000). Reliability, validity and clinical use of an Allen Diagnostic Module Activity. Presented at the American Occupational Therapy Association Annual Conference. Seattle, WA.

Henry, A. D., Moore, K., Quinlivan, M., & Triggs, M. (1998). The relationship of the Allen Cognitive Level Test to demographics, diagnosis, and disposition among psychiatric inpatients. *American Journal of Occupational Therapy, 52,* 638-643.

Holm, A., Michel, M., Stern, G. A., Hung, T., Klein, T., Flaherty, L., … Maletta, G. (1999). The outcomes of an inpatient treatment program for geriatric dementia and dysfunctional behaviors. *Gerontologist, 39,* 668-676.

Howell, T. (October 2014). Activity selection process for persons with dementia and caregivers. Presented at the 10th Annual Cognitive Symposium, Redondo Beach, CA.

Josman, N., & Katz, N. (1991). A problem-solving version of the Allen Cognitive Level Test. *American Journal of Occupational Therapy, 45,* 331-338.

Katz, N. (2006). *Routine Task Inventory–Expanded (RTI-E) manual.* Retrieved from http://www.allen-cognitive-network.org/images/stories/pdf_files/rtimanual2006.pdf

Katz, N., & Perelman, N. (1993). Cognitive levels and work recommendations: A study of chronic psychiatric patients in the community. *Work, 3,* 64-68.

Kehrberg, K. L., Kuskowski, M. A., Mortimer, J. A., & Shoberg, T. D. (1992). Validating the use of an enlarged, easier-to-see Allen Cognitive Level test in geriatrics. *Physical & Occupational Therapy in Geriatrics, 10,* 1-14.

Keller, S., & Hayes, R. (1998). The relationship between the Allen Cognitive Level Test and the Life Skills Profile. *American Journal of Occupational Therapy, 52*(10), 851–856. https://doi.org/10.5014/ajot.52.10.851

Koo, T. K., & Li, M. Y. (2016). A guideline of selecting and reporting intraclass correlation coefficients for reliability research. *Journal of Chiropractic Medicine, 15,* 155-163.

Kvedar, T., & Alonzi, D. (2014). Translating the tailored activity program in a chronic care hospital for dementia patients. Paper presented at the Cognitive Symposium sponsored by the Allen Cognitive Network. Redondo Beach, CA.

Lee, S. N., Gargiullo, A., Brayman, S., Kinsey, J. C., Jones, H. C., & Shotwell, M. (2003). Adolescent performance on the Allen Cognitive Levels Screen. *American Journal of Occupational Therapy, 57,* 342-346.

Levy, L. L. (2018). Cognitive information-processing memory. In N. Katz & J. Toglia (Eds.), *Cognition, occupation, and participation across the life span* (4th ed., pp. 105-128). Bethesda, MD: American Occupational Therapy Association.

Marom B., Jarus T., & Josman, N. (2011). The relationship between the Assessment of Motor and Process Skills (AMPS) and the Large Allen Cognitive Level (LACL) test in clients with stroke. *Physical & Occupational Therapy in Geriatrics, 24*(4), 33-50.

McAnanama, E. P., Rogosin-Rose, M. L., Scott, E. A., Joffe, R. T., & Kelner, M. (1999). Discharge planning in mental health: The relevance of cognition to community living. *American Journal of Occupational Therapy, 53,* 129-137.

McCraith, D. B., Austin, S. L., & Earhart, C. A. (2011). The cognitive disabilities model in 2011. In N. Katz (Ed.), *Cognition, occupation, and participation across the life span* (3rd ed., pp. 383-406). Bethesda, MD: American Occupational Therapy Association.

McCraith, D. B., & Earhart, C. A. (2018). Cognitive disabilities model: Creating fit between functional cognitive abilities and cognitive activity demands. In N. Katz & J. Toglia (Eds.), *Cognition, occupation, and participation across the life span* (4th ed., pp. 469-497). Bethesda, MD: American Occupational Therapy Association.

McCraith, D. B., & Henry, A. (2003). Usefulness of cognitive disabilities model in predicting community functioning among persons with mental disorders. Paper presented at the Allen Cognitive Symposium. Tampa, FL.

Moore, D. S. (1978). An occupational therapy evaluation of sensorimotor cognition: Initial reliability, validity, and descriptive data for hospitalized schizophrenic adults. Unpublished master's thesis, University of Southern California, Los Angeles, CA.

Ngoh, C. T., Lewis, I. D., & Connolly, P. M. (2005). Outcomes of inpatient geropsychiatric treatment: The value of assessment protocols. *Journal of Gerontological Nursing, 31*(4), 12-18.

Okamura, T., Takeshita, A., Teramoto, K., Aida, Y., & Kino, J. (2010). A comparison of the Allen Cognitive Level-5 Test (Japanese version) and Mini-Mental State-E (Japanese version) in elderly patients with cerebrovascular disorder. Unpublished manuscript, Division of Occupational Therapy, Department of Rehabilitation Sciences, Faculty of Health Care Sciences, Chiba-shi, Chiba, Japan.

Penny, N. H., Mueser, K. T., & North, C. T. (1995). The Allen Cognitive Level test and social competence in adult psychiatric patients. *American Journal of Occupational Therapy, 49,* 420-427.

Pollard, D., & Olin, D. W. (2005). *Allen's cognitive levels: Meeting the challenges of client focused services*. Monoma, WI: Selectone Rehab.

Raweh, D. V., & Katz, N. (1999). Treatment effectiveness of Allen's cognitive disabilities model with adult schizophrenic outpatients: A pilot study. *Occupational Therapy in Mental Health, 14*, 65-77.

Regier, N. G., Hodgson, N. A., & Gitlin, L. N. (2017). Characteristics of activities for persons with dementia at the mild, moderate, and severe stages. *Gerontologist, 57*(5), 987-997.

Roitman, D. M., & Katz, N. (1996). Predictive validity of the Large Allen Cognitive Levels Test using the Allen Diagnostic Module in an aged, non-disabled population. *Physical & Occupational Therapy in Geriatrics, 14*, 43-59.

Rojo-Mota, G., Pedrero-Perez, E. J., Huertas-Hoyas, E., Merritt, B., & MacKenzie, D. (2016). Allen Cognitive Level Screen for the classification of subjects treated for addiction. *Scandinavian Journal of Occupational Therapy, 24*, 290-298.

Scanlan, J. N., & Still, M. (2013). Functional profile of mental health consumers assessed by occupational therapists: Level of independence and associations with functional cognition. *Psychiatry Research, 208*, 29-32.

Schubmehl, S., Barkin, S. H., & Cort, D. (2018) The role of executive functions and psychiatric symptom severity in the Allen Cognitive Levels. *Psychiatry Research, 259*, 169-175.

Secrest, L., Wood, A. E., & Tapp, A. (2000). A comparison of the Allen Cognitive Level Test and the Wisconsin Card Sorting Test in adults with schizophrenia. *American Journal of Occupational Therapy, 54*, 129-133.

Shapiro, M. E. (1992). Application of the Allen Cognitive Level Test in assessing cognitive level functioning of emotionally disturbed boys. *American Journal of Occupational Therapy, 46*, 514-520.

Su, C.-Y., Tsai, P.-C., Su, W.-L., Tang, T.-C., & Tsai, A. Y.-J. (2011). Cognitive profile difference between Allen Cognitive Levels 4 and 5 in schizophrenia. *American Journal of Occupational Therapy, 65*, 453-461.

Thompson, K., Kulkami, J., & Serge, A. A. (2000). Reliability and validity of a new Medication Adherence Rating Scale (MARS) for the psychoses. *Schizophrenia Research, 42*, 241-247.

Velligan, D. I., Bow-Thomas, C. C., Mahurin, R., Miller, A., Dassori, A., & Erdely, F. (1998). Concurrent and predictive validity of the Allen Cognitive Levels Assessment. *Psychiatry Research, 80*, 287-298.

Velligan, D. I., True, J. E., Lefton, R. S., Moore, T. C., & Flores, C. V. (1995). Validity of the Allen Cognitive Levels Assessment: A tri-ethnic comparison. *Psychiatry Research, 56*, 101-109.

Warchol, K. (2004). An interdisciplinary dementia program model for long-term care. *Topics in Geriatric Rehabilitation, 20*, 59-71.

Wesson, J., Clemson, L., Brodaty, H., Lord, S., Taylor, M., Gitlin, L., & Close, J. (2013). A feasibility study and pilot randomised trial of a tailored prevention program to reduce falls in older people with mild dementia. *BMC Geriatrics, 13*, 89.

Wesson, J., Clemson, L., Brodaty, H., & Reppermund, S. (2016). Estimating functional cognition in older adults using observational assessments of task performance in complex everyday activities: A systematic review and evaluation of measurement properties. *Neuroscience and Biobehavioral Reviews, 68*, 335-360.

Wesson, J., Clemson, L., Crawford, J. D., Kochan, N. A., Brodaty, H., & Reppermund, S. (2017). Measurement of functional cognition and complex everyday activities in older adults with mild cognitive impairment and mild dementia: Validity of the Large Allen's Cognitive Level Screen. *American Journal of Geriatric Psychiatry, 25*(5), 471-482. http://dx.doi.org/10.1016/j.jagp.2016.11.021

Wesson J., & Giles, G. M. (2019). Understanding functional cognition. In T. J. Wolf, D. F. Edwards, & G. M. Giles (Eds.), *Functional cognition and occupational therapy: A practical approach to treating individuals with cognitive loss* (pp. 7–20). Bethesda, MD: AOTA Press.

White, S. M., Meade, S. A., & Hadar, L. (2007). OT cognitive adaptation: An intervention in time management for persons with co-occurring conditions. *Occupational Therapy Practice*, 9-14.

Ziv, N., Roitman, D. M., & Katz, N. (1999). Problem solving, sense of coherence and instrumental ADL of elderly people with depression and normal control group. *Occupational Therapy International, 6*, 243-256.

Routine Task Inventory– Expanded

Noomi Katz, PhD, OTR

The just-right challenge.
(Allen, 1987, p. 2)

Occupational therapists assess client functional cognition to assist with treatment planning, as well as planning for safe and effective discharge. Client level of independence has been a hallmark of the profession of occupational therapy. Of utmost importance is the selection of assessments that are easy to administer yet provide valid and reliable information that can be easily utilized clinically. The Routine Task Inventory–Expanded (RTI-E) is one such measure. This chapter will provide the reader insight into the development of the measure, its administration, and the utility of this assessment. A research-based case study at the end of the chapter provides the reader with a clear understanding of how the assessment can be easily and effectively used within clinical practice.

Theoretical Basis

The most recent development of the Allen Cognitive Model (ACM) was written by McCraith, Austin, and Earhart (2011). The current thinking, together with Claudia Allen's work, facilitated the next step from the ACM into the current Cognitive Disabilities Model (CDM). When the CDM was introduced, Allen (1985) defined cognitive disability as a "restriction in voluntary motor action originating in the physical or chemical structures of the brain and producing observable limitations in routine task behavior" (p. 31). This focus on disability rather than ability was in keeping with the conventions of the times.

Hemphill, B. J., & Urish, C. K. (Eds.). *Assessments in Occupational Therapy Mental Health: An Integrative Approach, Fourth Edition* (pp. 211-221). © 2020 Taylor & Francis Group.

Well into the 1990s, cognitive disabilities were the organizing constructs of the CDM (Allen, 1987; Allen & Blue, 1998; Allen, Earhart, & Blue, 1992). However, as the model evolved, the emphasis shifted to the concepts of cognition and function using terms such as *functional information-processing abilities* or *functional cognition* (Allen, Austin, David, Earhart, McCraith, & Riska-Williams, 2007; Pollard & Olin, 2005) instead of cognitive disability to describe the central construct of the CDM (McCraith et al., 2011).

Concepts/Construct

Two major concepts/constructs are essential to the CDM: cognitive levels and routine tasks (Allen et al., 1992; McCraith et al., 2011). Cognitive levels are the building blocks of person's conscious mind, as reflected in behavior. Routine tasks are the individual's occupational performance based on his or her cognitive level at a specific point in time.

Evaluation

According to the six-step cognitive functional evaluation (Hartman-Maeir, Katz, & Baum, 2009), the protocol of the CDM includes a cognitive screening, including the Allen Cognitive Level Screen–5 (ACLS-5) and Large Allen Cognitive Level Screen–5 (LACLS-5; Allen et al., 2007). Next, the occupational therapist chooses a measure to verify the ACLS-5 or LACLS-5 screening score with a general measure of cognition and executive function while engaged in occupation, which may include the choice of RTI-E or the Cognitive Performance Test (CPT; Burns, 2006; Levy & Burns, 2011). The difference between these two instruments is two-fold. First, the CPT is a performance test, while the RTI-E is a questionnaire. Second, the CPT consists of a battery of six simulated instrumental activities of daily living (IADL) tasks, whereas the RTI-E is a rating scale based on the observation of 30 tasks in 4 occupational areas (activities of daily living [ADLs], IADLs, communication, and work readiness). The RTI-E can be completed through the therapist's observation of the client, an interview with the client, or feedback from the caregiver, who can be a family member, a significant other, or other care provider, such as nursing staff or nursing assistant. The scores of both the CPT and RTI-E follow the hierarchy of the six cognitive levels developed by Allen et al. (1992).

The RTI-E is part of the evaluation process within the ACM and now the CDM. The RTI-E follows the basic tenet of the ACM/CDM model to assess functional cognition related to participation and engagement in daily occupations. The RTI-E provides the most valid measure of the actual day-to-day participation of the individual in four major occupational areas of life: ADLs, IADLs, communication, and work readiness, within which subareas are outlined and a scale of levels based on the Allen's six cognitive levels are measured.

History of Development

The RTI has been used as the standard since 1985 when it was prepared by Allen as the original RTI. The second iteration of the RTI (RTI-2; Allen et al., 1992) appeared to be unclear and too complicated for most practitioners and therefore was not used enough.

The RTI can be thought of as both an activity analysis and a functional evaluation instrument (Allen, 1985). As an activity analysis, its clinical utility is limited by the therapist's knowledge of cognitive disability theory (Allen, 1985). As a functional evaluation, it seems to make sense to caregivers; therefore, experience in living/working with the cognitively disabled may be the prerequisite for reliable use.

The original RTI has been expanded to include using adaptive equipment (on the physical scale) and child care (on the community scale); two additional scales were added: a communication scale and a work scale. The internal consistency, established by Heimann, Allen, and Yerxa (1989) for the original RTI, provided the confidence needed to extend the task analysis to other activities. Three sources of information can be used to complete a functional assessment: patient/client self-report, a family member or other caregiver's report, and observations of performance by a therapist. A self-report for an individual who is cognitively disabled is often unreliable and tends to underestimate the degree of difficulty in performing a task; therefore, an additional informant is necessary. In addition, discrepancies between self-report and observations, such as those found in legal proceedings, which often include a patient's self-report, can be helpful. For various reasons, family members and other caregivers may also under- or overestimate quality of performance, with most people placing more credibility in observations of performance.

Therapists conduct numerous observations of performance, usually more than what can be reasonably communicated in a progress note or team meeting. Preparing a comprehensive, fair, and objective report of a person with disabilities' ability to function is a complex and time-consuming assignment. The principle advantage of the format presented on the scoring sheet is that it helps to get an overview of the available information. As originally defined by Allen: "A cognitive disability is a restriction in sensorimotor actions originating in the physical or chemical structures of the brain, producing observable and assessable limitations in routine task behavior" (1985, p. 31). Like other assessments associated with the CDM, the RTI is intended to assess the degree to which this restriction interferes with everyday task performance through observation of task behavior.

Routine task behavior is defined here as occupational performance in the areas of self-care and instrumental activities at home and in the community, social communication through verbal and written comprehension and expression, and readiness for work relations and performance. The aim of the assessment of routine task behavior is to promote the safe, routine performance of an individual's valued occupations and to maximize participation in life situations. The assessment manual provides the RTI-E scales, a scoring sheet with a reporting form, and tables presenting a summary of research studies that provide initial reliability and validity data for the different versions of the RTI and references (Katz, 2006). Based on experience and research data, it seems the two areas that were added to the original RTI (communication and work readiness scales) are essential in the understanding of everyday functioning and occupational performance for a variety of populations for whom the instrument maybe appropriate. The RTI-E manual was prepared to provide practitioners and researchers with a clear protocol for administration and scoring so the assessment can be used consistently by practitioners and researchers. The RTI-E is intended for use by occupational therapy personnel. Administering the assessment requires knowledge of the CDM, interview skills, observation, and activity analysis skills.

The four areas of the RTI-E can be completed by calculating a mean score for each area. These scores correspond to the six levels of functional cognition. Although the theoretical levels developed by Allen and her colleagues range from 1 to 6, the entire range of scores is not included within each area of the RTI-E. The range of scores in each area is based upon the underlying theoretical understanding of the skills necessary for tasks included in each area. The range of possible scores are as follows: Physical scale-ADLs, 1 to 5; Community scale-IADLs, 2 to 6; Communication scale, 1 to 6; and Work Readiness scale, 3 to 6. A self-report describes the individual's view of the degree to which participation/engagement in routine task behaviors are restricted. The caregiver report describes the same information from the caregiver's perspective. The occupational therapist report describes the judgments of a therapist who has observed the individual perform at least four of the tasks within the area being scored. The entire RTI-E is available for the reader to use clinically and is found in Appendix C (Katz, 2006).

Psychometric Properties

A summary of the normative data, reliability, and validity are presented in Table 12-1. Research conducted utilizing the RTI-E including means and standard deviation are presented in Table 12-2.

Assessment Administration

The RTI-E is a rating scale based on observation that can be filled out by the client, a caregiver, or an occupational therapist. The scoring form provides has three columns for recording the score: self (S), caregiver (C), and therapist (T). If the RTI-E is completed by more than one source, a comparison can be made between these two perspectives, especially if one is the self-report from the client. This comparison may point to possible issues of self-awareness, which can be helpful in intervention planning and implementation.

Description of Environment

The RTI-E can be administered in any environment where the individual (i.e., client, occupational therapist, caregiver) has direct knowledge about client performance in the areas of ADLs, IADLs, communication, and work readiness.

Scoring

As can be seen in Appendix C, scoring is on a 6-point scale, according to ACLS. However, all six levels were not appropriate in all areas. Scoring on the ADL area ranges from 1 to 5, IADL from 2 to 6, communication from 1 to 6, and work readiness from 3 to 6. These ranges are in accordance with the concept and levels of the ACLS. Each area is scored separately, thus four final sum scores are obtained (see scoring sheet available in Appendix C). Administration can include all areas or selected areas, according to the client's abilities and situation.

Table 12-1

Routine Task Inventory–Expanded Research Summary

RTI Version	Method	Population	Results	Reference
RTI original 2 areas ADL, IADL Caregiver report	Establish psychometric properties	Psychiatry Dementia	Reliability: high interrater, test-retest, and internal consistency	Allen, 1985 Heimann et al., 1989 Wilson et al., 1989 Allen et al., 1992
RTI-Expanded 4 areas				Allen, 1989
Only IADL scale Self-report during interview	Group comparison and prediction of IADL performance	Elderly with depression ($n=31$) Healthy controls ($n=30$)	RTI & LACL $r=.70$ & MMSE $r=.63$ & GDS $r=-.60$ Sig differences between groups	Ziv et al., 1999
Only items that have parallel tasks on CPT Caregiver report and therapist observation	Group comparison and correlations of RTI and CPT	Dementia ($n=30$) Elderly healthy ($n=30$)	Sig differences between groups for both caregiver and therapist High correlations $r=.72$ to .94 with therapist; moderate with caregiver $r=.29$ to .56	Bar-Yosef et al., 1999
Only IADL scale Self-report during interview	Subgroup comparisons and correlations of RTI and KELS	Elderly in the community ($n=92$) 3 groups according to living situation Community, sheltered, day care	Sig correlation between RTI and KELS $r=.89$, $p<.000$ Sig difference on RTI between groups F=30.09, $p<.000$ Scheffe post hoc: day care group differs from the other 2 groups	Zimmavoda et al., 2002

(continued)

Table 12-1 (continued)

Routine Task Inventory–Expanded Research Summary

RTI Version	Method	Population	Results	Reference
3 areas except for work scale and safety item Self-report during interview Caregiver report	RTI in elderly stroke population, correlations with CPT	Elderly post stroke in the community ($n = 30$)	Sig moderate to high correlations between self and caregiver report on RTI areas except safety Sig correlations between RTI and CPT	Wachtel, 2003
All areas Therapist observation	RTI as outcome—correlations and explained variance by basic cognition and EF BADS & EFPT	Adult chronic schizophrenia ($n = 31$)	EF (BADS) explains RTI IADL and Communication variance beyond basic cognition (Cognistat) Sig correlations with EFPT components	Tadmor, 2004 Katz et al., 2005
3 areas: IADLs, communication, work readiness Caregiver report	OGI: EF treatment effectiveness RTI as outcome	Schizophrenia acute phase in day hospital ($n = 7$) pre ($n = 11$) post		Katz & Keren, 2011
RTI-2 (1992) 4 areas				Allen et al., 1992
All 4 areas Self-report during interview	ACL-90; RTI-2 Time I discharge Time II follow-up	Adult psychiatric inpatients ($n = 40$)	ACL & RTI Time II: IADL $r = .38$ $p < .016$ ADL $r = .20$ NS $r = .45$ for psychotic subgroup	McAnanama et al., 1999

(continued)

Table 12-1 (continued)

Routine Task Inventory–Expanded Research Summary

RTI Version	Method	Population	Results	Reference
All 4 areas Self with caregiver report during interview	Treatment effectiveness study: experimental CD ADM tasks vs. control sheltered workshop	Schizophrenic post acute experimental ($n=11$); control ($n=8$)	Sig change pre-post within group Sig difference between groups post; RTI & BPRS $r=.50\ p>.01$	Raweh & Katz, 1999
Not clear what areas were used Self-report during interview	Correlation with WCST	Adult men with schizophrenia ($n=33$)	Sig correlation WCST & RTI perseveration $r=-.59$; categories $r=.68$, $p<.01$	Secrest et al., 2000

RTI: Physical scale-ADLs; IADL; caregiver scoring.

RTI-Expanded: Physical scale-ADLs; Community scale- IADLs; Communication scale: Work readiness scale; Scoring options: S = self-report; C=caregiver report; T = therapist observation of performance.

RTI-2: Self-awareness disability; Situational awareness disability; Occupational role disability; Social role disability: Scoring options: S=self-report; C=caregiver report; O=observation of performance (therapists).

Abbreviations: ADLs = activities of daily living; ADM = Allen Diagnostic Module; ACL = Allen Cognitive Level; BADS = Behavioral Assessment of the Dysexecutive Syndrome; BPRS = Brief Psychiatry Rating Scale; CD = cognitive disabilities; CPT = Cognitive Performance Test; EF = executive function; EFPT = Executive Function Performance Test; GDS = Gordon Diagnostic Systems; IADL = instrumental activities of daily living; KELS = Kohlman Evaluation of Living Skills; LACL = Large Allen Cognitive Level; MMSE = Mini Mental State Examination; NS = not significant; OGI = Occupational Goal Intervention; WCST = Wisconsin Card Sort Test

Reprinted with permission from Katz, N. (2006). *Routine Task Inventory–Expanded (RTI-E)*. Retrieved from http://www.allen-cognitive-network.org/pdf_files/RTIManual2006.pdf

Table 12-2

Means and Standard Deviations With Source

Populations	Mean (SD)	Reference
Elderly with depression (n=31), healthy controls (n=30)	S 4.72 (.98) S 5.82 (.33)	Ziv et al., 1999
Elderly with dementia (n=30), elderly healthy (n=30)	T 3.43 (.90), C 3.02 (.66) T 5.23 (.48), C 5.34 (.35)	Bar-Yosef et al., 1999
Elderly in the community (n=92) 3 groups	S 5.77 (.40) 5.46 (.73) 4.0 (1.0)	Zimnavoda et al., 2002
Elderly post stroke in the community (n=30)	S 3.84 (1.18)	Wachtel, 2003
Adult chronic schizophrenia (n=31)	T 4.07 (.51)	Tadmor, 2004 Katz et al., 2005
Adults with schizophrenia acute phase in day hospital (n=17) pre (n=11) post	C 4.35 (.82) pre C 4.63 (.86) post	Katz & Keren, 2011
Adult psychiatric inpatients (n=40)	S 4.81 (.45)	McAnanama et al., 1999
Schizophrenic post acute E (n=11), control (n=8)	C 5.16 (.69) 4.53 (.73) pre C 5.41 (.50) 4.67 (.72) post	Raweh & Katz, 1999
Adult men with schizophrenia (n=33)	No data	Secrest et al., 2000

Reprinted with permission from Katz, N. (2006). *Routine Task Inventory–Expanded (RTI-E)*. Retrieved from http://www.allen-cognitive-network.org/pdf_files/RTIManual2006.pdf

Intervention Planning Based on Assessment Results

The major premise of the intervention approach based on Allen's CDM is a thorough assessment of functional cognition. This assessment includes a basic screening using the ACLS-5 or LACLS-5 and verification of the patient's cognitive level through use of an Allen Diagnostic Module (2nd Edition) task (Earhart, 2006), the RTI-E, or the CPT, as defined in a simulated functional task or in actual daily behavior. Following the assessment process, the accumulated data are the basis for intervention planning and implementation. The intervention should be accompanied by careful observations and adaptation to the process of change/no change, whether there is improvement or decline. Strongly emphasized by Allen, improvement may be evident not through change in cognitive level but rather through improving/enlarging the tasks and activities at the same level.

Case Study

The Occupational Goal Intervention (OGI; Katz & Keren, 2011; Keren, Gal, Degan, Yakoel, & Katz, 2008) utilized the RTI-E as a measure of functional performance in a study of clients with schizophrenia at a day treatment center. The study compared three treatment methods: a functional method (the OGI), a neuropsychological method (Frontal/Executive Program [FEP]), and a classic occupational therapy intervention (the Activity Training Approach). A quasi-experimental design was used with 18 adult participants, aged 20 to 38 years, who were randomly assigned to 1 of the 3 groups. Testing was performed before treatment, after treatment, and at the 6-month follow-up. Instruments assessed executive functions using the Behavioral Assessment of the Dysexecutive Syndrome (Wilson, Alderman, Burgess, Emslie, & Evans, 1996) and the Executive Function Performance Test (Baum, Morrison, Hahn, & Edwards, 2003); activity and participation were assessed using the RTI-E and the Activity Card Sort (Baum & Edwards, 2008). Participants received 18 treatment sessions over a period of 6 to 8 weeks. The results showed that in three components of the RTI-E (IADLs, communication, and work readiness), the OGI group's relative improvement was significant and higher than the Activity Training Approach group, whereas the FEP group showed no change at all on functional tasks.

The case studies from this client group (Keren et al., 2008) demonstrated that the client treated with the FEP program improved in formal executive functions but not in everyday life functions, whereas the client treated according to the OGI program improved in the daily life activities, which were important to them. This client had a desire to address these life areas. The client's RTI-E score was a cognitive level of 4.7, enabling the client to work on an activity program that was systematic and tangible. According to Allen's model:

> [I]ndividuals who function at cognitive level 4 initiate and complete familiar activities such as grooming, dressing, making a sandwich, or playing a card game at a slower than normal pace. These individuals take pleasure in following routines or procedures with known outcomes. They may note obvious errors or problems that prevent the completion of tasks, but they do not typically initiate problem solving. (McCraith et al., 2011, p. 390)

Translation of the Routine Task Inventory–Expanded to Other Languages

The RTI-E was translated into various languages, such as into Hebrew for research and for clinical use in Israel. Recently, the assessment was translated to Portuguese in Brazil by Patrícia Cotting. This Brazilian occupational therapist conducted research by collecting data on older adult clients in Sao Paulo, Brazil.

Another approach undertaken by Pirta Niemi, an occupational therapist from Finland, utilized the RTI-E as part of a thesis for a degree program. This practitioner translated the RTI-E to Finnish (with permission) and created a project for the occupational therapists who worked in the Oulu area. The project was to organize an educational program about the use of the RTI-E as an assessment tool and as a part of the Allen CDM. The thesis was a project for the Oulu University of Applied Sciences. The objective was to improve local professional expertise and the development of the occupational therapists in assessing functional cognitive abilities. The aim was after involvement in the program, participants would possess basic knowledge about the Allen CDM and the RTI-E assessment. Research addressed quality of the educational program, how informative the program was, and functionality and usability of knowledge gained by the occupational therapists. The educational program included a lecture about the basic theories and principles of the Allen CDM and the RTI-E. An assessment of a person with traumatic brain injury was shown through case video, and the RTI-E assessment tool was analyzed in small groups. Based on the verbal and written feedback gathered from the participants, the need for an official translation of the assessment tool was identified that would facilitate the usability of the instrument and the model. Participants stated their desire for an advanced course, including content on the assessment and model. This strategy for the provision of new information to build knowledge in different parts of the world appeared to be very beneficial for the occupational therapy profession globally.

In all translations, the procedure included translation to the new language and back translation to English, which was checked by an expert in the RTI-E administration.

Suggested Further Research

A recommendation included the revision of the current RTI-E for the older adult population and for persons who are unemployed. The inclusion of the areas of work preparation and community participation (e.g., leisure, volunteering) could assist in the evaluation of RTI-E populations who are already retired or are unable to work in a traditional employment situation and could provide important information regarding daily function.

Summary

The RTI-E (Katz, 2006) was developed as part of the Allen CDM. This assessment is unique in the breadth of information provided by rating persons' abilities in major life activities in four areas including basic ADLs, IADLs, communication, and readiness for work. At the same time, the measure adheres to the system of cognitive levels, enabling a match between theoretical understanding, actual performance and treatment guidelines, and providing the "just-right challenge" to treatment, according to appropriate guidelines (Allen et al., 1992; McCraith et al., 2011).

The RTI-E has been utilized and studied in various populations and was found to be a reliable and valid instrument. However, many of the studies are not recent and the extent of the clinical usage of the assessment is unclear. Occupational therapists are encouraged to utilize the instrument in clinical practice and, if possible, to collect data to further establish assessment validity.

References

Allen, C. K. (1985). *Occupational therapy for psychiatric diseases: Measurement and management of cognitive disabilities*. Boston, MA: Little, Brown and Company.

Allen, C. K. (1987). Activity: Occupational therapy's treatment method (Eleanor Clarke Slagle lecture). *American Journal of Occupational Therapy, 41*, 563-575.

Allen, C. K. (1989). Routine Task Inventory–Expanded (RTI-E). Unpublished manuscript.

Allen, C. K., Austin, S. L., David, S. K., Earhart, C. A., McCraith, D. B., & Riska-Williams, L. (2007). *Manual for the Allen Cognitive Level Screen-5 (ACLS-5) and Large Allen Cognitive Level Screen-5 (ACLS-5)*. Camarillo, CA: ACLS and LACLS Committee.

Allen, C. K., & Blue, T. (1998). Cognitive disabilities model: How to make clinical judgments. In N. Katz (Ed.), *Cognitive rehabilitation: Models for intervention in occupational therapy* (pp. 225-279). Bethesda, MD: American Occupational Therapy Association.

Allen, C. K., Earhart, C. A., & Blue, T. (1992). *Occupational therapy treatment goals for the physically and cognitively disabled*. Bethesda, MD: American Occupational Therapy Association.

Bar-Yosef, C., Katz, N., & Weinblatt, N. (1999). Reliability and validity of the Cognitive Performance Test (CPT) in Israel. *Physical and Occupational Therapy in Geriatrics, 17*, 65-79.

Baum, C., & Edwards, D. (2008). *Activity Card Sort*. Bethesda, MD: American Occupational Therapy Association.

Baum, C., Morrison, T., Hahn, M., & Edwards, D. (2003). *Executive Function Performance Test: Test protocol booklet.* Retrieved from http://www.ot.wustl.edu/about/resources/executive-function-performance-test-efpt-308

Burns, T. (2006). *Cognitive Performance Test (CPT).* Pequannock, NJ: Maddak.

Earhart, C. A. (2006). *Allen Diagnostic Module: Manual* (2nd ed.). Colchester, CT: S&S Worldwide.

Hartman-Maeir, A., Katz, N., & Baum, C. (2009). Cognitive-Functional Evaluation (CFE) for individuals with suspected cognitive disabilities. *Occupational Therapy in Health Care, 23,* 1-23.

Heimann, N. E., Allen, C. K., & Yerxa, E. J. (1989). The Routine Task Inventory: A tool for describing the functional behavior of the cognitively disabled. *Occupational Therapy Practice, 1,* 67-74.

Katz, N. (2006). *Routine Task Inventory–Expanded (RTI-E).* Retrieved from http://www.allen-cognitive-network.org/pdf_files/RTIManual2006.pdf

Katz, N., Felzen, B., Tadmor, I., & Hartman-Maeir, A. (2005). The Behavioral Assessment of the Dysexecutive Syndrome (BADS) in schizophrenia and its contribution to functional outcome. *Neuropsychological Rehabilitation, 17*(2), 192-205.

Katz, N., & Keren, N. (2011). Effectiveness of an occupational goal intervention (OGI) for clients with schizophrenia. *American Journal of Occupational Therapy, 63,* 1-10.

Keren, N., Gal, H., Degan, R., Yakoel, S., & Katz, N. (2008). Treatment of executive function deficits in individuals with schizophrenia: Presentation of two treatment methods with case examples. *Israeli Journal of Occupational Therapy, 17,* H97-H117. (English Abstract E64-e65).

Levy, L., & Burns, T. (2011). Cognitive disabilities reconsidered: Rehabilitation of adults with dementias. In N. Katz (Ed.), *Cognition, occupation and participation across the life span* (3rd ed., pp. 407-441). Bethesda, MD: American Occupational Therapy Association.

McAnanama, E., Rogosin-Rose, M., Scott, E., Joffe, R., & Kelner, M. (1999). Discharge planning in mental health: The relevance of cognition to community living. *American Journal of Occupational Therapy, 53,* 129-137.

McCraith, D., Austin, S., & Earhart, C. (2011). The cognitive disabilities model in 2011. In N. Katz (Ed.), *Cognition, occupation and participation across the life span* (3rd ed., pp. 206, 397-398). Bethesda, MD: AOTA Press.

Pollard, D., & Olin, D. W. (2005). *Allen's Cognitive Levels: Meeting the challenges of client focused services.* Monona, WI: Selectone Rehab.

Raweh, D. V., & Katz, N. (1999). Treatment effectiveness of Allen's cognitive disabilities model with adult schizophrenic outpatients: A pilot study. *Occupational Therapy in Mental Health, 14,* 65-77.

Secrest, L., Wood, A. E., & Tapp, A. (2000). A comparison of the Allen Cognitive Level Test and the Wisconsin Card Sorting Test in adults with schizophrenia. *American Journal of Occupational Therapy, 54,* 129-133.

Tadmor, I. (2004). *The relationship between executive functions, cognitive functions and occupational performance in people with chronic schizophrenia.* Unpublished thesis, Hebrew University Jerusalem, Jerusalem, Israel.

Wachtel, N. (2003). *Examining awareness to functional cognitive level among elderly living in the community following stroke.* Unpublished thesis, Hebrew University Jerusalem, Jerusalem, Israel.

Wilson, B. A., Alderman, N., Burgess, P. W., Emslie, H., & Evans, J. J. (1996). *Behavioral assessment of the dysexecutive syndrome (BADS).* Bury St. Edmunds, England: Thames Valley Test Company.

Wilson, S. D., Allen, C. D., McCormack, G., & Burton, G. (1989). Cognitive disability and routine task behaviors in a community-based population with senile dementia. *Occupational Therapy Practice, 1,* 58-66

Zimnavoda, T., Weinblatt, N., & Katz, N. (2002). Validity of the Kohlman Evaluation of Living Skills (KELS) with Israeli elderly individuals living in the community. *Occupational Therapy International, 9,* 312-325.

Ziv, N., Roitman, D., & Katz, N. (1999). Problem solving, sense of coherence and instrumental ADL of elderly people with depression and normal control group. *Occupational Therapy International, 6,* 243-256.

Contextual Memory Test

Emily Raphael-Greenfield, EdD, OTR/L, FAOTA
Joan Toglia, PhD, OTR/L, FAOTA
Ashley Hartman, MS, OTR/L

If any one faculty of our nature may be called more wonderful than the rest, I do think it is memory. There seems something more speakingly incomprehensible in the powers, the failures, the inequalities of memory, than in any other of our intelligences. The memory is sometimes so retentive, so serviceable, so obedient; at others, so bewildered and so weak; and at others again, so tyrannic, so beyond control! We are, to be sure, a miracle every way; but our powers of recollecting and of forgetting do seem peculiarly past finding out.
(Jane Austen, *Mansfield Park*, 1775-1817)

The aim of this chapter is to explain the background and procedures for the Contextual Memory Test (CMT), a unique and easy test of personal awareness of memory limitations, the use of strategies employed by people to remember everyday objects, as well as a client's response to cueing to enhance strategy use and recall. This assessment is not diagnostic, rather it can supplement more conventional measures of assessing memory (Toglia, 1993). The strengths of this assessment include the following:

- Based on theory of memory
- Easily transportable test that requires less than 10 minutes to administer
- Screens for memory impairment
- Provides a quantified measure of strategy use and awareness
- Links assessment results with suggestions for rehabilitation specialists, including identifying potential safety issues and possible strategy use

The assessment has been used with a variety of physical dysfunction and mental health diagnoses, including clients with traumatic brain injury, cerebrovascular disease, dementia, Parkinson's disease, as well as depression, alcohol use disorders, and schizophrenia. This chapter will also explore its limitations and make recommendations for further use of the CMT with clients with mental health disorders.

Hemphill, B. J., & Urish, C. K. (Eds.). *Assessments in Occupational Therapy Mental Health: An Integrative Approach, Fourth Edition* (pp. 223-237). © 2020 Taylor & Francis Group.

Theoretical Basis

As Jane Austen's description of memory suggests memory affects all of our thinking, including learning from past experiences and acquiring new information. Memory allows people to be independent, and memory impairments seriously impact daily functioning. Toglia (1993) describes the feeling of a lack of control over oneself, one's life, and one's environment that stems from memory loss. Memory problems also impact participation in many forms of health care services, including occupational therapy rehabilitation, because the client forgets to attend therapy sessions, does not absorb or carry over things learned in previous sessions, and may be at risk for serious injury in the home environment (Gil & Josman, 2001).

Memory dysfunction is described according to etiology, diagnoses, and memory symptoms. There are common symptoms of amnesia that are often present in clients seen by occupational therapists in physical disability and mental health settings, including problems with immediate and delayed recall, differences in recognition and recall, preservation of procedural memory, and sensitivity to retrieval cues. There are similarities and differences among patients with amnesia, including type of memory modality affected and metamemory abilities (Toglia, 1993). There are differences between primary and secondary amnesia. Secondary amnesia consists of a primary memory deficit (primary amnesia) accompanied by other cognitive problems, including initiation, attention, organization, abstract thinking, and flexibility. In clinical practice secondary memory deficits are more common than primary amnesia (Toglia, 1993).

In addition to memory problems following brain injury there is growing evidence that patients with mental health and substance-related disorders experience memory problems. Impaired cognitive function is now considered a core feature of schizophrenia (Harvey & Keefe, 1997; Moritz & Woodward, 2006; So, Toglia, & Donohue, 1997; Toglia, 1993). Executive function impairments are present across all symptom groups including schizophrenia, alcohol use disorders, and neurocognitive disorders (Gil & Josman, 2001; Lysaker, Bryson, Lancaster, Evans, & Bell, 2002). Working and episodic memory impairments are especially notable in schizophrenia and considered a key feature (Bonner-Jackson, Haut, Csernansky, & Barch, 2005; Guimond, Beland, & Lepage, 2018; Guo, Ragland, & Carter, 2018; Murty, McKinney, DuBrow, Jalbrzikowski, Haas, & Luna, 2018; Wongupparaj, Kumari, & Morris, 2015). Memory impairments were found to be prominent in people with schizophrenia's disorganized symptoms, whereas attentional and psychomotor impairments were common in both disorganized and negative symptom groups (Hill, Ragland, Gur, & Gur, 2001).

Other apparent cognitive deficits associated with schizophrenia include inhibition/control and learning (Konstantakopoulos et al., 2011). Memory problems are also associated with people who have alcohol use disorders (Finn & Hall, 2004; Sullivan, Rosenbloom, & Pfefferbaum, 2000). Impairment in memory ability, including immediate/delayed recall and recognition, as well as metamemory capacity are associated with neurocognitive disorders such as Alzheimer's disease (Gil & Josman, 2001). In the study of 60 elderly patients, 30 patients diagnosed with Alzheimer's disease were matched with 30 well elderly patients in Israel. The researchers found significant differences between the two groups in memory performance, improvement in memory under cued conditions, and overestimation of memory ability (Gil & Josman, 2001).

It appears that the memory deficits in schizophrenia cannot be attributed to avolition, distraction by psychotic symptoms, or psychotropic medications (Duffy & O'Carroll, 1994). There is some evidence that memory tests rather than tests of executive function are better predictors of instrumental activities of daily living (IADL) performance in patients with schizophrenia (Godbout, Limoges, Allard, Braun, & Stip, 2007). Godbout et al. (2007) demonstrated that patients with positive symptoms of schizophrenia were more impaired on a behavioral test of IADLs, which included planning a three-course meal while staying within a budget, buying ingredients and cooking them quickly, and synchronizing the timing of the dishes. The patients with negative symptoms exhibited greater impairment on tests of executive function. In addition, the researchers found that actual meal preparation relies more heavily on episodic memory than executive function.

Unlike individuals with brain injuries, people with schizophrenia experience problems in semantic memory (e.g., general knowledge of concepts, categories, and meanings), in episodic memory (e.g., personally experienced events), and in an inefficient use of encoding strategies (Bonner-Jackson et al., 2005; So et al., 1997). There is research documenting semantic memory impairment within individuals diagnosed with schizophrenia in terms of both concepts and events. For example, Chan, Chiu, Lam, Pang, and Chow (1999) reported a breakdown in the recall of a restaurant script wherein the participants were able to remember the general sequence but could not recall specific detail of the restaurant script. Different theories exist about why people with schizophrenia are inefficient encoders, including abnormalities in the frontal cortex, temporal lobes, hippocampus, and other areas of functional brain activation, but there is growing evidence that they can benefit from rehabilitation that targets encoding strategies (Bonner-Jackson et al., 2005; Godbout et al., 2007; Guimond et al., 2018; Guo et al., 2018; Murty et al., 2018).

So et al. (1997) researched the CMT with a sample of 23 chronic patients with undifferentiated and paranoid schizophrenia. Findings indicated that negative symptoms and not positive symptoms correlated with memory impairments, specifically alogia and attentional impairments. They also discovered that patients with paranoid schizophrenia performed better than those diagnosed as undifferentiated. Another of their findings was that the contextually cued situation resulted in improvement in immediate and delayed recall, but the improvement was quite small and must be interpreted with caution. In the study, positive and negative symptoms interfered with recall. The results found evidence of improvement in those who could identify their memory strategies. Some participants did employ memory strategies, such as categorizing, but they did not articulate that this was one of the strategies they employed (So et al., 1997). Toglia (1993) has observed that both patients with brain injuries and patients with schizophrenia employ a strategy of memorizing the details of each object. So et al. (1997) were uncertain if their findings reflected a lack of awareness of strategy use, a lack of capacity to express it, or a lack of ability to use the strategy.

Key concepts and theories that form the background for the CMT include the following:

- The Stage Model of Memory (short-term memory, active rehearsal, long-term memory, meaningful chunks, retrieval strategies)
- The Information-Processing Framework of Memory (effortful processing, automatic processing)
- Knowledge Structures in Memory
- Different Types of Long-Term Memory
- Metamemory (Toglia, 1993)

The Stage Model of Memory

The Stage Model of Memory provides a description of the normal memory process. Sensory receptors receive and register information. A small part of the sensory memories are retained as short-term or working memory. Active rehearsal must be employed to transfer these memories to long-term storage (Toglia, 1993). Short-term memory is the capacity to actively retain a small amount of information (7 [±2] meaningfully related chunks of information) for a brief amount of time, usually 20 to 30 seconds. More familiar information is easier to chunk than new information. When a person rehearses or repeats the information, it can be encoded and maintained in long-term memory, which can be kept in storage for hours, days, or years. Long-term memory has limitless capacity. Retrieval is the process by which long-term memory is searched, and information is transferred to working memory for use. The retrieval of information that is seldom used requires effort and is slow compared to the quicker recovery of more commonly used information. Memory impairment in this model is thought to reside in a higher rate of forgetting or an inability to move information from the short-term to long-term memory storage.

The Information-Processing Framework of Memory

The Information-Processing Framework of Memory expands upon the Stage Model. Rather than viewing the memory process as composed of separate stages, this model views input, storage, and retrieval as dynamic and interrelated. Long-term memory of information appears to depend on an active strategic approach to learning. There are three techniques that appear to be linked with deep memory processing and retention in long-term memory storage: elaboration (adding to presented information), visualization, and organization (chunking information). For example, changing the task demands can enhance encoding, presenting information that is to be remembered within a specific context (Toglia, 1993). Encoding deficit theories account for one explanation of memory problems. There are two types of encoding difficulties: failure of effortful processing and failure of automatic processing. Teaching clients with brain injuries how to attend to meaningful attributes of new information has improved their recall; the same approach has been successfully employed with clients with schizophrenia. The failure to automatically attend to contextual cues has been shown to significantly influence retrieval. The CMT uses the following definition of context: recognition of a background theme from the knowledge of typecast categories and events (Toglia, 1993).

Knowledge Structures in Memory

A third model of memory postulates that information is chunked and retained in large schemas that are organized around categories and events, which are used during encoding and retrieval. This schema or previously assimilated knowledge acts as internal guides for people, helping them know what to look for. This model suggests that people automatically relate and organize new and unfamiliar data with past experiences, which suggests the use of scripts. Research has shown that recall is decreased when organizational cues are absent, and learning is enhanced when previous knowledge is stimulated. Clinical work with patients with memory impairment has demonstrated that when they are given cues or strategies, both recall and retrieval improve (So et al., 1997; Toglia, 1993). This suggests that memory impairments are related to the unprompted commencement of strategies rather than a deficit related to a particular stage of memory.

Different Types of Long-Term Memory

Short-term memory is tested by means of immediate recall tasks. If there is a limited amount of information (7±2 items) presented, there can be exact recall. Long-term memory is studied by means of delayed recall tasks. Clients are asked to recall information minutes to hours after presentation. There are a number of different types of long-term memory. Examples of these types of long-term memory are visual; verbal or declarative (e.g., remembering facts, events, and general information); episodic (e.g., recall of personally experienced events); semantic (e.g., storage of general knowledge and concepts); procedural or action (e.g., ability to reproduce an action sequence or a memory for actions); and prospective (e.g., remembering to do something in the future). Unlike declarative knowledge, which is learned through observation alone, procedural knowledge is not searched for in long-term memory and is learned through practice and feedback (Toglia, 1993).

Metamemory

Some clients with memory impairments also exhibit problems with metamemory, which includes knowledge of the difficulty of a task as well as insight into oneself as a learner. Research has demonstrated that improved perception of one's memory function is correlated with improved memory capacity, especially in those situations involving learning new information. Differing brain injury lesions result in different types of self-awareness of memory problems. Clients with brain injury tend to overestimate their memory abilities, whereas healthy controls tend to underestimate their memory abilities (So et al., 1997). Clients with depression overestimated their memory problems (Toglia, 1993). There is increasing evidence that individuals with schizophrenia may overestimate performance (Moritz, Woodward, Cuttler, Whitman, & Jason, 2004).

The majority of the literature on awareness has focused on awareness of illness or awareness of cognitive symptoms within the context of an interview. Studies have shown that awareness of illness is independent from clinical awareness of cognitive or memory performance in individuals with schizophrenia (Gilleen, Greenwood, & David, 2011; Gonzalez-Suarez et al., 2011). In other words, a person may not acknowledge an illness but may recognize difficulties in remembering. Conversely, a person may acknowledge their illness without recognizing difficulties in memory. Several models of awareness highlight the disassociation that can occur in awareness across different domains, as well as within and outside the context of performance (Toglia & Maeir, 2018).

Impairment in metamemory in clients with schizophrenia has been examined both during the first episode and for those who are chronic (Irak & Capan, 2018; Moritz, Woodward, & Chen, 2006); however, the literature in this area is scarce. So et al. (1997) studied patients diagnosed with schizophrenia. Results indicated both over- and underestimation of the results on the CMT. If clients have difficulty accurately assessing task difficulty, the researchers suggested clients may not be able to modify learning strategies in order to encode new information (So et al., 1997). This premise was supported by Gilleen, Greenwood, and David (2014), who found a relationship between memory performance and awareness in individuals across three diagnostic groups, including schizophrenia. Diminished awareness of memory problems may make it more difficult for a person to accept the need for compensation or participate in rehabilitation.

Occupational Therapy Assessment of Memory Impairment

There is scant literature within occupational therapy on the assessment of memory impairment within everyday functioning. The CMT was developed to explore in adults with memory impairment awareness of and use of cognitive strategies. The CMT was used as a memory screen for clients with memory problems (Toglia, 1993). Most other memory tests were not developed to guide rehabilitation specialists nor are they reflective of everyday functioning. Memory rehabilitation literature does stress the importance of awareness of memory capacity and the ability to use strategies to encode and learn new knowledge.

Established memory tests, such as the Wechsler Memory Scale, quantify the existence and severity of memory difficulties. These standardized tests assist with diagnosing and determining the location of the brain lesion, as well as providing a baseline for measuring change; however, they do not provide information on where to begin rehabilitation. The ecological validity, or the ability of these tests to predict everyday memory problems, is also limited (Toglia, 1993). This may relate to the tasks included in the conventional memory tests, which use meaningless word lists or abstract designs rather than everyday objects to assess verbal and visual memory separately to pinpoint the area of brain dysfunction.

The distinctive features of the CMT include its theoretical basis in memory awareness and strategies; its use of a theme or script to detect if patients spontaneously use the theme to help them remember (and what happens if they are not using a theme to be told the theme by the examiner); its inclusion of a patient's metamemory awareness, which provides an important starting point for rehabilitation; and its use of drawings of meaningful and functional objects as a way to measure memory capacity for everyday functioning (Toglia, 1993).

Psychometric Properties

The CMT has been standardized for adults aged 18 years and older with a neurological disorder with memory impairment, including patients with traumatic brain injury, cerebrovascular accident, dementia, multiple sclerosis, Parkinson's disease, brain tumor, AIDS, epilepsy, and chronic alcohol use disorders (Toglia, 1993). Studies have also been conducted comparing typical children to those with cochlear implant (Engel-Yeger, Durr, & Josman, 2010) and to those with traumatic brain injury (Kizony, Tau, Bar, & Engel-Yeger, 2014; Josman, Berney, & Jarus, 2000). Reliability and validity studies are needed for adolescents with these types of memory disorders. The CMT was piloted with patients with schizophrenia (So et al., 1997) and used but not reported on in the literature with patients who have memory complaints with the following psychiatric diagnoses: anxiety disorders, bipolar disorder, and depression. Reliability and validity studies of these psychiatric populations are needed, as are studies of children and adolescents with memory disorders.

Reliability

Reliability was examined separately for the CMT's recall scores, prediction scores, and strategy scores. Reliability for the recall scores was examined using parallel form, test-retest, and Rasch analysis (Toglia, 1993). Forty-two participants with brain injury were randomly administered both the Morning and Restaurant versions with the same directions; the second version was conducted between three and 36 hours later. With this parallel format, reliability estimates ranged from 0.73 to 0.81. Test-retest reliability resulted from correlating the scores of immediate recall with delayed recall. These quasi test-retest reliability scores ranged from 0.85 to 0.94 for the group with brain injury and from 0.74 to 0.87 for the control group. The Rasch method produced two measures of estimating reliability for the CMT: person separation reliability (0.75 to 0.80) and item separation reliability (0.92 to 0.96). To determine the reliability of the prediction scores, 62 participants with brain injury were asked to predict how many objects of 20 they would be able to recall. When the difference between the immediate recall score and estimated score were correlated across two administrations, its value was 0.90, which means that the prediction score is highly reliable. To establish the reliability of the strategy scores, the total strategy scores on both the Restaurant and Morning forms were correlated and established at 0.75 (Toglia, 1993).

Concurrent Validity

Concurrent validity was derived by correlations between the recall scores on the CMT and the Rivermead Behavioral Memory Test. Both the CMT and Rivermead Behavioral Memory Test were conducted with 33 individuals with brain injury. The Rivermead Profile and Screening Score were correlated with the immediate, delayed, and total CMT scores. The CMT immediate, delayed, and total recall scores were correlated from 0.08 to 0.84 to Rivermead scores (Toglia, 1993). Kizony and Katz (2002) found that CMT performance in individuals with cerebrovascular disease was moderately related to IADL performance, as measured by the Assessment of Motor and Process Skills. This comparison supported the use of CMT to measure functional performance. Discriminant validity has been established within several different pediatric populations (Engel-Yeger et al., 2010; Josman et al., 2000; Kizony et al., 2014).

Sensitivity

The ability of an instrument to differentiate among different groups and to detect change is referred to as its *sensitivity* and is another way to measure its validity. Discriminate function analysis was used to determine the ability of the CMT to distinguish between individuals with brain injury (brain-injured group) and nondisabled individuals (control group). Using immediate and delayed scores, the discriminant function analysis correctly identified 332/375 nondisabled participants and 134/159 individuals with brain injury. This established the sensitivity of the CMT as 0.843 (Toglia, 1993). The sensitivity of the CMT was 0.837 when the discriminant function used the immediate and delayed scores, as well as the total strategy score. The sensitivity of the CMT was 0.846 when the discriminant function used the immediate and delayed scores, the total strategy score, and the discrepancy score (Toglia, 1993). A significant difference was found between control participants ($N = 310$) and participants with brain injury ($N = 62$) in their capacity to estimate how many items they would be able to immediately recall. Almost all of the individuals in the brain injury group overestimated their performance, whereas two thirds of the individuals in the control group underestimated their performance. Those individuals with a small discrepancy between the predicted score and immediate recall scores performed better than those with large discrepancies between the two scores (control group: $r = -.43$, $p < .001$; brain injury group: $r = -.40$, $p = .001$; Toglia, 1993).

Another area of difference between the two groups was found in the total strategy scores (TSS). The average TSS for the control group was 10.5 (standard deviation [SD] = 2.8); the average TSS for the brain injury group was 5.5 (SD = 4.8). Most of the individuals in the control group utilized subcategories of objects as well as event sequences to recall, whereas most of the individuals in the brain injury group could not describe how they remembered the objects (Toglia, 1993). There were also differences between the two groups in the order with which they recalled items. Pairs of items that were recalled together were examined for both groups: the number of pairs for the control group was 4.06, whereas the number of pairs for the brain injury group was 1.13. Finally, the control group more rapidly recalled items that were central to the theme and were associated with each other, whereas these association strategies and associations were not made in the brain injury group. These findings strongly suggest that memory problems are composed of both a decrease in the amount of information remembered as well as a reduction in the strategies employed to remember objects (Toglia, 1993).

In addition to brain injury, discriminative validity of the CMT has been supported in older people with and without Alzheimer's disease (Gil & Josman, 2001), in individuals with schizophrenia compared to healthy controls (So et al., 1997), and in typical children aged 8 years and older who were compared to those with cochlear implant (Engel-Yeger et al., 2011) and those with brain injury (Josman et al., 2000; Kizony et al., 2014). The results support the clinical usefulness of the CMT with these populations.

Assessment Administration

Area of Occupation/Performance Skills/ Performance Patterns/Client Factors Assessed

In the CMT, the objects that must be remembered are associated with the *Occupational Therapy Practice Framework: Domain and Process, Third Edition,* domain of the occupations of Activities of Daily Living (ADLs) and Instrumental Activities of Daily Living (IADLs; American Occupational Therapy Association [AOTA], 2014). This occupation-based information is presented with contextual cues, which is meant to be motivating, meaningful, and functional in contrast with the word lists of traditional memory tests, which are organized by affective or semantic categories. It is hoped that memory is stimulated by this daily context rather than unrelated objects (So et al., 1997).

The *Framework* domain of client factors includes the subcategories of body functions (specific mental functions) and body structures (i.e., structures of the nervous system), which are assessed by the CMT (AOTA, 2014). The CMT relies on visual memory skills and may not accurately reflect the memory of those with strong auditory memory skills. The CMT tests for three areas: recall (i.e., immediate and delayed of line-drawn objects); strategy use (i.e., the ability to describe strategy use and ability to use contextual information, which is provided by the examiner); and metamemory or self-awareness of memory capacity by general questioning, prediction of memory capacity before the task, and estimation of memory capacity after the task (So et al., 1997; Toglia, 1993). Participants in the CMT must have the following intact body functions/structures: follow two-step directions, recognize objects, and communicate verbally or in writing. Problems with moderate to severe visual agnosia, unilateral inattention, and aphasia may preclude participation in the CMT, although anomic aphasia (the inability to name objects) can be compensated for by description of the object's function or appearance, and expressive language deficits can be adapted for by using recognition instead of free recall format (Toglia, 1993).

The Performance Skills of the *Framework* (AOTA, 2014) are assessed by the CMT. These include the following process and social interaction skills, which are impacted by memory capacity and metamemory impairments: Process Skills (heeds, chooses, uses, inquires, continues, searches, locates, gathers, organizes, restores, adjusts, accommodates, and benefits) and Social Interaction Skills (regulates, questions, replies, discloses, transitions, matches language, clarifies, empathizes, heeds, accommodates, and benefits).

Description of Environment/ Description of Supplies/Materials Required

The test should be administered in a distraction-free, well-lit, quiet room. The test administrator will need the following: a pencil or pen, the CMT test booklet, the 2 picture cards, a stopwatch, and the 40 recognition cards. If a patient uses glasses for reading or near vision, they should be worn during the assessment. There are two comparable versions of the CMT: the Restaurant version, which is reflective of a typical restaurant scene, and the Morning version, which is reflective of what a person does in the home environment after getting up and preparing to leave in the morning. The test contains 2 cards that contain 20 line drawings of typical objects found in each of these themes and presented out of order (Toglia, 1993). The two cards are considered equivalent in levels of difficulty. The Restaurant version is usually presented first to make the assessment more consistent. There are also 40 single cards that are presented one at a time (determined by the numbers on the back) in an unpaced fashion that contain pictures of objects, some of which were included on the two stimulus cards presented earlier to the patient. This section tests for recognition memory if cued recall is not useful for facilitating retrieval (Toglia, 1993).

Administration

The test can be administered in two parts, Part I (noncontext) and Part II (context). Part I is presented to the patient without telling them that the objects relate to a theme. Part II is only administered if the patient scores below the norm on Part I; its purpose is to determine if recall behavior is improved by providing a background theme. Part II provides the cue about the theme to the patient before viewing the items. If a patient's memory is not significantly improved by provision of the theme, cued recall and recognition with 40 single cards are presented individually (Toglia, 1993).

Part I of the test begins with a series of standard questions about the patient's memory capacity, which is referred to as the Memory Questionnaire. This questionnaire seeks information about the patient's perception of changes to their memory, their current recall ability, and their frequency of forgetting. The Memory Questionnaire can be shown to the patient with their verbal answers recorded by the examiner or if they are capable, it can be filled out independently. Patients should be encouraged to guess an answer on Questions 1 through 9, if they are not sure. The patient is next shown one of the noncontext picture cards for 90 seconds by placing it on the table in the patient's midline. The examiner should observe the patient's behavior during the entire 90-second period to detect if there are any problems with attention, visual perception, or language. Immediately after removing the 20-object card, the patient is asked to recall as many objects as possible, in any order. The examiner should record all answers (even if incorrect), indicate repetitious answers, and probe for more specific answers if vague, overly general responses are provided. After the patient is engaged in another activity for 15 to 20 minutes, the patient is asked to recall as many items as possible from the stimulus card. A series of standard questions to assess awareness of memory capacity, as well as memory strategies, is administered after both immediate and delayed recall.

Part II is administered only under two conditions: the patient scored below the norm for recall or if they demonstrated poor strategy use. The time interval between Part I and II can be a minimum of 2 hours and maximum of 36 hours. Specific time frames have been established for those patients with specific head injuries but not with other diagnoses (Toglia, 1993). Part II is run similarly to Part I, which gives the patient 90 seconds to study the picture card, except there are no questions asked prior to administration and cues are provided about the context. If the Restaurant version was used for Part I, the Morning version should be used for Part II. As in Part I, after a 15- to 20-minute interval, delayed recall is administered. If the patient persists in scoring below the norm, cued recall and recognition can be administered (Toglia, 1993), although the cued recall and recognition memory procedures were not included in the original field testing. The recognition memory step can also be used to enable those patients with moderate to severe expressive language deficits succeed with the free recall task. The cards are presented one at a time in midline in an unhurried fashion and placed face-up on top of each other.

Scoring

There are scores for recall, cued recall, recognition, awareness, and strategy use. Raw scores are recorded in the test booklet for immediate and delayed recall and totaled for the Total Recall (raw score). Patients are not penalized for incorrect answers. Observations made by the examiner during study time or recall are checked off on the behavior list under Observations in the test booklet. Incorrect items are counted as "Confabulations #" on the Summary of Findings worksheet in the booklet. Raw recall scores are converted into standard scores and compared to normative performance, and standard scores are classified into the following categories: within normal limits (WNL), suspect, mild, moderate, or severe (Toglia, 1993). The cued recall score equals the delayed recall score plus items recalled during strategy questioning and verbal cues minus the incorrect times mentioned during strategy questioning and cues. The total recognition score is calculated by subtracting the number of false positives, which is identified as the number of incorrect identifications by patient and from the true positives (correct identifications). The cued recall and recognition scores are recorded in the Retrieval Cues section of the Summary of Findings worksheet and are compared with the delayed recall scores.

Awareness is examined by looking at differences in the ability to judge memory performance before and after the CMT task, as well as an analysis of responses to general interview questions compared to specific predictions and estimations of memory performance. Scores are based on the following three subscores: prediction (overestimation, underestimation, or accurate) and the Prediction Discrepancy Score, which is prediction minus immediate recall; estimation of performance following recall (overestimation or underestimation) and Estimation Discrepancy, which is estimated score minus immediate recall score; and response to general questioning, which is scoring the patient responses to Questions 1, 2, 5 through 9. The maximum score is 29, which indicates that the patient reports no memory problems to a minimum score of 7 and 8, which indicates that the patient reports significant memory problems. Following Recall, Questions 10 through 12 are scored and recorded in the After Memory Task Section to measure the patient's ability to judge their performance accurately.

Strategy use is measured in three different ways: effect of context, TSS, and the order of recall. To assess the effect of context the patient's recall scores from the context and noncontext, conditions are compared. If the patient receives a score on the context version, which is more than one standard error of measure above the score on the noncontext version, then the patient will likely benefit from cues for strategy (e.g., if food items are recalled together). The TSS is obtained from the patient's answers to Questions 15 and 16 about their strategy use. The TSS is calculated by adding up the four responses to questions 15A, 15B, 16A, and 16B; the maximum TSS score is 12. If the patient provides vague responses, the examiner should probe for more specific answers. The examiner should give the patient the highest possible score possible within the rating criteria. It is important to note that the TSS is a reflection of the patient's ability to verbalize a strategy. The TSS score is recorded in the Summary of Findings section on the worksheet, good (9 to 12), questionable (5 to 8), and poor (0 to 4), along with relevant observations (Toglia, 1993). The examiner should also examine the order of recall to determine whether items are recalled in clusters or categories. The order of recall can suggest use of strategies that the client was unaware of or did not verbalize.

The link between CMT assessment results and treatment is derived from an examination of the combination of awareness, strategy use, and recall across the context and noncontext versions. Two individuals can have the same impaired recall scores; however, differences in how the person responds to awareness questions, estimates their performance, uses strategies, and a contextual cue have different implications for treatment. For example, a client that recalls only 3/20 items but denies memory difficulties both before and immediately after performance, lacks use of strategies, and does not benefit from a contextual cue may not be a good candidate for a strategy-based treatment approach. On the other hand, if the same client shows some awareness of recall difficulties immediately after the memory task, responds to the context cue, and shows attempts to use strategies, they may be a good candidate for a strategy-based treatment approach. The CMT manual describes how different result patterns in these areas provide different treatment implications (Toglia, 1993).

Case Study

George was referred for an evaluation of his memory by an occupational therapist as part of the routine services provided within the psychosocial rehabilitation program at a large, urban homeless shelter for men with psychiatric disorders. George is 39-year-old man who previously worked as a purchasing manager for almost 20 years, since graduating high school. He completed a technical degree in architectural drafting, but stated that when drafting became computerized, he had difficulty finding a job in the field. George is an avid chess player, which he states requires him to have a good memory. George is diagnosed with having severe depression and anxiety with frequent hospitalizations for suicidal ideation. He also reports a history of alcohol abuse and an acknowledgment that drinking worsens his depression.

Through the use of the CMT, it was discovered that the client slightly underestimates his memory performance both prior to completing the task and after (prediction discrepancy = 3, estimation of performance discrepancy = 2), suggesting a tendency to slightly underestimate performance. George's noncontext recall scores indicate suspected memory dysfunction (immediate recall = 12, delayed recall = 11, total recall = 23); however, context recall scores were within normal limits (immediate recall = 16, delayed recall = 15, total recall = 31).

George stated that he used spatial visualization as a way to assist him with the task during both study and recall of noncontext objects. He stated that he "pictured where each object was located on the sheet." While this strategy may be beneficial while playing chess, it was generally ineffective for the task at hand. During the context test, George was able to improve his memory performance by utilizing the theme to create a story timeline. George stated, "First, I am greeted by the waitress, then I hang my coat on the coatrack…"

Because George's memory performance significantly improved between noncontext and context testing, interventions aimed at improving memory strategies may be beneficial. The client's underestimation of his memory performance is typical of those with depression. Improving the client's ability to use memory strategies and his confidence in his memory performance, in conjunction with metamemory rating scales, may lead to more accurate insight into the use of recall strategies and improved performance.

Suggested Further Research

The limitations of the CMT include the following:

- It is not diagnostic.
- The assessment is not a complete evaluation of memory dysfunction and must be used in conjunction with other cognitive assessments.
- It may not detect slight memory deficits.
- This assessment is not appropriate for individuals with moderate/severe aphasia or visual perceptual deficits (Toglia, 1993).

The ability of the CMT to predict everyday memory problems or ecological validity still needs to be researched, as well as its ability to predict patient's responses to rehabilitation and its ability to differentiate between patients with different types of memory problems (Kizony & Katz, 2002; Toglia, 1993). Toglia (1993) has suggested that the use of real objects as well as the CMT's focus on strategy use and awareness of memory problems may be better predictors of function than the conventional memory tests, which have poor ecological validity. Other areas for future research on the CMT include the continuing collection of normative data that balances ethnic diversity and different educational levels for adults aged 18 years and older and for young adults starting at 12 years of age. Interrater reliability on scoring strategy responses continues to be studied, as well as computerized scoring, and the effect of context within different diagnostic groups (Toglia, 1993). Changes in the administration of the CMT also warrant study, such as asking patients to recall spatial locations of the items, providing the context cue during the study period rather than prior, and creating more specific contextual cues.

In addition, a test-teach-retest dynamic format has been suggested (Toglia, 2011). In this format, the examiner reviews initial performance with the client (test phase) and assists the client in self-checking errors and self-generating strategies that could be helpful for memory (teach phase). The alternate version of the test immediately follows (retest phase) to examine the ability to carryover and effectively utilize the strategies that were discussed. Studies using the Wisconsin Card Sorting Test suggest that the test-teach-retest format of dynamic assessment may be useful in predicting learning potential and rehabilitation outcome in individuals with schizophrenia (Wiedl, Wienobst, & Schottke, 2001).

Further reliability and validity studies of the CMT are needed for the following populations with memory complaints: children and adolescents with neurological disorders; adults with positive and negative symptoms of schizophrenia; adults with anxiety, bipolar, and depressive disorders (Engel-Yeger et al., 2010; Josman et al., 2000; Kizony et al., 2014; Toglia, 1993). One published study of patients with schizophrenia and the CMT exists (So et al., 1997). These authors recommended further research that increased the sample size, extended the duration time of the study, randomized the uncued and cued parts of the assessment, selected patients with schizophrenia who did not also have comorbidities with substance-related disorders, and used a more objective rating scale of positive symptoms. It was also recommended that patients with schizophrenia be studied in terms of those with positive and negative symptoms as well as in comparison with patients with brain injury (So et al., 1997).

New Directions and Updates

Recently, a web-based version of the CMT was developed (CMT-2) and is in a pilot testing phase. The online CMT-2 is similar to the original version (Toglia 1993), and includes immediate and delayed recall of 20 objects related to a scene as well as questions that investigate the person's awareness of memory abilities and strategy use. The greatest difference is that colored photos of objects have replaced the black and white drawings; some items have been updated or replaced, and the test is administered on a tablet or computer. In addition, two scenes specifically designed for children have been added, including a school scene and a children's morning version. At this time, the CMT-2 does not have an option for testing recognition memory. The website includes frequently asked questions that review administration procedures; however, familiarity with the original CMT test and initial manual is helpful for comprehensive understanding and use.

The CMT-2 automatically generates a quick score summary and a documentation summary in the areas of awareness, recall performance, and strategy use. Normative data on the CMT-2 across the lifespan from children aged 7 years to older adults has just begun. There is presently no cost involved in using the CMT-2. Further information can be obtained by visiting the website at https://cmt.multicontext.net.

Summary

The CMT is a standardized, norm-based, quick, engaging, and easy-to-administer occupational therapy functional assessment of memory capacity as well as personal awareness of memory limitations and strategy use. Although the assessment is most often utilized with patients with neurological impairments, it holds real promise as an assessment and rehabilitation implementation for patients with psychiatric disorders. However, more studies are needed for patients who demonstrate positive and negative symptoms of schizophrenia, anxiety, bipolar, and depressive disorders. Further research is also needed to broaden the normative data for young adults, aged 12 years and older, as well as adults.

References

American Occupational Therapy Association. (2014). Occupational therapy practice framework: Domain and process (3rd ed.). *American Journal of Occupational Therapy, 62*(6), 625-663.

Austen, J. (1814). *Mansfield park*. London, United Kingdom: Thomas Egerton.

Bonner-Jackson, A., Haut, K., Csernansky, J. G., & Barch, D. M. (2005). The influence of encoding strategy on episodic memory and cortical activity in schizophrenia. *Biological Psychiatry, 58*(1), 47-55.

Chan, A. S., Chiu, H., Lam, L., Pang, A., & Chow, L. (1999). A breakdown of event schemas in patients with schizophrenia: An examination of their script for dining at restaurants. *Psychiatry Research, 87*, 169-181.

Duffy, L., & O'Carroll, R. (1994). Memory impairment in schizophrenia: A comparison with that observed in the Alcoholic Korsakoff Syndrome. *Psychological Medicine, 24*, 155-165.

Engel-Yeger, B., Durr, D. H. & Josman, N. (2010). Comparison of memory and meta-memory abilities of children with cochlear implant and normal hearing peers. *Disability and Rehabilitation, Aug*, 1-8.

Finn, P. R., & Hall, J. (2004). Cognitive ability and risk for alcoholism: Short-term memory capacity and intelligence moderate personality risk for alcohol problems. *Journal of Abnormal Psychology, 113*(4), 569.

Gil, N., & Josman, N. (2001). Memory and metamemory performance in Alzheimer's disease and healthy elderly: The Contextual Memory Test (CMT). *Aging Clinical Experimental Research, 13*, 309-315.

Gilleen, J., Greenwood, K., & David, A. S. (2011). Domains of awareness in schizophrenia. *Schizophrenia Bulletin, 37*, 61-72.

Gilleen, J., Greenwood, K., & David, A. S. (2014). The role of memory in awareness of memory deficits in Alzheimer's disease, schizophrenia, and brain injury. *Journal of Clinical and Experimental Neuropsychology, 36*, 43-57.

Godbout, L., Limoges, F., Allard, I., Braun, C. M. J., & Stip, E. (2007). Neuropsychological and activity of daily living script performance in patients with positive or negative schizophrenia. *Comprehensive Psychiatry, 48*, 293-302.

Gonzalez-Suarez, B., Gomar, J. J., Pousa, E., Ortiz-Gil, J., Garcia, A., Salvador, R., … McKenna, P. J. (2011). Awareness of cognitive impairment in schizophrenia and its relationship to insight into illness. *Schizophrenia Research, 133*, 187-192.

Guimond, S., Beland, S., & Lepage, M. (2018). Strategy for Semantic Association Memory (SESAME) training: Effects on brain functioning in schizophrenia. *Psychiatry Research: Neuroimaging, 271*, 50-58.

Guo, J. Y., Ragland, J. D., & Carter, C. S. (2018). Memory and cognition in schizophrenia. *Molecular Psychiatry.* https://doi.org/10.1038/s41380-018-0231-1

Harvey, P. D., & Keefe, R. S. E. (1997). Cognitive impairment in schizophrenia and the implication of atypical neuroleptic treatment. *CNS Spectrum, 2*, 41-55.

Hill, S. K., Ragland, J. D., Gur, R. C., & Gur, R. E. (2001). Neuropsychological differences among empirically derived clinical subtypes of schizophrenia. *Neuropsychology, 15*, 492-501.

Irak, M., & Capan, D. (2018). Beliefs about memory as a mediator of relations between metacognitive beliefs and actual memory performance. *Journal of General Psychology, 145*(1), 21-44. https://doi.org/10.1080/002 21309.2017.1411682

Josman, N., Berney, T., & Jarus, T. (2000). Performance of children with and without traumatic brain injury on the Contextual Memory Test (CMT). *Physical and Occupational Therapy in Pediatrics, 19*(3/4), 39-51.

Kizony, R., & Katz, N. (2002). Relationships between cognitive abilities and the Process Scale and skills of the Assessment of Motor and Process Skills (AMPS) in patients with stroke. *OTJR: Occupation, Participation, and Health, 22*(2), 82-92.

Kizony, R., Tau, S., Bar, O., & Engel-Yeger, B. (2014). Comparing memory and meta-memory abilities between children with acquired brain injury and healthy peers. *Research in Developmental Disabilities, 35*(7), 1666-1673. https://doi.org/10.1016/j.ridd.2014.03.041

Konstantakopoulos, G., Ploumidis, D., Oulis, P., Patrikelis, P., Soumani, A., Papadimitrou, G. N., & Politis, A. N. (2011). Apathy, cognitive deficits and functional impairment in schizophrenia. *Schizophrenia Research, 133*, 193-198.

Lysaker, P. H., Bryson, G. J., Lancaster, R. S., Evans, J. D., & Bell, M. D. (2002). Insight in schizophrenia: Associations with executive functions and coping style. *Schizophrenia Research, 59*, 41-47.

Moritz, S., & Woodward, T. S. (2006). The contribution of metamemory deficits to schizophrenia. *Journal of Abnormal Psychology, 15*(1), 15-25. https://doi.org/10.1037/0021-843X.15.1.15

Moritz, S., Woodward, T. S., & Chen, E. (2006). Investigation of metamemory dysfunctions in first-episode schizophrenia. *Schizophrenia Research, 81*(2), 247-252.

Moritz, S., Woodward, T. S., Cuttler, C., Whitman, J. C., & Jason, M. (2004). False memories in schizophrenia. *Neuropsychology, 18*, 276-283.

Murty, V., McKinney, R. A., DuBrow, S., Jalbrzikowski, M., Haas, G. L., & Luna, B. (2018). Differential patterns of contextual organization of memory in first-episode psychosis. *Nature Partner Journals, 4*(3). https://doi.org/10.1038/s41537-018-0046-8

So, Y. P., Toglia, J., & Donohue, M. V. (1997). A study of memory functioning in chronic schizophrenic patients. *Occupational Therapy in Mental Health, 13*(2), 1-23.

Sullivan, E. V., Rosenbloom, M. J., & Pfefferbaum, A. (2000). Pattern of motor and cognitive deficits in detoxified alcoholic men. *Alcoholism: Clinical and Experimental Research, 24*, 611-621. https://doi.org/10.1111/j.1530-0277.2000.tb02032.x

Toglia, J. P. (1993). *Contextual Memory Test.* San Antonio, TX: Therapy Skill Builders.

Toglia, J. (2011). The dynamic interactional model of cognition in cognitive rehabilitation. In N. Katz (Ed.), *Cognition, occupation and participation across the life span: Neuroscience, neurorehabilitation and models of intervention in occupational therapy* (3rd ed., pp. 161-201). Bethesda, MD: AOTA Press.

Toglia, J., & Maeir, A. (2018). Self-awareness and metacognition: Effect on occupational performance and outcome across the lifespan. In N. Katz & J. Toglia (Eds.), *Cognition, occupation, and participation across the lifespan* (4th ed., pp. 143-163). Bethesda, MD: American Occupational Therapy Association. https://doi.org/10.7139/2017.978-1-56900-479-1

Wiedl, K. H., Wienobst, J., & Schottke, H. (2001). Estimating rehabilitation potential in schizophrenic subjects. In H. D. Brenner, W. Boker, & R. Genner (Eds.), *The treatment of schizophrenia: Status and emerging trends* (pp. 88-120). Seattle, WA: Hogrefe & Huber Publishers.

Wongupparaj, P., Kumari, V., & Morris, R. G. (2015). Executive function processes mediate the impact of working memory impairment on intelligence in schizophrenia. *European Psychiatry, 30,* 1-7.

Weekly Calendar Planning Activity

Joan Toglia, PhD, OTR/L, FAOTA
Suzanne White, MA, OTR/L, FAOTA

> *Your biggest dreams can become reality, not by brute-forcing the end-goal,*
> *but breaking it down into smaller, more manageable parts.*
> (Darkholme, 2014, p. 142)

The Weekly Calendar Planning Activity (WCPA) is a recently developed performance-based measure of executive function that requires entering a list of appointments into a weekly schedule while adhering to rules, monitoring time, and managing conflicts. Performance on the WCPA involves the integration and coordination of executive function skills, such as planning, organization, keeping track of information, inhibiting irrelevant information, and flexibility of thinking. The WCPA has broad applications and can be used with adolescents through older adults across a wide array of neurological, medical, and mental health conditions that show vulnerabilities to executive functioning. These include, but are not limited to, individuals with attention-deficit hyperactivity disorder (ADHD), schizophrenia, major depression, substance abuse, bipolar disorder, autism, learning disabilities, and mild cognitive disorder. The purpose of this chapter is to provide the reader with information related to the theoretical basis of the assessment, psychometric properties, and administration information, as well as a case study to facilitate increased understanding of use of this assessment in clinical practice.

Research has shown executive function impairments influence functional outcomes in successful psychosocial rehabilitation, social problem-solving ability, and community living (Rempfer, Hamera, Brown, & Cromwell, 2003; Revheim et al., 2006). Executive functioning interferes with the ability of people with schizophrenia to navigate obstacles, solve everyday problems, plan social or daily activities, and fully engage in their communities (Josman, Schenirderman, Klinger, & Shevil, 2009; Lepage, Bodnar, & Bowie, 2014). Measures of executive function have been more closely associated with functional status,

Hemphill, B. J., & Urish, C. K. (Eds.). *Assessments in*
Occupational Therapy Mental Health: An Integrative Approach,
Fourth Edition (pp. 239-259). © 2020 Taylor & Francis Group.

level of care, problem behaviors, and need for services in individuals with psychiatric conditions than with symptomology (e.g., psychosis, mood disturbance) or nonexecutive cognitive domains (Lipskaya, Jarus, & Kotler, 2011; Royall et al., 2002). The impact of executive function on independence, community living, and participation highlights the critical importance of addressing executive function performance within occupational therapy assessment and treatment (Cramm, Krupa, Missiuna, Lysaght, & Parker, 2013; Josman et al., 2009; Toglia & Katz, 2018).

The WCPA provides information on both the ability to successfully complete a specific instrumental activity of daily living (IADL) task, as well as on the process and quality of higher-level cognitive performance. The ability to follow a list and enter information into a weekly schedule is an important everyday life activity that is relevant to school, home, work, leisure, and social activities. Measures of accuracy and normative comparison for individuals aged 16 to 94 years are provided to identify the extent of performance deficits. In addition, the WCPA allows for the opportunity to observe and analyze error patterns, task efficiency, adherence to rules, use of strategies, and self-monitoring skills to provide a comprehensive understanding of the underlying nature of performance abilities and deficiencies (Lussier, Doherty, & Toglia, 2019; Toglia, 2015). Therefore, the WCPA also provides general information about performance deficits that extends beyond the calendar task and is likely to influence broader functioning in multitasking or complex situations. This in-depth analysis of performance provides information that is highly relevant to treatment. A preliminary dynamic test-teach-retest format that provides additional information on learning and carryover of strategies is also included in the WCPA test manual (Toglia, 2015). Responsiveness to a brief strategy-mediated intervention provides the team and the client with useful information on potential for learning that can influence medication and recovery plans.

Description of the Weekly Calendar Planning Activity

The WCPA includes two components: (1) entering a list of appointments into a calendar and (2) a semistructured interview and self-rating. Different versions of the WCPA are available (e.g., youth, middle school, college, adult) within the test manual to accommodate different ages and levels of ability, as well as to allow for retesting. The WCPA has three levels of ability. In Level I, the list of appointments is arranged in proper sequence so that appointment conflicts are not likely to occur. In Level II, the appointment list is out of order, and preplanning is required to avoid conflicts. In Level III, appointments are embedded within a paragraph format that includes extraneous and irrelevant information. In addition, a shorter 10-item appointment list is available for lower functioning clients or acute inpatient settings. Level II has more extensive normative data and is used most frequently.

All versions of the WCPA use the same instructions, weekly schedule, and require adherence to 5 rules: (1) the occupational therapist asking the client 3 irrelevant questions at 2-, 5-, and 10-minute intervals (or when the client is nearly finished if it appears they will finish before 10 minutes); (2) the client states time within 5 minutes of targeted time; (3) the occupational therapist marks on the recording form whether the client states when he or she is finished; (4) the client does not schedule appointments on the free day; and (5) the number of appointments the client crosses out as they are instructed to not cross out appointments on the calendar (Toglia, 2015). The weekly schedule contains subtle errors that provide the opportunity to observe how the client copes and deals with unexpected problems.

The second component of the WCPA includes a semistructured interview and self-rating administered immediately after the task to investigate strategy use and self-perceptions of task difficulty and performance (Lussier et al., 2019; Toglia, 2015). There are several videos available that provide an overview of the WCPA as well as illustrate administration and scoring (Toglia, 2017).

Theoretical Basis

Concepts/Construct

The WCPA is based on both current conceptualizations of executive function, as well as on the Dynamic Interactional Model (DIM) of cognition.

Executive Function

Executive functioning has been conceptualized as an interrelated set of cognitive abilities that coordinate and control the planning and monitoring of complex, goal-directed actions (Rabinovici, Stephens, & Possin, 2015). According to the Supervisory Attentional System model of executive function (Norman & Shallice, 1986), overlearned activities and routines are carried out automatically or are triggered by environmental cues, with minimal requirements for executive function or top-down control. Therefore, executive function impairments may be easily missed within everyday activities and familiar environments. A key role of executive function is to inhibit or override automatic responses to familiar situations. This top-down control allows a person to control impulses, plan, troubleshoot, or adapt to unexpected circumstances and changes. Therefore, executive function is particularly important in novel, complex, unstructured, or multitasking activities that require strategic thinking (Burgess et al., 2006; Chan, Shum, Toulopoulou, & Chen, 2008).

Other models of executive function emphasize the role of sustained attention and working memory in maintaining goal-directed behavior. When working memory or sustained attention is compromised, the individual may lose track of the goal and become distracted, sidetracked, or disorganized as he or she engages in an activity. Goal-directed actions may be replaced by habitual routines or automatic responses that are not relevant to the task, particularly in situations that require sustained attention and ability to keep track of multiple aspects of a task (Chan et al., 2008; Levine et al., 2011).

These conceptualizations of executive function guided the manipulation of WCPA activity characteristics so that greater demands were placed on executive function. Although the task of entering appointments into a calendar can be considered familiar and routine, task complexity and novelty are increased by the WCPA through introducing rule restrictions, conflicts in scheduling, and subtle unexpected problems. Rule restrictions, such as leaving a specified day free, require the ability to inhibit automatic responses and to plan ahead. Rules also increase the amount of information the person has to keep track of while simultaneously carrying out the task. Minor, unexpected problems, such as change in the calendar format from 15- to 30-minute time slots at the end of the day, also require the individual to think flexibly and adjust his or her strategies or task methods.

The WCPA is a simulated task that requires the person to adopt the perspective of another person's schedule. Some individuals with executive function dysfunction are only able to view the task from the context of their own lives. The familiarity of the calendar can trigger automatic responses. For example, a person may begin to fill out the calendar with his or her routines and appointments that are personally relevant but are not part of the task. This response was not observed in the cognitively healthy sample. Normally, executive function skills override automatic actions or habits and allow a person to adhere to task requirements or view situations from multiple perspectives. The capacity to maintain goals and intentions and to view situations from another person's perspective or think flexibly is important in social skills, such as empathy, compromising, or understanding hidden agendas (Decety & Moriguchi, 2007). In addition, the ability to adopt a simulated or "what if" perspective, flexibly view problems, and generate alternate solutions is an inherent part of successful coping and problem solving (Wilder-Willis, Shear, Steffen, & Borkin, 2002).

Although such difficulties may not be obvious or apparent within the context of everyday routines or structured activities, consistent evidence demonstrates a close and consistent association between executive function and academics, social and vocational outcomes, emotional control, and quality of life in individuals with schizophrenia (Kluwe-Schiavon, Sanvicente-Vieira, Kristensen, & Grassi-Oliveira, 2013).

Dynamic Interactional Model of Cognition

Although the current conceptualizations of executive function shaped the design and activity demands of the WCPA, the DIM influenced the focus on strategies and awareness. In the DIM, cognition is defined as the person's capacity to acquire and use information to adapt to environmental demands. Information processing skills, learning, and generalization are inherent within this conceptualization of cognition. Strategies and self-awareness represent core aspects of cognitive function that interact dynamically with activity demands, environmental influences (e.g., social, physical, cultural), and personal context during learning and performance. Independent occupational performance requires the ability to recognize one's limitations, self-monitor performance, and use efficient strategies (Toglia, 2018).

Cognitive dysfunction is conceptualized in terms of deficiencies in processing strategies and self-monitoring skills rather than by deficits in specific cognitive skills (Toglia, 2018). Therefore, assessment of people with cognitive impairments emphasizes both self-awareness and use of strategies, as reflected in the WCPA. The common behaviors and patterns of errors that interfere with performance on a number of different tasks are analyzed rather than impairments in specific cognitive skills. In addition, the activity demands and the environmental influences that increase and decrease cognitive perceptual symptoms during occupational performance are specified when describing cognitive dysfunction. These key concepts of the DIM and their relevance to the WCPA are further explained in the following sections.

Strategies

Cognitive strategies are considered a central aspect of normal cognition and occupational performance. They can be described as *mind tools,* or task methods, that help one control performance errors and cope with cognitively challenging situations (Toglia, Rodger, & Polatajko, 2012). Typically, a person automatically uses a variety of both internal and external strategies in complex tasks to increase the effectiveness of information processing and performance. Inefficient strategies (e.g., a haphazard approach, overfocusing on pieces, jumping into tasks without preplanning) can impede performance. People with mental health conditions, including depression (Channon & Green, 1999), schizophrenia

(Gsottschneider, Keller, Pitschel-Walz, Fröböse, Bäuml, & Jahn, 2011), and substance abuse (Daig et al., 2010) often demonstrate restricted or inefficient strategy use compared to healthy controls. There is often a failure to initiate and apply self-regulatory or monitoring behaviors, such as self-checking and revising solutions.

The ability to use strategies to keep track of things to do, follow a list, organize a schedule, recognize conflicts, and monitor errors is essential for everyday life, and analysis of such strategies is a key aspect of the WCPA. During the WCPA, observed strategy use is rated and then probed in an after-task interview. On the WCPA, cognitively healthy people used an average of four to five strategies. For example, strategies such as entering fixed appointments before variable appointments, crossing out the free day, checking off or crossing off appointments, using one's finger, and self-checking were frequently employed by cognitively typical youth and adults, which helped to facilitate performance.

As strategies help people monitor and control performance errors, analysis of strategy use also requires examination of error types and patterns. The types of errors observed during WCPA performance (e.g., omissions, rule breaks) frequently represent general difficulties underlying complex task performance and should be examined in other complex IADL tasks. Consistency in observed error types can provide an indication of the type of strategies that might be helpful for intervention (Toglia, 2018).

Self-Awareness

In addition to strategies, the DIM also views self-awareness as a key aspect of cognition. Self-awareness is viewed as a multidimensional construct that includes both a general knowledge of abilities and limitations that exist outside the context of activities, as well as online awareness, or awareness of performance within the context of an activity. Online awareness includes the ability to recognize errors, judge task difficulty, regulate emotions, monitor and adjust performance when needed, recognize effective actions or task methods that promote success, and self-evaluate performance (Toglia & Maeir, 2018). Awareness of function, cognition, and task performance may be distinct or disassociated from general awareness of symptoms or illness (Bayard, Capdevielle, Boulenger, Raffard, 2009; Donohoe et al., 2009; Gonzalez-Suarez et al., 2011). Studies have indicated that up to 80% of individuals with schizophrenia do not believe that they are ill; however, at the same time, up to 48% acknowledge deficits in cognitive functioning (Gonzalez-Suarez et al., 2011). This suggests that a person may deny his or her illness (be unaware of illness) but recognize that he or she has difficulties concentrating within a task (have online awareness). Online awareness can influence strategy use within a task and may be more related to actual performance than other aspects of awareness (Toglia, Johnston, Goverover, & Dain, 2010). If a person is unaware of errors within a task, such as failing to accurately organize pills within a medication organizer or paying the wrong amount for a bill, it can result in significant safety risks and limit functional independence (Toglia & Maeir, 2018).

Poor awareness of illness is particularly well documented in schizophrenia (Amador, Strauss, Yale, Flaum, Endicott, & Gorman, 1993; Lehrer & Lorenz, 2014) and was the focus of the majority of research in this area. Recent evidence suggests that discrepant self-assessment of functioning across social, vocational, and everyday activities is a strong predictor of real-world functioning in individuals with schizophrenia (Gould et al., 2015). Direct assessment of performance awareness within the context of functional activities has not been adequately studied in individuals with mental illness. The WCPA examines online awareness, including the ability to recognize errors, identify task challenges, and realistically appraise the client's performance through the combination of observation, semistructured interview, and self-ratings.

Learning

In the DIM, cognitive performance is viewed as modifiable and as a process of ongoing learning and change that takes place with experience. In addition to analysis of strategy use and self-monitoring skills, a dynamic approach that analyzes change and learning is also advocated (Haywood & Lidz, 2007). The WCPA includes an optional dynamic test-teach-retest method that examines the extent to which a person is able to modify performance with mediation or guidance by another person. The influence of the social environment or the role of others in facilitating or inhibiting cognition plays a central role in some theories of cognitive development (Feuerstein, Rand, & Hoffman, 1979; Vygotsky, 1978).

The test-teach-retest format examines responsiveness to a brief strategy-mediated intervention. It includes a mini intervention using mediation techniques that's sandwiched between a pre- and post-assessment. The WCPA is administered as usual to obtain a performance baseline. The after-task interview is replaced with mediation, using guided questions and prompts in a systematic manner to facilitate self-awareness of performance and generation of strategies. Following mediation, the WCPA is readministered using an alternate WCPA form to examine any performance changes (Toglia, 2015, 2018).

Dynamic assessment goes beyond observation and analysis of quality of performance as it also provides information on *modifiability of performance*, or the ability to learn and carry over strategies to a similar task. Use of the test-teach-retest format in people with mental illness is supported by several studies. For example, compared with traditional assessments, dynamic assessment differentiates subgroups of learners (Rempfer, McDowd, & Brown, 2012) and predicts rehabilitation outcome (Wiedl, Schottke, Green, & Nuechterlein, 2004) and work skill acquisition (Sergi, Kern, Mintz, & Green, 2005) in people with schizophrenia. The dynamic format of the WCPA is in preliminary stages and has not yet been empirically tested. It is included in the WCPA manual as it may provide the clinician with additional information on potential for learning that can influence treatment and recovery plans; however, it needs to be systematically examined.

Activity and Environment

To understand cognitive function and occupational performance, one needs to fully analyze interactions among the person, activity, and environment. If activity and environmental demands change, self-monitoring abilities and the type of cognitive strategies needed for efficient performance may change as well (Toglia, 2018).

Activity Demands

Strategy use and self-monitoring skills are best observed when the activity is at the optimal level of challenge. If an activity is too easy for the person, strategies are not needed. On the other hand, if the activity is too difficult, the high cognitive load reduces the processing resources needed to effectively use strategies or monitor performance. Therefore, the WCPA includes different levels of ability. The variations in activity demands allow the examiner to choose the activity level that is most appropriate for the individual's abilities.

Consistent with the DIM, studies on the WCPA support the premise that manipulation of activity characteristics or demands changes performance. The addition of irrelevant information in Level III results in a decrease in average accuracy scores across both younger and older age groups. This indicates that the ability to accurately complete a task, such as placing appointments in a calendar, varies depending on activity characteristics. Therefore, it is critical to specify activity conditions when reporting assessment results because an emphasis on activity conditions (e.g., amount of irrelevant information, format of presentation, number of choices) has broad implications for function across different activities (Toglia, 2018).

Environment

The WCPA needs to be considered in the context of the client's prior functioning, personality, culture, and experiences. One limitation of the WCPA is that it is performed at one point in time, out of context, and in a single environment. A comprehensive profile of functioning requires that the WCPA be examined along with other occupational therapy assessments that examine performance skills, performance patterns, and areas of occupation across different environments.

Psychometric Properties

Normative Data

Normative data and percentiles for WCPA scores are provided in the manual for Level II ($n = 435$) across 4 age groups (16 to 21, 18 to 39, 40 to 64, and 65 to 90 years) and Level III across 3 age groups (18 to 39, 40 to 64, and 65 to 87 years) from ages 18 to 87 years ($n = 175$). Comparison of a clinical population with that of a cognitively healthy population provides an indication of the degree to which performance such as accuracy, efficiency, or strategy use is typical. Normative data for adolescents (ages 16 to 21 years) for the youth version were collected in the St. Louis area (Toglia & Berg, 2013), and normative data for ages 12 to 18 years were collected on the middle school version in Israel (Zlotnik & Toglia, 2018).

Normative data for adults were collected in the Greater New York city area; thus, additional normative data across a wider range of geographical regions is needed. Normative data for Level II ($n = 433$) have also been collected in Israel for adults aged 18 years and older. WCPA accuracy scores and the number of appointments entered were consistent with U.S. data, demonstrating support for stability of the normative data across countries and cultures. However, cross-cultural comparisons found significant differences in time and strategy use, suggesting that these variables are partially influenced by culture (Toglia, Lahav, Ben Ari, & Kizony, 2017).

Normative data on adults for the WCPA 10-item shortened version are currently in progress. Normative data have not been collected for Level I. Based on other normative data, it is assumed that healthy adults would not have difficulty with this version.

Reliability and Validity

The WCPA total accuracy scores have been demonstrated to have interrater reliability of scoring with an intraclass correlation coefficient of 0.99 (Weiner, Toglia, & Berg, 2012). The WCPA's discriminative validity has been established between community youths and at-risk youths (Toglia & Berg, 2013), younger and older healthy adults (Toglia et al., 2017), college students with and without ADHD (Lahav, Ben-Simon, Inbar-Weiss, & Katz, 2018), typical adolescents and those with epilepsy (Zlotnik, Schiff, Ravid, Shahar, & Toglia, 2018) or traumatic brain injury (Doherty, Dodd, & Berg, 2017), and between healthy adults and those with multiple sclerosis (Goverover, Toglia, & DeLuca, 2019) or acquired brain injury (Lussier & Toglia, 2019).

At-risk youth ($n = 113$) made more errors, used fewer strategies, and broke more rules than the community youth group ($n = 49$; Toglia & Berg, 2013). Consistent with literature on executive functioning, moderate relationships were found between academic performance and WCPA performance in at-risk youths, supporting construct validity. A study on college students with and without ADHD ($n = 157$) aged 20 to 30 years in Israel found that those with ADHD required significantly more time to complete the task, missed more appointments, used fewer strategies, and expressed difficulty more often (Lahav et al., 2018). Similarly, older adults were not only less accurate and less efficient than younger adults, but they also used less strategies and followed fewer rules during the task. As a group, these studies and others cited above demonstrate that the WCPA discriminates between various populations that have been identified as having subtle executive function impairments.

Holmqvist, Holmefur, and Arvidsson (2019) studied test-retest reliability of the Swedish version of the WCPA (Level I) with 24 adults with psychiatric, neurodevelopmental, or mild intellectual disorders. The WCPA was administered 2 weeks apart, across three different time points. The intraclass correlation coefficients between the first two test occasions were weak, but were acceptable to excellent (0.65 to 0.91) between test occasions 2 and 3, leading authors to suggest using two consecutive WCPA baselines in this particular population. There was a considerable amount of random variation observed in the results, but little systematic variation, indicating no or possibly a small learning effect in the total number of accurately recorded appointments. The random variation observed in this study may be reflective of the heterogeneity of the population combined with a small sample size, as well as the intra-individual cognitive variability documented in neurodevelopmental disorders (Fagot, Mella, Borella, Ghisletta, Lecerf, & De Ribaupierre, 2018).

The WCPA (Level II) was used to measure change in a randomized metacognitive 4-week group intervention study with adults with psychiatric disabilities, based on the DIM approach (Kaizerman-Dinerman, Roe, & Josman, 2018). The WCPA was administered at three time points in each group (pre-intervention, post-intervention, and 12-week follow-up). The control group ($n = 41$) demonstrated stable scores in accuracy, strategy use, and efficiency across each time point (no significant differences). In contrast, the intervention group ($n = 43$) demonstrated significant increases in accuracy and strategy use across each of the three time points and significant increases in efficiency between pre to post intervention. These results were consistent with changes observed on other functional measures taken at the same time points and support the WCPA's concurrent validity. They also suggest that the WCPA can reliably measure change as a result of intervention (Kaizerman-Dinerman et al., 2018).

Assessment Administration

Area of Occupation/Performance Skills/ Performance Patterns/Client Factors Assessed

The WCPA provides information on ability to accurately complete an IADL task of entering appointments into a calendar while simultaneously examining underlying strategy use, performance errors, and client factors. Analysis of observed errors and strategies is similar to assessing deficiencies in process performance skills. Performance skills are defined by the *Occupational Therapy Practice Framework: Domain and Process, Third Edition,* as small units of goal-directed, observable actions that contribute to occupational performance (American Occupational Therapy Association [AOTA], 2014). The WCPA performance errors, such as omissions, decreased planning time, misplacement of appointments, or repetitions, represent the outcome of deficiencies in performance skills, including the failure to attend, notice/respond, pace, sequence, adjust, accommodate, or organize performance. Client factors assessed by the WCPA are focused on specific mental functions and higher-level cognitive abilities, including metacognitive skills such as self-recognition of errors, identification of task challenges, and self-perceptions of performance. The emphasis of the WCPA is on observed performance. Executive function impairments or client factors, such as working memory, inhibition, or flexibility of thinking, are reflected in WCPA performance errors or ineffective strategy use; however, they are not directly assessed or rated.

Description of Environment/ Description of Supplies/Materials Required

The WCPA is a tabletop assessment that is easily portable and can be used in a wide range of settings. The individual is seated at a table in a quiet environment. Administration involves the selection of an appointment list and the accompanying calendar score worksheet according to age (youth or adults) and ability level (Level I, II, or III or the short 10-item version). The client is presented with written instructions and rules, an appointment list or paragraph, a blank weekly calendar, a calendar sample page, blank paper, pens, two highlighters, and a watch or clock in clear sight. Examiner materials include the WCPA Recording Form, Calendar Scoring Worksheet, a stopwatch, the After-Task Interview Form, and an optional observation worksheet. All client and examiner testing forms are included on a flash drive that accompanies the test manual.

Administration

Directions are presented orally while the examiner points to the written Weekly Calendar Activity Instruction Sheet and calendar sample page. The client is asked to enter appointments in any order into the weekly schedule. He or she is shown how to mark the exact time needed by referring to a sample page. He or she is also asked to enter the entire appointment and to follow a list of 5 written rules.

The WCPA rules include the following: (1) once an appointment is entered into the calendar, it cannot be crossed out; (2) let the examiner know when it is a specified time; (3) leave a specified day free; (4) distracting questions from the examiner should not be answered during the activity; and (5) tell the examiner when finished. Each rule is reviewed, and the person is asked to repeat them to ensure understanding. The person is told that he or she will be timed, but that it is more important to be accurate than to go fast. He or she is instructed to be careful because some of the appointments could conflict with others. Once the activity begins, the examiner can restate the directions or point to the instruction sheet at any time but cannot answer questions. During the activity, the examiner asks three unrelated questions, such as "Do you know what the weather will be tomorrow?" at specific time intervals (2, 5, and 10 minutes) that the person is instructed to ignore.

The examiner observes and records planning and total time, as well as adherence to all five rules during the activity. The type and the frequency of observed strategies are also documented on a strategy checklist. Strategies are grouped according to those that increase attention to key features (e.g., underlining or highlighting), help a person keep track of information (e.g., repeating an item out loud, checking items off the list after entering them), simplification or organization (e.g., entering fixed appointments first), and self-monitoring (e.g., self-checking).

Self-recognition of errors in appointment entries as observed through self-correction attempts, verbal remarks, or clear nonverbal signs, such as shaking his or her head, are also recorded during the activity. Additional observations include how the individual manages unexpected problems or errors on the calendar and the frequency with which the client refers back to the instruction sheet. These observations are not included in scoring.

Immediately after the person is finished with the calendar activity, a semistructured interview is conducted in a discussion-like manner to examine the person's self-percep-tions of his or her performance. Sample questions include "Tell me how you went about doing this task." "Did you use any strategies or special methods?" "Did you encounter (or experience) any challenges while doing this task?" "Which parts of this activity were hardest? Easiest?"

Responses are carefully probed in a nonthreatening manner according to test guide-lines. The examiner has the option of asking the individual to self-rate his or her agree-ment to four statements on a scale of 1 (agree) to 4 (disagree), as well as to estimate both the time required and the number of accurate appointments entered. The individual's self-perceptions can be compared to that of the examiner or to actual performance (Toglia, 2015).

Scoring

The WCPA scores include the following: planning time (seconds), total time (minutes), adherence to rules (0 to 5), total number of strategies used (observed + reported), number of entered appointments (0 to 17 for adults, 0 to 18 for youth version, 0 to 10 for short version), accuracy of entered appointments, and efficiency. Efficiency is calculated for accuracy scores of 7 or higher and is based on a ratio of accuracy and time, as described in the test manual. Two people can have the same accuracy score but demonstrate different levels of efficiency.

Each of these scores are compared to a healthy normative sample aged 16 to 94 years by examining both the means and standard deviations for selected scores or by convert-ing all scores to a percentage, using tables in the appendix of the WCPA test manual. This information is particularly important for identifying the presence or extent of per-formance difficulties. A number of options are included to summarize scores, including an initial and follow-up comparison form and a visual performance profile grid that summarizes percentile scores so that patterns of performance can be quickly analyzed. Percentiles quickly provide an indication of how common or uncommon a score is in the normative sample.

The Calendar Scoring Worksheet (specific to the version selected) is used to identify and score the accuracy of appointments. As an option, the examiner can code the type of errors to provide additional insight into underlying performance difficulties. Type of errors are coded as R (repetition or appointments that are repeated), L (location or incor-rect placement of appointment), T (time or incorrect allotment of time for an appoint-ment), and I (incomplete or inaccurate appointment entry). Missing appointments are documented in a separate column. In addition, extraneous appointments or entered appointments that are not on the list are also documented separately. In addition to summarizing overall scores, an Error Analysis Summary Profile can be used to provide a quick visual representation of the frequency, number, and pattern of errors.

Responses to the after-task interview provide important qualitative information. This information is not scored but is used to confirm observations and to gain a better understanding of the person's self-perceptions. Self-ratings can provide objective information on self-awareness that can supplement responses to the interview. Self-ratings can either be totaled (4 to 16) or be averaged and subtracted from the examiner's ratings. Lower self-ratings indicate that the task is perceived as easy. Agreement between client and examiner ratings (discrepancy = 0) generally suggests good awareness. Larger discrepancies can suggest greater unawareness (Toglia, 2015).

Intervention Planning
Based on Assessment Results

The WCPA provides important information on how a client copes with challenges and performs a multistep complex activity, including the strategies used, types of performance errors, and the client's self-awareness and self-monitoring skills. This information provides a strong foundation for treatment planning.

Interpretation of performance requires careful consideration of a combination of quantitative scores, observations, and ratings during the task, as well as responses to after-task interview questions. For example, the same accuracy scores can have different implications for treatment depending on other aspects of performance, such as the time required to complete the task, adherence to rules, self-recognition of errors, and the strategies and task methods used. Key areas that are emphasized in the evaluation summary include calendar performance; performance profile and analysis of error types; strategy use, including frequency, type, and generation of strategies; and self-awareness, including self-recognition of errors, awareness of strategies used, identification of task challenges, perception of task difficulty, and estimations of time and accuracy.

Simultaneous consideration of all areas provides guidance for selecting and choosing treatment approaches or strategies. Consistent with the DIM model, occupational performance can be enhanced by changing the activity demands and environment and/or by modifying the person's strategies and self-monitoring skills. Although treatment may include a combination of these factors, interventions that include a focus on strategy use and self-monitoring skills are hypothesized to impact function more broadly across activities and contexts. The WCPA provides information that is helpful in guiding task adaptations and strategies to optimize performance, as well as in choosing and selecting a treatment approach. Examples of implications for treatment follow and are illustrated through a case presented at the end of this chapter.

Calendar Performance

Difficulties in the task of entering a list of appointments into a calendar may be an area of occupation addressed within occupational therapy treatment if it is relevant to the person's goals.

Score Profile and Error Analysis

Analysis of the patterns of scores and performance errors can guide occupational therapy intervention. A visual performance profile (Table 14-1) provides a quick overview of strengths and weaknesses across different WCPA scores. Varying patterns of high and low scores can suggest different intervention strategies. The sample that follows shows a performance profile with a low number of entered appointments; however, all appointments that were entered were accurate. This suggests that the person is able to manage details and follow instructions once items are attended to. Despite excessive time and strategy use, six appointments from the list were not entered into the calendar. This pattern indicates that performance could be facilitated by either task adaptations or the reduction of the number of items presented at one time or through training to increase strategy effectiveness and efficiency.

In contrast to the previous example, a performance profile that includes a high number of entered appointments (16/17) within the context of poor accuracy (8/17) suggests the need for strategies to accurately follow items on a list. Detailed analysis of types of appointment errors provides further information on underlying performance difficulties that can be targeted in treatment.

Strategy Use

Analysis of the frequency, type, and effectiveness of strategies used during the WCPA provides information on intervention strategies that might be useful. For example, if the person does not check off or cross out appointments after entering them, simple strategies to more effectively manage a list could be addressed in treatment. On the other hand, if a person quickly abandons strategies or uses an excessive number of strategies, performance may be enhanced through increasing strategy efficiency and enhancing awareness of task methods that are most successful. Studies have demonstrated that interventions focused on cognitive strategies have a significant effect on functional outcome in individuals with schizophrenia (Twamley, Savla, Zurhellen, Heaton, & Jeste, 2008; Wykes, Huddy, Cellard, McGurk, & Czobor, 2011), indicating the importance of addressing this area in treatment. Katz and Keren (2011) provide an excellent illustration of how a structured strategy intervention can be integrated within occupational therapy intervention.

Self-Awareness

Independent strategy use requires understanding task demands and challenges and recognizing strengths and weaknesses in performance. Complete unawareness of significant performance difficulties may suggest that treatment approaches that do not require awareness, such as adaptations of the task or environment by others or error-less learning, may be most appropriate (Toglia, Golisz, & Goverover, 2018). A client with partial awareness may be vaguely aware of challenges during the WCPA yet be unable to identify how it was challenging or fail to recognize errors. In this case, treatment may emphasize metacognitive strategies and include practice in anticipation or identification of task challenges, self-checking, and self-evaluation of performance. There is evidence that interventions using metacognitive training or guided self-determination can increase clinical insight in individuals with schizophrenia (Gawęda, Krezolek, Olbrys, Turska, & Kokoszka, 2015; Jørgensen et al., 2015; Lam et al., 2015). Given the importance of self-awareness to functional outcome, it is important to systematically address awareness of functional performance within occupational therapy treatment.

Table 14-1

Performance Profile

Percentile	Entered Appt.	Accurate Appt.	Rules Followed	Strategy Use	Efficiency	Planning Time	Total Time	Percentile
>95								>95
>75								>75
70								70
60								60
50			4					50
40				4				40
30								30
25								25
20								20
10		11						10
<5	11				205	610 sec	25 min 20 sec.	<5

From Toglia, J. (2015). *The Weekly Calendar Planning Activity (WCPA): A performance test of executive function.* Bethesda, MD: American Occupational Therapy Association, Inc. © 2015 J. Toglia. Reprinted with permission.

Treatment implications depend on careful and simultaneous consideration of WCPA performance error patterns, strategy use, and self-awareness. Similar performance errors with differences in self-awareness and strategy use may suggest different treatment approaches. The optional dynamic assessment, the test-teach-retest format, can be used to further investigate the person's online self-awareness and strategy use and can provide information on responsiveness to intervention techniques aimed at modifying skills in these areas.

Case Study

Nicholas is a 24-year-old Black man who currently resides in a homeless shelter in a large urban area. Nicholas's case manager referred him to occupational therapy to address his poor organizational skills and difficulty with keeping appointments and for assistance with obtaining his goals. He completed the 11th grade and worked in a volunteer position at a day care center. Currently, he is working in a part-time stipend job in maintenance at the shelter. He was diagnosed with bipolar disorder 1 year previously, although he experienced intermittent symptoms of mania throughout his childhood. His family history is filled with family members who used drugs, and he has lived with many different family members at various points in his life. He also experienced a great deal of physical abuse within his family system. He used and sold drugs himself, but he has been clean for the past year. In his free time at the shelter, he enjoys playing basketball, boxing, writing songs, and socializing with other residents and staff. His goals are to get his GED, get more job experience, and complete his housing placement package.

The WCPA-10 (short version) was administered as one component of the occupational therapy assessment, which also included an occupational profile, or exploration of interests, routines, habits, and goals. The WCPA-10 involves entering 10 appointments into a weekly schedule while adhering to rules and avoiding conflicts. It was administered to provide information on Nicholas's ability to cope with a cognitively challenging everyday activity that included the ability to plan ahead, recognize potential conflicts, make performance adjustments, simultaneously keep track of information, restrain impulsive responses, self-monitor performance, and use efficient task strategies.

Performance Results

Nicholas entered 10/10 appointments in 9 minutes and 47 seconds and followed 4/5 rules; however, only 3/10 appointments were accurate. Table 14-2 shows Nicholas's results as recorded on the Calendar Scoring Worksheet. In addition, Table 14-3 provides a summary of his WCPA scores. Although normative data for the WCPA-10 are not yet available, norms from the 17-item WCPA suggest that an accuracy of 3/10 is below the 5th percentile. Nicholas jumped into the task without planning ahead, as indicated by minimal planning time (20 seconds). He appeared rushed during the task and often did not read the entire errand before entering it into the calendar. He did not refer back to the written instructions during the task. Errors were related to incorrect location and time allotment of appointments. An error analysis summary is presented in Table 14-4.

Table 14-2

Case Sample: WCPA-10 Calendar Scoring Worksheet: Adult Level II (Version A)

Entered	Missing	Error	Accurate	SR	Appointments
✓		L		✓	Visit with cousin Mon. or Tues. between 1:00 and 2:00 PM or 1:30 and 2:30 PM or on Thurs. between 2:30 and 3:30 PM or 3:00 and 4:00 PM
✓			✓		Mon. anytime or Tues. AM: Call to renew prescription
✓		T		✓	Tues.: Lunch with friend from 1:00 to 2:00 PM
✓		L			Tues.: Phone conference before 2:00 PM (30 minutes)
✓		L			Mon. or Tues.: Medication picked up between 9:00 AM and 3:00 PM (30 minutes). Must have previously called to renew prescription
✓		L		✓	Thurs.: Dentist at 3:00 PM (1 hour)
✓		L		✓	Thurs.: Movies with friends from 7:00 AM to 11:00 PM
✓		T			Thurs. or Fri.: Dinner with coworkers, starting between 6:30 and 8:00 PM (2 hours)
✓			✓		Doctor: Mon. or Fri. afternoon at 2:00 PM (90 minutes)
✓			✓		Carpool: One afternoon at 3:00 PM (45 minutes)
10	0	7	3	4	

I = appointment name is entered inaccurately or partially; L = appointment is placed in the wrong location, day, or time slot; R = appointment is repeated or entered more than once; SR = self-recognition of errors; T = appointment is in the right location, but the time allotted is incorrect.

From Toglia, J. (2015). *The Weekly Calendar Planning Activity (WCPA): A performance test of executive function.* Bethesda, MD: American Occupational Therapy Association, Inc. © 2015 J. Toglia. Reprinted with permission.

Strategy Use

Strategies Used

Three strategies observed during performance included verbal rehearsal of key words/instructions aloud, occasional self-checking, and pausing to reread. Verbal rehearsal appeared to effectively help Nicholas keep track of the rules and appointments that were entered. Self-monitoring strategies, such as self-checking and pausing to reread, were not effective because of a tendency to read or recheck information only partially, without attending to details. Nicholas also reported that his strategy was to complete all the appointments for Thursday first because this was the busiest day; however, this was not an accurate or effective strategy due to appointment choices and conflicts.

Table 14-3

Case Sample: Overview of Performance on WCPA-10

WCPA-10 Scores	Score
Planning time (min:sec)	0:20
Total time (min:sec)	9:47
Number of rules followed (0 to 5)	4 (crossed out wording of one appointment)
Total number of strategies used (observed + reported)	4 (3 + 1)
Number of appointments entered (0 to 10)	10
Number of accurate appointments (0 to 10)	3
Appointments missing	0
Location error	5
Time error	2
Repetition error	0
Incomplete error	0
Total number of errors	7
Self-recognition of errors	4

From Toglia, J. (2015). *The Weekly Calendar Planning Activity (WCPA): A performance test of executive function.* Bethesda, MD: American Occupational Therapy Association, Inc. © 2015 J. Toglia. Adapted with permission.

Table 14-4

Case Sample: Error Analysis of Performance on the WCPA-10

	Missing	Repetition	Incomplete	Location	Time	Extraneous	Self-Recognition
0	X	X	X			None	
1							
2					X		
3+				X			X

From Toglia, J. (2015). *The Weekly Calendar Planning Activity (WCPA): A performance test of executive function.* Bethesda, MD: American Occupational Therapy Association, Inc. © 2015 J. Toglia. Reprinted with permission.

Strategy Generation (After-Task Interview)

Nicholas was able to generate strategies to help support future performance, including paying greater attention to the timing of appointments and creating his own calendar to schedule in the appointments.

Self-Monitoring and Awareness

During Task (Self-Recognition of Errors/Self-Checking)

Nicholas self-checked his work; however, he did not do so consistently nor did his final review of the calendar improve his performance. He self-recognized 4/7 errors and attempted to self-correct either by drawing lines, writing notes, or verbally explaining to the occupational therapist; however, correction attempts were not all accurate.

Identification of Task Challenges

When prompted on possible task challenges experienced, Nicholas acknowledged the following challenges: (1) the 8:00 PM end time on the calendar, (2) writing small, and (3) distracting questions asked by the therapist.

Overall Perceptions of Task Performance

Overall, Nicholas said the task was very easy and estimated that he entered all 10 appointments accurately.

Awareness of Task Methods

Nicholas was unable to verbalize any special methods he used during the task and stated that he had to remember everything to do and just followed the list after entering in Thursday appointments first. He was unable to identify other strategies or methods used. He indicated that he somewhat agreed with the statement that efficient task methods were used, suggesting that he did not fully recognize the ineffectiveness of his task strategies.

Summary

Nicholas has difficulty pacing, regulating, and monitoring ongoing performance. As a result, errors involving attending to details frequently occurred. Strengths include initiation, task completion, and ability to inhibit distractions, enter full errand names, and keep track of information even though written instructions were not referred to. Effective use of verbal rehearsal likely supported performance and his ability to keep track; however, Nicholas appeared to be unaware that he used this strategy. Although Nicholas was partially aware of errors within the task, he considerably overestimated the accuracy of his overall performance. Partial attempts at self-checking and strategy use reflect positive task behaviors; however, increased effectiveness of monitoring skills and strategies is needed for successful performance. The test-teach-retest format of the WCPA may be useful in determining performance modifiability and responsiveness to strategy intervention.

Recommendations

Based on the results from the WCPA, Nicholas may benefit from training to help pace his speed of performance, increase his self-monitoring skills and organization, and plan an effective strategy use for planning activities. It is recommended that treatment focus on enhancing awareness of task methods that promote success and improving self-recognition of task errors during actual performance as an initial step (rather than addressing general awareness of performance). If error recognition and monitoring within a task improve, realistic appraisal of overall performance is more likely to emerge. The ability to accurately follow a list is an important skill for both work and school and could be addressed directly through a variety of activities involving following lists. In addition, a program such as Let's Get Organized (White, 2007, 2017) may be useful in helping Nicholas learn strategies to manage and organize his own time and appointments.

Suggested Further Research

As a recently published instrument, further research using the WCPA is encouraged. There is a need to increase representation of normative data across different geographical locations and educational levels and establish sensitivity for identifying performance deficits and measuring change. Although there are initial studies of validity and reliability of the WCPA in adults with mental health conditions, there are many areas that could be further investigated. For example, differences in types and frequencies of performance errors, strategy use, self-awareness of performance, and their relationship to IADL and functional outcome across different mental health conditions can be studied. In addition, the dynamic test-teach-retest method needs to be systematically examined, including prediction of functional outcome or response to intervention, to determine the extent that clinicians agree that the dynamic format provides additional useful information for intervention that is above and beyond the typical method.

Summary

This chapter presented an overview of the WCPA, including the theoretical basis of the WCPA, administration, scoring, interpretation, and implications for treatment. The WCPA provides information on both the ability to successfully complete a weekly calendar task as well as on the process and methods used to manage unexpected time conflicts, monitor performance, and juggle multiple task components. The WCPA allows the practitioner to learn what strategies the client uses that are effective and which ones are ineffective or counterproductive.

The recovery process requires clients to take greater responsibility for managing ever-increasing activity levels and daily routines. Establishing more effective performance patterns requires executive function skills. The WCPA provides a practical starting point for cognitive and functional strategy-based treatment to aid the client in building more satisfying life patterns, routines, and habits. The knowledge from the WCPA guides the therapist in identifying effective strategies for multistep activities, organization, and time management. It also provides consideration of tools, such as lists, calendars, and appointment books, to manage daily tasks and time effectively. The results of the WCPA need to be combined with the client's occupational profile, personal goals, performance patterns, and information from other occupational therapy assessments to develop a comprehensive treatment plan. When executive function abilities and performance skills are embedded into a productive set of performance patterns, health and participation are enhanced (AOTA, 2014).

Acknowledgments

A special thanks is extended to Emily Raphael-Greenfield, EdD, OTR/L, FAOTA, and Ashley Hartman, MS, OTR/L, for their contributions to the case study and to Kim Havel, OTS, for her valuable input and assistance.

References

Amador, X. F., Strauss, D. H., Yale, S. A., Flaum, M. M., Endicott, J., & Gorman, J. M. (1993). Assessment of insight in psychosis. *American Journal of Psychiatry, 150*, 873-879.

American Occupational Therapy Association. (2014). Occupational therapy practice framework: Domain and process (3rd ed.). *American Journal of Occupational Therapy, 68*(Suppl. 1), S1-S48.

Bayard, S., Capdevielle, D., Boulenger, J. P., & Raffard, S. (2009). Dissociating self-reported cognitive complaint from clinical insight in schizophrenia. *European Psychiatry, 24*, 251-258.

Burgess, P. W., Alderman, N., Forbes, C., Costello, A., Coates, L. M., Dawson, D. R., ... Channon, S. (2006). The case for the development and use of "ecologically valid" measures of executive function in experimental and clinical neuropsychology. *Journal of the International Neuropsychological Society, 12*, 194-209.

Chan, R. C., Shum, D., Toulopoulou, T., & Chen, E. Y. (2008). Assessment of executive functions: Review of instruments and identification of critical issues. *Archives of Clinical Neuropsychology, 23*, 201-216.

Channon, S., & Green, P. S. (1999). Executive function in depression: The role of performance strategies in aiding depression and non-depressed participants. *Journal of Neurology, Neurosurgery, & Psychiatry, 66*, 162-171.

Cramm, H. A., Krupa, T. M., Missiuna, C. A., Lysaght, R. M., & Parker, K. H. (2013). Executive functioning: A scoping review of the occupational therapy literature. *Canadian Journal of Occupational Therapy, 80*, 131-140.

Daig, I., Mahlberg, R., Schroeder, F., Gudlowski, Y., Wrase, J., Wertenauer, F., ... Kienast, T. (2010). Low effective organizational strategies in visual memory performance of unmedicated alcoholics during early abstinence. *GMS Psycho-Social-Medicine, 7*, Doc07. https://doi.org/10.3205/psm000069

Darkholme, A. J. (2014). *Rise of the morningstar*. Mistero Publishing.

Decety, J., & Moriguchi, Y. (2007). The empathetic brain and its dysfunction in psychiatric populations: Implications for intervention across different clinical conditions. *BioPyschoSocial Medicine, 1*(22), 1-21.

Doherty, M., Dodd, J., & Berg, C. (2017). Validation of the Weekly Calendar Planning Activity with teenagers with acquired brain injury. *Archives of Physical Medicine and Rehabilitation, 98*, e130. https://doi.org/10.1016/j.apmr.2017.08.423

Donohoe, G., Hayden, J., McGlade, N., O'Grada, C., Burke, T., Barry, S., ... Corvin, A. P. (2009). Is "clinical" insight the same as "cognitive" insight in schizophrenia? *Journal of the International Neuropsychological Society, 15*, 471-475.

Fagot, D., Mella, N., Borella, E., Ghisletta, P., Lecerf, T., & De Ribaupierre, A. (2018). Intra-individual variability from a lifespan perspective: A comparison of latency and accuracy measures. *Journal of Intelligence, 6*(1), 16.

Feuerstein, R., Rand, Y. A., & Hoffman, M. B. (1979). *The dynamic assessment of retarded performers: The learning potential assessment device, theory, instruments, and techniques*. Baltimore, MD: University Park Press.

Gawęda, L., Krezolek, M., Olbrys, J., Turska, A., & Kokoszka, A. (2015). Decreasing self-reported cognitive biases and increasing clinical insight through meta-cognitive training in patients with chronic schizophrenia. *Journal of Behavior Therapy and Experimental Psychiatry, 48*, 98-104.

Gonzalez-Suarez, B., Gomar, J. J., Pousa, E., Ortiz-Gil, J., Garcia, A., Salvador, R., ... McKenna, P. J. (2011). Awareness of cognitive impairments in schizophrenia and its relationship to insight into illness. *Schizophrenia Research, 133*, 187-192.

Gould, F., McGuire, L. S., Durand, D., Sabbag, S., Larrauri, C., Patterson, T. L., ... Harvey, P. D. (2015). Self-assessment in schizophrenia: Accuracy of evaluation of cognition and everyday functioning. *Neuropsychology, 29*, 675-682.

Goverover, Y., Toglia, J., & DeLuca, J. (2019). The Weekly Calendar Planning Activity in multiple sclerosis: A top-down assessment of executive functions. *Neuropsychological Rehabilitation*. https://doi.org/10.1080/09602011.2019.1584573

Gsottschneider, A., Keller, Z., Pitschel-Walz, G., Fröböse, T., Bäuml, J., & Jahn, T. (2011). The role of encoding strategies in the verbal memory performance in patients with schizophrenia. *Journal of Neuropsychology, 5*, 56-72.

Haywood, H. C., & Lidz, C. S. (2007). *Dynamic assessment in practice: Clinical and educational applications*. New York, NY: Cambridge University Press.

Holmqvist, K. L., Holmefur, M., & Arvidsson, P. (2019). Test–retest reliability of the Swedish version of the Weekly Calendar Planning Activity—A performance-based test of executive functioning. *Disability and Rehabilitation*, 1-6.

Jørgensen, R., Licht, R. W., Lysaker, P. H., Munk-Jørgensen, P., Buck, K. D., Jensen, S. O. W., ... Zoffmann, V. (2015). Effects on cognitive and clinical insight with the use of guided self-determination in outpatients with schizophrenia: A randomized open trial. *European Psychiatry, 30*(5), 1-9.

Josman, N., Schenirderman, A. E., Klinger, E., & Shevil, E. (2009). Using virtual reality to evaluate executive functioning among persons with schizophrenia: A validity study. *Schizophrenia Research, 115*, 270-277.

Kaizerman-Dinerman, A., Roe, D., & Josman, N. (2018). An efficacy study of a metacognitive group intervention for people with schizophrenia. *Psychiatry Research, 270*, 1150-1156.

Katz, N., & Keren, N. (2011). Effectiveness of occupational goal intervention for clients with schizophrenia. *American Journal of Occupational Therapy, 65*, 287-296.

Kluwe-Schiavon, B., Sanvicente-Vieira, B., Kristensen, C. H., & Grassi-Oliveira, R. (2013). Executive functions rehabilitation for schizophrenia: A critical systematic review. *Journal of Psychiatric Research, 47*, 91-104.

Lahav, O., Ben-Simon, A., Inbar-Weiss, N., & Katz, N. (2018). Weekly Calendar Planning Activity for university students: Comparison of individuals with and without ADHD by gender. *Journal of Attention Disorders, 22*(4), 368-378.

Lam, K. C., Ho, C. P., Wa, J. C., Chan, S. M., Yam, K. K., Yeung, O. S., ... Balzan, R. P. (2015). Metacognitive training (MCT) for schizophrenia improves cognitive insight: A randomized controlled trial in a Chinese sample with schizophrenia spectrum disorders. *Behaviour Research and Therapy, 64*, 38-42.

Lehrer, D. S., & Lorenz, J. (2014). Anosognosia in schizophrenia: Hidden in plain sight. *Innovations in Clinical Neuroscience, 11*(5-6), 10-17.

Lepage, M., Bodnar, M., & Bowie, C. R. (2014). Neurocognition: Clinical and functional outcomes in schizophrenia. *Canadian Journal of Psychiatry, 59*(1), 5-12.

Levine, B., Schweizer, T. A., O'Connor, C., Turner, G., Gillingham, S., Stuss, D. T., ... Robertson, I. H. (2011). Rehabilitation of executive functioning in patients with frontal lobe brain damage with goal management training. *Frontiers in Human Neuroscience, 5*, 1-9.

Lipskaya, L., Jarus, T., & Kotler, M. (2011). Influence of cognition and symptoms of schizophrenia on IADL performance. *Scandinavian Journal of Occupational Therapy, 18*, 108-187.

Lussier, A., Doherty, M., & Toglia, J. (2019). Weekly Calendar Planning Activity. In T. Wolf, G. Giles, D. Edwards (Eds.), *Functional cognition for occupational therapy: A practical approach to treating individuals with cognitive loss*. Baltimore, MD: AOTA Press.

Lussier, A., & Toglia, J. (2019). Measuring functional cognition: Comparison of adults with acquired brain injury (ABI) and healthy controls on the Short Weekly Calendar Planning Activity (WCPA-10). *American Journal of Occupational Therapy, 73*(4 Suppl. 1), 7311500071p1.

Norman, D. A., & Shallice, T. (1986). Attention to action: Willed and automatic control of behaviour. In R. J. Davidson, G. E. Schwartz, & D. Shapiro (Eds.), *Consciousness and self-regulation: Advances in research and theory* (pp. 1-18). New York, NY: Plenum Publishing.

Rabinovici, G. D., Stephens, M. L., & Possin, K. L. (2015). Executive dysfunction. *Continuum, 21*, 646-659.

Rempfer, M. V., Hamera, E. K., Brown, C. E., & Cromwell, R. L. (2003). The relations between cognition and the independent living skill of shopping in people with schizophrenia. *Psychiatry Research, 117*, 103-112.

Rempfer, M. V., McDowd, J. M., & Brown, C. E. (2012). Assessing learning potential in people with schizophrenia using the Rey Osterrieth Complex Figure Test. *Open Journal of Psychiatry, 2*, 407-413.

Revheim, N., Schechter, I., Kim, D., Silipo, G., Allingham, B., Butler, P., & Javitt, D. C. (2006). Neurocognitive and symptom correlates of daily problem-solving skills in schizophrenia. *Schizophrenia Research, 83*, 237-245.

Royall, D. R., Lauterbach, E. C., Cummings, J. L., Reeve, A., Rummans, T. A., Kaufer, D. I., ... Coffey, C. E. (2002). Executive control function: A review of its promise and challenges for clinical research. *Journal of Neuropsychiatry and Clinical Neurosciences, 14*, 377-405.

Sergi, M. J., Kern, R. S., Mintz, J., & Green, M. F. (2005). Learning potential and the prediction of work skill acquisition in schizophrenia. *Schizophrenia Bulletin, 31*, 67-72.

Toglia, J. (2015). *The Weekly Calendar Planning Activity (WCPA): A performance test of executive function*. Bethesda, MD: American Occupational Therapy Association.

Toglia, J. (2017). Multicontext: Functional cognitive activities and resources for occupational therapy and cognitive rehabilitation. Retrieved from https://multicontext.net/

Toglia, J. (2018). The dynamic interactional model and the multicontext approach. In N. Katz & J. Toglia (Eds.), *Cognition, occupation, and participation across the lifespan* (4th ed., pp. 355-385). Bethesda, MD: American Occupational Therapy Association, Inc. https://doi.org/10.7139/2017.978-1-56900-479-1

Toglia, J., & Berg, C. (2013). Performance-based measure of executive function: Comparison of community and at-risk youth. *American Journal of Occupational Therapy, 67*, 515-523.

Toglia, J. P., Golisz, K. M., & Goverover, Y. (2018). Evaluation and intervention for cognitive perceptual impairments. In B. A. Boyd Schell & G. Gillen (Eds.), *Willard and Spackman's occupational therapy* (13th ed., pp. 901-941). Philadelphia, PA: Lippincott Williams & Wilkins.

Toglia, J., Johnston, M. V., Goverover, Y., & Dain, B. (2010). A multicontext approach to promoting transfer of strategy use and self-regulation after brain injury: An exploratory study. *Brain Injury, 24*, 664-677.

Toglia, J., & Katz, N. (2018). Executive functioning: Prevention and health promotion for at-risk populations and those with chronic disease. In N. Katz & J. Toglia (Eds.), *Cognition, occupation, and participation across the lifespan* (4th ed., pp. 129-140). Bethesda, MD: American Occupational Therapy Association, Inc. https://doi.org/10.7139/2017.978-1-56900-479-1

Toglia, J., Lahav, O., Ben Ari, E., & Kizony, R. (2017). Adult age and cultural differences in the Weekly Calendar Planning Activity (WCPA). *American Journal of Occupational Therapy, 71*(5), 7105270010p1-7105270010p8.

Toglia, J., & Maeir, A. (2018). Self-awareness and metacognition: Effect on occupational performance and outcome across the lifespan. In N. Katz & J. Toglia (Eds.), *Cognition, occupation, and participation across the lifespan* (4th ed., pp. 143-163). Bethesda, MD: American Occupational Therapy Association, Inc. https://doi.org/10.7139/2017.978-1-56900-479-1

Toglia, J., Rodger, S. A., & Polatajko, H. J. (2012). Anatomy of cognitive strategies: A therapist's primer for enabling occupational performance. *Canadian Journal of Occupational Therapy, 79*, 225-236.

Twamley, E. W., Savla, G. N., Zurhellen, C. H., Heaton, R. K., & Jeste, D. V. (2008). Development and pilot testing of a novel compensatory cognitive training intervention for people with psychosis. *American Journal of Psychiatric Rehabilitation, 11*, 144-163.

Vygotsky, L. S. (1978). *Mind in society: The development of higher psychological processes*. Cambridge, MA: Harvard University Press.

Weiner, N. W., Toglia, J., & Berg, C. (2012). Weekly Calendar Planning Activity (WCPA): A performance-based assessment of executive function piloted with at-risk adolescents. *American Journal of Occupational Therapy, 66*, 699-708.

White, S. (2007). Let's Get Organized: An intervention for persons with co-occurring disorders. *Psychiatric Services, 58*, 713.

White, S. (2017). Collaborative use of Weekly Calendar Planning Activity and Assessment of Time Management Skills. *SIS Quarterly Practice Connections, 2*(4), 16-18.

Wiedl, K. H., Schottke, H., Green, M. F., & Nuechterlein, K. H. (2004). Dynamic testing in schizophrenia: Does training change the construct validity of a test? *Schizophrenia Bulletin, 30*, 703-711.

Wilder-Willis, K. E., Shear, P. K., Steffen, J. J., & Borkin, J. (2002). The relationship between cognitive dysfunction and coping abilities in schizophrenia. *Schizophrenia Research, 55*, 259-267.

Wykes, T., Huddy, V., Cellard, C., McGurk, S. R., & Czobor, P. (2011). A meta-analysis of cognitive remediation for schizophrenia: Methodology and effect sizes. *American Journal of Psychiatry, 168*, 472-485.

Zlotnik, S., Schiff, A., Ravid, S., Shahar, E., & Toglia, J. (2018). A new approach for assessing executive functions in everyday life among adolescents with genetic generalised epilepsies. *Neuropsychological Rehabilitation*. https://doi.org/10.1080/09602011.2018.1468272

Zlotnik, S., & Toglia, J. (2018). Measuring adolescent self-awareness and accuracy using a performance-based assessment and parental report. *Frontiers in Public Health, 6*, 15. https://doi.org/10.3389/fpubh.2018.00015

The Executive Function Performance Test

Carolyn M. Baum, PhD, OTR/L, FAOTA
Timothy J. Wolf, OTD, PhD, OTR/L, FAOTA

The EFPT provides the clinician with the information to answer the following questions:
What specifically will the client need help with? Can the client initiate tasks?
Does the client need help with organization? Does the client need cues to sequence a task?
Will the client be safe in performing tasks? Does the client perseverate and need help to finish an activity?
(Baum & Wolf, 2013)

The occupational therapist approaches the measurement of cognition and function not just to know what a person can do but to know what to do to foster the individual's engagement in daily life, because occupation is a basic human need, a determinant of health, and a source of meaning (Christiansen, 1999; Hasselkus, 2011; Meyer, 1922; Reilly, 1962; Townsend, 1997). For this reason, occupational therapists are essential members of the health care team who address the cognitive issues people with neurological injuries, chronic diseases, and mental illness must manage in order to participate in their daily lives.

While cognitive function is often assessed using neurocognitive assessment that evaluates isolated cognitive loss, assessment using neurocognitive assessments is not adequate to determine changes in everyday life activities. Determination of an individual's capacity for real-world or everyday performance is of significant importance (Alderman, Burgess, Knight, & Henman, 2003; Fisher, 1998; Giles, 2005; Gioia & Isquith, 2004; Keil & Kaszniak, 2002; Levy & Burns, 2005; Morrison, Edwards, & Giles, 2015; Shallice & Burgess, 1991). Capacity is determined by having the person demonstrate that he or she can perform an activity. The information obtained by the occupational therapist from such assessments enables the therapist to work with individuals and their families to maximize function in those who have experienced change in cognitive functioning.

Occupational therapists assess cognition to determine the person's capacity to be safe, live alone, work, or do any task that is important and meaningful. Assessment may address the impact that executive function has on performance by examination of

Hemphill, B. J., & Urish, C. K. (Eds.). *Assessments in*
Occupational Therapy Mental Health: An Integrative Approach,
Fourth Edition (pp. 261-275). © 2020 Taylor & Francis Group.

a person's cognitive capacity in the performance of daily tasks. It is possible to observe key executive constructs in the performance of daily life (Baum, Connor, Morrison, Hahn, Dromerick, & Edwards, 2008; Baum & Edwards, 1993). These include initiation, the process that precedes the performance of a task (DePoy, Maley, & Stanraugh, 1990; Kaye, Grigsby, Robbins, & Korzun, 1990; Lezak, Howieson, Loring, Hannay, & Fischer, 2004); organization, the physical arrangement of the environment, tools, and materials to facilitate efficient and effective performance (Lezak et al., 2004; Weld & Evans, 1990); judgment (Goel, Grafman, Tajik, Gana, & Danto, 1997; Lezak, 1982); and completion (Goel et al., 1997). The Executive Function Performance Test (EFPT), a performance-based assessment of functional cognition, is used to assist the therapist in identifying the strategies necessary to help the individual with cognitive loss improve occupational performance and participation. This chapter provides an overview of the EFPT, including administration, psychometric properties, and a case study at the end of the chapter.

Theoretical Basis

The EFPT was constructed to identify the occupational performance issues faced by individuals with cognitive impairment. Development of the assessment was informed by the Person-Environment-Occupational-Performance model, which requires clinicians to address in practice the relationship among person factors (i.e., psychological, cognitive, sensory, motor, physiological), occupations (i.e., what individuals need and want to do to maintain themselves and engage in work, family, and community activities), and environment (i.e., social support, social capital, the physical environment, culture). Many of these elements are dependent on executive function as the person identifies and uses resources to function in their home, family, and community environments.

In general, rehabilitation professionals use two different methods to identify limitations of individuals with executive dysfunction. The first method, neuropsychological testing, was developed to identify and characterize the cognitive/behavioral effects of brain pathologies (Marcotte & Grant, 2009). Neuropsychological tests are structured and norm-referenced and allow individuals' performance to be compared to standardized data from demographically comparable persons. The clinical utility of neuropsychological testing is enhanced by the use of tests that assess different cognitive domains to compare and contrast distinct aspects of functioning to identify an individual's cognitive strengths and weaknesses.

The second method, performance-based assessment, was developed for a different purpose and based upon a different theory. Performance-based assessments measure a spectrum of cognitive abilities and focus on the interaction between the person, the activity, and everyday environments. A body of literature demonstrates how individuals with neurological injury may experience performance limitations in everyday life, even in absence of impairment on neuropsychological testing (Baddeley & Wilson, 1988; Lezak et al., 2004; Shallice & Burgess, 1991). Both neuropsychological and performance-based assessment are central to our understanding of executive function; performance-based measures enhance cognitive assessment and treatment planning because they identify those at risk of experiencing limitations in everyday activities.

There are several ecologically valid performance-based assessments that measure the capacity of a person to perform a structured everyday life activity, including the following: the Assessment of Motor and Process Skills (Fisher, 1993), the Kettle Test (Hartman-Maeir, Harel, & Katz, 2009), various versions of the Multiple Errands Test (Alderman et al., 2003; Dawson, Gaya, Hunt, Levine, Lemsky, & Polatajko, 2009; Knight, Alderman, &

Burgess, 2002; Morrison et al., 2015), and the Test of Actual Reality (Goverover, O'Brien, Moore, & DeLuca, 2010). While these measures reveal problems in cognitive and processing skills, the assessments do not record the person's capabilities when provided with progressive levels of support. This information is essential to the occupational therapist when developing a treatment plan. The EFPT (Baum et al., 2008; Baum, Morrison, Hahn, & Edwards, 2003) was developed to identify supports needed to help individuals with executive dysfunction perform daily tasks, and therefore fills a gap that other currently available assessments did not address.

Psychometric Properties

The EFPT has been translated into Hebrew, Swedish, French, and Italian. The assessment has been validated for individuals with neurological conditions (i.e., stroke, multiple sclerosis, schizophrenia, traumatic brain injury), all of which are known to put people at risk for executive dysfunction. An essential consideration for the occupational therapist is to identify when a person's daily life performance is affected by executive dysfunction so treatment can be oriented to help the person develop effective strategies. Furthermore, assessment can provide the therapist with information to educate the family and other caregivers so these individuals will understand that the behaviors of their loved one need to be supported as the actions are not willful. An important consideration regarding an assessment's measurement properties is that the findings relate to the measures performance in the sample that has been tested. Multiple studies have been conducted to establish the reliability and validity of the EFPT, and the findings will be reported here.

- *Standard error of measurement*: Not established because the EFPT is used to identify the level of support an individual needs to perform a task. The task cannot be repeated because a learning effect will occur.
- *Minimal detectable change*: As above.
- *Minimal clinically important difference*: As above.
- *Normative data*: Control participants were used in the stroke validity study (Baum et al., 2008), multiple sclerosis (Kalmar, Gaudino, Moore, Halper, & DeLuca, 2008), and traumatic brain injury (Baum et al., 2016). In all situations, the EFPT discriminated between controls and individuals with mild impairment. When people with mild and moderate impairment were scored, the EFPT discriminated between the stroke (Baum et al., 2008), multiple sclerosis (Kalmar et al., 2008), schizophrenia (Katz, Tadmor, Felzen, & Hartman-Maeir, 2007), and traumatic brain injury (Baum et al., 2016) groups.

Reliability

Test-retest: Not established because the EFPT is used to identify the level of support an individual needs to perform a task. The task cannot be repeated as there will be a learning effect.

Interrater reliability: Intraclass correlation coefficient for overall EFPT is as follows: stroke (0.91), cooking (0.94), bill paying (0.89), medication (0.87), and phone (0.79; Baum et al., 2008).

Internal consistency: In a population of individuals who had experienced a stroke, the EFPT Cronbach's alpha individual tasks ranged from 0.77 to 0.94 (Baum et al., 2008). Within a population of individuals diagnosed with schizophrenia, the Cronbach's alpha was 0.88 (Katz et al., 2007).

Validity

Criterion validity: Has established moderate correlation with neurological tests known to be measures of executive function, including the Delis-Kaplan Executive Function System Trail Making (Wolf, Barbee, & White, 2010), Wisconsin Card Sort, National Institutes of Health Toolbox Fluid Cognition, and National Institutes of Health Toolbox Crystalized Cognition (Carlozzi et al., 2017). Excellent correlations exist with the Assessment of Motor and Process Skills process scores (Cederfeldt, Carlsson, Dahlin-Ivanoff, & Gosman-Hedström, 2015). Correlation coefficients between the EFPT and the total Behavioral Assessment of the Dysexecutive Syndrome profile revealed moderate to high correlations (Katz et al., 2007).

Predictive validity: This was determined in a sample of persons with traumatic brain injury with the EFPT total task score predicting self-reported independence (Carlozzi et al., 2017).

Assessment Administration

The EFPT was developed initially from work conducted on the Kitchen Task Assessment to provide a performance-based, standardized assessment of cognitive function (Baum & Edwards, 1993). The EFPT was designed to examine executive functions in the context of performing a task. Executive functions are described as the (1) ability to exhibit flexible adaptive behavior, (2) use of appropriate problem-solving strategies as required for maintaining and updating goals, (3) capacity to monitor the consequences of actions, and (4) ability to use prior knowledge to correctly interpret future events (Miyake & Shah, 1999). The term *executive functions* also derives in part from the idea of top-down control by a central executive, as proposed in models of working memory (Baddeley, 2001) or of attentional control (Posner & Petersen, 1990). From a performance-based perspective, executive functions are called on when individuals make plans, initiate actions, and modify activities as problems are experienced or information from the environment changes. Executive functions are a group of cognitive processes that mediate goal-directed activity (Kaye et al., 1990; Stuss, 1992). Thus, executive functions are involved in task execution.

Description of Environment/ Description of Supplies/Materials Required

The EFPT tasks can be administered in a clinic's life skills area or within the client's home; three of the tasks can be administered in a client's room. In the absence of a kitchen, the test can be administered using a chef burner and water from a pitcher. All of the items are in placed in a box and can be used at the point of testing. Please refer to the test manual to identify the supplies and materials required.

The assessment provides the occupational therapist with the information to answer the following questions: What specifically will the client need help with? Can the client initiate tasks? Does the client need help with organization? Does the client need cues to sequence a task? Will the client be safe in performing tasks? Does the client perseverate and need help to finish an activity?

1. Begin the EFPT with the script and all of the pre-test questions (see the test manual).
2. Leave all of the items necessary for all of the tasks in the box on a table (the "materials table"). Put it on a lower table or stool if the person sits in a wheelchair. Bills and

mail should be mixed together in a zip-top bag. The account/checkbook should have checks included inside. All other items are loose in the box.

3. Ask the client to begin the task (use the script available in the test manual).

4. Offer assistance only after the client has made a good attempt to process the actions necessary to carry out the step. The cueing guidelines should be used.

5. Complete the cueing chart and behavior assessment chart for each task (Table 15-1).

6. Time each of the tasks and write down the time in minutes and seconds on each task sheet.

7. Complete the score sheet with the information from each task sheet.

The test manual should be consulted for the specific test administration and supplies. The manual includes all forms, labels to personalize the tasks, and scripts for administration of the assessment. The assessment and the training manual are available online for free. The materials include all of the assessment forms and a scoring sheet that can be placed in the medical record. Some hospital systems have asked that the scoring sheet be included in their electronic medical record, which is possible since the tool is available free of charge and is within the public domain. The authors of the manual request that when the material is downloaded, an email confirming the download is sent to the authors. The email request is an important consideration of the assessment process because the individual who downloads the assessment will then receive notice when the updated manual is available, when changes are made, and when tasks are added. The testing manual and complete assessment can be accessed at http://www.ot.wustl.edu/about/resources/executive-function-performance-test-efpt-308.

The EFPT informs about the client-centered factor cognition by observing the client's capacity to perform a task. The forms to record the person's performance are available within the test manual. The form specific to the oatmeal task can be reviewed in Table 15-1.

- The test administrator delivers the cues (see the training manual for complete instructions and a cue sheet) necessary to help the client avoid errors and complete the task. Even clients with severe cognitive loss who have to be given step-by-step verbal cues can complete this test because the need for support can be recorded throughout the task.

- If the client has difficulty with any aspect of any of the tasks, the occupational therapist must wait to give the client time to process before giving a cue. However, it is important to note the occupational therapist should not allow the client to make an error; the cue avoids the error.

- Unless the client is in danger (e.g., putting the pitcher of water down where it could fall off the table and break, putting a hot pad on the burner, touching the burner to see if it is on, placing his or her sleeve in the fire), do not intervene until the client shows he or she is not processing to move to the next step.

- Give two cues of each kind before progressing to the next cueing level.

- Give cues in a progressive fashion from verbal guidance to gestural guidance to direct verbal assistance to physical assistance. If the client is still unable to perform a step in a task, the examiner should do the step and then the client should be cued back to the next sequential step of the task.

- Once the occupational therapist has determined the client needs direct verbal cues in one aspect of the observation (e.g., organization, sequencing, safety and judgment), go ahead and give the verbal cues to finish the task without starting over each time at a verbal and then gestural level.

Table 15-1

Executive Function Performance Test: Form B

Task: Simple Cooking	Independent 0	Verbal Guidance 1	Gestural Guidance 2	Verbal Direct Instruction 3	Physical Assistance 4	Do for Participant 5	Score
Initiation: *Beginning the task.*							
Upon your request to start, participant moves to table to gather tools/materials for making oatmeal.							
Execution: *Carrying out the actions of the task through the use of organization, sequencing, and judgment and safety.*							
Organization: *Arrangement of the tools/materials to complete the task.* Participant retrieves the items needed (pan, pot holder, measuring cup, oats, instructions, spoon).							

(continued)

Table 15-1 (continued)

Executive Function Performance Test: Form B

Task: Simple Cooking	Independent 0	Verbal Guidance 1	Gestural Guidance 2	Verbal Direct Instruction 3	Physical Assistance 4	Do for Participant 5	Score
Sequencing: *Execution of steps in appropriate order.* Participant performs steps according to the directions, participant measures water, puts water into pan, turns on stove, sets heat according to what is needed, boils water, measures oats, puts oats into boiling water, stirs, turns off stove, uses pot holder to lift hot pan, and pours oats into bowl. Participant does not confuse steps (e.g., turns off stove before water boils, replacing oats in cupboard before measuring some out but may measure oats before boiling the water or put salt in the water before or as it boils).							
Judgment and Safety: *Avoidance of dangerous situation.* Participant prevents or avoids danger (e.g., turns water off, does not lay pot holder near burner, turns burner off, uses pot holder to lift hot pan).							

(continued)

Table 15-1 (continued)

Executive Function Performance Test: Form B

Task: Simple Cooking	Independent 0	Verbal Guidance 1	Gestural Guidance 2	Verbal Direct Instruction 3	Physical Assistance 4	Do for Participant 5	Score
Completion: *Termination of task.*							
Participant knows he or she is finished (e.g., pours oatmeal into bowl and moves away from pot). If participant washed dishes, he or she moves away from the sink, does not continue to scrape the pan, etc.							
Task Score _____ **Time** _____							

Adapted from Baum, C. M., Connor, L. T., Morrison, T., Hahn, M., Dromerick, A. W., & Edwards, D. F. (2008). Reliability, validity, and clinical utility of the Executive Function Performance Test: A measure of executive function in a sample of people with stroke. *American Journal of Occupational Therapy, 62*(4), 446-55.

- The occupational therapist will often combine different levels of cues (e.g., several verbal prompts, a gestural movement, a specific direction, assistance). The score of the degree of assistance must reflect the highest level of cue used to get the task done.
- The occupational therapist is instructed not to initiate conversations during the test and not to cheerlead (e.g., do not provide positive or negative feedback related to client performance).
- If the client has a physical limitation and cannot perform the step, the client may ask for help (e.g., opening the oatmeal, opening the envelope) and not be scored for needing a cue because the client has knowledge of what to do but has a physical limitation that is impeding performance, thus indicating a physical problem rather than a cognitive one.

Administration

The EFPT can be administered in a clinical, home, or community environment. The assessment measures the level of support (i.e., cueing required from another person) a person needs to complete four daily life tasks central to community living (Lysack, Neufeld, Mast, MacNeill, & Lichtenberg, 2003). These tasks include the following: (1) following instructions to make oatmeal, (2) taking the correct medication, (3) using the telephone, and (4) paying bills. The level of support the person requires is recorded for five cognitive component skills: (1) initiation, (2) organization, (3) sequencing, (4) judgment and safety, and (5) completion. This information is crucial to the generation of a treatment plan as well as how to effectively train the family (or other caregivers) on how to provide appropriate cognitive support. The following describes how these cognitive constructs are used in the EFPT:

- *Initiation*: The start of motor activity that begins a task. The individual moves to the materials table to collect items needed for the task.
- *Execution*: The proper completion of each step consisting of the following three requirements: organization, sequencing, and safety and judgment. The individual carries out the steps of the task.
- *Organization*: The physical arrangement of the environment, tools, and materials to facilitate efficient and effective performance of steps. The individual correctly retrieves and uses the items necessary for the task.
- *Sequencing*: The coordination and proper ordering of the steps that comprise the task, requiring a proper allotment of attention to each step. The individual carries out the steps in an appropriate order, attends to each step appropriately, and can switch attention from one step to the next.
- *Judgment and safety*: The employment of reason and decision-making capability to intentionally avoid physically, emotionally, or financially dangerous situations. The individual exhibits an awareness of danger by actively avoiding or preventing the creation of a dangerous situation.
- *Completion*: The inhibition of motor performance driven by the knowledge that the task is finished. The person does not perseverate and keep going. The individual indicates that the task is finished or moves away from the area of the last step.

Using these definitions, the rater analyzes the executive functions that mediate each task. Accordingly, the EFPT allows the rater to record the level of guidance (cueing) the person needs to perform the task. The levels range from independent (0), no cue required (1), indirect verbal guidance (2), gestural guidance (3), direct verbal instruction (4), physical assistance (5), and doing the step for the person (6). This valuable information can then be shared with team members, caregivers, and care providers.

The person administering the assessment will respond to the person's need for help to be successful in performing the task. It is very important that the test administrator accurately records the level of cue the person needs in the right category of the test. The test begins with a series of questions to determine the person's perception of his or her skills for the tasks. These answers may confirm the person's recognition of their capabilities or may raise questions about difficulties with awareness.

Scoring

Individual tasks sheets and the final scoring sheets are provided in the test manual. Table 15-2 and Figure 15-1 provide a description of how the occupational therapist can create a description of the assessment results. The gray score is the control score and the black is the client's score. The figure can be constructed with the example in the test material available online. A short summary is provided based upon the client's test results. This information can be reported at a case conference and placed in the client's medical record to document cognitive problems the client is having in performance of daily tasks and level of cueing required for safe and successful completion.

Intervention Planning Based on Assessment Results

The assessment provides the clinician with the information to answer the following questions: What specifically will the client need help with? Can the client initiate tasks? Does the client need help with organization? Does the client need cues to sequence a task? Will the client be safe in performing tasks? Does the client perseverate and need help to finish an activity? The therapist will be able to identify strategies needed by the client and identify environmental modifications that may be helpful for the client. The information provided from the EFPT will help other clinicians understand how to support successful interactions, and the data will identify information that will be essential in preparing caregivers to understand what is needed to support the client in carrying out daily tasks. The data will assist the treatment team in planning the appropriate level of support needed for client discharge.

Table 15-2

Executive Function Performance Test Scoring Summary Sheet

Constructs

Must review all four task sheets to count totals; the highest in each construct goes on this form.

Construct	Cooking	Telephone	Medication	Bills	Construct Score
Initiation					
Organization					
Sequencing					
Judgment and safety					
Completion					

Total Construct Score (should match Total Task Score, if not recheck):

Tasks

Add from the total on each task sheet.

Task	Task Score	Time
Cooking		
Telephone		
Medication		
Bills		
Total Task Score and Time:		

(continued)

Table 15-2 (continued)

Executive Function Performance Test Scoring Summary Sheet

Pre-Test Self-Efficacy Person's Report	No Help	Help	Can't Do
Cooking	0	1	2
Telephone	0	1	2
Medication	0	1	2
Bills	0	1	2

Actual Performance Administrator's Experience	No Help	Help	Can't Do
Cooking	0	1	2
Telephone	0	1	2
Medication	0	1	2
Bills	0	1	2

Potential Awareness Problem

	Yes	No
Accurately estimated need for help (if 100% match between pre-test and actual performance). If no, please specify:		
Overestimated need for help		
Underestimated need for help		

 # Estimated incorrectly: ___ **of 4** *(If greater than 1 of 4, mark yes below.)*

Possible awareness problem: _____ **Yes** _____ **No**

Adapted from Baum, C. M., Connor, L. T., Morrison, T., Hahn, M., Dromerick, A. W., & Edwards, D. F. (2008). Reliability, validity, and clinical utility of the Executive Function Performance Test: A measure of executive function in a sample of people with stroke. *American Journal of Occupational Therapy, 62*(4), 446-55.

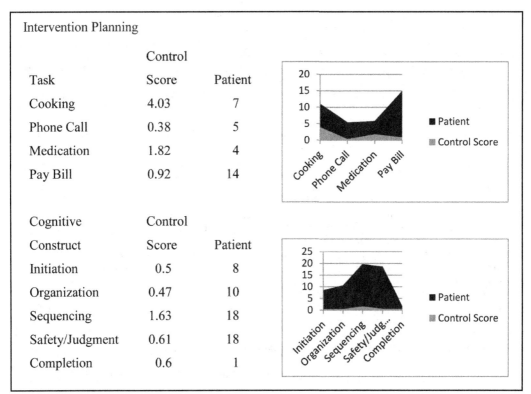

Intervention Planning

Task	Control Score	Patient
Cooking	4.03	7
Phone Call	0.38	5
Medication	1.82	4
Pay Bill	0.92	14

Cognitive Construct	Control Score	Patient
Initiation	0.5	8
Organization	0.47	10
Sequencing	1.63	18
Safety/Judgment	0.61	18
Completion	0.6	1

Figure 15-1. Intervention planning.

Summary

The EFPT is a valid performance-based assessment that provides the occupational therapist with a standardized method for a tool for recording cognitive issues that pose functional challenges and safety risks. This information is critical for treatment plan development, intervention implementation, enabling strategies, family/caregiver education, discharge disposition, and placement.

References

Alderman, N., Burgess, P. W., Knight, C., & Henman, C. (2003). Ecological validity of a simplified version of the multiple errands shopping test. *Journal of the International Neuropsychological Society, 9*(1), 31-44.

Baddeley, A. D. (2001). Is working memory still working? *American Psychologist, 56,* 851-864.

Baddeley, A., & Wilson, B. (1988). Frontal amnesia and the dysexecutive syndrome. *Brain and Cognition, 7,* 212-230.

Baum, C. M., Connor, L. T., Morrison, T., Hahn, M., Dromerick, A. W., & Edwards, D. F. (2008). Reliability, validity, and clinical utility of the Executive Function Performance Test: A measure of executive function in a sample of people with stroke. *American Journal of Occupational Therapy, 62,* 446-455.

Baum, C., & Edwards, D. F. (1993). Cognitive performance in senile dementia of the Alzheimer's type: The Kitchen Task Assessment. *American Journal of Occupational Therapy, 47,* 431-436.

Baum, C. M., Morrison, T., Hahn, M., & Edwards, D. F. (2003). *Test manual: Executive Function Performance Test.* St. Louis, MO: Washington University.

Baum, C. M., & Wolf, T. J. (2013). *The Executive Function Performance Test manual*. St. Louis, MO: Washington University. Retrieved from http://www.ot.wustl.edu/about/resources/executive-function-performance-test-efpt-308

Baum, C. M., Wolf, T. J., Wong, A. W. K., Chen, C. H., Walker, K., Young, A. C., ... Heinemann, A. W. (2016). Validation and clinical utility of the executive function performance test in persons with traumatic brain injury. *Neuropsychological Rehabilitation, 27*, 603-617.

Carlozzi, N. E., Tulsky, D. S., Goodnight, S., Heaton, R. K., Casaletto, K. B. , Wong, A. W. K., ... Heinemann, A. W. (2017). Construct validity of the NIH toolbox cognition battery in individuals with stroke. *Rehabilitation Psychology, 62*(4), 443-454. https://doi.org/10.1037/rep0000195

Cederfeldt, M., Carlsson, G., Dahlin-Ivanoff, S., & Gosman-Hedström, G. (2015). Inter-rater reliability and face validity of the Executive Function Performance Test (EFPT). *British Journal of Occupational Therapy, 78*, 563-569.

Christiansen, C. H. (1999). The 1999 Eleanor Clark Slagle Lecture. Defining lives: Occupation as identity: An essay on competence, coherence, and the creation of meaning. *American Journal of Occupational Therapy, 53*, 547-558.

Dawson, D. R., Gaya, A., Hunt, A., Levine, B., Lemsky, C., & Polatajko, H. J. (2009). Using the Cognitive Orientation to Occupational Performance (CO-OP) with adults with executive dysfunction following traumatic brain injury. *Canadian Journal of Occupational Therapy, 76*, 115-127.

DePoy, E., Maley, K., & Stanraugh, J. (1990). *Executive function and cognitive remediation: A study of activity preference. Occupational therapy approaches to traumatic brain injury*. New York, NY: Haworth Press.

Fisher, A. G. (1993). The assessment of IADL motor skills: An application of many-faceted Rasch analysis. *American Journal of Occupational Therapy, 47*, 319-329.

Fisher, A. G. (1998). Uniting practice and theory in an occupational framework. 1998 Eleanor Clarke Slagle Lecture. *American Journal of Occupational Therapy, 52*, 509-521.

Giles, G. M. (2005). A neurofunctional approach to rehabilitation following severe brain injury. In N. Katz (Ed.), *Cognition and occupation across the life span: Models for intervention in occupational therapy* (pp. 139-166). Bethesda, MD: AOTA Press.

Gioia, G. A., & Isquith, P. K. (2004). Ecological assessment of executive function in traumatic brain injury. *Developmental Neuropsychology, 25*, 135-158.

Goel, V., Grafman., J., Tajik, J., Gana, S., & Danto, D. (1997). A study of the performance of patients with frontal lobe lesions in a financial planning task. *Brain, 120*, 1805-1822.

Goverover, Y., O'Brien, A. R., Moore, N. B., & DeLuca, J. (2010). Actual reality: A new approach to functional assessment in persons with multiple sclerosis. *Archives of Physical Medicine and Rehabilitation, 91*, 252-260.

Hartman-Maeir, A., Harel, H., & Katz, N. (2009). Kettle test—A brief measure of cognitive functional performance. Reliability and validity in stroke rehabilitation. *American Journal of Occupational Therapy, 63*, 592-599.

Hasselkus, B. R. (2011). *The meaning of everyday occupation*. Thorofare, NJ: SLACK Incorporated.

Kalmar, J. H., Gaudino, E. A., Moore, N. B., Halper, J., & DeLuca, J. (2008). The relationship between cognitive deficits and everyday functional activities in multiple sclerosis. *Neuropsychology, 22*, 442-449.

Katz, N., Tadmor, I., Felzen, B., & Hartman-Maeir, A. (2007). Validity of the Executive Function Performance Test in individuals with schizophrenia. *OTJR: Occupation, Participation and Health, 27*, 44-51.

Kaye, K., Grigsby, J., Robbins, L. J., & Korzun, B. (1990). Prediction of independent functioning and behavior problems in geriatric patients. *Journal of the American Geriatric Society, 38*, 1304-1310.

Keil, K., & Kaszniak, A. W. (2002). Examining executive function in individuals with brain injury: A review. *Aphasiology, 16*, 305-335.

Knight, C., Alderman, N., & Burgess, P. W. (2002). Development of a simplified version of the multiple errands test for use in hospital settings. *Neuropsychological Rehabilitation, 12*, 231-255.

Levy, L. L., & Burns, T. (2005). Cognitive disabilities reconsidered: Rehabilitation of older adults with dementia. In N. Katz (Ed.), *Cognition and occupation across the life span: Models for intervention in occupational therapy.* (pp. 347-388). Bethesda, MD: AOTA Press.

Lezak, M. D. (1982). *Neuropsychological assessment* (2nd ed.). New York, NY: Oxford University Press.

Lezak, M. D., Howieson, D. B., Loring, D. W., Hannay, H. J., & Fischer, J. S. (2004). *Neuropsychological assessment*. New York, NY: Oxford University Press.

Lysack, C. L., Neufeld, S., Mast, B. T., MacNeill, S. E., & Lichtenberg, P. A. (2003). After rehabilitation: An 18-month follow-up of elderly inner-city women. *American Journal of Occupational Therapy, 57*, 298-306.

Marcotte, T. D., & Grant, I. (Eds.). (2009). *Neuropsychology of everyday functioning*. New York, NY: Guilford Press.

Meyer, A. (1922). The philosophy of occupation therapy. *Archives of Occupational Therapy, 1*, 1-10.

Miyake, A., & Shah, P. (1999). *Models of working memory: Mechanisms of active maintenance and executive control*. Cambridge, United Kingdom: Cambridge University Press.

Morrison, M. T., Edwards, D. F., & Giles, G. M. (2015). Performance-based testing in mild stroke: Identification of unmet opportunity for occupational therapy. *American Journal of Occupational Therapy, 69*(1), 1-5.

Posner, M. I., & Petersen, S. E. (1990). The attention system of the human brain. *Annual Review of Neuroscience, 13*, 25-42.

Reilly, M. (1962). Occupational therapy can be one of the great ideas of 20th century medicine. *American Journal of Occupational Therapy, 16*, 1-9.

Shallice, T., & Burgess, P. W. (1991). Deficits in strategy application following frontal lobe damage in man. *Brain, 114*, 727-741.

Stuss, D. T. (1992). Biological and psychological development of executive functions. *Brain and Cognition, 20*, 8-23.

Townsend, E. (1997). Occupation: Potential for personal and social transformation. *Journal of Occupational Science, 4*, 18-26.

Weld, E., & Evans, I. (1990). Effects of part versus whole instructional strategies on skill acquisition and excess behavior. *American Journal of Mental Retardation, 94*, 377-386.

Wolf, T. J., Barbee, A. R., & White, D. (2010). Executive dysfunction immediately after mild stroke. *OTJR: Occupation, Participation and Health, 31*, S23-S29.

Part V
Behavioral Assessments

Assessments Used Within the Model of Human Occupation

Celeste Januszewski, OTD, OTR/L, CPRP
Lisa Mahaffey, PhD, OTR/L, FAOTA

> *Values, interests, personal causation, roles, habits, performance capacity and the environment*
> *may produce a complex dynamic in which some factors support and*
> *others constrain a particular behavior, emotion, or thought. It is always the summation of*
> *their total contributions to the dynamic whole that results in the outcome.*
> (Kielhofner, 2008, p. 26)

Practitioners who use the Model of Human Occupation (MOHO; Taylor, 2017) as a key part of their conceptual practice framework find that although they can use a variety of assessments to gather information, the MOHO assessment tools are particularly well suited to gathering the information related to occupational adaptation and participation. Occupational therapy services are provided through a process that builds and forms an understanding of the person as an occupational being. The practitioner and the client, as well as other people who are significant in the client's life when needed, complete and review assessment tools that support the creation of the occupational profile. The occupational profile highlights the person's valued occupations along with the beliefs, responsibilities, and daily patterns that characterize participation in those occupations. The occupational profile also includes the person's perceived barriers and touches on one's need and capacity for adaptation in order to overcome those barriers. Based on the occupational profile, the individual, family, and practitioner work as a team to focus on any additional assessments needed to more thoroughly understand the person factors that create barriers to participation. The resulting analysis of performance, along with the profile, is combined with a thorough review of the supports and barriers that exist in the environments where the person participates in their occupations (American Occupational Therapy Association [AOTA], 2014). Intervention goals are arrived at through a collaborative process that draws upon supports to address both the person and the environmental barriers, resulting in goals that are meaningful to the person, their family, and the practitioner. The MOHO assessment tools continue to evolve and are constantly undergoing a

Hemphill, B. J., & Urish, C. K. (Eds.). *Assessments in Occupational Therapy Mental Health: An Integrative Approach, Fourth Edition* (pp. 279-305). © 2020 Taylor & Francis Group.

rigorous psychometric process that is attentive not only to the dependability of the information, but also to its usefulness within the occupational therapy process. An up-to-date database of worldwide research and evidence on MOHO assessment tools is available through the MOHO website (https://www.moho.uic.edu).

The chapter begins with a brief review of the MOHO concepts and then summarizes several MOHO assessments that are commonly used in mental health occupational therapy practice. This review of the MOHO concepts is only a brief introduction. Therapists who plan to use the assessments will need, at minimum, a basic understanding of the MOHO theory. Therapists with an understanding of the MOHO will feel more confident when interpreting and applying the results of the assessments as they make daily practice decisions. Readers are referred to *Kielhofner's Model of Human Occupation, Fifth Edition* (Taylor, 2017), where both the theory and the assessments are covered in more depth.

Theoretical Basis

Occupational Adaptation and Dimensions of Doing

Individuals are actors who engage in occupations in a variety of contexts over time. Identifying with specific roles, engaging in interesting activities, being connected with the temporal patterns of life, meeting responsibilities, and fulfilling personal expectations and values are all aspects of our lives as occupational beings. According to the MOHO, when individuals maintain patterns of occupational participation within the environments that reflect a sense of who they are as occupational beings, the end result is a sense of *occupational adaptation*, which involves the "construction of a positive occupational identity and achieving occupational competence over time" (Kielhofner, 2008, p. 121). Occupational identity and competence are influenced by our experiences, including illness and impairment, and these experiences can require individuals to reframe their sense of who they are or what occupations they enact in their daily lives. Several MOHO assessments explore an individual's sense of occupational competence and occupational identity.

Engaging in occupations involves three levels of doing: *occupational participation, occupational performance*, and *occupational skill* (Taylor, 2017). These concepts describe different levels at which one can examine doing (Haglund & Henriksson, 1995). Occupational participation refers to engagement in work, play, or activities of daily living (ADLs) that are desired and necessary for well-being according to a person's sociocultural context. Occupational participation is influenced by environmental and cultural contexts, as well as by individual person factors, such as motivation and motor capacities. Occupational participation can include maintaining a home, being an employee, or being a member of a social community. The actions required to participate at this broad level make up the next level of doing, occupational performance. Examples of occupational performance associated with occupational participation include preparing a meal, making a sale to a customer, and playing a game of cards. Performing occupations such as these requires a discrete set of purposeful actions, or occupational skills, that arise during an individual's engagement in goal-directed activities. These observable skills are a function of the interaction between the environment and an individual's personal characteristics. The motor, process, and social interaction skills (Taylor, 2017) associated with making a sale to a customer include manipulating money, sequencing actions to ring up the purchase on the register, and speaking with the customer (Table 16-1). MOHO's conceptualization of skill is reflected in the *Occupational Therapy Practice Framework: Domain and Process, Third Edition* (AOTA, 2014).

Table 16-1

Levels of Doing

Levels of Doing	Example
Occupational participation	• Salesperson
Occupational performance	• Make a sale to a customer
Occupational skills	• Speak with a customer • Sequence actions to use the register • Manipulate money
Adapted from Taylor, 2017.	

MOHO assessments support an evaluative process that considers all the levels of doing, participation, performance, and skills, within the context of the person's environment. This evaluative process helps a practitioner pinpoint supportive aspects of the person's doing, as well as the impact of specific areas of difficulty at all levels.

Individual Person Factors

The practitioner is required to have an understanding of what the *Framework* (AOTA, 2014) refers to as the person factors of occupational participation in order to accurately grasp the individual's occupational adaptation and to articulate the areas of support and difficulty in the different levels of doing (AOTA, 2014). The MOHO organizes person factors under the headings of volition, habituation, and performance capacity. Note that the MOHO considers how an individual's subjective experience of living in the body influences how the person performs and interacts with the world. Attempting to understand a person's "view from the inside" (Kielhofner, 2008, p. 83) can be especially powerful when working with individuals who experience positive psychotic symptoms, such as hallucinations and delusions (Table 16-2).

Environmental Factors

All aspects of the environment, including man-made and natural spaces, objects, other community members, and local customs, offer either an opportunity or a barrier to participating in meaningful and culturally relevant occupations. The MOHO recognizes that the environment is comprised of both physical and social elements. The physical environment includes spaces and objects; spaces can be both built and natural, whereas objects include things that people interact with or use while engaging in a variety of activities. Social groups and occupational forms make up the social aspect of the environment. Social groups can be formal or informal, and have related expectations for behavior within that group. Occupational forms include the actions and manners that characterize a certain activity and are connected to the meaning of the activity (Taylor, 2017). Each aspect of the environment can provide resources or opportunities for engagement in occupations or can demand and constrain specific actions. Each environment impacts an individual in a different way, depending on that person's volition, habitation, and performance capacity.

Table 16-2

Person Factors

Volition	• Motivation for occupation • Feelings, thoughts, and decisions about engaging in occupation	
	• Personal causation	• A person's sense of personal effectiveness while performing an activity
	• Values	• Importance and worth of that activity
	• Interests	• Enjoyment and satisfaction from engaging in that activity
Habituation	• Pattern of occupation • Recurrent patterns of engagement and interaction that organize daily life	
	• Habits	• How routine activities are performed, typical use of time, style of performance
	• Roles	• Internalized roles that create expectations for occupational performance
Performance Capacity	• Communication/interaction skills, motor skills, process skills • A person's physical and mental components, as well as the subjective experience of living within one's body	

Adapted from Parkinson et al., 2006 and Taylor, 2017.

The process of occupational adaptation, participation and performance, individual person factors, and the environment, as articulated by the MOHO, allows an occupational therapist to understand how a variety of factors influences an individual's engagement in occupations.

• • • • • • • • • • • • • • • • • •
Model of Human Occupation Assessments

A wide range of assessments based on the MOHO theory (Taylor, 2017) in more than 20 languages is available through the online resource MOHO Web at https://www.moho.uic.edu (Model of Human Occupational Clearinghouse, 2019). All assessments and manuals are available for immediate use in digital form. Assessments can be completed, scored, and stored online via a secure, confidential MOHO Web account or can be downloaded, printed, and completed with pen/pencil. The MOHO Web includes a database to search for up-to-date worldwide research and evidence on MOHO assessments and a selection tool to guide the practitioner to the appropriate assessment based on criteria including age, purpose of assessment, and MOHO domain. The MOHO assessments presented here are recommended for use with individuals with psychosocial dysfunction and are grouped by administration approach:

- Self-report
  - Occupational Self-Assessment (OSA) version 2.2
  - Occupational Self-Assessment Short-Form (OSA-SF)
  - Child Occupational Self-Assessment (COSA) version 2.2

Table 16-3

Sample of Statements Grouped by Model of Human Occupation Concept

MOHO Concept	OSA (Total 21 Statements) OSA-SF (Total 12 Statements)	COSA (Total 25 Statements)
Occupational performance	• Managing my finances • Getting where I want to go	• Following classroom rules • Dressing myself
Habituation	• Relaxing and enjoying myself • Getting done what I need to do	• Getting enough sleep • Doing things with my friends
Volition	• Doing activities I like • Working toward my goals	• Choosing things I want to do • Getting my homework done

- Interview
  - Occupational Performance History Interview (OPHI-II)
  - Occupational Circumstances Assessment Interview and Rating Scale (OCAIRS) version 4.0
- Observation
  - Volitional Questionnaire (VQ) version 4.1
  - Pediatric Volitional Questionnaire (PVQ) version 2.1
  - Assessment of Communication and Interaction Skills (ACIS) version 4.0
- Mixed report assessments
  - Model of Human Occupation Screening Tool (MOHOST) version 2.0
  - Short Child Occupational Profile (SCOPE) version 2.2
  - Residential Environment Impact Scale (REIS) version 4.0
- Additional resources based on MOHO concepts

Self-Report Assessments

Occupational Self-Assessment and Child Occupational Self-Assessment

To truly engage in client-centered therapy, it is vital to explore people's perceptions of their ability to engage in what is meaningful to them. The OSA (Baron, Kielhofner, Iyenger, Goldhammer & Wolenski, 2006), the OSA-SF (Popova, Ostrowski, Wescott, & Taylor, 2019), and the COSA (Kramer, ten Velden, Kafkes, Besu, Federico, & Kielhofner, 2014) are evaluation tools and outcome measures based on the MOHO principle that people's view of how well they perform an activity (Competence) and how important that activity is to them (Value) impacts their occupational performance (Taylor, 2017). The OSA/COSA contain a series of statements in straightforward language about everyday activities that relate to MOHO concepts (Table 16-3).

The OSA/COSA self-assessments offer people an opportunity to reflect on their capability to participate in a variety of everyday occupations and to prioritize those occupations that they find meaningful. The therapist and client are then able to collaborate to identify goals for client-centered occupational therapy intervention.

Psychometric Properties

The OSA (Baron et al., 2006) has been shown to be reliable for assessment with individuals aged 18 years and older. The evidence indicates that the OSA has good internal validity and is sensitive and able to differentiate between individuals in terms of Occupational Competence and Values (Kielhofner, Forsyth, Kramer, & Iyenger, 2009). The OSA-SF (Popova et al., 2019) has been found to be a valid and reliable measure for use with adults in acute care and acute inpatient rehabilitation. The original OSA contained a self-assessment of the environment, which was found to contain too few items to be considered a sound measure and is in the process of being revised (Baron et al., 2006). When readministered and used as an outcome measure, the OSA has the "ability to detect increases and decreases in self-reported Competence and Value for everyday activities over time" (Kielhofner, Dobria, Forsyth, & Kramer, 2010, p. 19).

The COSA (Kramer et al., 2014) is intended for use with school-aged children aged 6 to 17 years. Evidence suggested that the COSA has high internal validity and good content, structural, and substantive validity, with "theoretically meaningful representations of the constructs of occupational Competence and Value for everyday activities" (Kramer, Kielhofner, & Smith, 2010, p. 631). A study that readministered the COSA suggested that children's perceptions remained consistent over time (Ohl, Crook, MacSaveny, & McLaughlin, 2015).

Assessment Administration

Description of Environment

When administered in a quiet, private space, the OSA/COSA allows for reflective thought and ensures confidentiality. In some cases, it was preferable for the person to be given the assessment forms to complete on their own and to return the completed forms to be discussed with the therapist. Administration time varies widely, dependent on the methods used to administer. The OSA-SF was specifically designed for fast-paced, acute environments, and is estimated to take 7 to 15 minutes to complete.

Administration

The OSA/COSA is administered in three steps: (1) the individuals first rate a series of statements as to how well they think they perform the activity; (2) the individuals then rate each statement as to how much they value the activity; and (3) the individuals and therapists review the match between the activity and value to identity priorities to address in treatment.

To ensure that the OSA truly reflects the person's viewpoint, therapists are required to provide guidance solely through answering questions about the form or referring to the manual to clarify the meaning of terms. The COSA differs in that it encourages dialogue throughout the assessment, including open-ended questions at the end of the assessment, to gain a broad understanding of a younger person's perspectives. The COSA is available in three formats: (1) similar to the OSA using words to rate statements; (2) using symbols rather than words to rate statements; and (3) a card sort version that can be structured in a game-type format (Kramer et al., 2014; Table 16-4).

Suggested accommodations to ensure accessibility of the COSA include flexibility in the scheduling, presentation, and response format (Kramer, Heckmann, & Bell-Walker,

Table 16-4

Self-Assessment Rating Scales

	OSA and OSA-SF	COSA Words	COSA Symbols
Competence	I have a lot of difficulty doing this.	I have a big problem doing this.	☹☹
	I have some difficulty doing this.	I have a little problem doing this.	☹
	I do this well.	I do this OK.	☺
	I do this extremely well.	I am really good at doing this.	☺☺
Values	This is not so important to me.	Not really important to me	★
	This is important to me.	Important to me	★★
	This is more important to me.	Really important to me	★★★
	This is most important to me.	Most important to me	★★★★

Adapted from Baron et al., 2006; Kramer et al., 2014; and Popova et al., 2019.

2012). To compare the effectiveness of therapy, the OSA, OSA-SF, and COSA can be readministered at discharge to measure changes in a person's responses to competence and value ratings. The results can be used to chart progress and to develop discharge recommendations.

Scoring

None of the OSA, OSA-SF, or COSA self-assessments are meant to result in a score; rather the intent is that the results are discussed with the individual, interpreted by the therapist based on MOHO theory, and then an appropriate method to report the findings to others is identified. The OSA assessment results can be plotted on key forms that translate the ratings to obtain numerical scores that describe an individual's level as compared to others or as a measure of change in their perception of competence and value over time. The key form scores can also be used to examine the effectiveness of a program or intervention across groups of individuals (Baron et al., 2006). The OSA-SF scores are designed to be used to support individuals to identify and prioritize goal areas. The COSA Occupational Profile Form provides a visual summary of the individual's self-report of competence and values (Kramer et al., 2014). For an example of the OSA/COSA used in practice, see the case studies at the end of this chapter.

Interview Assessments

Interview assessments enable a therapist to establish therapeutic rapport, gain an understanding of a person's life story for the Occupational Profile, and elicit goals for treatment. Two commonly used MOHO interview assessments are the OPHI-II (Kielhofner et al., 2004) and the OCAIRS (Forsyth et al., 2005). Both assessments are semi-structured interviews that invite individuals to reflect on their lives and past and current occupational participation to frame treatment goals and interventions. They are intended to be flexible instruments that can easily be adapted to meet the needs of a specific person or situation and have been shown to be appropriate for use with adolescents, adults, and older adults who have the cognitive and emotional ability to participate in an interview.

Occupational Performance History Interview

The OPHI-II (Kielhofner et al., 2004) is used to gain people's perspectives about the details of their life history, the impact of current challenges, and their goals for the future to ensure client-centered intervention. The occupational therapist chooses questions to elicit narratives (stories) that provide an opportunity for the person to reflect upon past and current occupational participation in work, play, and self-care. These narratives enable individuals to "integrate their past, present, and future into a coherent whole" (Kielhofner et al., 2004, p. 9). The therapist then groups, rates, and documents the information gained according to three MOHO concepts: occupational identity, occupational competence, and occupational settings (environment).

Psychometric Properties

Psychometric analysis of the first version of the OPHI using Rasch measurement theory (Wright & Masters, 1982) revealed that there were three underlying constructs of occupational adaptation; as a result, the three subscales of occupational competence, occupational identity, and the occupational environment were created (Mallinson, Mahaffey, & Kielhofner, 1998). An international study of the OPHI-II provided evidence of the internal consistency and construct validity across cultures of the three rating scales of the OPHI-II (Kielhofner, Mallinson, Forsyth, & Lai, 2001) and provided the calibrations for the development of the OPHI-II keyforms (Kielhofner, Dobria, Forsyth, & Basu, 2005). In addition, aspects of the OPHI, particularly the narrative slope, was shown to predict future function, as well as service outcomes (Bar, Majadla, & Bart, 2015; Ennals & Fossey, 2009; Levin, Kielhofner, Braveman, & Fogg, 2007).

Assessment Administration

Description of Environment

It is recommended that the OPHI-II interview be conducted in a quiet, private space that allows for reflective thought and ensures confidentiality. Administration time varies widely, dependent upon the individual's motivation to engage in the interview and therapist's clinical judgment as to areas to explore.

Administration

Prior to administering the OPHI-II, it is essential that the therapist be familiar with the themes and questions of the OPHI-II in order to conduct the interview in an engaging, conversational manner. The OPHI-II manual contains a framework of recommended questions to gather the necessary information; however, the therapist is expected to improvise to meet the specific needs of the person. The questions are grouped into themes: occupational roles, daily routine, occupational settings (environment), activity/occupational choices, and critical life events. These themes can be covered in any order that fits the situation (Table 16-5).

The final step in the administration of the OPHI-II is the plotting of the person's life history narrative, either drawn by the individual or in collaboration with the therapist. This plot line reflects the person's perspectives of their critical life events and provides a graphic portrayal of their past, present, and hopes for the future. Individuals have reported the narrative slopes to be motivational and helpful for understanding one's life history (Apte, Kielhofner, Paul-Ward, & Braveman, 2005).

Table 16-5

Sample of Occupational Performance History Interview Items Grouped by Model of Human Occupation Concept

MOHO Concept	Assesses	Sample OPHI-II Items
Occupational identity	A person's sense of self as an occupational being and level of self-awareness	• Expects success • Accepts responsibility • Has interests
Occupational competence	What the person does	• Maintains satisfying lifestyle • Meets personal responsibility standards • Organizes time responsibly
Occupational settings (environment)	The impact of the physical and social environment	• Home-life occupational forms • Major productive role physical space • Leisure social groups

Adapted from Kielhofner et al., 2004.

Scoring

The OPHI-II scales are used to convert the narrative data gained from the interview into three rating scales measuring the MOHO concepts of occupational identity, occupational competence, and occupational settings (environment). Each of these concepts has a 4-point rating scale of occupational functioning including specific criteria for each rating and contains items about both past and current occupational participation. The past ratings capture previous experiences that a person can draw upon to face occupational challenges, and the current ratings identify the factors that are presently impacting occupational performance. The OPHI-II keyforms are used to obtain measures to monitor progress and evaluate intervention success. Keyforms for each rating scale, developed using Rasch measurement (Wright & Masters, 1982), convert the ordinal ratings to interval measures and provide the therapist with an individual measure and error. The perspectives gained through the interview, along with the narrative life history slope, OPHI-II rating scales, and keyforms, are used by the individual and the therapist to identify occupational goals for intervention.

Occupational Circumstances Assessment Interview and Rating Scale

The OCAIRS (Forsyth et al., 2005) provides both qualitative (interview responses) and quantitative (ratings on items) information about individuals' perceptions of their life and occupational participation. Like the OPHI-II, the OCAIRS interview questions are based on MOHO concepts and have a similar interview format. However, the OCAIRS differs in that it is intended to be completed in a shorter time frame and question sets are targeted to three specific practice settings: mental health, forensic mental health, and physical disabilities. Unlike the OPHI-II, ratings are assigned to each concept area and are used to guide the goal setting and intervention process.

Psychometric Properties

The OCAIRS version 4.0 format and content reflect research conducted on the previous versions of the assessment (Brollier, Watts, Bauer, & Schmidt, 1989; Haglund & Henriksson, 1994; Haglund, Thorell, & Walinder, 1998a, 1998b; Lai, Haglund, & Kielhofner, 1999). Collectively, these studies found that the OCAIRS had evidence of good interrater reliability. OCAIRS scores have also been shown to discriminate between patients who are in need of occupational therapy services and those who are not, as well as between those with varying severities of psychiatric disorder (Haglund et al., 1998a, 1998b). The OCAIRS is a commonly used assessment instrument in both specialized and general psychiatric care (Haglund, 2000; Smith & Mairs, 2014) and is recognized internationally as a cross-cultural assessment of occupational functioning (Chui, Wong, Maraj, Fry, Jecker, & Jung, 2016; Daremo, Kjellberg, & Haglund, 2010, 2015; Haglund & Forsyth, 2013; Morley, 2014).

Assessment Administration

Description of Environment

When conducted in a quiet, private space, the OCAIRS interview allows for reflective thought and ensures confidentiality. The OCAIRS can be completed, with practice, in as little as 20 to 30 minutes (Forsyth et al., 2005).

Administration

It is recommended that the therapist be familiar with the OCAIRS rating scales and descriptors prior to conducting the interview to facilitate gathering pertinent information. The therapist first establishes rapport with the client by explaining the purpose of the interview and what it might entail. The interview begins with familiar demographic questions to put the interviewee at ease, and then the OCAIRS interview questions are used to elicit information in 12 areas based on MOHO concepts. The OCAIRS interview is intended to be a conversation, and the therapist is expected to adapt the wording and sequence of the questions to the situation at hand. Time is often a limiting factor, and the therapist chooses when to curtail responses or eliminate questions or if there is a need to ask for elaboration on a specific item (Table 16-6).

Scoring

Each of the 12 OCAIRS items is rated on a 4-point scale according to how it facilitates, allows, inhibits, or restricts participation in occupation. The rating scale form has descriptive statements to assist the therapist in making a rating decision. The therapist rates an item using clinical judgment based on the available information and the item's overall impact on the person's occupational participation. Based on the findings from the evaluation process, the therapist completes the OCAIRS summary form with item ratings and a narrative of the individual's perceptions of their occupational performance for each area. The therapist uses this information to collaborate with the individual to develop goals and a plan for occupational therapy intervention.

Observation Assessments

Self-report and interview assessments rely on a person's ability, skills, and motivation to reflect on one's occupational participation. Therapists use systematic observation guided by theory to assess individuals who are unable to communicate their strengths and challenges through other means. Commonly used MOHO assessments based on observation are the VQ (de las Heras, Geist, & Kielhofner, 2007), the PVQ (Basu et al., 2008), and the ACIS (Forsyth, Salamy, Simon, & Kielhofner, 1998).

Table 16-6

Occupational Circumstances Assessment Interview and Rating Scale Sample Questions From Mental Health Interview Form

Areas of Information	Sample OCAIRS Questions
Roles	• What are your major responsibilities? (Parent? Spouse? Worker? Homemaker?) • How well are you able to (for each role mentioned)?
Habits	• Describe a typical weekday. • Are you satisfied with your current daily routine?
Personal causation	• What things in your life do you do well or are you proud of? • What is the biggest challenge you are currently facing?
Values	• What do you value most in your life? • What about your life reflects these values?
Interests	• Is (your major occupational role) something you enjoy? • What about it interests or satisfies you?
Skills	• Are you able to do the things you want or need to do? • If no, what limits your ability to do things?
Goals	• Do you ever set goals/make plans for the future? • Have you followed through on any of them?
Interpretation of past experiences	• Overall, do you feel you have had the typical ups and downs in your life, or do you feel your life has been exceptionally better or worse than typical?
Physical environment	• In the area where you live, are there things to do/places to go that interest you?
Social environment	• Do you spend a lot of time alone? • Who do you spend most of your time with?
Readiness for change	• Tell me about a time when you experienced a big change in your life (moving, going away to school, death of a parent/spouse/child). Was it difficult to adjust?

Adapted from Forsyth et al., 2005.

Volitional Questionnaire/Pediatric Volitional Questionnaire

The VQ (de las Heras et al., 2007) and the PVQ (Basu et al., 2008) are intended to examine a person's motivation through the observation of behavior in a natural environment. The tools aim to provide two types of information: (1) an understanding of the person's inner motives and the corresponding sense of the MOHO concepts of personal causation, interests, and values; and (2) how the environment either enhances or challenges the person's sense of volition. The items seek to reveal how confident someone feels doing an activity, how important the activity is, and how enjoyable the activity is. The VQ/PVQ are based on the theory of volitional development first proposed by Reilly (1974). Volitional development begins with the exploration stage, in which an individual tries to do things in order to discover capacities, interests, and values. In the next stage, the competence stage, an individual begins to practice these capacities and to work toward goals. When new challenges are sought and accomplished, an individual is demonstrating the final stage, volitional achievement. It is suggested that therapists using the VQ/PVQ be familiar with MOHO concepts and review the Remotivation Process, an intervention based on the VQ and volitional development (de las Heras, Kielhofner, & Llerena, 2003).

Psychometric Properties

The VQ/PVQ are intended for those who are not able to report their own level of motivation or to offer additional insight into an individual's volition (Basu et al., 2008; de las Heras et al., 2007). The VQ is appropriate for use with older children, adolescents, and adults, including individuals with psychiatric disabilities (Chern, Kielhofner, de las Heras, & Magalhaes, 1996; de las Heras et al., 2007; Li & Kielhofner, 2004). The PVQ is intended for older children with developmental delays aged ages 2 to 7 years and is appropriate for children with a wide range of abilities (Anderson, Kielhofner, & Lai, 2005; Basu et al., 2008; Harris & Reid, 2005; Kiraly-Alvarez, 2015; Reid, 2005). Repeated studies and Rasch analyses have confirmed that VQ/PVQ items fall along the volitional development continuum (Agren & Kjellberg, 2008; Anderson et al., 2005; Chern et al., 1996; Li & Kielhofner, 2004; Liu et al., 2013; Miller, Ziviani, & Boyd, 2014), indicating that the assessments are sensitive and have good content validity.

Assessment Administration

Description of Environment

The VQ/PVQ observations can be formal, such as a structured activity during a therapy session, or informal, such as ADLs, mealtime, or free play. Observation can take place in any occupational setting, including home, school, clinic, or playground. It is recommended that the therapist observe the person more than once and while engaged in varied activities in different settings that are part of the individual's natural environment. Observation time is flexible, generally from 10 to 30 minutes.

Administration

For each observation, the therapist completes two forms: the Volitional Rating form and the Environmental Characteristics form. The VQ/PVQ Volitional Rating form outlines 14 behaviors that indicate a person's motivation within the 3 stages of volitional development: exploration, competency, and achievement (Table 16-7).

The focus of the observation is to capture the individual's motivation by looking at their desire, confidence, and satisfaction as they engage in activity. Throughout the observation, the therapist is encouraged to use their professional skills to provide visual, verbal, or gestural support as needed to enable the person to participate in the activity.

Immediately after the observation, the therapist completes the Environmental Characteristics form, a structured way to examine the observation setting and its effects on the individual's motivation to participate in activity. The therapist rates descriptors in four sections: spaces, objects, social environment, and occupational forms/tasks.

Scoring

The therapist assigns a rating to each item on the Volitional Rating form using a 4-point scale: spontaneous, involved, hesitant, or passive, according to the level of spontaneity compared to the support and encouragement the individual required to exhibit the behavior. When conducting an observation in more than one setting and volitional ratings differ across the settings, the therapist considers how the environmental characteristics differ across the settings. In this way, the therapist is able to identify the interests and values of a person who is unable to share this information and, simultaneously, describe the

Table 16-7

Samples of Volitional Questionnaire/ Pediatric Volitional Questionnaire Items According to Stage of Volitional Development

Stage of Volitional Development	Sample VQ/PVQ Item
Exploration	• Shows curiosity • Initiates actions/tasks • Tries new things
Competency	• Shows pride • Tries to correct mistakes • Tries to solve problems
Achievement	• Pursues an activity to completion • Seeks challenges • Seeks additional responsibilities

Adapted from Basu et al., 2008 and de las Heras et al., 2007.

environments that are most supportive and motivating for that person. This information supports a client-centered intervention-planning and goal-setting process. For an example of the VQ used in practice, see the case study of Noah at the end of this chapter.

Assessment of Communication and Interaction Skills

The ACIS (Forsyth et al., 1998) is designed to measure an individual's performance skills in occupational forms within a social group. The tool allows therapists to examine a person's strengths and challenges in interacting and communicating with others in the course of daily activities in three domains: physicality, information exchange, and relations.

Psychometric Properties

The ACIS is intended for use with adults with difficulty in the area of communication and interaction skills (Forsyth et al., 1998; Fuller, 2011) and has been used with children (Lim & Rodger, 2008). Using Rasch analysis, the ACIS demonstrates internal, construct, and person response validity and can effectively measure people with varying levels of abilities, including those with psychiatric disabilities (Forsyth, Lai, & Kielhofner, 1999). The ACIS is utilized internationally and has been found to be valid and reliable in varied translations (Bonsaksen, Myraunet, Celo, Granå, & Ellingham, 2011; Haglund & Thorell, 2004; Hsu, Pan, & Chen, 2008; Kjellberg & Haglund, 2015; Kjellberg, Haglund, Forsyth, & Kielhofner, 2003; Parkinson, Cooper, de las Heras de Pablo, & Forsyth, 2014; Petersen & Hartvig, 2008).

Table 16-8	
Assessment of Communication and Interaction Skills Sample Skill Items	
Domain	*Sample Skill Item*
Physicality	Contacts, gazes, maneuvers
Information exchange	Articulates, asks, speaks
Relations	Collaborates, focuses, respects
Adapted from Forsyth et al., 1998.	

Assessment Administration

Description of Environment

The ACIS was developed for use in a wide range of settings, with observations performed in contexts that are meaningful and relevant to the person's life. The total administration time for the ACIS varies from 20 to 65 minutes, with observation time ranging from 15 to 45 minutes and completion of the ratings from 5 to 20 minutes.

Administration

To administer the ACIS, the therapist observes the individual's communication and social interaction while engaging with others. The therapist begins by interviewing the individual (or a significant other) to determine appropriate and meaningful contexts for the observation(s). Context can range from a one-on-one conversation or while engaged with others in a parallel task or in an open situation, such as a party. The ACIS can also be administered during a therapeutic group, with the therapist as group leader or participant. The ACIS contains a single scale that consists of 19 skill items divided into 3 communication and interaction domains: physicality, information exchange, and relations (Table 16-8).

Scoring

Ratings are completed as soon as possible after the observation. Each item is rated on a 4-point scale, from competent (4) to deficit (1) according to what the therapist observes, without inferring the reason for the behavior. The focus is on the impact of the person's skills both on the progression of the social interaction and the occupational form and on the impact on the others with whom the person interacts. The ACIS does not adjust scores for the type of social group or task in which the person is observed. Rather, a format exists for classifying the context of observation and its degree of approximation to the kind of everyday social situations in which the individual performs or wants to perform. The data gathered through the ACIS details the person's strengths and challenges in communication and social interaction, and guides the goal-setting and intervention process.

Mixed Report Assessments

Therapists gather information in a variety of ways that include multiple structured assessments, as well as self-report, person and caregiver interviews, observation, consultation with interdisciplinary staff, and chart reviews. The MOHO assessments that combine information-gathering methods that can be used in mental health settings include the MOHOST (Parkinson, Forsyth, & Kielhofner, 2006), SCOPE (Bowyer et al., 2005), and REIS (Fisher et al., 2014). The MOHOST/SCOPE provide an overview of an individual's occupational functioning addressing the majority of MOHO concepts, whereas the REIS focuses on the effect of the environment, examining the impact of community residential facilities on its residents.

Model of Human Occupation Screening Tool

Developed by a therapist practicing in an acute care psychiatric setting, the MOHOST (Parkinson et al., 2006) is a flexible screening tool that identifies an individual's strengths and challenges while formally documenting occupational therapy knowledge. The MOHOST is also used to document an individual's progress toward their occupational therapy goals. The terms used in the MOHOST describe MOHO concepts in familiar words to easily convey findings to the individual, the family, and health care professionals. The MOHOST manual provides links to other MOHO assessments to gain a more in-depth understanding of the individual's occupational profile and needs. The manual includes a treatment-planning guide that offers examples of goals and intervention strategies specific to each MOHO concept.

Psychometric Properties

The MOHOST is intended to measure the occupational participation of a variety of individuals, in a variety of settings, in which the individual has the opportunity to engage in meaningful activities (Parkinson et al., 2006). Rasch analysis and classical test theory have found that the MOHOST items validly represent the construct of occupational participation, and therapists are able to use the MOHOST in a valid manner across a variety of intervention settings, including community-based, forensic, and acute mental health settings (Fitzgerald, 2011; Forsyth, Parkinson, Kielhofner, Kramer, Summerfield Mann, & Duncan, 2011; Hawes & Houlder, 2010; Kielhofner et al., 2009, 2010; Mitchell & Neish, 2007; Notoh, Yamada, Kobayashi, Ishii, & Forsyth, 2014; Pan et al., 2011; Parkinson, Chester, Cratchley, & Rowbottom, 2008; Parkinson et al., 2014). The MOHOST was found to be sensitive enough to detect changes in an individual's occupational participation between admission to and discharge from an inpatient unit (Kramer, Kielhofner, Lee, Ashpole, & Castle, 2009). A Rasch analysis of the MOHOST Single-Observation Form (MOHOST-SOF) found it can assess individuals with a range of mental health diagnoses, and can be used to measure individual client change in a clinic environment (Maciver et al., 2016). The MOHOST is being used in the United Kingdom to develop care pathways and evaluate payment-by-results clusters in mental health (Lee et al., 2011, 2013; Morley, Garnham, Forsyth, Lee, Taylor, & Kielhofner, 2011).

Assessment Administration

Description of Environment

Information for the MOHOST is gained in multiple environments through multiple sources. The length of time to gather information varies depending on the context and methods used. When a therapist is familiar with the MOHOST, it generally takes 10 to 20 minutes to write up the assessment. The MOHOST-SOF is found in the manual, and is designed to be completed in one session. An observation of an individual engaged in a single activity can be completed in 10 to 15 minutes (Maciver et al., 2016).

Table 16-9

Model of Human Occupation Screening Tool Items

Concept Area	MOHOST Items
Motivation for occupation (volition)	• Appraisal of ability • Expectations of success • Interest • Choices
Pattern of occupation (habituation)	• Routine • Adaptability • Roles • Responsibility
Communication and interaction skills	• Nonverbal skills • Conversation • Vocal expression • Relationships
Process skills	• Knowledge • Timing • Organization • Problem solving
Motor skills	• Posture and mobility • Coordination • Strength and effort • Energy
Environment	• Physical space • Physical resources • Social groups • Occupational demands

Adapted from Parkinson et al., 2006.

Administration

The MOHOST is a flexible tool that allows the therapist to use multiple data gathering methods to screen for a broad range of occupational participation issues and the impact of the environment on participation. Data are gained through conversations with the individual, informal and formal observation, discussions with caregivers and interdisciplinary team members, case history, current staff notes, and other formal assessments. The MOHOST contains 24 items arranged into 6 main concept areas (Table 16-9).

Scoring

The therapist relies on clinical judgment and the data gathered to complete the item rating scale, guided by specific criteria descriptors for each item. The 4-point rating scale indicates how occupational participation is facilitated or restricted by patient or environmental factors: facilitates, assists, inhibits, or restricts occupational participation. The information documented in the MOHOST can be used in discussion with the individual and the interdisciplinary team to assess the need for further evaluation and to guide goal setting and occupational therapy intervention services. For an example of the MOHOST used in practice, see the case study of Noah at the end of this chapter.

Short Child Occupational Profile

Initially based on the MOHOST (Parkinson, Forsyth, & Kielhofner, 2004), the SCOPE (Bowyer et al., 2005) was developed in collaboration with expert pediatric occupational therapists practicing internationally in a variety of settings, including inpatient mental health. A variety of information-gathering methods are used to assess many MOHO concepts to illustrate how a child's volition, motivation, skills, and environment impact their ability to participate in occupation. Rather than compare the child to "normed" developmental scales, as do other pediatric assessments, the SCOPE examines the unique factors of each child and uses the phrase *individual developmental trajectory* to hypothesize what capacities the child has the potential to acquire in the future. Unlike the MOHOST, the SCOPE uses the professional language of MOHO and does not simplify the terminology. A guide to explain the SCOPE and MOHO concepts to parents, teachers, and other professionals is included in the SCOPE manual, as well as interview guides, information on how to write goals and intervention plans based on SCOPE ratings, and forms and resources to document outcomes. The manual contains links to other MOHO assessments that therapists use to gain a more in-depth understanding of the child's occupational profile and needs.

Psychometric Properties

The SCOPE is designed to screen for occupational therapy services and to document progress toward occupational therapy goals and has been found to be sensitive enough to assess children and adolescents from birth to age 21 years with a variety of abilities and in a variety of settings (Bowyer et al., 2005). The SCOPE has construct validity and was used by clinicians across disciplines in a reliable manner (Bowyer, Kramer, Kielhofner, Maziero-Barbosa, & Girolami, 2007; Bowyer, Lee, Kramer, Taylor, & Kielhofner, 2012; Kramer, Bowyer, Kielhofner, O'Brien, & Maziero-Barbosa, 2009). Practitioners report the SCOPE to be "easy-to-rate, helps them to communicate with caregivers, and supports client-centered and occupational-focused practice" (Bowyer et al., 2005, p. 3).

Assessment Administration

Description of Environment

Similar to the MOHOST, information for the SCOPE is gained in multiple environments through multiple sources. The length of time to gather information is flexible, depending on the context and methods used. When a therapist is familiar with the SCOPE, it generally takes 10 to 20 minutes to complete the ratings and report.

Administration

The SCOPE is a flexible tool that uses multiple data-gathering methods to assess a child's occupational participation issues and the impact of their environment on participation. Data are gained through informal and formal observations; discussions with the child, caregivers, teachers, and interdisciplinary team members; case history and current staff notes; and other formal assessments. The SCOPE form contains 25 items arranged into 6 main concept areas (Table 16-10).

Scoring

Similar to the MOHOST, the therapist relies on clinical judgment and the data gathered to complete the SCOPE item rating scale, guided by specific criteria descriptors for each item. The 4-point rating scale indicates how a child's occupational participation is

Table 16-10	
Short Child Occupational Profile Items	
Concept Area	*SCOPE Items*
Volition	• Exploration • Expression of enjoyment • Preferences and choices • Response to challenge
Habituation	• Daily activities • Response to transition • Routine • Roles
Communication and interaction skills	• Nonverbal communication • Verbal/vocal expression • Conversation • Relationships
Process skills	• Understands and uses objects • Orientation to environment • Plans and makes decisions • Problem solving
Motor skills	• Posture and mobility • Coordination • Strength • Energy and endurance
Environment	• Physical space • Physical resources • Social groups • Occupational demands • Family routine
Adapted from Bowyer et al., 2005.	

facilitated or restricted by patient or environmental factors: facilitates, assists, inhibits, or restricts occupational participation. The ratings can be converted to numbers in scoring reassessments to measure direction of change in each SCOPE section. The information documented in the SCOPE can then be used in discussion with the child, caregivers and the interdisciplinary team to assess the need for further evaluation, and as a guide for goal setting and occupational therapy intervention services. For an example of the SCOPE used in practice, see the case study of Lacey at the end of this chapter.

Residential Environment Impact Scale

The REIS (Fisher et al., 2014) is a nonstandardized, semistructured assessment and consulting tool that examines the effect of the group home environment on its residents. The REIS was based on the MOHO concept the environment and occupation are "insepa-rable" and the relationship is "intimate and reciprocal" (Kielhofner, 2008, as cited in Fisher & Kayhan, 2012, p. 224). The REIS measures the opportunities, resources, and constraints that impact the residents' ability to fully participate in occupations of their choice.

Psychometric Properties

The REIS has been designed to be appropriate for use with any community residential dwelling serving individuals with a wide variety of health and disability circumstances, including group homes (Fisher et al., 2014). The REIS was used internationally as a consulting tool in a variety of settings, including hospital wards/units and nursing homes, to offer recommendations to improve the residents' occupational participation (Fisher & Kayhan, 2012). A validation study with individuals with mental illness or behavior health needs has been completed, and it concluded that the REIS was reliable and valid. An article detailing the measurement properties of the REIS version 4.0 has been submitted for publication (Harrison et al., 2014).

Assessment Administration

Description of Environment

The REIS is conducted on-site of the community residential dwelling. Time to administer the assessment is flexible according to the data-gathering methods chosen.

Administration

Prior to administration, the therapist obtains background information on the residence and arranges with staff for a visit. The REIS aims to give an overview of the impact of the environment on the residents and uses a flexible data-gathering method in this sequence: (1) walk through of the facility (with residents if possible); (2) observe three daily routines or activities; (3) interview residents; and (4) interview staff and/or administrators. The REIS consists of 20 items grouped into 4 concept areas (Table 16-11).

Scoring

Several formats for data gathering are provided to support data collection and scoring for both novice and experienced therapists. The therapist relies on one's professional judgment and the data gathered to complete the item rating scale, guided by specific criteria descriptors for each item. The 4-point rating scale indicates how occupational participation is impacted by environmental factors, from strongly supports (4) to strongly inhibits (1). The ratings are then used to identify the strengths and challenges of the residence and to formulate recommendations to improve opportunities for the residents to participate in occupation.

Additional Resources

In addition to the assessments discussed previously, several other MOHO resources are available that are appropriate for use in mental health practice. These resources can be downloaded at no cost from the MOHO Web (https://www.moho.uic.edu).

- Role Checklist (Oakley, 2006; Oakley, Kielhofner, Barris, & Reichler, 1986): Identifies an individual's perceptions of their level of participation in past and current roles, and roles they would like to engage in. Role Checklist V2 adds the individual's perception of the quality of their occupational performance, and has been found to be reliable with concurrent validity (Scott et al., 2014, 2017). An adapted child's version is available with pictures (Oakley, Bogues, & Wilson, 2006).

- Modified Interest Checklist (Kielhofner & Neville, 1983) and the Pediatric Interest Profiles (Henry, 2000): Gather data related to a person's interests.

Table 16-11

Residential Environment Impact Scale Items

Section	Items
Everyday space	• Accessibility of space • Adequacy of space • Home-like qualities • Sensory space • Visual supports
Everyday objects	• Availability of objects • Adequacy of objects • Home-like qualities • Physical attributes of objects • Variety of objects
Enabling relationships	• Availability of people • Enabling respect • Support and facilitation • Provision of information • Empowerment
Structure of activities	• Activity demands • Time demands • Appeal of activities • Routine • Decision making

Adapted from Fisher et al., 2014.

- Occupational Questionnaire (Smith, Kielhofner, & Watts, 1998): Identifies an individual's daily activity patterns, and documents occupational participation in half-hour intervals.
- Assessment of Occupational Functioning–Collaborative Version (Watts & Madigan, 1993): Identifies an individual's perceptions of their volition, habituation, and performance skills that influence their occupational participation.

Intervention Planning Based on Assessment Results: Case Studies

Client: Noah (Adult)

Model of Human Occupation Assessments: Occupational Self-Assessment, Volitional Questionnaire, Model of Human Occupation Screening Tool

Noah is a 53-year-old man with a history of bipolar disorder. Noah spent 6 years living in a nursing home because he lost his housing during a particularly long inpatient hospitalization for mania about 10 years ago. For the past 4 years, Noah was living in an apartment with wrap-around community-based services and was able to maintain his apartment with those services. One month ago, Noah was admitted to the hospital because he was experiencing symptoms of severe depression. He stayed for 1 week while the medical team adjusted his medications. While there, he met with an occupational therapist and completed the OSA. Noah's responses on the OSA indicated that he felt that he was capable of managing the day-to-day activities associated with caring for himself and his apartment when he was not severely depressed. He felt his biggest struggle at home was getting out of his apartment and doing things with people. Until now, he was unable to build a network of friends and, because of distance, he had little contact with his family. All of Noah's goals focused on community participation and increasing participation in roles that would help him build social capital. Upon discharge, Noah was referred for occupational therapy services through the assertive community treatment team to help him establish a system to manage his daily activities while his depression symptoms continue to resolve, and then to increase his participation in the community in which he lives.

Noah has a number of medical issues that complicate his recovery and contribute to his difficulty in balancing his home responsibilities with getting out in the community. Noah has debilitating arthritis in both of his knees and in his lower back that is, in part, the result of a work-related back injury that he sustained about 15 years ago. However, the arthritis is complicated by severe obesity that Noah claims happened during the time he was in the nursing home. Noah also complains of several intestinal issues and during this hospitalization he was diagnosed with diabetes mellitus and was advised to follow a restrictive diet and take medication.

During their first meeting, Noah provided the assertive community treatment team's occupational therapist with a copy of the OSA he completed in the hospital, pointing out the four items he felt were most problematic and most important for him. Noah said he felt overwhelmed with the diet changes and was very uncertain how he will increase exercise given the pain in his back and knees. In addition, he identified transportation and community mobility as major challenges to getting out and around the community. He stated he has a bus pass but walking to the bus stop and climbing on the bus was very painful and that many bus stops require he walk to his final destination. Most importantly, he wants to add the roles of friend, student, and worker to his life so he can feel productive and build both social and monetary capital. Historically, Noah worked jobs that have a high level of physical effort, so he has no idea what kind of work he can do with his current physical barriers. Noah agreed to complete an OPHI interview. He also agreed to attend a cooking group activity at the drop-in center so that the therapist could observe his physical and interactive skills while doing something he identified as pleasurable with others. The therapists used the VQ because, although Noah said it was pain that interfered with his going out, there were indications that other volitional issues were impacting his decisions. The therapist pulled all the information together and reported it to the team using the MOHOST.

Based on the results of the OSA, VQ, interview, and the MOHOST, Noah identified several aims. The most important aim was to have a productive routine that included social engagement in the form of work or volunteering, taking a class, and doing things with friends. Noah is aware that he will have to learn how to balance his self-care and home maintenance tasks with the responsibilities of these new roles without depleting his energy and while managing his pain.

The assertive community treatment team worked with Noah's Medicaid managed care company to secure a scooter for community mobility. They also established paratransit services so he can have door-to-door transportation services. The occupational therapist worked with Noah to enroll in a drawing class at the local library, something he loves and is good at, and a volunteer position at the YMCA where he is teaching basic drawing skills to children in the after school program. The therapist taught Noah to use a five-step system for problem solving and helped him use the computers at the apartment building to find alternative solutions. They used this problem-solving process to find new approaches to cleaning, laundry, shopping, and meal preparation that incorporated spatial organization, to make tool storage and use easier, and took advantage of energy-conservation techniques. Together, they identified a schedule that spread out the responsibilities, scheduled harder tasks during lower pain/higher endurance times, and included mandatory rest periods. They identified several activities that could be accomplished while sitting, such as finding recipes that fit his new diet needs, creating a recipe file, and weekly meal planning. Noah states that having the scooter and getting up every day with a plan has changed his life and brought back some sense of purpose and joy. Noah is beginning to work with a dietician to help with weight loss and is thinking about vocational counseling.

Client: Lacey (Pediatric)

Model of Human Occupation Assessments: Child Occupational Self-Assessment, Short Child Occupational Profile

Lacey, a 10-year-old girl, admitted to a therapeutic day program to address the psychological challenges that were interfering with her ability to complete her schoolwork or get along with her peers in her classroom. Lacey lives with her mom and her brother, who is 2 years older. Her biological father sees her and her brother often; however, Lacey refuses to stay with him overnight or spend time with him without her brother present. Lacey and her brother were physically and sexually abused by a stepfather when Lacey was 7 years old. When her mom found out, she kicked the stepfather out and filed charges. He has since been prosecuted and remains in jail. Lacey was seeing a counselor but she has struggled with school and developing friendships since that year. Lacey was referred to the occupational therapist when the teacher noticed that she was jumping, slamming her pencil box, and generally gravitating to activities that provided her with a lot of heavy sensory input (e.g., swinging, spinning). Lacey was working with her counselor and with her mom to address her post traumatic stress disorder and post-trauma issues. After observing Lacey in the classroom and out in the playground area, the therapist completed the COSA with Lacey to identify her concerns and goals.

Lacey completed the COSA sorting task to learn about occupational therapy and to identify some goals for her school year. Lacey was confident in her ability to do all her self-care items. She identified some problems with getting enough sleep, getting her chores done, and taking care of her things. At this time, she is most focused on problems she feels impact her school performance but also create challenges for her at home. During the discussion guided by the COSA, Lacey and the therapist agreed that they would start with goals addressing her inability to maintain focus and finish her tasks, especially when they get harder to do. Lacey also expressed a desire to work on her difficulty finding solutions for problems that come up at school and at home and to find better ways to communicate her ideas to others. Lacey states that her mom and teachers get mad at her when she loses focus. Her classmates make fun of her for a number of things, including things about her personal appearance and her inability to sit still. Because she tends to quit activities when they get hard for her, her friends no longer ask her to play with them. The teasing has been going on for a few years and at first she tried ignoring it, but now she gets so mad that she feels out of control and starts yelling and has occasionally struck out at people. She states she feels very sad when no one will play with her at school or at home.

Based on the results of the COSA, plus data gained from the an assessment of her sensory sensitivities and other informal observations and discussions with Lacey, her mom, her teacher, and her counselor, the therapist completed the SCOPE to help pinpoint personal and environmental barriers to school participation and building friendships. The occupational therapist, along with Lacey, worked with the teacher and Lacey's mom to explore some creative ways for her to complete her school and home tasks. Lacey and her teacher now review each assignment, identifying places where she can take a quick break to incorporate quiet but effective sensory activities. The therapist worked with Lacey and her teacher to modify her desk space and her schoolroom to help decrease the visual and auditory distractions. Lacey, with support from the teacher and therapist, presented information on changes in the classroom and the sensory-based tools she was using to her classmates. They also taught the other children about the tools and gave them the opportunity to try them out too. Lacey is excited to apply her new skills to other areas of her life, particularly getting better sleep. The therapist and the teacher, along with Lacey's mom, have been helping Lacey recognize and respond more effectively to the social cues of others. Two of her peers have agreed to be friends with Lacey, and they now include her in their group at recess and lunch. The occupational therapist and counselor have set up a lunch group for the girls to talk about growing up, developing friendships, and becoming young women. This group allows Lacey to practice her new skills with support. She is also learning to understand feedback from her friends and to express her feelings and ideas. Her new friends say they did not realize how fun Lacey could be. They recently invited Lacey to a sleepover, and both Lacey and her mom stated that she had a good time and did really well. The lunch group leaders have introduced all the girls to the idea of creating mental health toolboxes. Lacey states that it really helps to look at her list of strategies in her toolbox when she is not sure about what she should do.

Summary

The MOHO is an occupational therapy conceptual practice framework that identifies person and environmental factors that impact successful occupational adaptation. It is a highly developed model with a substantial evidence base. "It has been argued that MOHO is the most widely cited and utilized occupation-based focused practice model in the world" (MOHO Clearinghouse, 2019). Occupational therapists in a behavioral health setting can use MOHO concepts and MOHO-based assessment tools during the evaluation process to generate an occupation profile of an individual and gain an in-depth understanding of their occupational needs. For further information, therapists are encouraged to read *Kielhofner's Model of Human Occupation, Fifth Edition* (Taylor, 2017), where both the theory and the assessments are covered in more depth, and to visit the MOHO Web for up-to-date publications and scholarship at https://www.moho.uic.edu.

References

Agren, K., & Kjellberg, A. (2008). Utilization and content validity of the Swedish version of the Volitional Questionnaire (VQ-S). *Occupational Therapy in Health Care, 22,* 163-176.

American Occupational Therapy Association. (2014). Occupational therapy practice framework: Domain and process (3rd ed.). *American Journal of Occupational Therapy, 68*(Suppl. 1), S1-S48.

Anderson, S., Kielhofner, G., & Lai, J. S. (2005). An examination of the measurement properties of the Pediatric Volitional Questionnaire. *Physical and Occupational Therapy in Pediatrics, 25,* 39-57.

Apte, A., Kielhofner, G., Paul-Ward, A., & Braveman, B. (2005). Therapists' and clients' perceptions of the Occupational Performance History Interview. *Occupational Therapy in Health Care, 19,* 173-192.

Bar, M. A., Majadla, S. J., & Bart, O. (2015). Managing everyday occupations as a predictor of health and life satisfaction among mothers of children with ADHD. *Journal of Attention Disorders.* Retrieved from http://journals.sagepub.com/doi/abs/10.1177/1087054715601211?journalCode=jada

Baron, K., Kielhofner, G., Iyenger, A., Goldhammer, V., & Wolenski, J. (2006). *The Occupational Self-Assessment (version 2.2).* Chicago, IL: Model of Human Occupation Clearinghouse.

Basu, S., Carey, P. D., Hollins, N. L., Helfrich, C., Blondie, M., Hoffman, A., ... Blackwell, A. (2008). *Pediatric Volitional Questionnaire PVQ (version 2.1).* Chicago, IL: Model of Human Occupation Clearinghouse.

Bonsaksen, T., Myraunet, I., Celo, C., Granå, K. E., & Ellingham, B. (2011). Experiences of occupational therapists and occupational therapy students in using the Assessment of Communication and Interaction Skills in mental health settings in Norway. *British Journal of Occupational Therapy, 74,* 332-338.

Bowyer, P., Kramer, J. M., Kielhofner, G., Maziero-Barbosa, V., & Girolami, G. (2007). Measurement properties of the Short Child Occupational Profile (SCOPE). *Physical and Occupational Therapy in Pediatrics, 27*(4), 67-85.

Bowyer, P. L., Kramer, J., Kielhofner, G., Ploszaj, A., Ross, M., Schwartz, O., & Kramer, K. (2005). *A user's manual for the Short Child Occupational Profile (SCOPE) (version 2.2).* Chicago, IL: Model of Human Occupation Clearinghouse.

Bowyer, P., Lee, J., Kramer, J., Taylor, R. R., & Kielhofner, G. (2012). Determining the clinical utility of the Short Child Occupational Profile (SCOPE). *British Journal of Occupational Therapy, 75,* 19-28.

Brollier, C., Watts, J. H., Bauer, D., & Schmidt, W. (1989). A concurrent validity study of two occupational therapy evaluation instruments: The AOF and OCAIRS. *Occupational Therapy in Mental Health, 8*(4), 49-59.

Chern, J., Kielhofner, G., de las Heras, C., & Magalhaes, L. (1996). The Volitional Questionnaire: Psychometric development and practical use. *American Journal of Occupational Therapy, 50,* 516-525.

Chui, A. L., Wong, C. I., Maraj, S. A., Fry, D., Jecker, J., & Jung, B. (2016). Forensic occupational therapy in Canada: The current state of practice. *Occupational Therapy International, 23,* 229-240.

Daremo, Å., Kjellberg, A., & Haglund, L. (2010). *Values of different assessments when measuring occupational performance in mental health.* Retrieved from http://www.diva-portal.org/smash/record.jsf?pid=diva2%3A291792&dswid=2938

Daremo, Å., Kjellberg, A., & Haglund, L. (2015). Occupational performance and affective symptoms for patients with depressive disorder. *Advances in Psychiatry.* Retrieved from https://www.hindawi.com/journals/apsy/2015/438149/

de las Heras, C. G., Geist, R., & Kielhofner, G. (2007). *A user's manual to the Volitional Questionnaire (VQ) (version 4.1).* Chicago, IL: Model of Human Occupation Clearinghouse.

de las Heras, C. G., Kielhofner, G., & Llerena, V. (2003). *A user's manual for remotivation process: Progressive intervention for individuals with severe volitional challenges (version 1.0).* Chicago, IL: Model of Human Occupation Clearinghouse.

Ennals, P., & Fossey, E. (2009). Using the OPHI-II to support people with mental illness in their recovery. *Occupational Therapy in Mental Health, 25,* 138-150.

Fisher, G., Forsyth K., Harrison, M., Angarola, R., Kayhan, E., Noga, P. L., ... Irvine, L. (2014). *Residential Environment Impact Scale (REIS) (version 4.0).* Chicago, IL: Model of Human Occupation Clearinghouse.

Fisher, G., & Kayhan, E. (2012). Developing the Residential Environment Impact Survey instruments through faculty practitioner collaboration. *Occupational Therapy in Health Care, 26,* 224-239.

Fitzgerald, M. (2011). An evaluation of the impact of a social inclusion programme on occupational functioning for forensic service users. *British Journal of Occupational Therapy, 74,* 465-472.

Forsyth, K., Deshpande, S., Kielhofner, G., Henriksson, C., Haglund, L., Olson, L., ... Kulkarni, S. (2005). *A user's manual for the Occupational Circumstances Assessment Interview and Rating Scale (OCAIRS) (version 4.0).* Chicago, IL: Model of Human Occupation Clearinghouse.

Forsyth, K., Lai, J., & Kielhofner, G. (1999). The Assessment of Communication and Interaction Skills (ACIS): Measurement properties. *British Journal of Occupational Therapy, 62,* 69-74.

Forsyth, K., Parkinson, S., Kielhofner, G., Kramer, J., Summerfield Mann, L., & Duncan, E. (2011). The measurement properties of the Model of Human Occupation Screening Tool and implications for practice. *New Zealand Journal of Occupational Therapy, 58*(2), 5-13.

Forsyth, K., Salamy, M., Simon, S., & Kielhofner, G. (1998). *The Assessment of Communication and Interaction Skills (ACIS) (version 4.0)*. Chicago, IL: Model of Human Occupation Clearinghouse.

Fuller, K. (2011). The effectiveness of occupational performance outcome measures within mental health practice. *British Journal of Occupational Therapy, 74*, 399-405.

Haglund, L. (2000). Assessments in general psychiatric care. *Occupational Therapy in Mental Health, 15*(2), 35-47.

Haglund, L., & Forsyth, K. (2013). The measurement properties of the Occupational Circumstances Interview and Rating Scale-Sweden (OCAIRS-S V2). *Scandinavian Journal of Occupational Therapy, 20*, 412-419.

Haglund, L., & Henriksson, C. (1994). Testing a Swedish version of OCAIRS on two different patient groups. *Scandinavian Journal of Caring Sciences, 8*, 223-230.

Haglund, L., & Henriksson, C. (1995). Activity: From action to activity. *Scandinavian Journal of Caring Sciences, 9*, 227-234.

Haglund, L., & Thorell, L. (2004). Clinical perspective on the Swedish version of the assessment of communication and interaction skills: Stability of assessments. *Scandinavian Journal of Caring Sciences, 18*, 417-423.

Haglund, L., Thorell, L., & Walinder, J. (1998a). Assessment of occupational functioning for screening of patients to occupational therapy in general psychiatric care. *Occupational Therapy Journal of Research, 18*, 193-206.

Haglund, L., Thorell, L., & Walinder, J. (1998b). Occupational functioning in relation to psychiatric diagnoses: Schizophrenia and mood disorders. *Journal of Psychiatry, 52*, 223-229.

Harris, K., & Reid, D. (2005). The influence of virtual reality play on children's motivation. *Canadian Journal of Occupational Therapy, 72*(1), 21-29.

Harrison, M., Forsyth, K., Fisher, G., Murray, A. L., Angarola, R., Henderson, S., & Irvine, L. (2014). *The measurement properties of the Residential Environmental Impact Scale (version 4.0)*. Chicago, IL: MOHO Clearinghouse.

Hawes, D., & Houlder, D. (2010). Reflections on using the Model of Human Occupation Screening Tool in a joint learning disability team. *British Journal of Occupational Therapy, 73*, 564-567.

Henry, A. D. (2000). *Pediatric interest profiles: Surveys of play for children and adolescents, kid play profile, preteen play profile, adolescent leisure interest profile*. New York, NY: Psychological Corporation.

Hsu, W.-L., Pan, A.-W., & Chen, T.-J. (2008). A psychometric study of the Chinese version of the Assessment of Communication and Interaction skills. *Occupational Therapy in Health Care, 22*, 177-185.

Kielhofner, G. (2008). *Model of Human Occupation: Theory and application* (4th ed.). Baltimore, MD: Lippincott Williams & Wilkins.

Kielhofner, G., Dobria, L., Forsyth, K., & Basu, S. (2005). The construction of keyforms for obtaining instantaneous measures from the occupational performance history interview rating scales. *OTJR: Occupational Therapy Journal of Research, 25*, 23-32.

Kielhofner, G., Dobria, L., Forsyth, K., & Kramer, J. (2010). The Occupational Self-Assessment: Stability and the ability to detect change over time. *OTJR: Occupation, Participation, and Health, 30*, 11-19.

Kielhofner, G., Fan, C., Morley, M., Garnham, M., Heasman, D., Forsyth, K., … Taylor, R. (2010). A psychometric study of the Model of Human Occupation Screening Tool. *Hong Kong Journal of Occupational Therapy, 20*, 63-70.

Kielhofner, G., Fogg, L., Braveman, B., Forsyth, K., Kramer, J. M., & Duncan, E. (2009). A factor analytic study of the Model of Human Occupation Screening Tool of hypothesized variables. *Occupational Therapy in Mental Health, 25*, 127-137.

Kielhofner, G., Forsyth, K., Kramer, J. M., & Iyenger, A. (2009). Developing the Occupational Self-Assessment: The use of Rasch analysis to assure internal validity, sensitivity, and reliability. *British Journal of Occupational Therapy, 72*, 94-104.

Kielhofner, G., Mallinson, T., Crawford, C., Nowak, M., Rigby, M., Henry, A., & Walens, D. (2004). *Occupational Performance History Interview II (OPHI-II) version 2.1*. Chicago, IL: Model of Human Occupation Clearinghouse.

Kielhofner, G., Mallinson, T., Forsyth, K., & Lai, J. S. (2001). Psychometric properties of the second version of the Occupational Performance History Interview (OPHI-II). *American Journal of Occupational Therapy, 55*, 260-267.

Kielhofner, G., & Neville, A. (1983). The modified interest checklist. Chicago, IL: Model of Human Occupation Clearinghouse.

Kiraly-Alvarez, A. (2015). Assessing volition in pediatrics: Using the Volitional Questionnaire and the Pediatric Volitional Questionnaire. *The Open Journal of Occupational Therapy, 3*, Article 7. https://doi.org/10.15453/2168-6408.1176

Kjellberg, A., & Haglund, L. (2015). Utilization of the Swedish version of the Assessment of Communication and Interaction Skills. *British Journal of Occupational Therapy, 79*, 228-234.

Kjellberg, A., Haglund, A., Forsyth, K., & Kielhofner, G. (2003). The measurement properties of the Swedish version of the Assessment of Communication and Interaction skills (ACIS). *Scandinavian Journal of Caring Sciences, 17,* 271-277.

Kramer, J., Bowyer, P., Kielhofner, G., O'Brien, J., & Maziero-Barbosa, V. (2009). Examining rater behavior on a revised version of the Short Child Occupational Profile (SCOPE). *OTJR: Occupation, Participation and Health, 29,* 88-96.

Kramer, J., Heckmann, S., & Bell-Walker, M. (2012). Accommodations and therapeutic techniques used during the administration of the Child Occupational Self-Assessment. *British Journal of Occupational Therapy, 75,* 495-502.

Kramer, J., Kielhofner, G., Lee, S. W., Ashpole, E., & Castle, L. (2009). Utility of the Model of Human Occupation Screening Tool for detecting client change. *Occupational Therapy in Mental Health, 25,* 181-191.

Kramer, J. M., Kielhofner, G., & Smith, E. V. (2010). Validity evidence for the child Occupational Self-Assessment. *American Journal of Occupational Therapy, 64,* 621-632.

Kramer, J., ten Velden, M., Kafkes, A., Besu, S., Federico, J., & Kielhofner, G. (2014). *The user's manual for Child Occupational Self-Assessment (COSA) (version 2.2).* Chicago, IL: Model of Human Occupation Clearinghouse.

Lai, J. S., Haglund, L., & Kielhofner, G. (1999). Occupational case analysis interview and rating scale. *Scandinavian Journal of Caring Sciences, 13,* 267-273.

Lee, S. W., Forsyth, K., Morley, M., Garnham, M., Heasman, D., & Taylor, R. R. (2013). Mental health payment-by-results clusters and the Model of Human Occupation Screening Tool. *OTJR: Occupation, Participation and Health, 33,* 40-49.

Lee, S. W., Morley, M., Taylor, R. R., Kielhofner, G., Garnham, M., Heasman, D., & Forsyth, K. (2011). The development of care pathways and packages in mental health based on the Model of Human Occupation Screening Tool. *British Journal of Occupational Therapy, 74,* 284-294.

Levin, M., Kielhofner, G., Braveman, B., & Fogg, L. (2007). Narrative slope as a predictor of work and other occupational participation. *Scandinavian Journal of Occupational Therapy, 14,* 258-264.

Li, Y., & Kielhofner, G. (2004). Psychometric properties of the Volitional Questionnaire. *The Israel Journal of Occupational Therapy, 13,* E85-E98.

Lim, S. M., & Rodger, S. (2008). An occupational perspective on the Assessment of Social Competence in Children. *British Journal of Occupational Therapy, 71,* 469-481.

Liu, L., Pan, A., Chung, L., Gau, S., Kramer, J., & Lai, J. (2013). Reliability and validity of the Paediatric Volitional Questionnaire–Chinese version. *Journal of Rehabilitation Medicine, 45,* 99-104.

Maciver, D., Morley, M., Forsyth, K., Bertram, N., Edwards, T., Heasman, D., ... Willis, S. (2016). A rasch analysis of the Model of Human Occupation Screening Tool Single Observation Form (MOHOST-SOF) in mental health. *British Journal of Occupational Therapy, 79*(1), 49-56. https://doi.org/10.1177/0308022615591173

Mallinson, T., Mahaffey, L., & Kielhofner, G. (1998). The Occupational Performance History Interview: Evidence for three underlying constructs of occupational adaptation. *Canadian Journal of Occupational Therapy, 65,* 219-228.

Miller, L., Ziviani, J., & Boyd, R. N. (2014). A systematic review of clinimetric properties of measurements of motivation for children aged 5-16 years with a physical disability or motor delay. *Physical & Occupational Therapy in Pediatrics, 34,* 90-111.

Mitchell, R., & Neish, J. (2007). The use of a ward-based art group to assess the occupational participation of adult acute mental health clients. *British Journal of Occupational Therapy, 70,* 215-217.

Model of Human Occupational Clearinghouse. (2019). MOHO Web. Retrieved from http://www.moho.uic.edu

Morley, M. (2014). Evidencing what works: Are occupational therapists using clinical information effectively? *British Journal of Occupational Therapy, 77,* 601-604.

Morley, M., Garnham, M., Forsyth, K., Lee, S. W., Taylor, R. R., & Kielhofner, G. (2011). Developing occupational therapy indicative care packages in preparation for mental health payment by results. *Mental Health Occupational Therapy, 16,* 15-19.

Notoh, H., Yamada, T., Kobayashi, N., Ishii, Y., & Forsyth, K. (2014). Examining the structural aspect of the construct validity of the Japanese version of the Model of Human Occupation Screening Tool. *British Journal of Occupational Therapy, 77,* 516-525.

Oakley, F. (2006). Role checklist. Chicago, IL: Model of Human Occupation Clearinghouse.

Oakley, F., Bogues, K., & Wilson, R. (2006). *Role Checklist: Adapted for children.* Chicago, IL: Model of Human Occupation Clearinghouse.

Oakley, F., Kielhofner, G., Barris, R., & Reichler, R. K. (1986). The Role Checklist: Development and empirical assessment of reliability. *Occupational Therapy Journal of Research, 6*(3), 157-170.

Ohl, A., Crook, E., MacSaveny, D., & McLaughlin, A. (2015). Test-retest reliability of the Child Occupational Self-Assessment (COSA). *American Journal of Occupational Therapy, 69,* 1-4.

Pan, A., Fan, C., Chung, L., Chen, T., Kielhofner, G., Wu, M., & Chen, Y. (2011). Examining the validity of the Model of Human Occupation Screening Tool: Using classical test theory and item response theory. *British Journal of Occupational Therapy, 74*, 34-40.

Parkinson, S., Chester, A., Cratchley, S., & Rowbottom, J. (2008). Application of the Model of Human Occupation Screening Tool (MOHOST assessment) in an acute psychiatric setting. *Occupational Therapy in Health Care, 22*(2-3), 63-75.

Parkinson, S., Cooper, J. R., de las Heras de Pablo, C. G., & Forsyth, K. (2014). Measuring the effectiveness of interventions when occupational performance is severely impaired. *British Journal of Occupational Therapy, 77*, 78-81.

Parkinson, S., Forsyth, K., & Kielhofner, G. (2004). *A user's manual for the Model of Human Occupation Screening Tool (MOHOST).* Chicago, IL: Model of Human Occupation Clearinghouse.

Parkinson, S., Forsyth, K., & Kielhofner, G. (2006). *Model of Human Occupation Screening Tool (MOHOST) (version 2.0).* Chicago, IL: Model of Human Occupation Clearinghouse.

Petersen, K., & Hartvig, H. (2008). A process for translating and validating Model of Human Occupation assessments in the Danish context. *Occupational Therapy in Health Care, 22*, 139-149.

Popova, E. S., Ostrowski, R. K., Wescott, J. J., & Taylor, R. R. (2019). Development and validation of the Occupational Self-Assessment–Short Form (OSA–SF). *American Journal of Occupational Therapy, 73*(3), 7303205020p1-7303205020p10.

Reid, D. (2005). Correlation of the Pediatric Volitional Questionnaire with the Test of Playfulness in a virtual environment: The power of engagement. *Early Child Development and Care, 175*, 153-164.

Reilly, M. (1974). An explanation of play. In M. Reilly (Ed.), *Play as exploratory learning* (pp. 117-149). Thousand Oaks, CA: Sage.

Scott, P. J., Cacich, D., Fulk, M., Michel, K., & Whiffen, K. (2017). Establishing concurrent validity of the Role Checklist version 2 with the OCAIRS in measurement of participation: A pilot study. *Occupational Therapy International.* https://doi.org/10.1155/2017/6493472

Scott, P. J., McFadden, R., Yates, K., Baker, S., & McSoley, S. (2014). The Role Checklist V2: QP: Establishment of reliability and validation of electronic administration. *British Journal of Occupational Therapy, 77*(2), 96-102. https://doi.org/10.4276/030802214X13916969447272

Smith, J., & Mairs, H. J. (2014). Use and results of MOHO global assessments in community mental health: A practice analysis. *Occupational Therapy in Mental Health, 30*, 381-389.

Smith, N. R., Kielhofner, G., & Watts, J. H. (1998). *Occupational questionnaire.* Chicago, IL: Model of Human Occupation Clearinghouse.

Taylor, R. R. (Ed.). (2017). *Kielhofner's Model of Human Occupation: Theory and application.* Philadelphia, PA: Wolters Kluwer.

Watts, J., & Madigan, M. (1993). Assessment of occupational functioning—Collaborative version. Retrieved from https://www.moho.uic.edu

Wright, B. D., & Masters, G. N. (1982). *Rating scale analysis: Rasch measurement.* Chicago, IL: MESA Press.

The Assessment of Occupational Functioning– Collaborative Version

Christine Raber, PhD, OTR/L
Janet Watts, PhD, OTR Retired

Before I can tell my life what I want to do with it, I must listen to my life telling me who I am.
(Palmer, 1999, p. 2)

The Assessment of Occupational Functioning–Collaborative Version (AOF-CV) is a theory- and research-based, semistructured screening tool appropriate for use in a variety of contexts. It is designed to efficiently collect a broad range of complex, interrelated qualitative information on key components of the Model of Human Occupation (MOHO) that supports or hinders occupational performance and to identify areas needing more in-depth evaluation. The AOF-CV incorporates research-based changes and is formatted for either therapist administration or self-administration with therapist follow-up. Watts and Madigan (1993) developed the current collaborative version after using the original AOF with various groups, experimenting with a self-administered format, and further instrument development research. The original AOF (Watts, Kielhofner, Bauer, Gregory, & Valentine, 1986) was based directly on the original MOHO, and although this model was revised, the AOF-CV continues to be compatible with the current model's theory and practice (Kielhofner, 2008). This chapter will present an overview of the AOF-CV; a discussion of its relationship to MOHO and the *Occupational Therapy Practice Framework: Domain and Process, Third Edition* (American Occupational Therapy Association, 2014); a summary of instrument development and psychometric properties; assessment administration and intervention planning using a case study; and recommendations for future research.

Hemphill, B. J., & Urish, C. K. (Eds.). *Assessments in
Occupational Therapy Mental Health: An Integrative Approach,
Fourth Edition* (pp. 307-319). © 2020 Taylor & Francis Group.

Theoretical Basis

The MOHO (Kielhofner, 2008) provides the conceptual framework for this evaluation. This model conceptualizes human occupation as being composed of volition, habituation, and performance capacities, with these capacities being interrelated aspects of the whole person. Volition comprises personal causation, values, and interests. Habituation comprises roles and habits. Performance capacities incorporate both objective physical and mental components, as well as subjective experiences. Occupational performance capacity is the demonstrated ability to perform motor, process, communication, and interaction skills in the context of occupational performances.

The MOHO draws on systems theory to describe humans' occupational functioning as flexibly assembled in such a way that the person, the task, and the environment all contribute to the dynamics of occupation (Kielhofner, 2008). Thus, the human system continually creates its structure through the ongoing interaction of the person, occupation, and environment. The parts of the system are related heterarchically, meaning that "each component contributes something to the total dynamic" (Kielhofner, 2008, p. 25). Put another way:

> Values, interests, personal causation, roles, habits, performance capacity, and the environment may produce a complex dynamic in which some factors support and others constrain a particular behavior, emotion, or thought. It is always the summation of their total contributions to the dynamic whole that results in the outcome. (Kielhofner, 2008, p. 26)

While the MOHO incorporates much more complexity, these core concepts serve as a basis for discussing the AOF-CV, which relates to the MOHO in the following ways:
- It deals with a group of core concepts (i.e., aspects of the volitional, habituation, and performance capacities), not the entire model in its complexity.
- It focuses on the person more than the task or environment.
- It addresses structure more than process.
- It provides screening-level information, not detailed data about all model elements.
- It was developed to systematically ask questions about the person's volition, habituation, and occupational performance skills.

The AOF-CV assesses the structure of the volition subsystem by questioning the following:
- A person's beliefs about his or her abilities and sense of control (i.e., personal causation)
- A person's convictions about occupations, beliefs about how time should be used, and the related goals (i.e., values)
- A person's favorable dispositions toward certain occupations (i.e., interests)

Structure of the habituation subsystem is assessed in the AOF-CV by examining the aspects of roles and habits.

Occupational performance skills questions are general and yield information about how individuals perceive their performances of movement, dealing with processes, and social communication and interaction. These were originally conceptualized as part of a performance subsystem; however, these are addressed as performance capacities in the current model.

Psychometric Properties

The AOF-CV offers a theory-based, self-report assessment with established psychometric properties. It was developed as an initial screening tool to be supplemented with other history taking assessments and direct observation. Thus, it was designed to be as efficient as possible, while yielding clinically useful information. The history of its development is outlined within this chapter. As a screening tool yielding criteria ratings specific to the client, normative data were not used to develop this assessment.

The AOF-CV is the current, refined version of the original AOF. Reliability and validity estimates for the AOF-CV have been developed through systematic studies (Baber, 1988; Brollier, Watts, Bauer, & Schmidt, 1988a, 1988b; Elliott & Newman, 1993; Hopkins & Schmidt, 1986; McGuigan, 1993; Morgan, 1988; Viik, Watts, Madigan, & Bauer, 1990). The original AOF was developed as a semistructured interview and rating scale for a therapist who needed a brief, comprehensive, theory-based evaluation that could help establish treatment priorities for physically disabled or older residents. Research on the original AOF with 83 community-based and institutionalized older individuals provided initial support for dimensionality, with AOF items corresponding consistently with MOHO components. It also provided preliminary support for reliability and validity, as well as guidance for revisions. Test-retest and interrater reliabilities for total scores were generally acceptable, with a few low item scores. Concurrent validity was supported by correlations with the Life Satisfaction Index–Z (Wood, Wylie, & Sheafor, 1969) and by the demonstrated ability to distinguish between institutionalized and community-based participants. However, the Geriatric Rating Scale correlations were mixed (Plutchik, Conte, Lieberman, Bakur, Grossman, & Lehrman, 1970). Those research findings informed the first revision of the AOF (Brollier et al., 1988b).

Watts, Brollier, Bauer, and Schmidt (1988a) compared the AOF (first revision) to the revised Occupational Circumstances Assessment Interview and Rating Scale (Kaplan & Kielhofner, 1989) in a study of 41 patients with schizophrenia and 5 occupational therapists who had used both instruments. The occupational therapists found the instruments to be clinically valuable and provided suggestions for refinements (Watts et al., 1988a). Concurrent validity was supported (Brollier et al., 1988a) by correlations with the Global Assessment Scale (Endicott, Spitzer, Fleiss, & Cohen, 1976). Quantitative and qualitative data from 11 experts supported the AOF's (first revision) content validity (Brollier et al., 1988b), and this study's findings informed the second AOF revision (Watts et al., 1988b).

The validity of the AOF-CV (second revision) was examined in several studies. Morgan (1988) studied the ability of the AOF (second revision) to distinguish between 25 healthy older residents in a retirement home and 25 intermediate care facility residents. The total score and component scores for personal causation, roles, habits, and skills differed significantly, whereas value and interest scores did not, adding further support for validity and utility of the AOF with older individuals. Baber's (1988) research supported concurrent validity of the AOF (second revision) in relation to the Quality of Life Index (Ferrans & Powers, 1985) in a study with 30 individuals who were physically disabled and recently out of rehabilitation. The AOF (second revision) personal causation, interests, roles, and skills components correlated moderately to strongly with conceptually similar Quality of Life Index items, but there were no conceptually similar Quality of Life Index habit items and the values correlation was not statistically significant. Additionally, using the Alcohol Dependence Scale, Viik et al. (1990) established preliminary validity for use of the AOF (second revision) with 48 participants with alcohol use disorder (Skinner & Horn, 1984).

In 1991, the AOF-CV (research version) was created to:

- Clarify communication among diverse English-speaking cultures (i.e., Australian Aboriginal and non-Aboriginal populations)
- Simplify items
- Reformat the rating sheet
- Add administration guidelines
- Combine related questions
- Reword items to be compatible with optional self-administration

Research on the AOF-CV (research version) examined content validity, appropriateness of terminology across cultures, and which patients could effectively use it in the self-administration format (Elliott & Newman, 1993; McGuigan, 1993). McGuigan (1993) considered content validity by surveying experts from several English-speaking countries (i.e., Australia, Canada, New Zealand, the United States), asking them to match AOF-CV items to the model components from which they were derived. This yielded a similar pattern to that established in previous research (Brollier et al., 1988b). Qualitative findings suggested that, although the language of the instrument seemed to pose no problems, there was a need to interpret items relative to cultural values (McGuigan, 1993). For example, one person commented on the cross-cultural difficulties of the item "Do you feel in control of your life?" because, with Maori and Pacific Islanders, the good of the group takes precedence over the good of the individual (McGuigan, 1993).

Elliott and Newman (1993) explored the utility and effectiveness of AOF-CV (research version) self-administration with 27 psychiatric patients. The study found that higher Mini-Mental State (Folstein, Folstein, & McHugh, 1975) scores (>27), educational level, and verbal ability indicated which patients may complete it independently with limited follow-up. Overall, 89% of the questions were effectively answered independently, and therapist follow-up required an average of 12 minutes. Therapists noted that patients gained useful insights from the process. Thus, the study supported AOF-CV (research version) utility when used as a self-assessment with therapist follow-up (Folstein et al., 1975). The instrument was refined in 1993 based on findings from McGuigan's (1993) and Elliott and Newman's (1993) research to produce the current AOF-CV (Watts & Madigan, 1993). Finally, 20 anonymous online surveys electronically submitted between June 2004 and July 2005 indicated that the AOF-CV was uniformly useful; overall usefulness and ease of use were rated superior by all.

Assessment Administration

The AOF-CV is a semistructured, self-report screening instrument based on MOHO that collects information about clients' perceptions of their strengths and limitations in the areas of values, personal causation, interests, roles, habits, and skills. It does not directly address underlying performance capacities (e.g., musculoskeletal constituents) or environmental variables. It yields an occupational profile, numerical ratings for each item, and information for the occupational analysis; it is recommended as an initial screening tool. It consists of a 1-page administration protocol, a 1-page cover sheet that asks about recent employment history and reasons for job changes, a 22-question interview schedule coded to model components, and a 5-point rating scale.

Area of Occupation/Performance Skills/ Performance Patterns/Client Factors Assessed

The AOF-CV most directly addresses the *Framework* areas of occupation, performance skills, performance patterns, and client factors. It does not specifically address context. Table 17-1 correlates the most directly related concepts; however, many other domain areas are diffusely addressed by the AOF-CV.

The AOF-CV initiates a client-centered approach to the evaluation stage of the occupational therapy process. It contributes critical information toward the development of the occupational profile and the analysis of occupational performance. It also stimulates a collaborative client/therapist dialogue and client self-reflection. The process of completing the AOF-CV yields a broad picture of client needs, concerns, and problems while focusing on issues related to the domain of occupational therapy. As a screening tool, the data yield useful information to guide the selection of additional assessments to be using in the evaluation process.

Description of Environment/ Description of Supplies/Materials Required

When administered as a self-report, the primary environment requirements are a quiet space, a table and chair, and a writing instrument. Instructions are provided to the client regarding how to self-administer the AOF-CV, and the self-administration process includes a follow-up session with the therapist to review the client's report, which necessitates a comfortable, well-lit environment that provides privacy for the discussion. Similarly, when administered as an interview by the therapist, the environment should be conducive to interviewing, including being a comfortable, private space that promotes discussion and minimizes interruption. In clinical settings, the AOF-CV can easily be administered in client rooms and therapy spaces designed for interviews and private interactions between the client and therapist.

Supplies required are copies of the assessment and writing instrument. Access to a comfortable space to write, such as a table or desk, and a chair is recommended for self-administration. The AOF-CV is available at no cost on the MOHO Clearinghouse website (https://www.moho.uic.edu), which is a valuable resource for using MOHO in practice. The AOF-CV is found under the Products tab on the homepage and is listed as "Free Resources."

Administration

The AOF-CV can be used either as a paper-and-pencil self-report with therapist follow-up or as a semistructured interview. It should be used only with clients who are capable of responding thoughtfully to an interview. The interviewer should have good interview skills and knowledge of the MOHO.

For client administration with therapist follow-up, the therapist simply asks the patient to complete the interview form. The therapist then reviews the responses, probing or clarifying as needed, and rates the items. Probing and clarification are indicated if the specified questions elicit:

- No reply
- A request for clarification

Table 17-1

Occupational Therapy Practice Framework and Related Assessment of Occupational Functioning– Collaborative Version Concepts

Framework *Category*	AOF-CV *Related Components*
• *Area of occupations*: Activities of daily living, instrumental activities of daily living, rest and sleep, education, work, play, leisure, and social participation	• *Interest*: Discrimination, range • *Values*: Enacted through selection of meaningful activities
• *Client factors*: (1) values, beliefs, and spirituality; (2) body functions; and (3) body structures that reside within the client that influence the client's performance in occupations • *Body functions/global mental functions*: Energy and drive → motivation, interests, values • *Body functions/specific mental functions*: Higher-level cognitive functions → time management, problem solving • *Body functions/specific mental functions*: Language → receptive and expressive spoken language	• *Values*: Demonstrated through personal goals; enacted through selection of meaningful activities • *Values*: Temporal orientation expressed as awareness of past, present, and future events, and beliefs about how time should be used • *Values*: Social appropriateness/personal standards • *Personal causation*: Belief in internal control, confidence in a range of skills and competence at personally relevant tasks, hopeful anticipation for success • *Interest*: Pursuit • *Problem solving*: Observed during interview and/or completion of self-assessment • *Occupational performance skills*: Observation of receptive and expressive communication during interview/follow-up
• *Performance skills*: Motor, process, communication/interaction	• *Occupational performance skills*: Motor and communication/interpersonal skill performance
• *Performance patterns*: Habits, routines, roles	• *Habit*: Time use, pattern organization, social acceptability, flexibility • *Occupational role*: Array of life roles • *Occupational role*: Understanding role demands and obligations • *Occupational role*: Balance, comfort, security

- An answer suggesting the interviewee misunderstood the question
- A superficial response
- Any other indications of miscommunication, whether by the interviewer or client

Using the interview form as a self-assessment tool with therapist follow-up may not only enhance accuracy over either an interview or self-assessment used alone, but it may also permit more time for the client's unpressured, uninhibited self-reflection; integrally involve the client in the therapy planning process; and save time. The self-assessment combined with the therapist follow-up has the potential to improve both assessment effectiveness and efficiency. For therapist administration, the therapist follows the interview format, using parenthetical probes or clarifications as needed. Responses are noted on the interview schedule and provide the information needed to mark the rating form. Time required for a therapist-administered interview is 20 to 30 minutes, and less than 15 minutes is allotted for client self-report (Forsyth et al., 2008).

Scoring

A descriptive 3-point rating scale is used to rate interpersonal and communication skills and is based on either the therapist's experience conducting the entire interview or on the therapist's review and use of follow-up questions to interview the patient. The therapist then uses recorded information gathered in the self-assessment or the therapist-generated interview to rate the 20 items using the rating form. Each item is rated using the following 5-point ordinal scale:

- 5 = very highly
- 4 = highly
- 3 = moderately
- 2 = little
- 1 = very little

Ratings of 3 and lower may suggest a need for further assessment of that area and may guide assessment choice. The score sheet is organized in major categories of volition, habituation, and occupational performance skills, with specific items associated with the category listed, as illustrated in Table 17-2. All ratings contribute to the occupational profile and are interpreted in this context, with no total score yielded from the AOF-CV.

Case Study

Contributed by Sandra M. Newman, MS, OTR/L

Tom is a 35-year-old man who sustained a right hand crush injury at work. His right hand is his dominant hand. He fractured his ring finger and dislocated his middle finger. The tips of his small finger and ring finger were amputated. He began outpatient hand therapy when the temporary pins were removed from his fingers 2 months after the accident. Tom has a history of substance abuse.

Tom has lived with his significant other, Debbie, for 7 years and they have two young children. They had been living on the West Coast, but Debbie wanted to move east to be closer to Tom's family. Tom was not eager to be located near his family but believed that the West Coast was not the best place to raise his children because it did not provide a healthy environment for children. He was employed installing/finishing floors prior to the move and took great pride in his detailed work in some luxurious homes. After the move, he performed temporary work until he found a similar job just 1 month prior to his injury. Debbie works in an office, and Tom's sister provides day care for the children.

Qualitative Information/Occupational Profile

Tom completed the AOF-CV as self-administered with therapist follow-up.

Table 17-2

Tom's Assessment of Occupational Functioning– Collaborative Version Ratings[a]

Volition

Values	5	4	3	2	1
Meaningfulness			X		
Occupational goals		X			
Personal standards		X			
Temporal orientation		X			
Personal Causation	**5**	**4**	**3**	**2**	**1**
Belief in control			X		
Belief in skill			X		
Belief in efficacy			X		
Expectancy of success		X			
Interests	**5**	**4**	**3**	**2**	**1**
Discrimination		X			
Pattern	X				
Potency				X	

Habituation

Roles	5	4	3	2	1
Balance				X	
Internalized expectations				X	
Perceived incumbency				X	
Habits	**5**	**4**	**3**	**2**	**1**
Degree of organization				X	
Social appropriateness			X		
Rigidity/flexibility			X		
Occupational Performance Skills	**5**	**4**	**3**	**2**	**1**
Motor			X		
Process				X	
Communication/interpersonal				X	

Key: 5 = Very highly   4 = Highly   3 = Moderately   2 = Little   1 = Very little

[a]The ratings were made by Tom's therapist after completion of the AOF-CV, with 1 meaning "very little" and 5 meaning "very highly." Thus, higher ratings indicate more commitment to or engagement in the specified concept. Scores of 1 to 3 suggest possible areas for more detailed evaluation.

Values

Tom reported deriving meaning from spending time with his children. His short-term goals involved finding activities for his children, himself, and Debbie. He believed that he could make better use of his time and that he was not as attentive to the children as he could be. His long-term goal was to be self-employed so he could spend more time with his family.

Personal Causation

Tom believed that he had limited control over his life. His family is very opinionated about how he should run his life and raise his children. He believes that Debbie is immature and spoiled. Since they moved east, Debbie sides with his family when conflicts arise. The hand injury has compounded the friction between them because he is unable to work full-time and has to rely on his family more. In the past, he has taken great pride in his woodworking skills and now has doubts about his ability to return to that line of work.

Interests

Tom likes to read, fish, hike, and ride his bike. He also expressed an interest in learning how to play the guitar or violin. Due to his hand injury, he is unable to pursue many of his interests, so he spends most of his time reading about various topics online. He also believes that taking care of the problems in his relationship with his significant other is a priority.

Roles

Tom's current roles are father, partner, and homemaker. Since he injured his hand, he no longer fulfills the role of a worker. Since he has not worked, he enjoys spending more time with his children and performing domestic tasks, such as cooking. Although he wants to return to work, he is taking advantage of this time off to decrease the stress of daily responsibilities on Debbie and to work on their relationship.

Habits

Prior to the injury, Tom's daily routine involved getting up, fixing breakfast for his family, and then going to work. After work, he would spend time with his children and help out with any housework. Although his children still go to his sister's home for day care, he is able to spend more time with them since the injury. Because Debbie works, he does most of the housework and has dinner ready when she comes home. He does not understand why Debbie does not appreciate his efforts or why his family is critical of how he spends his time.

Occupational Performance Skills

Although his injury is to his dominant hand, Tom has the ability to use his right thumb and index finger to perform light self-care and homemaking. He is able to lift or hold only light objects. He is concerned about how much use he will regain in his hand in order to return to his previous line of work, which involved lifting tools like hammers and power saws and operating them with precision.

Occupational Analysis

Tom is a young man with many interests and goals. Prior to his hand injury, he already felt limited by the lack of control over his life. His limitations were exacerbated by the injury, which left him with range of motion and strength deficits in his dominant hand. He lost his role as a worker, which previously gave him much pride and satisfaction. He no longer pursued his interests and did not spend his time in goal-related activities. Thus, education in time management was planned to facilitate a balance of his interests, values, and roles. Identifying short-term goals and providing the means to successfully achieve them may enhance his confidence in his abilities and give him a sense of accomplishment. During the rehabilitative process, it is anticipated that he will feel that he has regained control over his life. His ultimate goal is to return to work and pursue his long-term goal of being self-employed.

Treatment Implications

Treatment goals include the following:
- *Values*: Assist Tom with identifying and prioritizing his short- and long-term goals and set realistic time frames for each.
- *Personal causation*: Provide hand therapy to increase the functional use of his right hand. Successful engagement in work-related activities should increase Tom's sense of efficacy. He needs to rely less on his family in order to gain control of his life. He expressed an interest in moving out of state to be away from his family, but he needs to regain adequate use of his hand and return to work first.
- *Interests*: Explore his many interests and pursue the ones that are compatible with his values, his limited use of his right hand, and his financial constraints.
- *Roles*: Identify the sources of conflict in his relationship with his significant other and work on resolving the issues. Explore constructive ways to increase the attention he gives to his children. Identify the skills required to return to work and provide opportunities to practice those skills.
- *Habits*: Identify ways that his time could be better spent. Provide a daily schedule to reduce wasted time and increase time spent in goal-oriented tasks.
- *Occupational performance skills*: Provide graded activities that are related to returning to work in order for Tom to regain confidence in his abilities and realize his limitations.

Response to Treatment

During therapy, Tom participated in graded activities to experience both success and the appropriate challenge. Whenever possible, he was given choices to enhance his sense of personal control. One of his short-term goals that involved his values and interests was to go on a camping trip with his family. He planned a successful outing, which improved his confidence in his parent and partner roles. He took great pride in his ability to set up the tent despite the limited use of his right hand. In another activity, he used his woodworking skills to construct a model wooden car for his son. He especially enjoyed mixing paints to achieve the exact desired colors for the model. It reminded him of his expertise in mixing stains when he previously finished hardwood floors. He gained a sense of competency and improved self-esteem by completing the activity. During therapy, he developed a sense of hope that he had the potential to achieve his goals, including returning to work.

Suggested Further Research

Reported uses of the AOF and the AOF-CV include a wide range of clinical applications. The AOF is used in mental settings in Sweden (Eklund, 1996a, 1996b, 1999; Eklund & Hansson, 1997) to assess perceived functioning in daily activities in people living with serious mental illness. Therapists have used the AOF to assess clients living with other chronic conditions and the impact of occupational therapy interventions (Grogan, 1994; Lycett, 1992; Widen-Holmqvist et al., 1993). The AOF-CV is used in preventative and wellness applications, including with college students experiencing psychosocial stressors (Nolan & MacCobb, 2006) and a participant in a NASA experiment that required 12 weeks of bedrest (Hatfield, 2008). Additionally, the AOF-CV was translated into Japanese and French (Marcoux, n.d.; Yamada & Ishii, 2008). Of note, the Self-Assessment of Occupational Functioning (Henry, Baron, Mouradian, & Curtin, 1999) has similarities to the AOF and AOF-CV but is a different assessment, with the most recent literature on the Self-Assessment of Occupational Functioning being a reported translation into Brazilian Portuguese (Tedesco, Nogueira-Martins, de Albuquerque Citero, & Iacoponi, 2010).

In a study examining therapist-reported uses of MOHO assessments (Lee, Taylor, Kielhofner, & Fisher, 2008), use of the AOF-CV was cited as less than 10% ($n=256$), and approximately 65% of therapists in the study using the MOHO were unaware of the AOF-CV (response: "I don't know") and 35% were aware of the AOF-CV but reported that they "don't use" the assessment, indicating a need for increased resources to educate therapists about this assessment.

While the AOF-CV, and its predecessor the AOF, is used with an interesting range of populations and diagnoses, no recent research has systematically examined these applications and additional potential clinical uses. Systematic descriptions of clinical uses are needed to further identify needs for ongoing AOF-CV research to answer these questions:

- How useful is the AOF-CV in developing an occupational profile that guides successful outcomes in occupational therapy treatment?
- Are there populations, diagnoses, and/or treatment settings in which the AOF-CV is more (or less) effective and/or useful to guide occupational therapy interventions and program development?
- Does the AOF-CV align with current MOHO constructs?
- What are these linkages, and how could the AOF-CV be further developed to ensure validity with the latest version of the MOHO?
- What components and specific items of the AOF-CV are most and least useful when completing the occupational therapy evaluation and developing interventions?
- Do interventions guided by data from the AOF-CV result in substantive functional outcomes?
- Is the AOF-CV useful in measuring client perceptions of functional outcomes of occupational therapy services?

Additional psychometric testing of the AOF-CV could strengthen its intra- and interrater reliability, and studies could be designed to explore methods to assess factors impacting reliability of the assessment. As reports on use of the AOF-CV has been limited in the past decade, areas of further inquiry include clinical utility in a range of settings, the examination of converting self-administration from paper-and-pencil format to electronic/online administration, while keeping the option for paper-and-pencil, which would be useful for settings lacking internet access. One benefit of the AOF-CV is that it provides the client and therapist with a dynamic understanding of perceptions about occupational performance, which may not be captured through other interview assessments. Comparing quality of occupational profiles generated by AOF-CV data with other methods of developing occupational profiles would be beneficial, especially because the *Framework* reinforces the creation of the occupational profile as central to the evaluation and intervention process. Examining outcomes of therapy when the AOF-CV is used as a screening tool, with selection of additional MOHO assessments, could be used to further strengthen the evidence of clinical utility of the AOF-CV in guiding interventions and attaining client-centered outcomes. As the ratings on the AOF-CV are subjective and could be operationalized more thoroughly, findings from recommended studies could be used to further strengthen the rating scale, as well as the entire assessment. Finally, the MOHO Clearinghouse offers access to an international community of therapists using the MOHO and associated assessments in practice and research. Therapists interested in advancing the research on AOF-CV are encouraged to access this community to identify options for collaboration.

Summary

This chapter presented an overview of the AOF-CV, demonstrated its basis in research and compatibility with occupation-based theory and practice, and illustrated its use. The AOF-CV arose from a clinical need, and its development was informed by both instrument development research and therapist feedback regarding its clinical value. Its strengths lie in how it efficiently generates a breadth of critical information for treatment and discharge planning, its applicability to varied settings, the reflection it stimulates within clients, its ability to identify salient psychosocial issues regardless of the diagnosis or client situation, and the collaborative relationship it stimulates between client and therapist.

References

American Occupational Therapy Association. (2014). Occupational therapy practice framework: Domain and process (3rd ed.). *American Journal of Occupational Therapy, 68*(Suppl. 1), S1-S48.

Baber, K. P. (1988). *Construct validity inferences about the Assessment of Occupational Functioning for persons with physical disabilities.* Unpublished master's thesis, Virginia Commonwealth University/Medical College of Virginia, Richmond, VA.

Brollier, C., Watts, J. H., Bauer, D., & Schmidt, W. (1988a). A concurrent validity study of two occupational therapy evaluation instruments: The AOF & OCAIRS. *Occupational Therapy in Mental Health, 8*(4), 49-59.

Brollier, C., Watts, J. H., Bauer, D., & Schmidt, W. (1988b). A content validity study of the assessment of occupational functioning. *Occupational Therapy in Mental Health, 8*(4), 29-47.

Eklund, M. (1996a). Patient experiences and outcome of treatment in psychiatric occupational therapy: Three cases. *Occupational Therapy International, 3*, 212-239.

Eklund, M. (1996b). Working relationship, participation, and outcome in a psychiatric day care unit based on occupational therapy. *Scandinavian Journal of Occupational Therapy, 3*, 106-113.

Eklund, M. (1999). Outcome of occupational therapy in a psychiatric day care unit for long-term mentally ill patients. *Occupational Therapy in Mental Health, 14*(4), 21-45.

Eklund, M., & Hansson, L. (1997). Stability of improvement in patients receiving psychiatric occupational therapy: A one-year follow-up. *Scandinavian Journal of Occupational Therapy, 4*, 15-22.

Elliott, K. R., & Newman, S. M. (1993). *A concurrent validity study of the 1991 research version of the Assessment of Occupational Functioning.* Unpublished master's thesis, Virginia Commonwealth University/Medical College of Virginia, Richmond, VA.

Endicott, J., Spitzer, R., Fleiss, J., & Cohen, J. (1976). The Global Assessment Scale: A procedure for measuring overall severity of psychiatric disturbance. *Archives of General Psychiatry, 33*, 766-771.

Ferrans, C., & Powers, M. (1985). Quality of Life index: Development and psychometric properties. *Advances in Nursing Science, 8*, 15-21.

Folstein, M. F., Folstein, S. E., & McHugh, P. R. (1975). Mini-Mental State: A practical method for grading the cognitive state of patients for the clinician. *Journal of Psychiatric Research, 12,* 189-198.

Forsyth, K., Kielhofner, G., Bowyer, P., Kramer, K., Ploszaj, A., Blondis, M., ... Parkinson, S. (2008). Assessments combining methods of information gathering. In G. Kielhofner (Ed.), *Model of Human Occupation: Theory and application* (4th ed., pp. 288-310). Baltimore, MD: Wolters Kluwer.

Grogan, G. (1994). The personal computer: A treatment tool for increasing sense of competence. *Occupational Therapy in Mental Health, 12,* 47-70.

Hatfield, A. F. (2008). *Mental health maintenance: Psychiatric occupational therapy for a participant in the NASA 12 week bedrest study.* Unpublished research study, University of Toledo, Toledo, OH.

Henry, A. D., Baron, K. B., Mouradian, L., & Curtin, C. (1999). Reliability and validity of the self-assessment of occupational functioning. *American Journal of Occupational Therapy, 53,* 482-488.

Hopkins, S. E., & Schmidt, W. C. (1986). *A comparison and concurrent validity examination of two evaluation instruments used with psychiatric patients.* Unpublished master's thesis, Virginia Commonwealth University/ Medical College of Virginia, Richmond, VA.

Kaplan, K., & Kielhofner, G. (1989). *Occupational Case Analysis Interview and Rating Scale.* Thorofare, NJ: SLACK Incorporated.

Kielhofner, G. (2008). *Model of Human Occupation: Theory and application* (4th ed.). Baltimore, MD: Wolters Kluwer.

Lee, S. W., Taylor, R., Kielhofner, G., & Fisher, G. (2008). Theory use in practice: A national survey of therapists who use the Model of Human Occupation. *American Journal of Occupational Therapy, 62,* 106-117.

Lycett, R. (1992). Evaluating the use of an occupational assessment with elderly rehabilitation patients. *British Journal of Occupational Therapy, 55,* 343-346.

Marcoux, C. (n.d.). *Translated MOHO assessments.* Retrieved from http://www.cade.uic.edu/moho/resources/translations.aspx

McGuigan, P. M. (1993). *Content validity of the 1991 research version of the Assessment of Occupational Functioning.* Unpublished master's thesis, Virginia Commonwealth University/Medical College of Virginia, Richmond, VA.

Morgan, R. (1988). *The Assessment of Occupational Functioning: Use as an elderly screening tool.* Unpublished master's thesis, University of Indianapolis, Indianapolis, IN.

Nolan, C., & MacCobb, S. (2006). Uni-Link: A mental health service initiative for university students. *World Federation of Occupational Therapists Bulletin, 54,* 53-59.

Palmer, P. J. (1999). *Let your life speak: Listening to the voice of vocation.* San Francisco, CA: Jossey-Bass.

Plutchik, R., Conte, M. A., Lieberman, M., Bakur, M., Grossman, J., & Lehrman, N. (1970). Reliability and validity of a scale for assessing the functioning of geriatric patients. *Journal of American Geriatrics Society, 18,* 491-500.

Skinner, H. A., & Horn, J. L. (1984). *Alcohol Dependence Scale (ADS) user's guide.* Toronto, Ontario, Canada: Addiction Research Foundation.

Tedesco, S. A., Nogueira-Martins, L. A., de Albuquerque Citero, V., & Iacoponi, E. (2010). Translation and validation to Brazilian Portuguese of self-assessment of occupational functioning scale. *Mundo da Saúde, 34,* 230-237.

Viik, M. K., Watts, J. H., Madigan, M. J., & Bauer, D. (1990). Preliminary validation of the assessment of occupational functioning with an alcoholic population. *Occupational Therapy in Mental Health, 10,* 19-33.

Watts, J. H., Brollier, C., Bauer, D., & Schmidt, W. (1988a). A comparison of two evaluation instruments used with psychiatric patients in occupational therapy. *Occupational Therapy in Mental Health, 8*(4), 7-27.

Watts, J. H., Brollier, C., Bauer, D., & Schmidt, W. (1988b). The Assessment of Occupational Functioning: The second revision. *Occupational Therapy in Mental Health, 8*(4), 61-88.

Watts, J. H., Kielhofner, G., Bauer, D. F., Gregory, M. D., & Valentine, D. B. (1986). The assessment of occupational functioning: A screening tool for use in long-term care. *American Journal of Occupational Therapy, 40,* 231-240.

Watts, J. H., & Madigan, M. J. (1993). *Assessment of Occupational Functioning–Collaborative Version.* Retrieved from http://www.cade.uic.edu/moho/products.aspx?type=free

Widen-Holmqvist, L., de Pedro-Cuestra, J., Holm, M., Sandsrom, B., Hellbolm, A., Stawiarz, L., & Bach-y-Rita, P. (1993). Stroke rehabilitation in Stockholm: Basis for late intervention in patients living at home. *Scandinavian Journal of Rehabilitation Medicine, 25,* 173-181.

Wood, V., Wylie, M. L., & Sheafor, B. (1969). An analysis of a short self-report measure of life satisfaction: Correlation with rater judgments. *Journal of Gerontology, 24,* 465-469.

Yamada, T., & Ishii, Y. (2008). *A manual for the Assessment of Occupational Functioning–Collaborative Version (AOF-CV)* [in Japanese]. Tokyo, Japan: The Japanese Society of Occupational Behavior.

18

Role Assessments Used in Mental Health

Victoria Schindler, PhD, OTR, BCMH, FAOTA

Social roles which define the social position of an individual within a given social system are based on enduring relations with other people and provide both a sense of identity and behavioral guidance.
(Kuntsche, Knibbe, & Gmel, 2009, p. 1263)

The assessments presented in this chapter address social roles and the task and interpersonal components of those roles. In addition to the assessments, this chapter will present a treatment intervention and research that incorporated the assessments. The assessments address nine roles and the tasks and interpersonal skills that are the foundation to these roles. These assessments and the intervention are within a set of guidelines for clinical practice entitled *Role Development*. This set of guidelines for practice is designed to provide practitioners with the theoretical background that forms the basis for the assessment and intervention and with instructions to administer the assessments and to implement the intervention.

Roles are patterns of behavior and the foundation of all social behavior, and they are commonly referred to as *social roles*. Social roles are life roles that are the foundation of our relationships with our families, friends, work, and community. The most common and desired social roles in our society are partner/spouse, parent, and worker/student, accompanied by other roles such as community member and friend. Enacting roles that are important and meaningful to us produces contentment, joy, and satisfaction (Kielhofner, 2007; Mosey, 1986; Parsons, 1951b; Van Naarden Braun, Yeargin-Allsopp, & Lollar, 2006; Wolfensberger, 2000).

Roles can be learned in a functional or dysfunctional manner. An individual can be highly adept at performing many aspects of a role or can be lacking in skills or motivation to perform a role successfully and consistently. To enact a role effectively, individuals need a repertoire of task and interpersonal skills, and these skills are the foundation of roles (Liberman, Wallace, Blackwell, Eckman, Vaccaro, & Kuehnel, 1993; Mosey, 1986).

Hemphill, B. J., & Urish, C. K. (Eds.). *Assessments in Occupational Therapy Mental Health: An Integrative Approach, Fourth Edition* (pp. 321-339). © 2020 Taylor & Francis Group.

The development of roles can be disrupted in individuals diagnosed with a mental illness. The more disabling the mental illness, the more it affects the learning of and ability to sustain social roles (Anthony, 1993; Wolfensberger, 2000). Individuals diagnosed with mental illness often have deficits in learning and/or maintaining the task and interpersonal skills necessary to enact positive, socially acceptable roles (Anthony, 1993; Anzai, Yoneda, & Kumagai, 2002; Liberman et al., 1993; Torres, Mendez, & Merino, 2002). Research has reported a reduction in social roles among men and women with common mental disorders (Van Naarden Braun et al., 2006; Weich, Sloggett, & Lewis, 2001). For individuals at risk for psychosis, research has documented impaired social and role functioning and lower scores on tests measuring memory, executive function, language, and processing speed (Lencz et al., 2006). However, the literature has also documented the importance of social roles for individuals diagnosed with mental illness. Social roles serve as a link to community integration, family relationships, and peer support (Hunt & Stein, 2012), and improvements in role functioning are seen in response to treatment and to environmental change (Cornblatt et al., 2007).

For individuals diagnosed with mental illness, commonly available treatments, such as medication and psychosocial interventions (Lehman & Steinwachs, 1998), alleviate symptoms and promote involvement in activity and social interactions. However, psychosocial interventions may not address the development of social roles or the specific skills that are the foundation to these roles. Additionally, the development of social roles has typically had a subordinate position in discussions of mental health recovery (Hunt & Stein, 2012). Additional treatment methods focused on social roles and their underlying skills, which also have empirical support, are required to develop these skills and roles (Lehman & Steinwachs, 1998; Roy-Byrne, Sherbourne, & Craske, 2003). Intervention that directly addresses the skills and components of roles can improve the likelihood of acquiring social roles (Van Naarden Braun et al., 2006). One such method is treatment based on a set of guidelines for clinical practice. Sets of guidelines for practice describe the assessment and intervention methods necessary to promote change within a specific theoretical foundation. Practitioners trained in the use of a set of guidelines for practice are then able to use their skills and knowledge to facilitate positive growth and change in their clients (Mosey, 1996).

Role Development (Schindler, 2004a, 2004b), a set of guidelines for clinical practice, has been developed to provide direction for health care practitioners to assist individuals diagnosed with mental illness to learn social roles and their underlying task and interpersonal skills. Role Development is operationally defined as an intervention based on a theoretical set of guidelines for practice that address the development of meaningful social roles and the skills that are the foundation of these roles. Role Development is a theory-based, individualized intervention in which the practitioner and client work collaboratively to identify and develop the client's social roles and the skills associated with these roles.

As with all sets of guidelines for practice, Role Development guidelines link theory to practice and consist of four parts: theoretical base, function/dysfunction continuums, behaviors indicative of function and dysfunction, and methods to promote positive change. The theoretical base of Role Development provides a description of an individual's need to learn and feel competent and successful in social roles. It describes how learning takes place, the learning of typical and atypical roles, and the therapeutic tools that assist in the process of developing roles. The continuums and the behaviors indicative of function and dysfunction provide a means to evaluate an individual's skills (task and interpersonal) and roles (e.g., worker, student, group member, friend). The postulates to promote positive change describe specific methods to assist an individual to develop skills and roles (Mosey, 1986; Schindler, 2004b).

Role Development:
A Set of Guidelines for Clinical Practice
Theoretical Basis

Concepts/Constructs

The theoretical base for the Role Development set of guidelines for practice was derived primarily from the Role Acquisition frame of reference (Mosey, 1986), with secondary sources from the seminal literature on role theory (Durkheim, 1938; Mead, 1964; Parsons, 1951b; Sarbin, 1954), social learning theory (Bandura, 1977), and skill development (Anthony, 1993; Kielhofner, 2007; Liberman et al., 1993). The theoretical basis of Role Development addresses the following five principles: (1) the nature of the individual, (2) what needs to be learned, (3) how learning takes place, (4) typical and atypical development, and (5) appropriate tools.

The Nature of the Individual

All individuals have inherent needs to explore and interact with their social and physical environments and to experience a sense of competency and mastery in various aspects of daily living within these environments. This is especially true in aspects of the environments that interest the individual. These interests develop from exploration and from the worth placed on them by the individual's significant others, family, and cultural group (Kielhofner, 2007; Mosey, 1986).

What Needs to Be Learned

An individual's goals, interests, and societal and cultural orientation specify what one learns and categorizes into social roles (Durkheim, 1938; Mead, 1964). Skill competence has also been viewed as an integral part of role satisfaction and manifestation (Liberman et al., 1993; Sarbin, 1954). The foundation of all roles is task and interpersonal skills. To enact a role effectively, individuals need a repertoire of task and interpersonal skills. Task skills are those skills that address one's sensorimotor, cognitive, and psychological functions as they relate to the completion of tasks. Task skills that are basic to roles include paying attention, following directions, and solving problems related to a task. Interpersonal skills are those skills that address one's cognitive, psychological, and social functions as they relate to interactions with others. Interpersonal skills basic to roles include initiating and sustaining a conversation and expressing one's ideas and feelings. Task and interpersonal skills are learned and refined as one participates in social roles. The social roles one may learn in the Role Development set of guidelines include worker, student, friend, and group member (Black, 1976; Liberman et al., 1993; Pollock & McColl, 1998).

How Learning Takes Place

Learning of task and interpersonal skills and social roles occurs according to two processes: the socialization process and the application of the principles of learning. The socialization process describes the agents and the setting that facilitate the learning of a role. The agents are the individuals responsible for collaborating with the client regarding what is to be learned, providing feedback, and rewarding positive growth. An agent can be a positive role model who consistently and clearly defines expectations, provides constructive feedback, and rewards positive growth or can be a negative role model who neglects this process or engages in this process in a destructive or harmful manner. For example, a parent who gently and consistently teaches a child appropriate moral and societal values would be viewed as a positive agent. To the contrary, a parent who ignores or neglects these teachings or teaches them in a way that is contrary to society's norms (e.g., teaching a child that the use of illegal drugs is acceptable) would be viewed as a negative agent. The ideal settings for the learning of adequate socialization are settings in which relevant behavior is elicited, evoked, required, and permitted (Bandura, 1977; Mosey, 1986; Parsons, 1951b; Sarbin, 1954).

In Role Development, the agent is clearly a facilitator. As a facilitator, the agent adheres to several principles. First, the agent assumes that the individual has knowledge of needs regarding roles and skills. The individual, in collaboration with the agent, sets the agenda for therapy. Second, the agent accepts the individual's report as relevant information. Hence, it is of the utmost importance to develop a plan that incorporates the individual's stated desires, goals, and feedback. The final assumption is that the agent does not promote change but rather creates an environment to facilitate change (Pollock & McColl, 1998).

Settings in the socialization process should provide enough stimulation to generate interest, and the practice of skills should be encouraged. For example, an ideal setting is one that is safe and has enough activities and interactions to stimulate exploration, competency, and mastery. A setting that is deprived, unsanitary, or harmful is not conducive to learning (Mosey, 1986; Parsons, 1951a).

Learning also occurs through the use of the *principles of learning*. These principles are psychological tenets that serve as a foundation to learning. A summation of these principles is as follows (Mosey, 1986):

- Learning is influenced by an individual's inherent capacities, age, sex, interests, culture, and motivation.
- Learning is more likely to occur when learning goals are set by the individual and when the individual understands what is to be learned and the rationale for learning.
- Learning is increased when the individual is an active participant in learning and when learning begins at the individual's current level and proceeds at a comfortable rate.
- Frequent repetition, trial and error, reinforcement and feedback, and a supportive environment are important aspects of the learning process.
- Anxiety affects learning differently, and conflicts and frustrations must be recognized and addressed.

Typical and Atypical Development

Typical development occurs when an individual interacts in an environment that promotes exploration, competency, and mastery. There are an adequate number of agents, and the agents are positive role models. The settings have an appropriate amount of stimulation and incentives to encourage the learning of social roles. The individual is motivated to explore and develop new roles in a satisfying manner. In *atypical development*, the number of agents may be inadequate or some of the agents may be unable or unwilling to encourage appropriate learning. Settings may be deprived or harmful. Atypical development could also occur due to a major life disruption, such as illness or the loss of a role partner (Matsutsuyu, 1971; Mosey, 1986; Parsons, 1951a).

Typically, the learning of roles follows a normal developmental progression (Parsons, 1951a; Pollock & McColl, 1998; Sarbin, 1954). This typical development of roles can become severely hindered by a diagnosis of mental illness. The more disabling the mental illness, the more it impacts on the learning of social roles (Cornblatt et al., 2007; Heard, 1976; Hunt & Stein, 2012).

Appropriate Tools

The tools used to evaluate performance and promote change include the nonhuman environment (i.e., everything in an environment other than the individuals), therapeutic use of self, the teaching-learning process (i.e., teaching activities required for independent living), purposeful activities, activity analysis and synthesis (i.e., the process of developing, examining and selecting suitable activities), group dynamics, therapeutic groups, and activity groups. Tools should emphasize active participation in activities as opposed to passive participation or random activity. Activities should be real and tangible as opposed to abstract. In order to be successful in a variety of roles, one must be involved in doing the skills or components of these roles (Fidler, 1969; Parsons, 1951b; Rogers, Sciarappa, & Anthony, 1991; Van Naarden Braun et al., 2006).

Function/Dysfunction Continuums

This set of guidelines for practice describes two categories of function/dysfunction continuums: skills and social roles. Skills are task skills and interpersonal skills. The skills involve coordination among an individual's motor, sensory/perception, process, psychological, communication/interaction, and social functions. Social roles include the following: worker, student, group member, friend, family member, parent, community member, health maintainer, and home maintainer. The task and interpersonal skills are necessary components for participation in social roles (Mosey, 1986; Schindler, 2004b).

Behaviors Indicative of Function/Dysfunction

The behaviors indicative of function and dysfunction are the assessments used to evaluate the specific skills and roles. There is an assessment for the task skills and interpersonal skills and for each role within the function/dysfunction continuums (i.e., worker, student, group member, friend, family member, community member, health maintainer, home maintainer).

Postulates to Promote Positive Change

The postulates to promote positive change are the specific methods to engage the individual in the development of roles and skills. The postulates describe the way in which the practitioner selects and adapts activities, arranges and modifies the therapeutic environment, and uses therapeutic use of self to promote change (Mosey, 1986; Schindler, 2004b).

History of Development

The Development of Role Development Guidelines

From its inception, the sources for the Role Development guidelines included Role Acquisition, a frame of reference developed by Mosey (1986), as the primary source, and some of the seminal literature on role theory (Durkheim, 1938; Mead, 1964; Parsons, 1951b; Sarbin, 1954), social learning theory (Bandura, 1977), and skill development (Anthony, 1993; Kielhofner, 2007; Liberman et al., 1993). For the revision of this chapter, Role Development was updated to include current literature on role strain theory (Plaisier et al., 2008), role enhancement theory (Cornblatt et al., 2007; Hunt & Stein, 2012; Weich et al., 2001), and social role valorization (Wolfensberger, 2000).

A historical review of role theory began in the 1930s and continues to evolve today. The concept of role originated in drama (Landy, 1991) and evolved to describe roles in society. Structural functionalism and symbolic interactionism contributed to this description. Structural functionalism views roles as the expected behaviors of an individual's status or position in a social structure. Symbolic interactionism, to the contrary, states that human behavior is attributable more to an individual's unique characteristics and perceptions than to an overlying social structure (Blumer, 1969). Social learning theory (Bandura, 1977) also had an impact on the development of role theory with concepts such as modeling, reinforcement, punishment, and consequences. Wolfensberger (2000) developed Social Role Valorization, a theory that addresses how society devalues individuals such as the mentally ill, the poor, and prisoners—individuals who have few roles or negative roles, such as criminals. Current thinking compares and contrasts the concepts of role enhancement and role strain. Role enhancement suggests that having multiple roles fosters positive health (Plaisier et al., 2008). Multiple roles can equip a person to positively address and cope with a wide variety of situations and to compensate for disappointment in one role by succeeding in other roles (Cornblatt et al., 2007; Hunt & Stein, 2012; Weich et al., 2001). Plaisier et al. (2008) reported results from a longitudinal study that supported a positive effect of the social roles of partner, parent, and worker on higher levels of mental health and lower risks of mental disorders. Kuntsche et al. (2009) found that men and women with the same three roles were less likely to have behaviors associated with heavy or risky alcohol consumption. This contrasts with role strain, which suggests that multiple roles can cause stress due to scarcity of time, energy, and skill to devote to each role to achieve satisfying results (Plaisier et al., 2008). A reduction in social roles was reported among men and women with common mental disorders, although it is not known whether role strain was the cause of the disorders (Weich et al., 2001).

Psychometric Properties
Reliability of the Task Skills Scale and the Interpersonal Skills Scale

At the time of initial development of the Role Development guidelines, a study was conducted to establish the interrater reliability, internal consistency, and test-retest reliability of the Task Skills Scale (TSS) and Interpersonal Skills Scale (ISS; Mosey, 1986; Schindler, 2004b). The results were described in detail in a previous edition of this book and are summarized here.

To assess interrater reliability, bivariate correlations were conducted on every item in every scale for all four raters (TSS: eight items; ISS: eight items). The ISS had correlations ranging from 0.70 to 0.88: interacts comfortably with peers (0.70); interacts comfortably with staff (0.73); communicates accurately and expresses self clearly (0.75); controls impulsive, offensive, or annoying behavior (0.75); keeps all statements appropriate to context (0.79); ability to initiate, respond to, and sustain verbal interactions (0.80); uses appropriate nonverbal behavior and tone of voice (0.83); and cooperates as a member of a group (0.88).

The TSS had correlations ranging from 0.81 to 0.93: tolerates frustration (0.81); ability to organize task in a logical manner (0.86); willingness to engage in doing tasks (0.87); rate of performance (0.88); attention to detail (0.88); ability to follow directions (0.90); ability to maintain concentration on task (0.90); and physical capacity (0.93). Alpha coefficients were conducted to determine internal consistency. Alpha coefficient was 0.99 ($n = 32$) for the TSS and 0.99 ($n = 32$) for the ISS.

To assess test-retest reliability, bivariate correlations were conducted on each of the eight items in the TSS and the ISS. The ISS had correlations ranging from 0.82 to 1.0: interacts comfortably with peers (0.82); interacts comfortably with staff (0.84); communicates accurately and expresses self clearly (0.89); controls impulsive, offensive, and/or annoying behavior (0.90); keeps all statements appropriate to context (0.85); ability to initiate, respond to, and sustain verbal interactions (1.0); uses appropriate nonverbal behavior and tone of voice (0.86); and cooperates as a member of a group (0.89).

The TSS had correlations ranging from 0.81 to 0.93: tolerates frustration (0.93); ability to organize task in a logical manner (0.81); willingness to engage in doing tasks (0.87); rate of performance (0.82); attention to detail (0.87); ability to follow directions (0.82); ability to maintain concentration on task (0.93); and physical capacity (0.93).

Validity of the Task Skills Scale and the Interpersonal Skills Scale

A study was conducted to determine if convergent validity existed between the TSS and the ISS and other scales that were similar in content and format to these two scales.

Convergent validity was tested between the TSS and the Occupational Therapy Task Observation Scale (OTTOS; Margolis, Harrison, Robinson, & Jayaram, 1996). The OTTOS assesses the task and general behaviors of individuals diagnosed with mental illness. The OTTOS has 10 descriptors of task performance (Part 1) and 5 descriptors of general behaviors (Part 2). Each item is scored on a range of 0 (maximal dysfunction) to 10 (no evidence of dysfunction). The OTTOS has established interrater reliability, and convergent validity was established with the Comprehensive Occupational Therapy Evaluation Scale and the Milwaukee Evaluation of Daily Living Skills. The Spearman rho correlation test was used to determine nonparametric correlations between the TSS and the OTTOS. The correlation between the total mean score for the TSS and the total mean score for the OTTOS was statistically significant ($r = .709$; $p \leq .01$). The correlation between the total mean score for the TSS and the total mean score for the Task Behavior subscale of the OTTOS was statistically significant ($r = .813$; $p \leq .01$). The correlation between the total mean score for the TSS and the total mean score for the General Behavior subscale of the OTTOS was statistically significant ($r = .370$; $p \leq .05$; Goldman, Rodriguez, Saunders, Shiman, & Soloman, n.d.; Margolis et al., 1996).

Convergent validity was tested between ISS and the Specific Level of Functioning Assessment Scale (SLOF; Schneider & Struening, 1983). The SLOF consists of 43 behavioral items grouped into six subscales: physical functioning, personal care skills, interpersonal relationships, social acceptability, activities of community living, and work skills. The SLOF uses a rating of 1 to 5, with 1 being highly atypical and 5 being highly typical. Several measures of reliability and validity have been established on this assessment tool. Interrater reliability, internal consistency, construct validity, and convergent validity were established. Convergent validity was established with the Global Assessment of Functioning Scale. The Spearman rho correlation test was used to determine nonparametric correlations between the ISS and the SLOF (for the purpose of this study, two of the subscales of the SLOF were used: interpersonal relationships and social acceptability). The correlation between the total mean score for the ISS and the total mean score for the SLOF was significant ($r = .761$; $p \leq .01$). The correlation between the total mean score for the

Interpersonal Relationships subscale of the SLOF and the total mean score for the ISS was significant ($r = .749$; $p \le .01$). The correlation between the total mean score for the Social Acceptability subscale of the SLOF and the total mean score for the ISS was significant ($r = .44$; $p \le .01$; Goldman et al., n.d.; Schneider & Struening, 1983).

Documented Use of Role Development Guidelines

Since the inception of the Role Development guidelines (Schindler, 2004a), several research studies have either been conducted on the set of guidelines or have used the TSS and ISS as pre-test–post-test measures. Three research studies conducted on the Role Development guidelines were described in detail in the first edition of this text and are summarized below. Two additional studies incorporated the TSS and ISS as pre-test–post-test measures with mental health populations and are described later. For all studies, participants completed written informed consent.

Study A: Research Conducted at a Maximum-Security Psychiatric Facility

The purpose of this study (Schindler, 2004a, 2004b, 2008) was to examine if adults diagnosed with schizophrenia who resided in a forensic setting demonstrated improved task and interpersonal skills and social roles when involved in an individualized inter-vention based on the Role Development guidelines compared to an intervention based on a multidepartmental activity program. Participants were 84 adult men aged 18 to 55 years, with 42 participants each in the experimental and comparison groups. Eighteen rehabilitation department staff participated in the Role Development training (15.5 hours) and implementation.

The study used a repeated measures pre-test–post-test design with an experimental group (Role Development program) and a comparison group (multidepartmental activity program). Participants in both groups were assessed with 4 instruments, including the TSS and ISS, on admission to the study and at 4, 8, and 12 weeks of participation in the study. Qualitative measures included client interviews and staff focus groups.

Data analysis indicated that participants in the program based on the Role Development guidelines showed statistically significant improvement ($p \le .05$) in the development of task skills, interpersonal skills, and role functioning, especially after 4 weeks of treatment, in comparison to participants in the multidepartmental activity program. Qualitative data from staff focus groups and client interviews supported the findings.

Study B: Research Conducted at a Community Mental Health Center

Two studies (Schindler & Baldwin, 2005) were conducted to examine if adults diag-nosed with severe and persistent mental illness who attended a community mental health center demonstrated improved task and interpersonal skills and social roles when involved in a program based on Role Development guidelines. The first study was a pilot study as a precursor to the second study. Both studies used a single-subject case study quantitative and qualitative design with pre-test and post-test follow-up at 8 weeks.

The first study (i.e., the pilot study) included two participants. The second study consisted of six men and four women. The same assessments used in Study A were used as pre-test–post-test measures in Study B. Case study reports documented that the two clients in the pilot study demonstrated improvement in the majority of scores from pre-test to post-test. Results of the second study demonstrated a statistically significant improvement in role functioning ($p \leq .02$), interpersonal skills ($p \leq .02$), and task skills ($p \leq .05$; Schindler & Baldwin, 2005).

Study C: Research Conducted on a Program for Adults With Higher Education and/or Employment Goals

The purpose of this study was to evaluate the effectiveness of a program for adults with higher education and/or employment goals. The study used a one-group pre-test–post-test design. Instruments included the TSS and the ISS at pre-test and post-test (1 academic year). Participants were 69 adults (53% men, 47% women) aged 18 to 50 years diagnosed with a mental health or autism spectrum diagnosis.

The intervention was a program that consisted of mentoring and classroom modules. Mentoring was the collaborative effort of the mentor and participant to identify higher education or employment goals and to develop and implement occupation-based interventions unique to the client to achieve these goals. Modules were weekly presentations of academic and vocational topics for success in higher education or employment. They were implemented in a classroom format using lecture and small group experiences (Schindler & Sauerwald, 2013).

Task Skills Scale

Pre-test scores ranged from 16 to 40, with a mean of 23.42. Post-test scores ranged from 23 to 40, with a mean of 26.99. Change in mean from pre-test to post-test was 3.57. Comparison of pre-test to post-test scores using a related-samples Wilcoxon signed-ranks test reported statistical significance at $p \leq .000$.

Interpersonal Skills Scale

Pre-test scores ranged from 18 to 34, with a mean of 23.01. Post-test scores ranged from 20 to 38, with a mean of 26.91. Change in mean from pre-test to post-test was 3.90. Comparison of pre-test to post-test scores using a related-samples Wilcoxon signed-ranks test reported statistical significance at $p \leq .000$.

Study D: Research Conducted on a Supported Education Program for College Students

The purpose of this study was to evaluate the effectiveness of a supported education mentoring program for college students. The study used a one-group pre-test–post-test design. Instruments included the TSS and the ISS at pre-test and post-test (1 academic year). Participants were 25 college students (72% men, 28% women) aged 18 to 44 years, diagnosed with a mental health or autism spectrum diagnosis.

The intervention was designed to assist college students in building academic, social, and psychological skills to succeed in higher education. The program consisted of one-to-one mentoring, which is defined as the collaborative effort of the mentor and student to develop goals and implement interventions to achieve these goals. Common goals include time management/organization, study skills, writing skills, social skills, healthy living, residential life, and leisure time. The goals were systematically addressed each week through interventions implemented in a sequenced, strategic manner (Schindler, Cajiga, Aaronson, & Salas, 2015).

Task Skills Scale

Pre-test scores ranged from 14 to 32, with a mean of 20.85. Post-test scores ranged from 16 to 35, with a mean of 22.46. Change in mean from pre-test to post-test was 1.62. Comparison of pre-test to post-test scores using a related-samples Wilcoxon signed-ranks test reported lack of statistical significance at $p \leq .135$. However, one of the eight items achieved statistical significance (ability to organize tasks, $p \leq .013$), which may reflect the predominant task addressed in the mentoring process—time management and organization.

Interpersonal Skills Scale

Pre-test scores ranged from 15 to 32, with a mean of 21.91. Post-test scores ranged from 19 to 36, with a mean of 24.99. Change in mean from pre-test to post-test was 3.08. Comparison of pre-test to post-test scores using a related-samples Wilcoxon signed-ranks test reported statistical significance at $p \leq .009$.

Assessment Administration

Area of Occupation/Performance Skills/ Performance Patterns/Client Factors Assessed

The Role Development guidelines address many areas within the *Occupational Therapy Practice Framework: Domain and Process, Third Edition* (American Occupational Therapy Association [AOTA], 2014). Several of the Areas of Occupation are addressed because the guidelines are based on the development of social roles and include the following: instrumental activities of daily living (e.g., home maintainer, health maintainer); education (e.g., student); work (e.g., worker); and social participation (e.g., parent, family member, friend, community member, group member).

The Role Development guidelines also address the Performance Skills because the TSS and ISS contain many of the items in the Performance Skills, including the following: (1) motor skills, (2) process skills, and (3) social interaction skills. The Role Development guidelines also addresses the performance patterns because the roles within this part of the *Framework* (AOTA, 2014) directly relate to the nine roles in the guidelines. Lastly, the Role Development guidelines address the Body Functions category of Client Factors because the components of the TSS and ISS include many of the Specific and Global Mental Functions (e.g., higher-level cognitive, attention, memory, temperament, personality).

Description of Environment/ Description of Supplies/Materials Required

Task Skills Scale

The TSS assesses eight skills related to completion of tasks (see Appendix D). Individuals are observed and then rated on a scale of 1 to 5, with 1 being the lowest level of functioning and 5 being the highest level of functioning.

Interpersonal Skills Scale

The ISS assesses eight skills related to cognitive, psychological, and social functioning within interpersonal interactions (see Appendix D). Like the TSS, individuals are observed and then rated on a scale of 1 to 5, with 1 being the lowest level of functioning and 5 being the highest level of functioning.

Role Scales

Individual scales were developed for nine roles (e.g., worker, student, friend, group member, parent, family member, community member, health maintainer, home maintainer). Each of these scales describes behavior within the specific role and uses the same 1 to 5 rating scale as the TSS and the ISS (see Appendix D).

Administration

Individuals are observed in an activity that elicits the behavior outlined on the scale. Observations are conducted for at least 30 minutes or for the length of time necessary to observe all of the behaviors on the scale. The rater should be as inconspicuous as possible, and the environment should be comfortable for the individual being rated. The rater observes all behaviors prior to selecting the rating, and bases the ratings only on the current behaviors observed. The rater only incorporates nonobserved behavior into the rating when this information is otherwise unobtainable through observation (e.g., client report or documentation of group/class/work attendance). The rater does not allow information about behaviors not observed (e.g., report from other individuals) to influence clinical judgment. If completing a post-test, the rater should not look at the pre-test scores for the client. Raters write information in each of the comments to support the quantitative score. Comments can then be written in a narrative summary, which is also beneficial when comparing/contrasting behavior from pre-test to post-test.

Scoring

When completing the scales, the practitioner writes his or her name, the name of the client, and the date in the spaces provided. Each scale is provided with a rating scale from 1 to 5. A rating of 1 indicates the individual is performing significantly below essential performance standards, and a rating of 5 indicates the individual is performing significantly above essential performance standards. A rating of 3 indicates the individual is meeting essential performance standards. If an individual is doing what is required for adequate performance in the behavior or interaction, a rating of 3 is assigned. If the individual is performing somewhat below standards, a rating of 2 is assigned. If the behavior is significantly below standards, a rating of 1 is assigned. In contrast, if the individual is performing somewhat above standards, a rating of 4 is assigned. If the individual is performing significantly above standards, a rating of 5 is assigned.

Intervention Planning Based on Assessment Results

To implement the Role Development guidelines, the practitioner follows a set of instructions that are summarized briefly. First, the practitioner conducts an initial interview with the client to determine the roles and skills (i.e., areas of occupation, performance skills, patterns [roles]) the client chooses to address. Then, the practitioner observes the client in settings that elicit the roles and skills and completes the appropriate assessments for skills and roles based on the observation and interview. Next, the practitioner develops a treatment plan in collaboration with the client. The practitioner and the client discuss the types of activities and interactions in which the client could participate in order to develop the task and interpersonal skills (i.e., performance skills) that compose the desired role (within performance patterns). At least weekly, and more often if necessary, the practitioner and the client meet for approximately 15 to 30 minutes to discuss the client's progress with the treatment intervention and develop a plan for the following week. The practitioner documents a weekly progress report based on this meeting. Modifications to the treatment plan are made accordingly (AOTA, 2014).

Case Study

J. is a 29-year-old, single, White man. He is a full-time college student and is currently in his junior year. He lives on campus with three roommates during the academic year and travels 1 hour to his parents' home each weekend to work stocking shelves at a department store where he has worked for 2 years. He was diagnosed with schizoaffective disorder at age 21 years and has been prescribed a variety of antipsychotic and antidepressant medications. A common side effect of various medications he has been prescribed is insomnia followed by oversleeping.

At the start (pre-test) and end (post-test) of the 2019-2020 academic year, J. was assessed with the TSS, ISS, and School Behavior Scale (to assess functioning in the student role). The ratings follow with comments summarized at the end of each scale.

J. was enrolled in the Skills for Success program, a supported education program (Soydan, 2004) developed and conducted by a master's level occupational therapy program to assist college students in building academic, social, and psychological skills to succeed in higher education. The program consists of one-to-one mentoring, which pairs master's level occupational therapy students with undergraduate students with a mental health, learning disability, or autism spectrum disorder under the supervision of occupational therapy faculty. Mentoring is defined as the collaborative effort of the occupational therapy student and participant to develop goals and implement interventions to achieve these goals. Common goals include time management/organization, study skills, writing skills, social skills, healthy living, residential life, and leisure time. The goals are systematically addressed each week through interventions implemented in a sequenced, strategic manner. The TSS (Table 18-1), ISS (Table 18-2), and the School Behavior Scale (Table 18-3) are three assessments used as pre-test–post-test measures to evaluate the effectiveness of the program. The tables provide the pre-test–post-test measures for J.

Table 18-1

Task Skills

Task Behavior	Initial Rating (Fall 2019)	Final Rating (Spring 2020)
1. *Willingness to engage in doing tasks.* Is the level of readiness, eagerness, or enthusiasm to engage in tasks compatible with what would be the typical expectation for the tasks? Is the level of prompting or encouragement needed compatible with what would be the typical expectation for the tasks?	3	3
2. *Physical capacity.* Are posture, strength, gross and fine motor coordination, and endurance compatible with what would be the typical expectation for the tasks?	3	3
3. *Ability to maintain concentration on task.* Is the level of attention to tasks and number of breaks satisfactory so that the tasks are completed within time periods compatible with the typical expectation for the tasks?	3	3
4. *Ability to organize task in a logical manner.* Is the level of organization satisfactory so that there is evidence of planning for tasks prior to beginning, including having all the items needed for task completion close at hand, and considering what should be done first, second, and so forth?	2	2
5. *Ability to follow directions.* Is the level of following directions compatible with the typical expectation for the tasks regarding comprehension of directions, following directions without assistance, and returning to directions to check whether tasks are being done correctly?	2	3
6. *Rate of performance.* Is the rate of performance compatible with the typical expectation for the tasks regarding working at a steady pace so as not to be excessively slow in performing a task so that little is accomplished in comparison to others, or excessively fast so that quality is sacrificed? Is the rate of performance compatible with the typical expectation for the tasks being completed correctly and on time?	3	3
7. *Attention to detail.* Is the level of attention to detail compatible with the typical expectation for the tasks so that there is the required amount of detail without too little or excessive detail and is considerate of aspects of a task that are more or less important?	3	3
8. *Tolerates frustration.* Is the level of frustration tolerance reflective of an ability to emotionally and socially address frustration with tasks when confronted with a problem, mistake, delay, or setback?	2	3

(continued)

Table 18-1 (continued)

Task Skills

Initial Comments: J. is willing to engage in tasks but must be prompted. He has a difficult time concentrating and is often forgetful of what tasks/assignments need to be addressed. J. is able to organize tasks if the mentor initiates the assignment, and he follows directions appropriately. However, he overlooks important details (e.g., APA format for a paper). J. does not become upset when confronted with conflict, but rather becomes very quiet and uses avoidance strategies to remove himself from the situation.

Final Comments: Overall, J. has demonstrated only minimal improvement in task behaviors (increase of 1 point in two items). J. can now follow directions for certain assignments with less reliance on the mentor. J still utilizes avoidance techniques to tolerate frustration; however, he was able to develop solutions to problems that arose with a group presentation, which is a significant improvement for him. Generally, J. has remained the same in his other task behaviors. His ongoing symptoms of his diagnosis and insomnia have made it difficult for him to sustain improvement week to week. He has short periods of improvement and then declines due to symptoms.

Adapted with permission from Mosey, A. C. (1986). *Psychosocial components of occupational therapy*. New York, NY: Raven Press.

Table 18-2

Interpersonal Skills

Interpersonal Behavior	Initial Rating (Fall 2019)	Final Rating (Spring 2020)
1. *Ability to initiate, respond to, and sustain verbal interactions.* Does the level of interaction reflect the expectation for spontaneously initiating a conversation with another person, spontaneously responding to others, carrying on a conversation, and participating in the normal give-and-take of conversation?	2	4
2. *Keeps all statements appropriate to context.* Does the level of interaction reflect the expectation for following the thread of discussion, making statements that are appropriate and relevant to the subject matter?	3	3
3. *Communicates accurately and expresses self clearly.* Does the level of interaction reflect the expectation for communicating in a way that is sensible to the listener, communicating accurate statements, and expressing ideas in a straightforward manner?	2	3
4. *Interacts comfortably with staff.* Does the level of interaction reflect the expectation for requesting or receiving attention or assistance, and interacting in a way that is friendly and respectful?	3	3

(continued)

Table 18-2 (continued)

Interpersonal Skills

Interpersonal Behavior	Initial Rating (Fall 2019)	Final Rating (Spring 2020)
5. *Interacts comfortably with peers.* Does the level of interaction reflect the expectation for the appropriate amount of interaction, friendliness and respectfulness, consideration of the needs of others, collaboration with peers, and acceptance of help from peers?	1	3
6. *Uses appropriate nonverbal behavior and tone of voice.* Does the level of interaction reflect the expectation for maintaining space between others, tone of voice, and the level in which nonverbal gestures are consistent or appropriate to verbal content or context of the situation?	3	3
7. *Cooperates as a member of a group.* Does the level of interaction reflect the expectation for group interaction including acting independently and collaboratively where cooperation is required, and appropriately accepting being the winner or the loser in a competitive group situation?	2	3
8. *Controls impulsive, offensive, or annoying behavior.* Does the level of interaction reflect the expectation for regulating and managing emotions and behaviors so as not to act out toward self or others in a negative or harmful manner; intentionally irritate, torment, tease, or cause anguish to others; or be verbally degrading or abusive to others?	3	3

Initial Comments: J. has difficulty initiating conversations about subjects other than his health or school work. He follows the discussion appropriately, but jumps from one topic to another without finishing. J. will agree to mentor recommendations even when he does not understand or plan to complete the recommendation. J. is able to interact with staff appropriately but does not interact with peers or group members. He remains quiet and only speaks when prompted.

Final Comments: Overall, J. has improved in four of eight interpersonal behaviors, reflecting a 6-point increase in scores. He interacts with peers and group members with more ease; he is able to communicate the needs of the task; and he is able to give opinions. He communicates and expresses himself with more clarity. His overall demeanor with his peers has changed, and he is more comfortable. In his group projects, he works like a team player, accomplishing his assigned tasks and often organizing what is required. However, he still is not completely comfortable interacting with people outside his comfort zone.

Adapted with permission from Mosey, A. C. (1986). *Psychosocial components of occupational therapy.* New York, NY: Raven Press and Rogers, E. S., Sciarappa, K., & Anthony, W. A. (1991). Development and evaluation of situational assessment instruments and procedures for persons with psychiatric disabilities. *Vocational Evaluation and Work Adjustment Bulletin, 24,* 61-67.

Table 18-3

School

School Behavior	Initial Rating (Fall 2019)	Final Rating (Spring 2020)
1. *Class attendance.* Does the school behavior reflect the expectation for class attendance, arrival to class, and remaining in class for the duration of class periods?	2	2
2. *Group behavior.* Does the school behavior reflect the expectation for paying attention and participating in tasks, discussions, and interactions?	2	3
3. *Relationship with teachers.* Does the school behavior reflect the expectation for following the teacher's instructions, approaching the teacher for guidelines or assistance when needed, adapting to the style of the teacher, and acting independently as appropriate?	3	3
4. *Relationship with classmates.* Does the school behavior reflect the expectation for the level and quality of interaction with classmates, including being friendly and respectful, considerate of the needs of others, working collaboratively with peers, and accepting help from peers?	2	2
5. *Academic performance.* Does the school behavior reflect the expectation for grades that are at or above the level one would expect given the individual's apparent abilities, that are consistent across subjects and/or grading periods, that demonstrate the amount of effort required, and that demonstrate responsibility for one's own academic performance?	2	3
6. *Participation in academic evaluations.* Does the school behavior reflect the expectation for studying for tests, giving appropriate attention to each item, and managing test anxiety and preoccupation with grades?	2	3

Initial Comments: J. reports that he has a history of periodic absence from class due to symptoms of his diagnosis and insomnia. J. has anxiety about participating in groups and is often quiet and inattentive. He interacts appropriately with teachers. J. has no interaction with classmates and has little motivation to begin projects and assignments. J. does not study for tests.

Final Comments: Overall, J. has improved in three of six school areas reflecting a 3-point increase in scores. He still has difficulty consistently attending classes due to symptom recurrence. Improvement has been observed in his group behavior. He is more attentive to group members and increased collaboration in a group project. J. continues to interact appropriately with professors, but also continues to avoid or show anxiety when interacting with classmates. J.'s academic performance has increased on written assignments. Additionally, he has improved in the area of participation in academic evaluations. From the beginning of the semester, he has utilized Quizlet for study preparation, which he is now using for every examination.

Adapted with permission from Mosey, A. C. (1986). *Psychosocial components of occupational therapy.* New York, NY: Raven Press.

Summary

The results of the pre-test–post-test measures indicate minimal positive improvement in task behaviors and moderate improvement in interpersonal behaviors and school behaviors. The comments on the scales support the quantitative ratings. Interventions tailored to address study skills, writing skills, social skills, and time management and organization led to positive improvements, but the ongoing recurrence of symptoms related to J.'s diagnosis and insomnia limited the amount of improvement. However, J. has demonstrated perseverance to continue to achieve his undergraduate degree.

Suggested Further Research

Areas of future inquiry/research include additional use of the scales in research studies as a means to assess client development of task and interpersonal skills and social roles. With increased use of the role scales, reliability and validity studies could be conducted. The scales closely reflect areas of the *Framework* (AOTA, 2014), and therefore could be used to assess intervention aimed at developing areas of occupation, performance skills, performance patterns (roles), and client factors.

Summary

This chapter described the assessment tools used with the Role Development guidelines for practice. The Role Development guidelines were described, including the theoretical base, the function/dysfunction continuums, the behaviors indicative of function/dysfunction, and the postulates to promote positive change. The history of the Role Development guidelines was described, and psychometric properties of the assessments were provided. Research studies based on the Role Development guidelines and related studies that used assessments associated with the guidelines were described. The assessment tools, including the TSS, the ISS, and the Role Scales, were described. Methods to administer the scales were outlined, as well as their application to the *Framework* (AOTA, 2014). Finally, a case example using the assessment tools was provided.

References

American Occupational Therapy Association. (2014). Occupational therapy practice framework: Domain and process (3rd ed.). *American Journal of Occupational Therapy, 68*(Suppl. 1), S1-S48.

Anthony, W. A. (1993). Recovery from mental illness: The guiding vision of the mental health system in the 1990's. *Innovations & Research, 2*(3), 17-24.

Anzai, N., Yoneda, S., & Kumagai, N. (2002). Training persons with schizophrenia in illness self-management: A randomized controlled trial in Japan. *Psychiatric Services, 53*, 545-547.

Bandura, A. (1977). *Social learning theory.* Englewood Cliffs, NJ: Prentice-Hall.

Black, M. M. (1976). The occupational career. *American Journal of Occupational Therapy, 30*, 225-228.

Blumer, H. (1969). *Symbolic interactionism: Perspective and method.* Englewood Cliffs, NJ: Prentice-Hall.

Cornblatt, B. A., Auther, A. M., Niendam, T., Smith, C. W., Zinberg, J., Bearden, C. E., & Cannon, T. D. (2007). Preliminary findings for two new measures of social and role functioning in the prodromal phase of schizophrenia. *Schizophrenia Bulletin, 33*, 688-702.

Durkheim, E. (1938). *The rules of sociological method.* Chicago, IL: University of Chicago Press.

Fidler, G. S. (1969). The task-oriented group as a context for treatment. *American Journal of Occupational Therapy, 32*, 305-310.

Goldman, D., Rodriguez, C., Saunders, D., Shiman A., & Solomon, A. (n.d.). *Convergent validity between the Interpersonal Skills Scale and the Specific Level of Functioning Scale (SLOF) and the Task Skills Scale and the Occupational Therapy Task Observation Scale (OTTOS)*. Unpublished master's thesis, Richard Stockton College of New Jersey, Galloway, NJ.

Heard, C. (1976). Occupational role acquisition: A perspective on the chronically disabled. *American Journal of Occupational Therapy, 31,* 243-247.

Hunt, M. G., & Stein, C. H. (2012). Valued social roles and measuring mental health recovery: Examining the structure of the tapestry. *Psychiatric Rehabilitation Journal, 35,* 441-446.

Kielhofner, G. (2007). *Model of Human Occupation: Theory and application* (4th ed.). Baltimore, MD: Lippincott Williams & Wilkins.

Kuntsche, S., Knibbe, R. A., & Gmel, G. (2009). Social roles and alcohol consumption: A study of 10 industrialised countries. *Social Science & Medicine, 68,* 1263-1270.

Landy, R. J. (1991). The dramatic basis of role theory. *Arts in Psychotherapy, 18,* 29-41.

Lehman, A. F., & Steinwachs, D. M. (1998). At issue: Translating research into practice: The Schizophrenia Patient Outcomes Research Team (PORT) treatment recommendations. *Schizophrenia Bulletin, 24*(1), 1-10.

Lencz, T., Smith, C. W., McLaughlin, D., Auther, A., Nakayama, E., Hovey, L., & Cornblatt, B.A. (2006). Generalized and specific neurocognitive deficits in prodromal schizophrenia. *Biological Psychiatry, 59,* 863-871.

Liberman, R. P., Wallace, C. J., Blackwell, G., Eckman, T. A., Vaccaro, J. V., & Kuehnel, T. G. (1993). Innovations in skills training for people with serious mental illness: The UCLA social and independent living skills modules. *Innovations & Research, 2*(2), 46-59.

Margolis, R. L., Harrison, S. A., Robinson, H. J., & Jayaram, G. (1996). Occupational Therapy Task Observation Scale (OTTOS): A rapid method for rating task group psychiatric patients. *American Journal of Occupational Therapy, 50,* 380-385.

Matsutsuyu, J. (1971). Occupational behavior: A perspective on work and play. *American Journal of Occupational Therapy, 25,* 291-294.

Mead, G. H. (1964). *On social psychology.* Chicago, IL: The University of Chicago Press.

Mosey, A. C. (1986). *Psychosocial components of occupational therapy.* New York, NY: Raven Press.

Mosey, A. C. (1996). *Applied scientific inquiry in the health professions: An epistemological orientation* (2nd ed.). Bethesda, MD: American Occupational Therapy Association.

Parsons, T. (1951a). Illness and the role of the physician: A sociological perspective. *American Journal of Orthopsychiatry, 21,* 452-460.

Parsons, T. (1951b). *The social system.* Glencoe, IL: The Free Press.

Plaisier, I., Beekman, A., Bruijn, J., Graaf, R., Have, M., Smith, J., & Penninx, B. (2008). The effect of social roles on mental health: A matter of quantity or quality? *Journal of Affective Disorders, 111,* 261-270.

Pollock, N., & McColl, M. (1998). Assessment in client-centered occupational therapy. In M. Law (Ed.), *Client-centred occupational therapy* (pp. 89-105). Thorofare, NJ: SLACK Incorporated.

Rogers, E. S., Sciarappa, K., & Anthony, W. A. (1991). Development and evaluation of situational assessment instruments and procedures for persons with psychiatric disabilities. *Vocational Evaluation and Work Adjustment Bulletin, 24,* 61-67.

Roy-Byrne, P. P., Sherbourne, C. D., & Craske, M. G. (2003). Moving treatment research from clinical trials to the real world. *Psychiatric Services, 54,* 327-332.

Sarbin, T. R. (1954). Role theory. In G. Lindzey (Ed.), *Handbook of social psychology* (pp. 223-225). Cambridge, MA: Addison-Wesley.

Schindler, V. P. (2004a). A role development intervention for persons with schizophrenia. *Psychiatric Services, 55,* 88-89.

Schindler, V. P. (2004b). Occupational therapy in forensic psychiatry: Role development and schizophrenia. *Occupational Therapy in Mental Health, 20,* 3-4.

Schindler, V. (2008). Role assessments used in mental health. In B. Hemphill (Ed.), *Assessments in occupational therapy in mental health* (2nd ed.). Thorofare, NJ: SLACK Incorporated.

Schindler, V. P., & Baldwin, S. A. (2005). Role development: Application to community-based clients. *Israeli Journal of Occupational Therapy, 14*(1), E3-E8.

Schindler, V. P., Cajiga, A., Aaronson, R., & Salas, L. (2015). The experience of transition to college for students diagnosed with Asperger's disorder. *Open Journal of Occupational Therapy, 3,* Article 2.

Schindler, V. P., & Sauerwald, C. (2013). Outcomes of a 4-year program with higher education and employment goals for individuals diagnosed with mental illness. *Work: A Journal of Prevention, Assessment and Rehabilitation, 46,* 325-336.

Schneider, L. C., & Struening, E. L. (1983). SLOF: A behavioral rating scale for assessing the mentally ill. *Social Work Research and Abstracts, 19,* 9-21.

Soydan, A. (2004). Supported education: A portrait of a psychiatric rehabilitation intervention. *American Journal of Psychiatric Rehabilitation, 7*, 227-248.

Torres, A., Mendez, L. P., & Merino, H. (2002). Improving social functioning in schizophrenia by playing the train game. *Psychiatric Services, 53*, 799-801.

Van Naarden Braun, K., Yeargin-Allsopp, M., & Lollar, D. (2006). A multi-dimensional approach to the transition of children with developmental disabilities into young adulthood: The acquisition of adult social roles. *Disability & Rehabilitation, 28*, 915-928.

Weich, S., Sloggett, A., & Lewis, G. (2001). Social roles and the gender difference in rates of the common mental disorders in Britain: A 7-year, population-based cohort study. *Psychological Medicine, 31*, 1055-1064.

Wolfensberger, W. (2000). A brief overview of social role valorization. *Mental Retardation, 38*, 105-123.

Australian Therapy Outcome Measures for Occupational Therapy
A Measure of Global Client Outcomes

Carolyn A. Unsworth, BAppSci(OccTher), PhD, OTR

Every line is the perfect length if you don't measure it.
(Rubin, 1987, p. 1)

To remain viable, occupational therapy services must be evidence based. The profession cannot gather evidence without reliable, valid, and responsive assessment instruments. Therefore, it is essential that occupational therapists have a range of outcome measures from which to choose. An outcome measure is an instrument developed and standardized for use by therapists. The instrument can assist the therapist in determining whether the desired therapeutic outcomes were achieved (Laver-Fawcett, 2007). These measures can be used to document client progress and can be used in research to determine if changes were attributable to participation in occupational therapy. This chapter describes the development and use of one outcome measure, the Australian Therapy Outcome Measures for Occupational Therapy (AusTOMs-OT) and details the research that supports the properties and clinical use. The AusTOMs-OT scales were designed using the *International Classification of Functioning, Disability and Health* (ICF; World Health Organization [WHO], 2001) terminology and theoretical concepts and can be used with clients of all ages and diagnoses with improving and deteriorating conditions to measure outcomes in terms of function, participation, and well-being in less than 5 minutes. The client case study of Peter, who has schizophrenia, is used to illustrate how AusTOMs-OT can be used with people who have mental health problems. Areas for further research are proposed to promote research that monitors client progress over time and measures therapy outcomes. Strong evidence can be gathered to support occupational therapy practice if professionals have a selection of measures to choose from to suit particular needs. The AusTOMs-OT provides reliable and valid data from the therapist perspective that can contribute to the demonstration of the effectiveness of occupational therapy services.

Hemphill, B. J., & Urish, C. K. (Eds.). *Assessments in Occupational Therapy Mental Health: An Integrative Approach, Fourth Edition* (pp. 341-356). © 2020 Taylor & Francis Group.

Theoretical Basis

Concepts/Constructs

The AusTOMs-OT includes outcome measurement scales. Outcome measures are different from assessments, although the purpose of these two approaches to measuring client status can overlap. The main difference is that the primary aim of an assessment is to assist the therapist and client to determine the occupational performance problems the client is experiencing and what the client wants to work on in therapy. In contrast, an outcome measure primarily aims to capture client status at two points in time in order to determine if change has occurred over the course of a therapy program. Research can then determine if any change is attributable to client participation in that program. While many assessments can be used in research to document change over time, outcome measures are designed primarily for this purpose. Occupational therapists can use the AusTOMs-OT to demonstrate client change over time in everyday clinical practice and in research.

The AusTOMs-OT was developed using Classical Measurement Theory (Anastasi, 1982; Nunnally, 1978). Within these frameworks, a measure needs to have established reliability and validity and a method of interpreting the scores. Good validity ensures that the outcome measure tests what it intended to, while good reliability ensures the measures are repeatable (DeVellis, 1991; Nunnally, 1978). Consistent with most measures used in clinical practice in occupational therapy, the AusTOMs-OT uses norms as a means of referencing scores obtained. Client scores on the AusTOMs-OT can be compared against other clients who have the same diagnosis (e.g., using the WHO's [2004] *International Classification of Diseases and Related Health Problems, 10th Revision* [ICD-10], codes to determine how much progress the client is making and if this might be attributable to the type and length of therapy offered).

In addition to being based on Classical Measurement Theory as a method of measurement development, the AusTOMs-OT was based on the concepts as presented in the ICF (WHO, 2004). The ICF, a taxonomy of the consequences of disease, provides a useful framework for therapists to identify where to focus their outcome data collection. Of the four domains measured in AusTOMs-OT, three are from the ICF: Impairment, Activity Limitation, and Participation Restriction. The fourth AusTOMs-OT domain of Distress/Well-Being is embedded across the ICF. The domain of central importance in the AusTOMs-OT, and providing the headings for each scale, is that of Activity Limitation. The importance of Activity Limitation (using ICF terminology) and occupation (using American Occupational Therapy Association [AOTA, 2014] language) is central to all occupational therapy theories.

History of Development and Previous Versions/ Important Changes to Note in Current Version

The AusTOMs-OT was developed based on measures that were originally developed in the United Kingdom. In 1997, Enderby and John published *Therapy Outcome Measures for Speech and Language Pathology*. In 1998, Enderby, John, and Petherham published *Therapy Outcome Measures Manual: Physiotherapy, Occupational Therapy, Rehabilitation Nursing*. The measures were developed to suit the needs of British therapists and funding models. The scale headings included a mix of diseases and diagnoses that could be used by therapists from across disciplines. A team of Australian researchers then consulted with Enderby and John and set about developing sets of scales that could be used by therapists internationally and for each of the three disciplines of occupational therapy, speech pathology, and physiotherapy. A research grant was secured from the Australian Commonwealth Department of Health and Aging to develop these measures. This chapter documents the use of the occupational therapy measures.

The AusTOMs-OT scales were developed and refined over a 2-year period. The general documentation concerning development can be found in Perry et al. (2004), with the specific details in the AusTOMs-OT manual, which can be downloaded for free at www. austoms.com and is also summarized here. The development of the AusTOMs-OT commenced with a focus group discussion with a range of academic occupational therapists to identify occupation-specific scales based on the constructs as outlined in the ICF (WHO, 2004). Following this, several focus groups drafted each scale. Occupational therapists from a variety of practice settings and representing practice with diverse groups of clients participated. Once drafted, the scales were provided to occupational therapists across Australia using a modified Delphi process. The measures were revised using the feedback and were provided to therapists for a second review. At this point, the research team negotiated with several clinical sites to collect AusTOMs-OT data after ethical approval was obtained to collect data. The occupational therapists at these sites were trained to use AusTOMs-OT, and reliability data were collected. The AusTOMs-OT scales were then tested over a 6-month period. Data were collected by more than 40 occupational therapists for more than 450 clients (Unsworth, 2005; Unsworth & Duncombe, 2005; Unsworth, Duckett, Duncombe, Perry, Skeat, & Taylor, 2004).

The first edition of AusTOMs-OT was published in 2004 (Unsworth & Duncombe). In the second edition, published in 2007 (Unsworth & Duncombe), the AusTOMs-OT scales remained largely unchanged, although some editorial changes were made to improve clarity. A training DVD was added, and a new data collection form was developed. Given that the measures had been used internationally for almost 3 years, the AusTOMs-OT team was able to reflect on the emails sent and questions asked and used these to provide additional question and answer information in the second edition of the manual. An additional four case studies were added to the original six in the manual. Two Australian clinicians and one clinician each from the United Kingdom and Sweden contributed the additional case studies. ICD-10 codes (WHO, 2004) replaced the original etiology and disorder codes that were used to classify clients in the first edition, and finally, the reference list was updated. The third edition of the AusTOMs-OT was undertaken when a reprint was required in 2014. This was an opportunity for the AusTOMs-OT team to further clarify some descriptions in the manual. Information from several more published studies was included (Abu-Awad, Unsworth, Coulson, & Sarigiannis, 2014; Fristedt, Elgmark, & Unsworth, 2013; Unsworth, 2008; Unsworth, Bearup, & Rickard, 2009). In 2014, a website was created to provide information about the measures and enable the AusTOMs-OT manual, scales, and reference list to be freely downloaded (www.austoms.com). The AusTOMs-OT has been translated into Swedish, Arabic, and Japanese, and Chinese and Turkish translations are currently underway.

Psychometric Properties

Normative Data

Because client data obtained on the AusTOMs-OT may be compared against scores obtained by the population, the measures can be described as norm-referenced. However, while normed tests often provide the range of scores expected for members of the population from different genders or age groups, the AusTOMs-OT assumes that all people without difficulty will score a 5 on each scale for each of the four AusTOMs-OT domains. Therefore, it is not relevant to provide tables of normed data for the AusTOMs-OT. As noted in the AusTOMs-OT manual, when developing the Distress/Well-Being domain, one therapist suggested that only the Dalai Lama could score a 5 (Unsworth & Duncombe, 2014). This turned out to be a helpful comment as this is not the case. We would expect that all people who are managing their level of concern to achieve this score. Therefore, when scoring the Distress/Well-Being domain, it is important that therapists do not overinflate their expectations of what is required to score a 5.

Reliability

A study with 53 occupational therapists was conducted to examine the test-retest and interrater reliability of all 12 AusTOMs-OT scales (Morris et al., 2005). A panel of experts prepared written case vignettes, and therapists were then asked to rate these vignettes on completion of an AusTOMs-OT training course at the sites where we planned the initial occupational therapy data collection. The test-retest reliability of clinician's ratings for these vignettes were calculated 4 weeks after the initial training by measuring the agreement between ratings made at training sessions and ratings made at follow-up sessions. The percentage of agreement over time and between clinicians was calculated, and for most scales, a 60% to 100% agreement was found for test-retest and interrater reliability. While these results provided preliminary evidence of reliability, the data collected did not allow for more robust data analyses (e.g., the use of intraclass correlation coefficients [ICCs]). More recently, a detailed test-retest and interrater reliability study was undertaken with Scale 7 (Self Care; Scott, Unsworth, Fricke, & Taylor, 2006). Seven occupational therapists rated 15 written case studies on two occasions on the four domains of the Self Care scale. The results showed that the Self Care scale had moderate to high interrater reliability with ICCs of more than 0.79 for the three domains of Activity Limitation, Participation Restriction, and Distress/Well-Being and more than 0.70 for Impairment. Test-retest reliability was also reported to be moderate to high, with ICCs of 0.88 for Activity Limitation, 0.81 for Participation Restriction, 0.94 for Distress/Well-Being, and 0.74 for Impairment. The findings of this study support the reliability of the AusTOMs-OT Self Care scale; however, detailed studies such as this one need to be conducted for the other 11 AusTOMs-OT scales.

In addition, interrater reliability and test-retest reliability of the Swedish translation of the AusTOMs-OT measures was reported (Fristedt et al., 2013). Fifteen occupational therapists rated 11 case study clients 2 times separated by 2 weeks. Intrarater reliability was calculated for each of the 15 therapists across all 12 scales. The intrarater reliability was found to be high for nearly all the therapists (ICCs > 0.745). Test-retest and interrater reliability was also studied for Scale 7 (Self Care) and Scale 5 (Transfers), with ICCs ranging from 0.705 to 0.902 for test-retest reliability and from 0.762 to 0.904 for interrater reliability.

Validity

The development of the AusTOMs-OT involved occupational therapy researchers and clinicians at each step of the way, thus promoting validity. Occupational therapists across Australia contributed to developing the scale descriptors for the 12 scales. Consumers (i.e., clients with disabilities, along with client advocates) reviewed the scales and adjusted the Participation Restriction and Distress/Well-Being domains. The construct (concurrent) validity of the AusTOMs-OT measures was established by comparing client data with data from the EuroQol-5D (EQ-5D; Unsworth et al., 2004). The EQ-5D (Brooks, 1996) is a short, simple-to-administer, generic measure of health status, and this measure provides a descriptive profile of client problems on five dimensions as well as an overall score for client self-rated health and generates a single index value that can be used in the clinical and economic evaluation of health care and in population health surveys. Unlike the AusTOMs-OT, the EQ-5D was a client-rated scale; therefore, while a relationship between the two sets of scores was anticipated, this was not expected to be particularly high. Thirty-eight occupational therapists and 67 clients provided data on the AusTOMs-OT and EQ-5D (Unsworth et al., 2004). Spearman rank order correlation coefficients were used to analyze the relationships between scores from the two tools. Moderate to strong statistically significant correlations between the AusTOMs-OT and EQ-5D were found across all four domains, ranging from 0.612 to 0.748. These data provide evidence that the AusTOMs-OT, similar to the EQ-5D, measured global health outcomes.

Sensitivity

As the main objective of an outcome measure is to determine if the client has changed over time, key features are its sensitivity to change and the minimal clinically important difference (MCID; Unsworth, Coulson, Swinton, Cole, & Sarigiannis, 2015). To investigate sensitivity to change, data were collected with 466 clients at 12 metropolitan and rural health care facilities using the 12 AusTOMs-OT scales. There was significant change over time in client scores on the 4 domains of all 12 AusTOMs-OT scales (Unsworth, 2005). The Wilcoxon signed-rank tests for the 12 scales ranged from $Z = -2.280$ to $Z = -12.186$ and were all statistically significant ($p < .05$). Further data collection is required to investigate scale sensitivity with clients in different settings or who have specific disorders. For example, it needs to be confirmed if each of the scales were sensitive to change when used with clients living in the community with a mental health problem or with adults in psychiatric facilities. However, results to date demonstrated strong sensitivity.

To establish the MCID for AusTOMs-OT, criterion- and distribution-based approaches were adopted (Unsworth et al., 2015). Using a criterion approach, 30 international clinicians were surveyed about their perceptions of the MCID. Using a distribution-based approach, the MCID was calculated as half of the standard deviation of the AusTOMs-OT raw scores for a sample of 787 clients. Just over half the clinicians surveyed indicated that a 1-point change represented the MCID for AusTOMs-OT for three domains (Activity Limitation, Participation Restriction, and Distress/Well-Being), and 0.5-point change showed MCID for the Impairment domain. The data analyzed for the distribution-based calculation indicated that the half standard deviation ranged from 0.51 to 0.61. Using both approaches, the authors concluded that a change on the four domains of the AusTOMs-OT of between 0.51 and 1 point shows MCID. For ease of clinical interpretation, it was recommended that a 1-point shift be conservatively adopted as the MCID across domains for all scales.

Assessment Administration

There are 12 AusTOMs-OT scales in total. These represent all the groups of occupations in which an individual may engage across productivity, self-care, and leisure, as outlined in *Occupational Therapy Practice Framework: Domain and Process, Third Edition* (AOTA, 2014). The scales and their definitions are as follows:

- *Scale 1. Learning and Applying Knowledge*: Learning and applying the knowledge that was learned. This includes sensory experiences (e.g., watching, touching, listening), foundation learning (e.g., copying, rehearsing, learning to write), and knowledge application (e.g., solving problems and making decisions).

- *Scale 2. Functional Walking and Mobility*: The ability to move by walking, wheeling oneself, or crawling, either at home or in the community, in order to carry out everyday functions. Use of stairs, ramps, and escalators and high-level mobility activities, such as skipping, hopping, climbing, jumping, and running. While this may include using equipment such as crutches, a walker, or a manual wheelchair with which the individual pushes him- or herself, it excludes using powered wheelchairs or scooters, which are covered under Scale 6 (Using Transport).

- *Scale 3. Upper Limb Use*: Use one or both upper limbs during activities of daily living, including gross and fine manipulative skills and hand and arm use. This may include lifting and moving a heavy object while walking; picking up and using a pencil; grasping, using, and releasing objects such as keys, buttons, or taps; throwing and catching an object; and pushing, pulling, twisting, and turning objects.

- *Scale 4. Carrying Out Daily Life Tasks and Routines*: The ability to undertake simple and complex daily life tasks (e.g., initiating a task, organizing and managing time [time budget], choosing appropriate space and materials, monitoring endurance, sustaining performance to complete a task). This may include the ability to manage a variety of tasks in a given time.

- *Scale 5. Transfers*: The ability to move or transfer one's body position with the intent of achieving an outcome. Includes bed mobility, changing body position, and transfers (e.g., standing, kneeling, getting in and out of a car, getting in and out of the bath, adjusting position in a wheelchair).

- *Scale 6. Using Transport*: Ability to be a passenger or driver (meet and hold a licence if required); use public, private, or commercial transport (i.e., bus, train, tram, car, van, truck, taxi, scooter, wheelchair, bicycle, aircraft, watercraft), which includes safe and appropriate use of a restraint. This scale includes seating and using transportation as a driver or passenger. It does not include transferring into and out of a vehicle (see Scale 5 [Transfers]) or managing money to use public transport (see Scale 9 [Domestic Life—Managing Resources]).

  - Exception: Driver vs. public transport user. If the client has never been a driver, just rate the client in relation to public transportation use and using transportation as a passenger. If you are unsure if the client will be a driver or public transportation user, do not rate using this scale until you have made this decision with the client. Rate the scale when you are ready to work toward the goal of being a transportation user or driver.

- *Scale 7. Self Care*: Consists of washing and drying one's body, caring for one's body (e.g., cutting nails), toileting, grooming (e.g., shaving, brushing hair, applying makeup, cleaning teeth), dressing and undressing, eating and drinking, and looking after one's health (e.g., taking medication).

- *Scale 8. Domestic Life—Home*: Completing regular household activities, such as preparing and serving meals; cleaning and laundry; storing food and managing garbage; house and garden maintenance; pet care (e.g., exercising the dog); and using and maintaining household appliances. Domestic life also includes being concerned about the well-being of others in the house (e.g., children, spouse) and assisting household members with their self-care.

- *Scale 9. Domestic Life—Managing Resources*: Shopping and acquiring services to assist management of domestic life and managing one's own money and economic resources, including using money to purchase goods or pay bills, budgeting, and using banking services.

- *Scale 10. Interpersonal Interactions and Relationships*: Basic and complex communication. Includes interacting with and maintaining and managing people in a contextually, culturally, and socially appropriate manner. This involves such things as showing tolerance and appropriate physical contact/forming and terminating relationships and following social rules. Interactions can be formal (e.g., employer), transactional within a community (e.g., salesperson), informal (e.g., family and friends), or intimate (e.g., sexual). These interactions can occur in familiar or unfamiliar situations or in situations of conflict or change and involve verbal and nonverbal communication (e.g., devices, sign language, body language).

- *Scale 11. Work, Employment and Education*: Involvement in all aspects of paid or unpaid, full-time, part-time, or casual employment, including, but not limited to, seeking, engaging, maintaining, and terminating employment roles and monitoring one's own work performance. Unpaid employment refers to employment with formal work expectations of start and finish times and defined roles and responsibilities. This contrasts with more informal participation in community service organizations and charity or volunteer activities (included in Scale 12 [Community Life, Recreation, Leisure and Play]), and may include informal education (e.g., home schooling), preschool education, school education, vocational training, or higher education. Engaging in education has an expectation of attendance and has defined roles and responsibilities.

- *Scale 12. Community Life, Recreation, Leisure and Play*: The ability to engage in community life. This involves investigating, choosing, performing, and participating in community associations (e.g., social clubs, ethnic groups), ceremonies (e.g., weddings, funerals), and religious or spiritual activities in any environment. This involves engaging in any activity for fun or enjoyment, including play (e.g., informal or organized play), leisure, or recreational activity (e.g., informal or organized sports, arts and culture, crafts, hobbies, socializing).

Each of the 12 scales is assessed across 4 domains: Impairment, Activity Limitation, Participation Restriction, and Distress/Well-Being. This means that the client is assessed in relation to his or her severity of impairments for each scale selected, the performance in activity related to the scale, global level of participation, and global level of well-being. The Impairment and Activity Limitation domains of the AusTOMs-OT are specific to the scale selected. The ranges of behaviors or factors that illustrate the levels of difficulty clients experience were provided for each scale. The Impairment domain describes structural (anatomical) or functional (physiological or psychological) difficulties that a client may have. For example, there may be difficulties with movement, cognitive abilities, or psychological status. When rating the Impairment domain, the occupational therapist needs to consider all the impairments the client currently experiences and the severity of these compared to all other clients. The Activity Limitation domain measures a client's level of ability and difficulty in performing activities. When a client experiences difficulties in the performance or execution of a task, he or she is experiencing an activity limitation. When rating the Activity Limitation domain, the therapist needs to consider all the components of the activity as described in the scale definition that are relevant to the client's age and living circumstances.

The Participation Restriction and Distress/Well-Being domains are identical across all scales. These domains are not related to each scale (e.g., the client's level of distress/well-being is not just related to work, education, and employment as rated on Scale 11) but are global constructs related to all areas of the client's life. Therefore, an occupational therapist making a rating for a client using the AusTOMs-OT will need to rate the Participation Restriction and Distress/Well-Being domains once, even if using several AusTOMs-OT scales for that client. The Participation Restriction domain examines, overall, the limitation that a client may experience in real-life, daily situations. Such limitations include roles within vocational, educational, and social contexts. For example, a plumber who experiences depression may not be able to work while he or she recovers. This is a restriction of his or her vocational role. An individual's participation in an activity is facilitated or restricted by a range of individual, environmental, and societal issues. The Distress/Well-Being domain describes a client's level of concern. Concern, when used in the AusTOMs-OT, may be evidenced by a client's anger, frustration, apathy, or depression.

Description of Environment/ Description of Supplies/Materials Required

The AusTOMs-OT is a therapist-scored outcome measure. The occupational therapist rates the client on the selected AusTOMs-OT scales in any environment after completing the usual initial interview and assessments that are always conducted when the therapist first meets the client. The AusTOMs-OT can be scored away from the client after completion of a routine interview and initial assessment. The occupational therapist makes discharge ratings in the same manner, either when the client completes a goal or is discharged from occupational therapy.

No equipment is needed to administer the AusTOMs-OT, as it is scored following administration of the usual assessments undertaken by the therapist. No training is needed to use the AusTOMs-OT. Occupational therapists read the manual, practice, discuss with other therapists, and then commence scoring clients. A score form template is also available on the website; however, many occupational therapists prefer to upload their AusTOMs-OT scores directly into their client management software. While a training DVD was made to accompany the second edition of the AusTOMs-OT, this became difficult to distribute and was not deemed necessary as the manual guides therapists to administer the measures.

Administration

After reading through the manual, practicing the 10 case studies, and practicing with a few clients, an occupational therapist is ready to begin collecting data. If possible, it can also be very helpful to have team discussions about scoring the AusTOMs-OT and score a couple of clients together to ensure that all therapists have understood the scoring approach and calibrated scores against one another. This is especially important for therapists with less experience. Feedback from clinicians suggested that while experienced therapists have seen clients with a range of severity levels of impairments, activity limitations, participation restrictions, and distress/well-being, less experienced therapists have not. This means that selecting a score on the continuum from best to worst may be harder for these therapists. Discussing and scoring real client examples has assisted less experienced therapists to calibrate scores against more experienced therapists, thus improving the reliability of scores. The process of score clients can be documented as follows:

1. Assess the client using usual methods (e.g., an initial interview, Canadian Occupational Performance Measure, and other standardized assessments).
2. Establish goals as usual.
3. Select AusTOMs-OT scales that reflect current goals.
4. Make an initial rating for each scale, for each domain.
5. Implement occupational therapy program.
6. Reevaluate client goals as needed.
7. Rate the client a second time on AusTOMs-OT scales when goals are met/client is discharged.
8. If a new goal is set, rate the client on the relevant AusTOMs-OT scale.
9. On the conclusion of the therapy program, check all scales have been scored at start and finish.
10. Use AusTOMs-OT scores to track change over time for individuals or groups and in quality assurance or research projects on service provision outcomes.

Scoring

The first decision to make when scoring a client with the AusTOMs-OT is which of the 12 scales to select. This decision is relatively easy because the scales selected should reflect the goals that the client and clinician have set. Usually, the client and clinician will set one to three goals; therefore, one to three scales will be chosen by the therapist to score. However, if more goals are set, more scales can be selected. The important thing to remember is that once a goal has been reached and a new goal is set, then the AusTOMs-OT must be scored a second time and a new scale scored related to the new goal. Each AusTOMs-OT scale is scored on the four domains of: Impairment, Activity Limitation, Participation Restriction, and Distress/Well-Being. Therefore, a client is given a profile of four scores for every scale selected. Each domain is scored between 0 and 5, where 0 is a problem and 5 is without problems. Half points can be awarded. Hence, there are 6 defined points and 5 half points, providing an 11-point scale. There is a generic scoring system for each of the four domains, and these are further defined in relation to each of the 12 scales. This is not the case for the domains of Participation Restriction and Distress/Well-Being as these are generic constructs and can be scored the same, no matter how many scales are selected. Therefore, this score is only given once at the time of scoring, no matter how many scales are selected. This point is reinforced again in the case study that follows. The core scoring system for the four domains are as follows:

- *Impairment of Either Structure or Function (as appropriate to age)*: Impairments are problems in body structure (anatomical) or function (physiological) as a deviation or loss.
  - 0 = The most severe presentation of impairment
  - 1 = Severe presentation of this impairment
  - 2 = Moderate/severe presentation
  - 3 = Moderate presentation

- 4 = Mild presentation
- 5 = No impairment of structure or function

- *Activity Limitation (as appropriate to age)*: Activity limitation results from the difficulty in the performance of an activity. Activity is the execution of a task by the individual.
  - 0 = Complete difficulty
  - 1 = Severe difficulty
  - 2 = Moderate/severe difficulty
  - 3 = Moderate difficulty
  - 4 = Mild difficulty
  - 5 = No difficulty

- *Participation Restriction (as appropriate to age)*: Participation restrictions are difficulties the individual may have in the manner or extent of involvement in his or her life situation. Clinicians should ask themselves: "Given their problem, is this individual experiencing disadvantage?"
  - 0 = Unable to fulfill social, work, educational, or family roles. No social integration. No involvement in decision making. No control over environment. Unable to reach potential in any situation.
  - 1 = Severe difficulties in fulfilling social, work, educational, or family roles. Very limited social integration. Very limited involvement in decision making. Very little control over environment. Can only rarely reach potential with maximum assistance.
  - 2 = Moderately severe difficulties in fulfilling social, work, educational, or family roles. Limited social integration. Limited involvement in decision making. Control over environment in one setting only. Usually reaches potential with maximum assistance.
  - 3 = Moderate difficulties in fulfilling social, work, educational, or family roles. Relies on moderate assistance for social integration. Limited involvement in decision making. Control over environment in more than one setting. Always reaches potential with maximum assistance and sometimes reaches potential without assistance.
  - 4 = Mild difficulties in fulfilling social, work, educational, or family roles. Needs little assistance for social integration and decision making. Control over environment in more than one setting. Reaches potential with little assistance.
  - 5 = No difficulties in fulfilling social, work, educational, or family roles. No assistance required for social integration or decision making. Control over environment in all settings. Reaches potential with no assistance.

- *Distress/Well-Being (as appropriate to age)*: The level of concern experienced by the individual. Concern may be evidenced by anger, frustration, apathy, or depression.
  - 0 = High and consistent levels of distress or concern.
  - 1 = Severe concern, becomes distressed or concerned easily. Requires constant reassurance. Loses emotional control easily.
  - 2 = Moderately severe concern. Frequent emotional encouragement and reassurance required.
  - 3 = Moderate concern. May be able to manage emotions at times, although may require some encouragement.

- ∘ 4 = Mild concern. Able to manage emotions in most situations. Occasional emotional support or encouragement needed.
- ∘ 5 = Able to cope with most situations. Accepts and understands own limitations.

Intervention Planning Based on Assessment Results

AusTOMs-OT is an outcome measure rather than an assessment, and therefore does not play a strong role in guiding intervention planning. However, the following case study of Peter illustrates how the AusTOMs-OT can be used to record the outcomes of an occupational therapy program. This case study is from the AusTOMs-OT manual (Unsworth & Duncombe, 2014) and has been further developed for use in this chapter.

Case Study

Peter has schizophrenia, which has until recently been very stable. Because he had been well for about 5 years, he decided to try cutting back his medication to see if he would be all right without it. Shortly after this, he experienced a psychotic episode (April) and was admitted for 2 days to an acute psychiatric facility and then discharged home. That was 1 week ago.

His case manager, Alize, is an occupational therapist. Alize and Peter decided to focus on his goals of getting back to work and his leisure activities. Therefore, Alize chose to rate Peter on AusTOMs-OT Scales 11 and 12.

Alize had noted that Peter is 42 years old and works for a printer. He has never married but has a good network of family (three siblings) and two friends who he sees monthly. He seems stable again now that he is back on medication and says he experiences infrequent paranoid thoughts, and that the ones he does experience are manageable. This is similar to his level of impairment prior to the recent psychotic episode. He is currently working with his case manager to return to work. A work site assessment revealed that Peter was able to manage his usual work tasks but that fatigue made him slower than usual. He did not need any extra rest breaks. At this time, the case manager also noted that he seemed to require frequent reassurance that he was doing well and that things would return to the way they had been. Although he was fulfilling most of his usual roles, he seemed quite subdued and lacking in confidence, to the extent that he needed some prompts to make choices about what he wanted to achieve from therapy.

Please refer to Figure 19-1 to consider the dynamic interaction among the therapy goals, individual, and the environment.

Peter returned to work, and after 3 weeks (May), the case manager reassessed him and found that he was completing all his usual work tasks in a timely fashion. However, Peter complained that this seemed to be at the expense of his social life as he was very tired in the evenings and had not been seeing friends or family much. He stated that he was currently only engaging in leisure activities if a friend came and took him out or if one of his siblings called and organized something to do. For example, to go swimming, he needed his sister to accompany and supervise him for safety. He stated that he lacked confidence and was embarrassed about having stopped his medication and that he felt he needed more support from the case manager than their regular meeting every 3 weeks. The case manager then set a new goal of increasing leisure time activities.

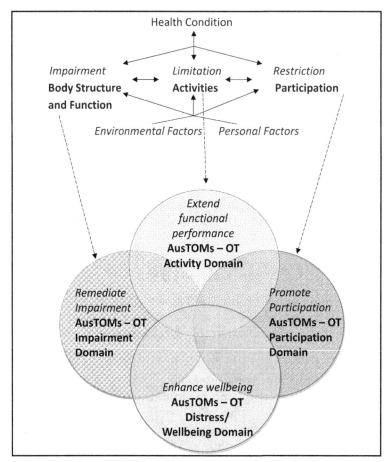

Figure 19-1. Relationships of therapy goals, ICF (WHO, 2001), and AusTOMs-OT.

After 2 months (July), Peter reported that things had settled very well and that the strategies he had developed with the case manager to increase his leisure activities had been useful. He reported that things seemed back to normal and that he was engaging in his regular leisure activities, which included swimming, having a couple of drinks and playing a game of darts with a friend at the pub, or having dinner with a sibling. He continued to meet the case manager every 3 weeks as he had done prior to his recent hospital admission to gain support and encouragement as needed.

In terms of scoring Peter using the AusTOMs-OT, Alize made the following notes. For the start scores for Scale 11 (Work, Employment and Education), Peter was only having infrequent paranoid thoughts, and his schizophrenia was mild. Therefore, a rating of 4 was appropriate in the Impairment domain for the Work, Employment and Education scale. His condition was stable for the duration of his therapy; therefore, his Impairment ratings remain as 4s for both scales at each assessment. Peter was performing slower than usual at work; thus, he scored a 4 in the Activity Limitation domain. Fatigue was making him slower than usual at work, consistent with a score of 3.5 for Participation Restriction. Peter required frequent support and reassurance, so he scored 2 for Distress/ Well-Being. In May, Alize found that Peter was completing all his usual work tasks in a timely fashion and reassessed him. He no longer experienced any limitation with regard to work; therefore, he scored a 5 in the Activity Limitation domain for Scale 11. However,

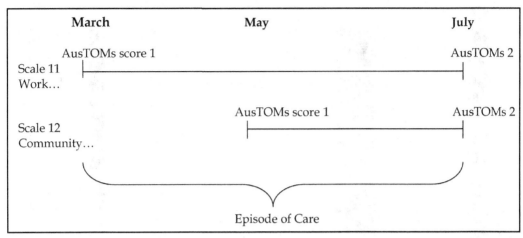

Figure 19-2. Scoring example using AusTOMs-OT with Peter.

Peter has limited social integration and is lacking in confidence, therefore scoring 2.5 in the Participation Restriction domain. He expressed a moderate level of concern about his situation, thus scoring 3 in the Distress/Well-Being domain.

At the same time as discharge ratings of the Work, Employment and Education scale were made, Peter and his case manager started to work on a new goal using Scale 12 (Community Life, Recreation, Leisure and Play). In assessing him for his new goal, the case manager gave Peter a score of 3 in the Activity Limitation domain as he still required his sister to take him swimming and to stay to supervise him. Peter's scores in the Participation Restriction and Distress/Well-Being domains (2.5 and 3, respectively) at the time of "admission" to this new goal are the same as those for "discharge" from his first goal because one action directly followed the other. In July, Alize made a final rating for Peter on the Community Life scale. He scored 5 in the Activity Limitation domain after reporting that things were back to normal and that he was engaging in his regular leisure activities. His participation in community life was no longer being restricted in any way by his disorder, so he scored a 5 for Participation Restriction. Although Peter achieved the two therapeutic goals he and his case manager set, he was not discharged from the service. He continues to see his case manager every 3 weeks for support and encouragement, so a rating of 4 is appropriate in the Distress/Well-Being domain. The process and timing for scoring Peter is noted in Figure 19-2, and his scores are summarized on an AusTOMs-OT score sheet in Figure 19-3.

Suggested Further Research

The AusTOMs-OT scales, as with all outcome measures, require ongoing validation and reliability studies. In particular, further interrater and test-retest reliability studies like the ones undertaken with Scale 7 (Self Care) are required with the other 11 scales. A recent study demonstrated the MCID for the AusTOMs-OT as 1 point, and research is currently underway to document the minimum detectable change as well as the standard error of measurement for AusTOMs-OT. There are many opportunities for occupational therapists to examine how the AusTOMs-OT scales can be used to support practice and promote an evidence base for therapy services. For example, while several studies have reported AusTOMs-OT data with clients who have age-related or neurological disabilities

AUSTOMS FOR OCCUPATIONAL THERAPY

Data Collection Form

AFFIX CLIENT RECORD STICKER HERE

ICD-10 CODES: **1.** F20   **2.**   **3.**

CARER: (e.g. husband, sister) NA but 3 siblings in close contact

TIME: (Total face to face contact with client or caregiver) 38 hours.

GROUP OR INDIVIDUAL THERAPY: Individual

TYPES OF THERAPY: **1.** Individual Meeting   **2.**   **3.**   **4.**   **5.**

AusTOMs Ratings

Scale No.	Goal Start Date	Impairment	Activity Limitation	Participation Restriction	Distress/ W. Client	Distress/ W. Carer	Goal End Date	Impairment	Activity Limitation	Participation Restriction	Distress/ W. Client	Distress/ W. Carer
11	5 March	4	4	3·5	2	1	7 May	4	5	2·5	3	1
12	7 May	4	3	2·5	3	1	10 July	4	5	5	4	1

Discharge Code (Please tick one):

1. Treatment complete ✓	**2.** Therapist ceased treatment
3. Client did not attend	**4.** Treatment stopped, transferred to other service
5. Acute episode (further event) but remained at facility	**6.** Treatment stopped, client self discharge
7. Deceased	**8.** Other (Specify)

Figure 19-3. Completed AusTOMs-OT score sheet for Peter. (Reprinted with permission from La Trobe University.)

(Abu-Awad et al., 2014; Unsworth, 2008; Unsworth et al., 2009; Unsworth & Duncombe, 2005), no publications have documented change over time for clients with mental health problems. Finally, although the AusTOMs-OT is widely used across the Asian Pacific, Canada, and Europe (particularly in the United Kingdom and Sweden), the measures are not as commonly used in the United States. Therefore, further research is required using the AusTOMs-OT scales with therapists in the United States.

Summary

Although occupational therapy researchers and clinicians have written about outcome measures for more than 2 decades (Foto, 1996; Fricke, 1993; Unsworth, 2000), it has only been over the past 5 to 10 years that health services and reimbursers/payers have demanded that therapy managers provide data as evidence to support the effectiveness of, and therefore continued funding for, occupational therapy services. The AusTOMs-OT has been used in research as well as clinical practice over the past 10 years both internationally and in a variety of therapy settings and has been shown to be a valid and reliable outcome measure. This chapter has documented some of the key features and information about the AusTOMs-OT and has provided a case study to illustrate how it can be used. Although further research is required to demonstrate the ongoing psychometric features of any outcome measure, the AusTOMs-OT has been shown to be suitable to determine how much change clients make during their participation in an occupational therapy program. Furthermore, the AusTOMs-OT measures the conduct of research such as randomized controlled trials to demonstrate that changes in client capacity, performance, and well-being are directly attributable to participation in the occupational therapy program.

References

Abu-Awad, Y., Unsworth, C. A., Coulson, M., & Sarigiannis, M. (2014). Using the Australian Therapy Outcome Measures for Occupational Therapy (AusTOMs-OT) to measure client participation outcomes. *British Journal of Occupational Therapy, 77*, 44-49.

American Occupational Therapy Association. (2014). Occupational therapy practice framework: Domain and process (3rd ed.). *American Journal of Occupational Therapy, 68*(Suppl. 1), S1-S48.

Anastasi, A. (1982). *Psychological testing* (5th ed.). New York, NY: MacMillan Publishing.

Brooks, P. (1996). EuroQol: The current state of play. *Health Policy, 37*, 53-72.

DeVellis, R. F. (1991). *Scale development: Theory and applications.* Thousand Oaks, CA: Sage Publications Inc.

Enderby, P., & John, A. (1997). *Therapy outcome measures for speech and language pathology.* San Diego, CA: Singular.

Enderby, P., John, A., & Petherham, B. (1998). *Therapy outcome measures manual: Physiotherapy, occupational therapy, rehabilitation nursing.* San Diego, CA: Singular.

Foto, M. (1996). Outcome studies: The what, why, how, and when. *American Journal of Occupational Therapy, 50*, 87-88.

Fricke, J. (1993). Measuring outcomes in rehabilitation: A review. *British Journal of Occupational Therapy, 56*, 217-221.

Fristedt, S., Elgmark, E. & Unsworth, C. A. (2013). The inter-rater and test-retest reliability of the self-care and transfer scales and intra-rater reliability of all scales of the Swedish translation of the Australian Therapy Outcome Measures for Occupational Therapy (AusTOMs-OT-S). *Scandinavian Journal of Occupational Therapy, 20*, 182-189.

Laver-Fawcett, A. (2007). The importance of accurate assessment and outcome measurement. In A. Laver Fawcett (Ed.), *Principles of assessment and outcome measurement for occupational therapists and physiotherapists: Theory, skills and application.* Chichester, United Kingdom: John Wiley & Sons.

Morris, M., Perry, A., Unsworth, C., Skeat, J., Taylor, N., Dodd, K., … Duckett, S. (2005). Reliability of the Australian Therapy Outcome Measures for quantifying disability and health. *International Journal of Therapy and Rehabilitation, 12*, 340-346.

Nunnally, J. C. (1978). *Psychological theory* (2nd ed.). New York, NY: McGraw-Hill.

Perry, A., Morris, M., Unsworth, C., Duckett, S., Skeat, J., Dodd, K., … Riley, K. (2004). Therapy outcome measures for allied health practitioners in Australia: The AusTOMs. *International Journal for Quality in Health Care, 16*, 285-291.

Rubin, M. (1987). *The boiled frog syndrome.* New York, NY: Alyson Publications.

Scott, F., Unsworth, C. A., Fricke, J., & Taylor, N. (2006). Reliability of the Australian Therapy Outcome Measures for Occupational Therapy (AusTOMs-OT) self-care scale. *Australian Occupational Therapy Journal, 53*, 265-276.

Unsworth, C. A. (2000). Measuring the outcome of occupational therapy: Tools and resources. *Australian Occupational Therapy Journal, 47*, 147-158.

Unsworth, C. A. (2005). Measuring outcomes using the Australian Therapy Outcome Measures for Occupational Therapy (AusTOMs-OT): Data description and tool sensitivity. *British Journal of Occupational Therapy, 68*, 354-366.

Unsworth, C. A. (2008). Using the Australian Therapy Outcome Measures for Occupational Therapy (AusTOMs-OT) to measure outcomes for clients following stroke. *Topics in Stroke Rehabilitation, 15*, 351-364.

Unsworth, C. A., Bearup, A., & Rickard, K. (2009). A benchmark comparison of outcomes for clients with upper limb dysfunction following stroke using the Australian Therapy Outcome Measures for Occupational Therapy (AusTOMs-OT). *American Journal of Occupational Therapy, 63*, 732-774.

Unsworth, C. A., Coulson, M., Swinton, L., Cole, H., & Sarigiannis, M. (2015). Determination of the minimum clinically important difference on the Australian Therapy Outcome Measures for Occupational Therapy (AusTOMs-OT). *Disability and Rehabilitation, 37*, 997-1003.

Unsworth, C., Duckett, S., Duncombe, D., Perry, A., Skeat, J., & Taylor, N. (2004). Validity of the AusTOM Scales: A comparison of the AusTOMs and EuroQol-5D. *Health and Quality of Life Outcomes, 2*, 1-12.

Unsworth, C. A., & Duncombe, D. (2004). *AusTOMs for occupational therapy.* Melbourne, Victoria, Australia: La Trobe University.

Unsworth, C. A., & Duncombe, D. (2005). A comparison of client outcomes from two acute care neurological services using self care data from the Australian Therapy Outcome Measures for Occupational Therapy (AusTOMs-OT). *British Journal of Occupational Therapy, 68*, 477-482.

Unsworth, C. A., & Duncombe, D. (2007). *AusTOMs for occupational therapy* (2nd ed.). Melbourne, Victoria, Australia: La Trobe University.

Unsworth, C. A., & Duncombe, D. (2014). *AusTOMs for occupational therapy* (3rd ed.). Melbourne, Victoria, Australia: La Trobe University.

World Health Organization. (2001). *International classification of functioning, disability and health (ICF).* Geneva, Switzerland: Author.

World Health Organization. (2004). *ICD-10: International classification of diseases and related health problems* (10th ed.). Geneva, Switzerland: Author.

Part VI
Learning Assessments

The Performance Assessment of Self-Care Skills

Margo B. Holm, PhD, OTR/L, FAOTA, ABDA
Joan C. Rogers, PhD, OTR, FAOTA

People may doubt what you say, but they will always believe what you do.
(Cass, as cited in Klunder, 2013, p. 7)

The Performance Assessment of Self-Care Skills (PASS), Version 4.1 (Rogers, Holm, & Chisholm, 2016) is a performance-based, criterion-referenced, observational instrument developed to assist practitioners in documenting functional status and change. The PASS 4.0 consists of 26 core occupations, categorized in 4 functional domains: functional mobility (FM), basic activities of daily living (BADLs), instrumental ADLs with a cognitive emphasis (CIADLs), and IADLs with a physical emphasis (PIADLs). The PASS manual includes a template for developing new tasks, and the authors gladly assist in task development (www.shrs.pitt.edu/ot/about/performance-assessment-self-care-skills-pass). Because the PASS is designed to identify the specific point of task breakdown, the amount and type of assistance needed, and the risks to safety during task performance, it facilitates treatment and discharge planning. Based on client needs and the reason for referral, practitioners can choose which PASS tasks are appropriate to administer to each client. Statistically, each task stands alone and is psychometrically sound. Therefore, a practitioner can administer one, five, or all tasks. However, two series of tasks (Money Management and Meal Preparation) are each meant to be administered as a series to increase their complexity. In this chapter, the conceptual foundations of the PASS are described, as well as the psychometric properties, administration, and utility for intervention planning. In addition to the home and clinic performance-based measures, self-report and proxy report versions of the PASS address habit and skill for the 26 core occupations (available at www.shrs.pitt.edu/ot/about/performance-assessment-self-care-skills-pass).

Hemphill, B. J., & Urish, C. K. (Eds.). *Assessments in Occupational Therapy Mental Health: An Integrative Approach, Fourth Edition* (pp. 359-370). © 2020 Taylor & Francis Group.

Theoretical Basis

Concepts/Constructs

The PASS combines two conceptual foundations of assessment: interactive assessment and graduated prompting. Interactive (dynamic) assessment (Feuerstein, Rand, & Hoffman, 1979; Missiuna, 1987; Tzuriel & Haywood, 1991) is associated with the Soviet psychologist Vygotsky (1896-1934; Vygotsky, 1978), who described a zone of proximal (potential) development as the difference between a client's independent performance on a test and the performance when the client is assisted or guided on a test. Therefore, the PASS, as an interactive assessment, consists of establishing a client's current level of performance without assistance, providing the type and amount of assistance required for improved performance, and documenting the outcome of the assisted task performance (Haywood, Tzuriel, & Vaught, 1991). Most testing prohibits an assessor from assisting a client during testing, but because the PASS uses interactive assessment, systematic assistance is encouraged when necessary. Moreover, the PASS data collection and rating forms include space to document the assistance provided.

The second conceptual foundation of the PASS is graduated prompting (Gold, 1980). Graduated prompting consists of a hierarchy of prompts that are used only when there is a breakdown in task performance and only in a specific sequence. The PASS hierarchy of assists takes into account the power of the assist, the cost of the assist based on the practitioner's time, and the level of intrusiveness to the client (Gold, 1980). The layout and design of the PASS data collection and rating forms reflect both conceptual foundations.

History of Development and Previous Versions/ Important Changes to Note in Current Version

The initial version of the PASS was developed in 1984, with subsequent major revisions occurring in 1989, 1994, and 2014. The PASS 4.0 (Rogers & Holm, 2014) updates include additional subtasks and an update of the data collection and scoring form. For example, the management of clothing during the toileting process was added to the Toilet Mobility and Management task. Most wording changes were for clarity rather than changes in the substance of the subtask. The data collection forms for each task were revised to make them easier to use for both data collection and scoring.

Psychometric Properties

Population

The PASS was originally designed for an adult population. However, the PASS has been used to document functional status and change in adolescents and adults from various diagnostic populations, including depression, bipolar disorder, dementia, mild cognitive impairment (MCI), schizophrenia, developmental delay, spinal cord injury, multiple sclerosis, head trauma, stroke, heart failure, parkinsonism, cardiac arrest, heart transplant, artificial heart, osteoarthritis, and macular degeneration (Chisholm, 2005; Chisholm, Toto, Raina, Holm, & Rogers, 2014; Finlayson, Havens, Holm, & Van Denend, 2003; Raina, 2005; Rogers, Holm, Beach, Schulz, & Starz, 2001). The assessment has also been used with healthy older adult populations in the United States and Canada. The PASS tasks have also been translated and culturally adapted, when appropriate, into Arabic, Spanish, French, Farsi, Hebrew, Portuguese, Japanese, Finnish, and Turkish.

Reliability

Test-retest reliability, with clients from a variety of diagnostic populations, was established using a 3-day interval. PASS-Clinic test-retest reliability was independence, $r = .92$; safety, 89% agreement; and adequacy, $r = .82$. PASS-Home test-retest reliability was independence, $r = .96$; safety, 90% agreement; and adequacy, $r = .97$. Interobserver reliability with a total of 5 different rater dyads observing 25 older adults from a variety of diagnostic populations was independence, 92%; safety, 93%; and adequacy, 90%. PASS-Home interobserver reliability was independence, 96%; safety, 97%; and adequacy, 88%. Therefore, decision consistency among practitioners observing the same client perform everyday tasks was good to excellent. PASS-Clinic and PASS-Home tasks also had good to excellent interobserver reliabilities.

Validity

Content validity of the PASS is based on a review of multiple self-report assessments of ADLs (Gurland, Kuriansky, Sharpe, Simon, Stiller, & Birkett, 1977; Lawton, Moss, Fulcomer, & Kleban, 1982; Pfeffer, 1987; Pfeiffer, 1975). The items from these instruments were then adapted and converted into performance-based tasks consisting of specific tasks, subtasks, and performance criteria. Construct validity of the PASS is gleaned from multiple investigations. Construct validity of the unidimensionality of the independence, safety, and adequacy scales of the PASS was established using exploratory factor analysis and Cattell's screen test (Cattell, 1966; Chisholm, 2005), which supported a dominant construct that met the unidimensionality assumption for each construct. Construct validity of the 26 core tasks was also confirmed in a study of older adult women with depression. Rasch analysis revealed that all PIADLs, CIADLs, BADLs, and FM (in that order) were more difficult for those who required inpatient treatment ($n = 60$; mean [standard deviation {SD}] age, 73.7 [7.1] years; 93% White) than those who required outpatient treatment ($n = 59$; mean [SD] age, 75.7 [4.1] years; 81% White; Chisholm, 2005).

Construct validity of the PASS was also confirmed using known group differences (Goldstein, McCue, Rogers, & Nussbaum, 1992; Holm & Rogers, 1990a, 1990b; McCue, Rogers, & Goldstein, 1990; Rogers, Holm, Goldstein, & Nussbaum, 1994). In another study, clients who were readmitted within 1 year of discharge demonstrated greater difficulty in task performance at discharge, especially in the CIADL and PIADL domains. Likewise, for female clients with depression, those with slower cognitive processing speeds ($n = 76$; mean [SD] age, 74.2 [5.9] years; 84% White) on the Trails B (a neuropsychological test of cognitive flexibility) showed significantly worse performance in CIADLs, BADLs, PIADLs, and FM (in that order) than those clients with depression and faster cognitive processing speeds ($n = 23$; mean [SD] age, 75.5 [4.7] years; 100% White; Chisholm, 2005).

Sensitivity

In 274 older women (mean [SD] age, 78.8 [5.1] years; 86% White), the PASS detected significant ($p < .001$) change in independence of performance over 6 months for FM, BADL, CIADL, PIADL tasks, and the overall constructs of independence and adequacy. Safety did not evidence change because participants remained consistently safe despite deteriorating independence and adequacy. In a study of 217 stroke survivors ($n = 94$ women; mean [SD] age, 64.4 [15.4] years; 93.5% White), the PASS was able to detect change in function between 24 hours post-stroke and 5 days, 3 months, 6 months, 9 months, and

12 months post-stroke for all 3 constructs (i.e., independence, safety, adequacy) and all 4 domains (i.e., FM, BADLs, CIADLs, PIADLs) of function. Significant changes ($p < .05$ or greater) were found for independence, safety, and adequacy, as well as FM and CIADLs. The PASS BADL and PIADL domain tasks measured improvement over time, but the changes were not significant.

Assessment Administration

The PASS measures three aspects of occupational performance: independence, safety, and adequacy, using separate rating scales. The PASS has two versions: the PASS-Clinic and the PASS-Home. Of the 26 core PASS occupations, 18 measure the types of assistance necessary for a client to return to (PASS-Clinic) or remain in (PASS-Home) the community. Specifically, the 26 core occupations of the PASS consist of 5 FM tasks, 3 BADL tasks, 14 CIADL tasks, and 4 PIADL tasks. Both versions of the PASS include the same occupations, subtask criteria, and directions. However, the task materials differ in each setting, with task materials being provided in the clinic and clients using many of their own task materials in their homes.

Description of Environment/
Description of Supplies/Materials Required

Conditions and Instructions

Each PASS task includes two types of directions: conditions and instructions. They include the context for the task (e.g., kitchen, bathroom, stairway), the materials (e.g., utility bills, prescription bottle, wallet with real dollars and coins), how they are to be arranged (e.g., centered in front of the client, on bed next to pillow, items available on the table), and the starting position of the client (e.g., seated at a table, positioned next to the foot of the bed, positioned at the bottom of the stairs). Instructions include the standardized wording to be given to the client, as well as cues to the practitioner (e.g., wait for response). The materials and equipment used in the PASS are common household items (e.g., flashlight, mixing bowl, paring knife), and specifications, when relevant (e.g., 1-quart sauce pan), are listed in the task conditions. Task items are purchased by the practitioner to develop the test kit. The PASS-Clinic kit requires more items than the PASS-Home kit because in the home clients use many of their own items. Both kits include some adaptive equipment (e.g., lighted magnifying glass, large button, display calculator), some of which may already be present in a clinic. It is recommended that the kit for the PASS-Home be transported in a small rolling suitcase.

Tasks, Subtasks, and Interactive Assessment

The 26 PASS core tasks (Table 20-1) consist of 164 criterion-referenced subtasks that the practitioner uses to rate task performance. Task subtasks vary between 2 and 13 subtasks, depending on the complexity of the task being observed. Once the set-up conditions and task materials are arranged, the practitioner begins by giving the client the standardized instructions. In the clinic, adaptive items that may be needed are arranged according to the standardized conditions. In the home, the standardized task materials are set up by the occupational therapist, but clients are prompted to use their own task materials and adaptive items as much as possible. Independence in task performance is rated using an

Table 20-1

Performance Assessment of Self-Care Skills
Tasks Categorized by Functional Domains

Domain	Tasks
FM	• Bed mobility • Stair use • Toilet mobility and management • Bathtub and shower mobility • Indoor walking
BADLs	• Oral hygiene • Trimming toenails • Dressing
CIADLs	• Shopping (money management) • Bill paying by check (money management) • Checkbook balancing (money management) • Mailing (money management) • Telephone use • Medication management • Obtaining critical information from the media (auditory current events) • Obtaining critical information from the media (visual current events) • Small repairs (home maintenance) • Home safety (environmental awareness) • Playing Bingo (leisure) • Oven use (meal preparation) • Stovetop use (meal preparation) • Use of sharp utensils (meal preparation)
PIADLs	• Clean-up after meal preparation (light housework) • Changing bed linens (heavy housework) • Sweeping (home maintenance) • Bending, lifting, and carrying out the garbage (heavy housework)

Abbreviations: BADLs = basic activities of daily living; CIADLs = IADLs with a cognitive emphasis; FM = functional mobility; IADLs = instrumental activities of daily living; PIADLs = IADLs with a physical emphasis.

interactive assessment approach. When the client is no longer able to proceed independently with a task (point of subtask breakdown), the practitioner begins the interactive assessment process using a nine-level system of graduated prompts to:

• Facilitate initiation, continuation, or completion of task performance
• Alert the client to safety concerns
• Address concerns about inefficiency in task process or concerns about task quality

When prompts are necessary, the type and number of prompts needed to continue task performance are recorded for each relevant subtask. This blending of interactive assessment and graduated prompting yields a documented profile of client performance that identifies the exact point of subtask breakdown and the type and number of prompts needed for successful task performance during the assessment. The profile of prompts is also beneficial for intervention and discharge planning because it identifies those prompts that enabled, improved, or resulted in successful task performance.

Table 20-2

Rating Scales for PASS Independence, Safety, and Adequacy

Score	Independence	Safety	Adequacy	
			Process	*Quality*
3	No assists given for task initiation, continuation, or completion	Safe practices were observed	Subtasks performed with precision and economy of effort and action	Optimal (performance matches the quality standards listed in each subtask)
2	No Level 7 to 9 assists given, but occasional Level 1 to 6 assists given	Minor risks were evident but no assistance provided	Subtasks generally performed with precision and economy of effort and action; occasional lack of efficiency, redundant or extraneous action; no missing steps	Acceptable (performance, for the most part, matches or nearly matches the quality standards listed in each subtask)
1	No Level 9 assists given; occasional Level 7 or 8 assists given OR Continuous Level 1 to 6 assists given	Risks to safety were observed and assistance given to prevent potential harm	Subtasks generally performed with lack of precision and/or economy of effort and action; consistent extraneous or redundant actions; steps may be missing	Marginal (performance, for the most part, does not match the quality standards listed in each subtask)
0	Level 9 assists given OR Continuous Level 7 or 8 assists given OR Unable to initiate, continue, or complete subtask or task	Risks to safety of such severity were observed that task was stopped or taken over to prevent harm	Subtasks are consistently performed with lack of precision and/or economy of effort and action so that task progress is unattainable	Unacceptable (performance does not match the quality standards listed in each subtask, perhaps with a few exceptions)

Scoring

Data Collection, Rating, and Scoring Forms

PASS task subtasks are rated on three distinct concepts: independence, safety, and adequacy of outcome. Each concept is scored on a predefined 4-point ordinal scale (Table 20-2 and Appendix E, PASS scoring grid). For each PASS task, the data collection and rating form includes a section for subtask criteria, independence data, independence scores for subtasks, safety data, and adequacy data (process and quality). Under subtask criteria, the observable criterion behaviors for each subtask are demarcated with a double underscore and are the relevant behaviors for rating task independence and adequacy process. The criterion behaviors demarcated with a single underscore define the adequacy-quality standard with which the criterion behaviors are to be carried out, with relevant examples for making that judgment in the parentheses that follow (see Table 20-2 and Appendix E).

Using the PASS Data Grids to Record Observations

For each subtask on the PASS 4.0 data collection and scoring form (see Table 20-3 and Appendix E) under independence data, a grid of the hierarchical prompts is used by the practitioner to place a check mark each time a prompt is given for the client to accomplish a subtask. The prompt hierarchy includes 10 levels of graduated prompts. When a task cannot be performed independently, the practitioner provides the least powerful/intrusive type of assistance to facilitate task performance, safety, and/or adequacy. The grid, organized by types of prompts, begins with the least assistive and progresses to the most assistive (see Table 20-3):

- (0) No assistance
- (1) Verbal supportive (encouragement)
- (2) Verbal non-directive
- (3) Verbal directive
- (4) Gestures
- (5) Task or environment rearrangement
- (6) Demonstration
- (7) Physical guidance
- (8) Physical support
- (9) Total assist

The next section of the grid is a column to score independence for each subtask using the PASS scoring grid.

Task safety is also anchored to each subtask. The practitioner again places a check mark in the safety data grid opposite the relevant subtask if any risks to safety are observed during task performance or if the practitioner is required to intervene because of a risk to the client or environmental safety. Therefore, the PASS helps to identify the specific aspect of task performance where safety concerns were evident. Likewise, task adequacy is also noted during task performance, and the adequacy data grid enables practitioners to place a check mark to identify task-adequacy problems related to the process and quality of subtask performance. Adequacy process is rated for the precision and economy of effort and completeness with which a subtask is performed (e.g., manipulates the flashlight parts, identifies the problem). Adequacy quality is rated based on subtask sample quality standards (e.g., adequately, correctly, within three tries). Therefore, each time a prompt is provided, the practitioner uses the data grid to note the level of assistance provided (independence), as well as to note whether the assist was given to improve task safety or the adequacy (process, quality) of the task outcome.

PASS Summary Scores

The PASS yields three summary scores: independence, safety, and adequacy. Independence is initially rated for each subtask of a PASS task using the PASS scoring grid, and the independence summary score for each task is the mean of all task subtask ratings. Safety for each PASS task is a single summary score that reflects total task safety. The safety summary score is based on the clinical judgment of the practitioner after referencing the PASS scoring grid. Adequacy is also a single summary score that reflects the combined process and quality data for the total task. When referencing the PASS scoring grid, if process and quality yield different scores, the lower of the two scores is used. Use of the lowest score was chosen so that clients are not put in a situation of risk through practitioner overestimation of task adequacy.

Table 20-3

Sample PASS Data Collection and Scoring Form: Medication Management

Task # C14: CIADL: Medication Management

Assistive Technology Devices (ATDs) used during task:

1.

2.

3.

Total # of ATDs used: _____

Subtasks	MOBILITY/ADL/IADL SUBTASKS	Assist level →	No Assistance 0	Verbal Supportive (Encouragement) 1	Verbal Non-Directive 2	Verbal Directive 3	Gestures 4	Task or Environment Rearrangement 5	Demonstration 6	Physical Guidance 7	Physical Support 8	Total Assist 9	Independence scores for subtasks	Unsafe Observations	PROCESS: Imprecision, lack of economy, missing steps	QUALITY: Standards not met / improvement needed
1 Med 1 C-P*	Reports next time first medication is to be taken correctly (based on testing time, matches direction on label)													▓		
2 Med 1 C-P	Opens first pill bottle with ease (by second try)															
3 Med 1 C-P	Distributes pills from first pill bottle into correct time slots for the next 2 days (all pills & all slots indicated; days indicated)													▓		
4 Med2 N-C-P*	Reports next time second medication is to be taken correctly (based on testing time, matches direction on label)													▓		
5 Med2 N-C-P	Opens second pill bottle with ease (by second try)															
6 Med2 N-C-P	Distributes pills from second pill bottle into correct time slots for the next 2 days (all pills and all slots indicated; days indicated)													▓		

INDEPENDENCE DATA | SAFETY DATA | ADEQUACY DATA

SUMMARY SCORES

ADEQUACY SCORE → [ ]

SAFETY SCORE → [ ]

INDEPENDENCE MEAN SCORE → [ ]

Intervention Planning Based on Assessment Results

As the PASS is criterion referenced, each task can stand alone statistically. Occupational therapy practitioners only need to select those tasks that are relevant to the needs and wants of the client. This is key to a client-centered approach. Because the money management and meal preparation task series are designed to be administered as a series, practitioners can use these to ascertain clients' abilities to carry out a complex sequence of tasks independently, safely, and adequately. In addition, if there is an everyday task vital to a client's lifestyle that is not included in the 26 PASS core occupations, the task development template can be used to develop a new task. The interactive assessment strategy used in the PASS allows practitioners to identify the point of task breakdown as well as assistance strategies that result in a better functional outcome. For example, Don, an 82-year-old man, hospitalized with a major depressive episode, wants to return home, but he requires verbal and physical cues to perform meal preparation, medication management, and toileting tasks. The PASS identified the points of task breakdown for each occupation: meal preparation (monitoring the stovetop: independence, safety, adequacy); turning off the burner in a timely manner (safety); medication management (sorting his medications correctly for day and time: independence, adequacy); and toileting (management of clothing: independence, safety, adequacy). This information is valuable for intervention and discharge planning. Because Don completed other subtasks in each of the PASS tasks independently, safely, and adequately, the occupational therapist knows exactly where to focus the intervention. As Don is eager to return home and because these tasks are critical to him returning home and residing in the community, the interventions will be relevant and focused. Finally, the greatest proportion of PASS tasks consist of IADL tasks. This makes the PASS unique among functional assessment instruments because it enables practitioners to address task performance that is necessary for successful community living.

Clinical Research Using the Performance Assessment of Self-Care Skills

The PASS has been used as an outcome measure in multiple research studies of clients with mental health and cognitive impairments. In clients with depression, several studies have examined patterns of concordance/discordance between self-reported habits (does do), skills (can do), and observed task performance of daily living tasks. This line of research is important because when practitioners interview clients about daily occupations, they need to be aware of the construct about which they are asking (habits vs. skills) and whether observing the client performing a task provides more accurate data that confirms a client's self-evaluation. In a study of older women with depression, their self-reported skills were better than their observed performance, which in turn was better than their self-reported habits (Rogers & Holm, 2000), indicating a lack of concordance among the methods used to gather data about daily occupations. If self-reports are the only measures used in this population, the impact of depression on self-perceptions, performance, and habits would be missed. In another study comparing older adult controls with older adults with depression and no cognitive impairment, and older adults with depression and MCI, similar results were found for the more complex CIADLs and PIADLs. The concordance between self-reported skills and performance was close to, or less than, chance but was better for self-reported habits, especially for those with depression and MCI. No significant differences were found among the groups or methods for FM or BADLs. The authors concluded that when performance-based assessment is not possible, self-reports of habits may be more accurate than those that focus on skills (Rogers et al., 2010). In a randomized, double-blind, placebo-controlled maintenance trial of older adults with depression, with random assignment to a maintenance antidepressant and a cognitive enhancer or a maintenance antidepressant and a placebo, the PASS was used as a functional outcome measure. A marginal benefit to CIADL tasks was observed for the group taking the maintenance antidepressant and the cognitive enhancer (Reynolds et al., 2011).

Two recent studies have identified the value of the PASS for distinguishing between clients with normal cognitive functioning and those with MCI. Rodakowski et al. (2014) administered eight CIADL tasks to older adults with normal cognition and to older adults diagnosed with MCI. The eight PASS tasks were shopping, bill paying, checkbook balancing, bill mailing, telephone use, medication management, critical information retrieval, and small device repair. The eight tasks significantly discriminated between those participants with normal cognition vs. MCI, but two tasks, shopping and checkbook balancing, were the most discriminating. Thus, practitioners can administer the two most discriminating CIADL tasks and provide data to the team when there is a question about a client's cognitive status. In a pilot study of clients with amnestic MCI (a-MCI) and age- and gender-matched controls, the authors examined differences between the two groups on the self-report Patient-Reported Outcomes Measurement Information System (PROMIS) measure and the 14 CIADL tasks of the PASS. Total PASS scores were significantly lower for the group with a-MCI than for the controls. Also, the PASS adequacy scores were significantly lower. However, there were no differences between the groups on the self-report PROMIS measure. The authors concluded that the PASS CIADLs can help to distinguish subtle performance issues for those with a-MCI compared to those with normal cognition (Ciro, Anderson, Hershey, Prodan, & Holm, 2015).

The PASS has also been used as an outcome measure in several studies of clients with bipolar disorder. Gildengers et al. (2007) found decrements in executive function and cognitive speed of processing in older adults with bipolar disorder results in poorer PASS IADL performance. Further, in 2008, Gildengers, Butters, Chisholm, Reynolds, and Mulsant found that use of a cognitive enhancer with clients with bipolar disorder did not improve their cognition or IADL performance. In a study comparing older adult clients with bipolar disorder and major depressive disorder, Gildengers et al. (2012) found that although those with bipolar disorder had great cognitive decline, there were no differences in performance of PASS CIADLs between the groups. In 2013, Gildengers et al. compared older adults with bipolar disorder and a comparator group with no cognitive or mental health diagnoses at two points in time: baseline and at a 2-year follow-up. Those with bipolar disorder showed lower cognitive function and IADL performance than the comparator group at both time points, which was attributed to long-standing neuroprogressive processes in the bipolar group, compounded by normal cognitive aging. This series of studies indicates that those with bipolar disorder are at risk for performance deficits in the more complex IADLs and that the trend continues over time. Practitioners need to focus on IADL performance in clients diagnosed with bipolar disorder.

Suggested Further Research

Further outcomes research is needed with various diagnostic populations to identify those occupations for which client performance is most dependent, unsafe, and inadequate. Likewise, further outcomes research is needed with various diagnostic populations to identify those occupations for which client performance is most independent, safe, and adequate for various levels of unsupported or supported community living.

Summary

The PASS is a valid and reliable performance-based observational instrument for assessing everyday tasks necessary for living in the community. The PASS yields scores for independence, safety, and adequacy of performance. Because it is criterion referenced and each task stands alone statistically, practitioners can select to administer the total instrument, a complex series of tasks, or only those tasks relevant to the client. The use of interactive assessment when administering the PASS enables practitioners to identify the point of task breakdown as well as types of assistance that enable improvement in task performance. Self-report and proxy-report versions of the PASS are also available (Rogers et al., 2003), as are two online shopping tasks (www.shrs.pitt.edu/ot/about/performance-assessment-self-care-skills-pass; www.otiadl.net).

References

Cattell, R. B. (1966). The screen test for the number of factors. *Multivariate Behavioral Research, 1*, 245-276.

Chisholm, D. (2005). *Disability in older adults with depression.* Unpublished doctoral dissertation, University of Pittsburgh, Pittsburgh, PA.

Chisholm, D., Toto, P., Raina, K. D., Holm, M. B., & Rogers, J. C. (2014). Evaluating capacity to live independently and safely in the community: Performance Assessment of Self-Care Skills (PASS). *British Journal of Occupational Therapy, 77*, 59-63.

Ciro, C. A., Anderson, M. P., Hershey, L. A., Prodan, C. I., & Holm, M. B. (2015). Instrumental activities of daily living performance and role satisfaction in people with and without mild cognitive impairment: A pilot project. *American Journal of Occupational Therapy, 69*, 6903270020p1-p10.

Feuerstein, R., Rand, Y., & Hoffman, M. B. (1979). *The dynamic assessment of retarded performers: The learning potential assessment device—theory, instruments and techniques.* Baltimore, MD: University Park Press.

Finlayson, M., Havens, B., Holm, M. B., & Van Denend, T. (2003). Integrating a performance-based observation measure of functional status into a population-based longitudinal study of aging. *Canadian Journal of Aging, 22*, 185-195.

Gildengers, A. G., Butters, M. A., Chisholm, D., Anderson, S. J., Begley, A., Holm, M., ... Mulsant, B. H. (2012). Cognition in older adults with bipolar versus major depressive disorder. *Bipolar Disorders, 14*, 198-205.

Gildengers, A. G., Butters, M. A., Chisholm, D., Reynolds, C. F., III, & Mulsant, B. H. (2008). A 12-week open-label pilot study of donepezil for cognitive functional and instrumental activities of daily living in late-life bipolar disorder. *International Journal of Geriatric Psychiatry, 23*, 693-698.

Gildengers A. G., Butters, M. A., Chisholm, D., Rogers, J. C., Holm, M. B., Bhalla, R. K., ... Mulsant, B. H. (2007). Cognitive functioning and instrumental activities of daily living in late-life bipolar disorder. *American Journal of Geriatric Psychiatry, 15*, 174-179.

Gildengers, A. G., Chisholm, D., Butters, M. A., Anderson, S. J., Begley, A., Holm, M., ... Mulsant, B. H. (2013). Two year course of cognitive and IADL function in older adults with bipolar disorder: Evidence for neuroprogression? *Psychological Medicine, 43*, 801-811.

Gold, M. W. (1980). *Try another way training manual.* Champaign, IL: Research Press.

Goldstein, G., McCue, M., Rogers, J. C., & Nussbaum, P. D. (1992). Diagnostic differences in memory test based predictions of functional capacity in the elderly. *Neuropsychological Rehabilitation, 2*, 307-317.

Gurland, B., Kuriansky, J., Sharpe, L., Simon, R., Stiller, P., & Birkett, P. (1977). The Comprehensive Assessment and Referral Evaluation (CARE). *International Journal of Aging and Human Development, 8*, 9-42.

Haywood, H. C., Tzuriel, D., & Vaught, S. (1991). Psychoeducational assessment from a transactional perspective. In H. C. Haywood & D. Tzurial (Eds.), *Interactive assessment* (pp. 38-63). New York, NY: Springer-Verlag.

Holm, M. B., & Rogers, J. C. (1990a). Functional assessment outcomes: Differences between settings. *Archives of Physical Medicine and Rehabilitation, 71,* 761.

Holm, M. B., & Rogers, J. C. (1990b). Functional performance differences between the health care setting and the home. *Gerontologist, 30,* 327A.

Klunder, W. (2013). *Lewis Cass and the politics of moderation.* Kent, OH: Kent State University Press.

Lawton, M. P., Moss, M., Fulcomer, M., & Kleban, M. H. (1982). A research and service oriented multilevel assessment instrument. *Journals of Gerontology, 37,* 91-99.

McCue, M., Rogers, J. C., & Goldstein, G. (1990). Relationships between neuropsychological and functional assessment in depressed and demented elderly. *Rehabilitation Psychology, 35,* 91-99.

Missiuna, C. (1987). Dynamic assessment: A model for broadening assessment in occupational therapy. *Canadian Journal of Occupational Therapy, 54,* 17-21.

Pfeffer, R. I. (1987). The functional activities questionnaire. In I. McDowell & C. Newell (Eds.), *Measuring health: A guide to rating scales and questionnaires* (2nd ed., pp. 92-95). New York, NY: Oxford University Press.

Pfeiffer, E. (1975). *Multidimensional functional assessment: The OARS methodology.* Durham, NC: Center for the Study of Aging and Development.

Raina, K. D. (2005). *Disability in older women with heart failure.* Unpublished doctoral dissertation, University of Pittsburgh, Pittsburgh, PA.

Reynolds, C. F., III, Butters, M. A., Lopez, O., Pollock, G. P., Dew, M. A., Mulsant, B., … DeKosky, S. T. (2011). Maintenance treatment of depression in old age: A randomized, double-blind, placebo-controlled evaluation of the efficacy and safety of Donepezil combined with antidepressant pharmacotherapy. *Archives of General Psychiatry, 68,* 51-60.

Rodakowski, J., Skidmore, E. R., Reynolds, C. F. III, Dew, M. A., Butters, M. A., Holm, M. B., … Rogers, J. C. (2014). Can performance of daily activities discriminate between older adults with normal cognitive function and those with mild cognitive impairment? *Journal of the American Geriatrics Society, 62,* 1347-1352.

Rogers, J. C., & Holm, M. B. (2000). Daily living skills and habits of older women with depression. *Occupational Therapy Journal of Research, 20,* 68S-85S.

Rogers, J. C., & Holm, M. B. (2014). *Performance Assessment of Self-Care Skills (4.0).* Pittsburgh, PA: Author.

Rogers, J. C., Holm, M. B., Beach, S., Schulz, R., Cipriani, J., Fox, A., & Starz, T. (2003). Concordance of four methods of disability assessment using performance in the home as the criterion method. *Arthritis and Rheumatism, 49,* 640-647.

Rogers, J. C., Holm, M. B., Beach, S., Schulz, R., & Starz, T. (2001). Task independence, safety, and adequacy among nondisabled and OAK-disabled older women. *Arthritis Care and Research, 45,* 410-418.

Rogers, J. C., Holm, M. B., & Chisholm, D. (2016). Performance Assessment of Self-Care Skills (Version 4.1). Pittsburgh, PA: Author. Available at pass@shrs.pitt.edu.

Rogers, J. C., Holm, M. B., Goldstein, G., & Nussbaum, P. D. (1994). Stability and change in functional assessment of patients with geropsychiatric disorders. *American Journal of Occupational Therapy, 48,* 914-918.

Rogers, J. C., Holm, M. B., Raina, K. D., Dew, M. A., Shih, M. M., Begley, A., … Reynolds, C. F. III. (2010). Disability in late-life major depression: Patterns of self-reported task abilities, task habits, and observed task performance. *Psychiatry Research, 178,* 475-479.

Tzuriel, D., & Haywood, H. C. (1991). The development of interactive-dynamic approaches to assessment of learning potential. In H. C. Haywood, & D. Tzurial (Eds.), *Interactive assessment* (pp. 3-37). New York, NY: Springer-Verlag.

Vygotsky, L. S. (1978). *Mind in society: The development of higher psychological processes.* Cambridge, MA: Harvard University Press.

The Comprehensive Occupational Therapy Evaluation

Jennifer Allison, OTD, OTR/L
Mary P. Shotwell, PhD, OT/L, FAOTA

We should continue to be the leaders in the area of occupation and performance-based assessment.
In the area of mental health, 37 years ago Sara Brayman and colleagues developed and published the
Comprehensive Occupational Therapy Evaluation.
(Brayman, Kirby, Misenheimer, & Short, 1976)

Many of the behaviors included on this scale were identified by A. Jean Ayres 60 years ago.
(Gillen, 2013, p. 648)

The Comprehensive Occupational Therapy Evaluation (COTE) is a rating scale that provides a snapshot of a client's functioning at a particular moment in time as measured during the performance of an activity. This criterion-referenced measure was designed to show a client's progress over time in terms of behaviors observed during individual or group intervention. This scale allows the therapist to quickly document relevant information and provides an easily referenced visual aide to demonstrate client progress. Consistent with client-centered care, the COTE uses the client's behavior as the benchmark for progress rather than comparing the client to norms or cut-off scores.

Articulating the unique focus of occupational therapy in the mental health setting continues to be relevant today. The American Occupational Therapy Association ([AOTA] 2016) included in the year 2016 fiscal priorities "to clearly articulate and promote the distinct value of occupational therapy" with one area of emphasis in mental health.

History of Development

Informed by a vocational checklist developed by A. Jean Ayres (1954), the COTE was developed at a private 50-bed acute inpatient psychiatric hospital in Greenville, South Carolina in 1975 by 5 occupational therapy practitioners, a psychiatrist, and a psychologist. The majority of the patients had diagnoses that included depression, anxiety, schizophrenia, and bipolar disorder. The average length of hospitalization was

Hemphill, B. J., & Urish, C. K. (Eds.). *Assessments in*
Occupational Therapy Mental Health: An Integrative Approach,
Fourth Edition (pp. 371-382). © 2020 Taylor & Francis Group.

11 days. Most of the patients were independent in basic activities of daily living (ADLs; Brayman & Kirby, 1982).

According to Brayman (personal communication, March 15, 2016), the first objective guiding development of the COTE was to identify factors addressed by occupational therapy in the inpatient psychiatric setting. The authors wanted to articulate the unique focus of occupational therapy in this milieu to explain the domains occupational therapy addressed to the physicians, other team members, and for reimbursement. Brayman contended several different disciplines, including nursing, social work, and recreational therapy, and completed documentation on general and interpersonal behavior. The addition of task behaviors to the COTE highlighted occupational therapy's focus on performance skills and engagement in occupation.

The second objective that guided the development of the COTE was definition of the behaviors to allow the observations of different therapists in a corresponding fashion. Clearly defined parameters of the 26 behaviors, subdivided into 5 levels of performance, printed on the instrument eliminated vague descriptions and decreased misinterpretation by the reader and the recording therapist.

The third objective of the COTE was to provide a framework for reporting observations during the course of daily activities. Due to the volume of information contained within the COTE and related descriptors of performance, a checklist form was developed to concisely report the client status and to compare performance of the client over time. This enabled the therapist to "… readily explain what occupational therapy addressed to the physician, the team, and for reimbursement" (Brayman, personal communication, March 15, 2016).

The final objective informing the development of the COTE was to provide a method of recording and retrieving data. The numeric assignments demonstrated, at a glance, a daily listing of client improvement and regression in 26 different behaviors. Changes in client performance, when compared across several days, or the course of a week, provided a basis for recommendations to change of a client treatment plan, evaluated treatment efficacy, and assisted in determining discharge (Brayman, 2008).

The COTE was first published in 1976 and revised and published in 1982, 1999, and 2008 (Brayman, 2008; Brayman & Kirby, 1982; Kunz & Brayman, 1999). Some revisions were due to typographical errors and scoring parameters being inaccurately stated. It should be noted in the three book publications of the COTE scale that the versions were slightly different; thus, these authors contacted Brayman directly to ensure accuracy and intent of the version. Appendix F contains the most current version of the tool, which addresses the original intent of the tool and includes changes in the graphic layout of the tool and the scoring form.

The first edition of the COTE, published in the *American Journal of Occupational Therapy* (Brayman et al., 1976), contained a recording form and a table of evaluative scale definitions. When republished in 1982 (Brayman & Kirby, 1982), complete descriptions of all 25 behaviors assessed by the instrument were included in the text. This was the first time descriptions of the behaviors appeared. Three appendices were included in this edition: Appendix W, which served as a recording form; Appendix X, which outlined evaluation scale definitions for all three sections of the COTE; and Appendix Y, which provided evaluation scale definitions for solely the task behavior section. Under the task behavior section, two separate subsections, activity neatness and attention to detail, were both listed under one heading (activity neatness or attention to detail). This appears to better align with the scoring sheet and to highlight opposite ends of a behavioral continuum in which the therapist would only pick one of the two items to rate.

In 1999, the COTE was republished in the first edition of this book (Kunz & Brayman). At that time, an additional item, conceptualization, described as the ability to abstract, was added under general behavior. In addition, some of the behaviors were redefined, reflecting professional changes in terminology. Further, behavioral criteria were tightened to assist in interrater reliability. This publication also presented the KidCOTE, which was developed in 1995 by Kunz at the University of Texas Medical Branch at Galveston. The KidCOTE included "27 behaviors that were divided into four specific areas—general behaviors, sensory motor performance, cognitive behaviors, and psychosocial behaviors" (Kunz & Brayman, 1999, p. 267). Although some of the constructs on the KidCOTE were similar to the constructs contained in the COTE, the KidCOTE further expands its focus to include psychosocial behaviors, such as self-management skills and a sensory motor performance section. As the KidCOTE was not included in the 2008 edition of the Hemphill text and as practitioners may not have access to the 1999 edition of the text, the instrument is once again included in this edition and is available in Appendix G.

In the second edition of this text, no notable changes to the measure were made; however, a few errors in the scoring descriptors were noted by the first author of this chapter. In 2008, the grid format of the recording form was also changed and provided 8 columns to capture 4 weeks of twice weekly occupational therapy sessions on one form, which enabled the clinician to examine trends in client behavior. In 2008, Brayman introduced the connection between the *Occupational Therapy Practice Framework: Domain and Process, Third Edition* (AOTA, 2014) and the COTE.

Theoretical Basis

Although Brayman (personal communication, March 15, 2016) stated that the COTE authors did not clearly articulate a theory that guided the development of the COTE, the instrument was informed by Fidler and Fidler (1963) and the 1970 Mosey text *Three Frames of Reference for Mental Health*. Brayman contended that the COTE was consistent with the occupational behavior theory of Mary Reilly, in that task behavior affected occupational performance and well-being. Brayman asserted that the premise of the measure was to determine a degree of engagement; the occupational therapy practitioner can ascertain where the client was challenged in occupational performance. Although the measure was developed prior to the Model of Human Occupation (MOHO) development as an occupational therapy practice model, the COTE addressed the performance capacities, which is a portion of the MOHO and also consistent with client factors identified within the *Framework* (AOTA, 2014).

In terms of the relationship to the *Framework* (AOTA, 2014), the COTE addressed client factors (e.g., body functions) and performance skills that impact occupation. For example, the client with difficulty concentrating may have experienced difficulty in areas of work or education. Similarly, the client who demonstrated difficulty with decision making could have experienced problems with instrumental ADLs and work.

Upon critical examination of the *Framework* (AOTA, 2014), it appeared that three domains of the COTE (i.e., general, interpersonal, and task behaviors) fall under the client factors and performance skill areas of the *Framework*. Body functions, of the three categories encompassed within client factors, were the most relevant category to the COTE. An example of body function documented in the COTE was concentration, included in the definition of attention. Within the *Framework*, attention was listed under the category of specific mental functions. With consideration of the performance skill domain of the *Framework*, the primary focus of the COTE was on process skills as well as social interaction skills that included phrases such as heeds, initiates, regulates, and expresses emotion. To a lesser degree, the COTE assessed motor performance skills but primarily focused on the performance skill domain.

The COTE has some basis in behaviorism as it is designed to measure client behaviors that help guide intervention as well as measuring outcomes of service. The COTE does not necessarily measure occupation, but rather, precursor behaviors to occupation that may facilitate or hinder engagement. The precursors were categorized into three areas: general behavior, interpersonal behavior, and task-specific behavior.

Concepts/Constructs

In the COTE, three constructs were represented in the domains of the measure:
1. General behavior, which included a snapshot of the client's appearance and what might be termed as outward manifestations of internal regulation, such as responsibility, sense of time, alertness, arousal, and affect
2. Interpersonal behavior, such as interaction with peers, independence, and assertiveness
3. Task behavior, which addresses engagement, interest, concentration, problem solving, and, to a lesser degree, motor coordination

Psychometric Properties

The COTE scale is a criterion-referenced measure; therefore, no normative data was assumed. Clients were compared to the criterion that described each behavior, and the ultimate purpose was to use the measure to describe client behavior and to show changes in behavior (progress or regression) over time. The measure was intended to identify the magnitude of problem behaviors that affect occupational performance. As a result, a higher score was more indicative of problems on the COTE. While the tool could benefit from further research with regard to validity and reliability, much of the initial work on reliability clearly demonstrated consistency between practitioners of current relevance.

Reliability

Interrater reliability of the initial version of the COTE was determined by computing percent agreement among the ratings of five different therapists. Ratings within 2 degrees were considered acceptable, and the percent agreement for 55 patients (in an inpatient psychiatric facility) ranged from 76% to 100% and averaged 95% for the total COTE score. Percent agreement for exact agreements ranged from 36% to 84% and averaged 63%. A subsequent review of interrater reliability between 2 occupational therapists and an occupational therapy aide was conducted at a 14-bed inpatient psychiatric unit in a large general hospital. Reliability data were reported on seven cases, and agreement ranged from 96% to 100%, with an average rating of 98% agreement (Brayman et al., 1976).

Brayman (2008) noted that the COTE was used as a tool to assess the competence of occupational therapists and occupational therapy assistants in observing and documenting patient behaviors. Results demonstrated that the percentage agreement between experienced occupational therapists and novice occupational therapists was not as high as the percent agreement between experienced therapists and experienced occupational therapy assistants. Brayman discovered that the percentage of agreement between experienced occupational therapy assistants and novice occupational therapy assistants was not as high as between novice therapists and novice assistants.

While working with four Level II occupational therapy fieldwork students, one of the authors (J. A.) sought to establish interrater reliability on the COTE prior to use of the tool as an outcome measure in a community-based mental health agency. During a 2-week period, each student used the COTE during check-in and during a regularly scheduled group activity. Each day, students met with the instructor and discussed and explained rationale for specific scores. On day 1, the scores on some items were as much as 3 points apart between raters. During discussion, students shared that scoring was being conducted on the client at different times during the group. For example, one rated the client at the beginning of group session, whereas another rated the client at the end of the group, which may have impacted the client score. As a result, the student raters agreed to score clients at the same point during a group activity to ensure that ratings occurred at the same point in time. The process of scoring and discussion scores was repeated for 5 days, at which time the scores were 100% in agreement for three of four students and 90% agreement with the fourth student. As a result, the group felt confident in using the COTE as an outcome measure as part of implementing a sensory-based protocol.

Validity

Because one of the key purposes of the COTE was to measure client progress and outcomes, the initial validity research regarding the measure consisted of exploring whether the tool demonstrated changes in client behavior over time. In order to explore whether the COTE scores showed change over time, a sample of 5 cases were randomly selected from a group of 400 patients discharged from a local inpatient psychiatric facility. Total COTE scores for the first and last days in occupational therapy were compared. The scores averaged 31 at initial evaluation and 17 at discharge, and the drop in the score agreed with observations of other professionals (as per chart review) about the client's progress in the acute hospital setting. A similar review in another facility comparing initial and discharge scores showed average admission scores of 33.5, with a discharge score of 22.25 and an average change of 10.8 points (Kunz & Brayman, 1999).

Brayman and Kirby (1982) sought to confirm the utility of the COTE to monitor client progress. Collaborating with an occupational therapy student in a psychiatric unit of a medical university hospital, a patient's total COTE scores decreased from the first to the last day in occupational therapy. To ensure trustworthiness of ratings conducted each day, the student scored the patient(s) on a new form daily to avoid potential influence of ratings on the previous day. The average score for the first day of occupational therapy was 20, with a range of 0 to 28. The average decrease in scores was 11 points, with a range of 0 to 57 (Brayman & Kirby, 1982). These studies indicated the potential of the COTE to demonstrate change in client performance, although further research regarding the measure is still warranted (Brayman & Kirby, 1982).

Related Research

Table 21-1 summarizes the literature where the COTE is discussed in several capacities. First, writings about the COTE were descriptive about the measure and its administration (Brayman, 2008; Brayman et al., 1976; Brayman & Kirby, 1982; Kunz & Brayman, 1999). A second theme found in the literature mentioned the COTE in studies that surveyed therapists

Table 21-1

Summary of Literature Regarding the Comprehensive Occupational Therapy Evaluation Score

Theme/Topic	Citations	Summary/Findings
Description of the measure	• Brayman et al., 1976 • Hemphill, 1980 • Brayman & Kirby, 1982 • Kunz & Brayman, 1999 • Brayman, 2008	• All references summarize the COTE's purpose, procedures, and scoring as well as suggesting what future research should be conducted on the measure.
Survey of occupational therapists regarding assessment use in which the COTE is mentioned	• Bartlow & Hartwig, 1989 • Haglund, Ekbladh, Thorell, & Hallberg, 2000 • Mohammed Alotaibi, Reed, & Shaban Nadar, 2009 • Duncan, Munro, & Nicol, 2009	• The COTE continues to be used in the United States and in other countries. • Settings for use include mental health and geriatrics. • There is also mention of the KidCOTE use.
Use of the COTE as a comparison tool in the development of a new measure	• Margolis, Harrison, Robinson, & Jayaram, 1996 • Ralston, Bell, Mote, Rainey, & Shotwell, 2001 • Wu, Wang, Chan, & Chen, 2010 • Li, Chen, & Deng, 2012	• Comparison with other observational measures in inpatient psychiatry shows significant correlations.
Relevance of the COTE in other countries	• Australia: Bartlow & Hartwig, 1989 • England: Duncan et al., 2009 • Taiwan: Wu et al., 2010 • India: Acharya & D'souza, 2012 • China: Li et al., 2012 • Spain: Bellido, Berrueta, Sanz, Lopez, & Sanchez, 2015	• In general, the COTE is relevant for use in other countries. • Most frequently, it was listed as being adapted for use in psychiatry settings.
Use of the COTE as a descriptive or outcome measure	• Bartlow & Hartwig, 1989 • Shotwell et al., 2001 • Bickes, DeLoache, Dicer, & Miller, 2001 • Wu et al., 2010 • Chisvo, Smith, Stewart, & Thill, 2011	• In general, the COTE has significant relationships to other measures of function and has been used to demonstrate statistically significant outcomes of occupational therapy.

about which assessment tools were used (Bartlow & Hartwig, 1989; Duncan et al., 2009; Mohammed Alotaibi et al., 2009). Interestingly, several studies were in countries other than the United States, which indicated that the COTE was used internationally. A related theme to international use of the COTE was mentioned in the investigation of application of this measure with occupational therapy practice in China as well as in Taiwan (Li et al., 2012; Wu et al., 2010). There was mention of the use of the COTE in Spain (Bellido et al., 2015). Brayman (personal communication, March 15, 2016) reported recent request for permission for the COTE to be translated into Spanish for in an inpatient psychiatric facility in Mexico.

The COTE was discussed in the literature regarding use as a comparison measure when developing related assessment tools. Of particular note was discussion of the use of the COTE as a comparison measure in developing the Occupational Therapy Task Observation Scale (OTTOS) in which Margolis et al. (1996) found significant correlations between the COTE and the OTTOS. Finally, and perhaps most importantly, was discussion of the use of the COTE as a descriptive or outcome measure in occupational therapy practice (Bartlow & Hartwig, 1989; Bickes et al., 2001; Chisvo et al., 2011; Shotwell et al., 2001; Wu et al., 2010). Although the COTE was mentioned in the past 30 years as a tool used in occupational therapy, the instrument was not without critics. Acharya and D'souza (2012) noted that the instrument appeared more appropriate for acute inpatient psychiatry and that the measure did not address role dysfunction.

Clinical Application and Relationship to the *Occupational Therapy Practice Framework*

Although the COTE has existed since 1975, the purpose has not changed. The purpose of the measure was to identify behaviors that might influence functional performance. In terms of the *Framework*, the COTE measured client factors, particularly psychosocial factors that might affect occupations. While the COTE seemed to endure in applicability to acute psychiatric settings, both authors used the COTE as a tool for documentation and outcomes research in several other clinical situations.

Like many university programs, the Brenau University Occupational Therapy Program placed students in Level I and Level II fieldwork in community-based programs for persons with cognitive impairments and mental health disorders. In addition, the university placed students in nontraditional fieldwork environments with well older adults, adolescents with behavioral health concerns, juvenile justice settings, shelters for persons who have experienced domestic violence or homelessness, individuals engaged in high school transition programming, sheltered workshop programs, social programs for persons with developmental disabilities, community-based mental health programs (day programs), and residential programs for older adults. The majority of these settings do not employ occupational therapists, and although the university has faculty who assist students at these field sites, students were challenged to articulate the unique value of occupational therapy in these settings.

The COTE assisted faculty and students in articulating which behaviors may signify need for occupational therapy intervention. Examples of how the COTE was used to monitor client progress and demonstrate positive outcomes included use of the COTE as follows: (a) exploring the effectiveness of a sensory-based protocol in a day program for people with chronic, persistent mental illness; (b) demonstrating the effectiveness of occupation-based vs. a psychoeducational intervention when working in a clubhouse for people with chronic, persistent mental illness as well as a similar study working with older adults with mild cognitive impairments; (c) implementing a "summer camp" program in a residential behavioral health facility for adolescents; (d) assisting job coaches in a high school vocational transition program in the area of problem solving challenging task/work behaviors; and (e) assisting clients with task behaviors and instructing the volunteers in a socialization program for persons with developmental disabilities. In several instances, persistent use of the COTE to document client progress and outcomes led to creation of several new occupational therapy practitioner positions.

Assessment Administration

Administration of the COTE required 15 to 20 minutes and about 5 minutes to total each of the 3 domains. Optimally, the practitioner observes the client while engaged in an activity and writes notes or directly assigns scores while observing the client.

Description of Environment/ Description of Supplies/Materials Required

The COTE is a fairly unobtrusive measure and is best performed while watching a client engaged in activity. This measure was initially developed in the 1970s in an inpatient psychiatric setting where craft and activity groups were common occurrences. Both authors of this chapter have used this measure to assess clients who were engaged in verbal, educational, and task/activity groups, and both authors have found the highest yield with the COTE while the client is engaged in an activity rather than passively being involved in a classroom environment, although many of the items can be graded during these activities as well. In short, the environment for performance of the assessment is not critical; most authentic results are likely to occur while the client is engaged in some form of activity, particularly activity that involves working with other clients.

The only material needed is the COTE scoring form and a copy of the descriptors for scoring. The original format included the descriptions on the back of the form for ease in communication with other team members and payers (Brayman, 2008). The current format includes one column, which was used during data collection by the first author at a community mental health center. Another format could contain two columns and might be used for twice-weekly intervention frequency or for a pre-test/post-test in which the COTE might be done at the initial period of intervention and then at some reevaluation at a later point. The pre-test/post-test version was used by the first author at a community mental health center during the implementation of a program that explored the effectiveness of a new sensory program. The second author of this chapter has worked with young adult students in a high school transition program, and she adapted the COTE form to record student progress over a 6-week period. According to Brayman (personal communication, March 15, 2016), any of the listed formats were acceptable as long as the criteria for scoring was maintained and accurately documented.

Administration

No specific instructions for administration of the COTE exist; however, one must advise the client that documentation of performance may occur during therapist observation of behavior. The occupational therapy practitioner should take notes while observing the client engage in a task or group activity. There is no time requirement for how long one should observe a client. In general, one should observe a client long enough to score all items on the COTE to best capture a description of the client's general, interpersonal, and task behaviors.

There were no specifications regarding whether the observer who is scoring the COTE should be the same practitioner who may be leading the therapy-related activities, but according to Brayman (personal communication, March 15, 2016), the COTE was intended to be scored by the practitioner who provided intervention, although professionals have used the measure in multiple capacities. For example, during several thesis research studies conducted at Brenau University, a licensed practitioner provided the intervention while student researchers scored the COTE. Conversely, other projects included the use of licensed practitioners who scored the COTE and occupational therapy students who provided the group intervention. Regardless of how the COTE was used during the intervention, if multiple practitioners or students used the COTE in a specific setting or rated the same clients, establishing interrater reliability prior to all practitioners (or students) scoring clients was highly recommended.

Scoring

Scores for each of the 26 behavior items ranged from 0 to 4, with 0 indicating normal behavior and 4 indicating severe behavior. After assigning each item a score, the practitioner totaled the score for each domain and for the grand total. The maximum total for the 3 subscores is 104. A higher score indicated more problems. The form did not describe (or label) what the range of totaled scores would be indicated to mean (e.g., 0 to 20 indicates normal functioning). The COTE was designed to provide a snapshot of an individual client's functioning during performance of an occupation or activity. Thus, per Brayman (personal communication, March 15, 2016), "… you only rate someone according to themselves … the person was not being compared to norms, nor to anyone else …"

Intervention Planning Based on Assessment Results: Utilizing *Occupational Therapy Practice Framework* Case Studies

Barry was a 59-year-old man who regularly attended a peer support program for adults with a chronic, persistent mental illness. He enjoys walking, listening to the radio, reading the newspaper, and completing word searches and word puzzles. Barry reported that he began hearing voices shortly after graduating from high school and was subsequently diagnosed with schizophrenia, paranoid type. He has been an active participant in the occupational therapy group sessions for the past 5 years.

The COTE is used as an assessment tool for reevaluation and serves as our daily documentation of occupational therapy services and as a tool to guide intervention at the community mental health center. Barry was reassessed twice over the course of 1 year using the weekly data provided by the COTE, the Occupational Performance History Interview-II (OPHI-II), and the Toglia Category Assessment (TCA). Typically, Barry's scores on the COTE were low across all three areas. From June to November, Barry's scores on the COTE began to increase. In addition, his scores on the TCA decreased across this time span (lower numbers indicated decreased problem-solving and reasoning skills). Through interviews conducted by two different Level I students and guided by the OPHI-II, Barry reported, in June, that he was independent in occupations such as cooking breakfast foods, cleaning the house, and washing his laundry. In November, he identified cooking, cleaning, and grooming/hygiene as areas he wanted to improve.

The COTE was administered during an activity group in which the consumers made a puzzle piece collage. Barry was noted rubbing wintergreen rubbing alcohol on his head, which is a behavior he engages in when the voices are loud and demanding, was late to group, and appeared disheveled for group. He started out seated facing the others in his group, but as group continued, Barry moved his chair around so he would not have to look at the other members. During the activity, Barry required several prompts to initiate and persist in the task with other group members. He stood up several times, pulled up his shirt, and rubbed his stomach. Barry was able to place glue on magazine pictures, but the pictures were glued and extended over the puzzle piece so that his piece could not be fit into the group puzzle. When asked if he could think of a way to make the pieces fit or to rearrange the pictures, Barry repeatedly twisted the puzzle piece around without trimming the excess or rearranging the pictures. He asked the therapist twice if she thought he was smart. He then said that he could not make it work and asked the therapist to fix the piece for him. Using his question as a prompt, the therapist took the opportunity to share the COTE with Barry and showed him the areas that were assessed in the COTE.

The therapist asked Barry if he noticed any changes in his behavior or if he was having a difficult time engaging in occupations in the last several months. Barry indicated that he was not sleeping as well as the voices were out of control in his head and made it hard for him to remember to take his medications. The therapist then reviewed with Barry the sensory preference checklist he completed and also made comments on what sensory strategies she saw during group that appeared to help calm him and allow him to engage with others and complete an activity. Together, they came up with a sleep hygiene schedule that included the use of sensory strategies throughout the day to facilitate engagement in his desired occupations and roles. They also examined his wellness recovery action plan, discussed which sensory strategies he found most effective, and incorporated those into his wellness recovery action plan, within his toolkit. Several sensory items, such as a partially inflated beach ball, ankle weights, stress balls, and intensely flavored candies and gum, were provided for Barry to keep in his wellness toolkit at the center, and one was provided for home that contained relaxation CDs, an essential oil pillow spray, and a glitter calming bottle that Barry had made in group.

Results of the occupational therapy reevaluation were shared with peer support staff. Two of the three staff members were new to the center, and the results of the COTE, gathered across 6 months, provided an objective measurement of Barry's changes in occupational engagement and performance. Barry's major areas of difficulty, as identified by the COTE, included appearance, nonproductive behavior, independence, engagement, problem solving, and frustration tolerance. This, coupled with similar results on the TCA, served to informally validate the data provided by the COTE.

Suggested Further Research

Brayman and Kirby (1982) noted that further research regarding the COTE reliability and validity was warranted; however, no information is evident in the scholarly literature. The authors recommended a factor analysis of the scale and relationship to the domains and overall total is in order. In addition, further research regarding interrater reliability of the tool when used by students as well as experienced therapists was suggested.

To further explore the construct validity of the tool, several types of studies were recommended:

- Studies employing concurrent validity by comparing the COTE to other measures to ensure measurement of what was intended to be measured
- Studies that compare typical or nondisabled populations on the COTE with people with disabilities to explore whether the COTE adequately identified problems

- Studies that explored the use of the COTE in populations other than persons with mental illness (there was some indication that the measure was being used in gerontology, yet no validity studies have demonstrated that the tool was appropriate for the population)
- Exploration of possible cut-off scores potentially indicative of a person's ability to live independently or safely

Summary

Developed in 1976, the COTE served as documentation of client performance during occupational therapy services provided during group and individual intervention sessions. This allowed the therapist to capture a large quantity of information regarding client factors, performance skills, and performance patterns demonstrated by each client during the session. When combined with an occupational profile, the COTE was quite useful in guiding intervention. The COTE also provided a structured framework that was valuable when teaching students and novice therapists to observe and identify aspects of the domain of occupational therapy, such as client factors, performance patterns, and performance skills pertinent to occupational performance. The instrument provided a means of documentation of observation in an expedient and organized manner.

The COTE provided the occupational therapy practitioner with several methods for using the assessment. It can be used as a pre/post measure to record the effectiveness of certain interventions and as an outcome measure when comparing the effectiveness of two different interventions for a specific client. It is an effective way to document a client's occupational performance during a specific occupation or activity. It allowed the practitioner to look at different domains of client performance with the same instrument and for the same client multiple times throughout the same day. The COTE also allowed one to capture a client's performance over time. This can assist the occupational therapist in comparing similarities and differences to reveal patterns that may be positively or negatively impacting the client's ongoing occupational performance.

Acknowledgments

The authors are indebted to Dr. Sara Brayman for her support, feedback, and guidance during the writing of this chapter. We are also grateful for her many years of service to the profession and for her significant contributions to the field of occupational therapy.

References

Acharya, V., & D'souza, D. D. (2012). Problem identification grid: Assessment tool for acute mental health settings. *Indian Journal of Occupational Therapy, 44*, 11-14.

American Occupational Therapy Association. (2014). Occupational therapy practice framework: Domain and process (3rd ed.). *American Journal of Occupational Therapy, 68*(Suppl. 1), S1-S48.

American Occupational Therapy Association. (2016). Centennial vision for occupational therapy priorities: Boldly navigating a changing world. Retrieved from http://www.aota.org/aboutaota/get-involved/bod/2016-centennial-vision.aspx

Ayres, J. A. (1954). A form used to evaluate the work behavior of patients: A preliminary report. *American Journal of Occupational Therapy, 8*, 73-74.

Bartlow, P., & Hartwig, C. (1989). Status of practice in mental health: Assessment and frames of reference. *Australian Occupational Therapy Journal, 36,* 180-192.

Bellido, M., Berrueta, M., Sanz, V. P., Lopez, G. T., & Sanchez, A. (2015). Adaptación española de las Comprehensive Occupational Therapy Scale (COTE) para pacientes psiquiátricos. TOG (A Coruna). Retrieved from http://www.revistatog.com/num22/pdfs/original5.pdf

Bickes, M. B., DeLoache, S., Dicer, J., & Miller, S. (2001). Effectiveness of experiential and verbal occupational therapy groups in a community mental health setting. *Occupational Therapy in Mental Health, 17,* 51-72.

Brayman, S. (2008). The Comprehensive Occupational Therapy Evaluation. In B. J. Hemphill-Pearson (Ed.), *Assessments in occupational therapy mental health: An integrative approach* (2nd ed., pp. 113-125). Thorofare, NJ: SLACK Incorporated.

Brayman, S. J., & Kirby, T. F. (1982). The Comprehensive Occupational Therapy Evaluation. In B. J. Hemphill (Ed.), *The evaluative process in psychiatric occupational therapy* (pp. 211-226). Thorofare, NJ: SLACK Incorporated.

Brayman, S. J., Kirby, T. F., Misenheimer, A. M., & Short, M. J. (1976). Comprehensive occupational therapy evaluation scale. *American Journal of Occupational Therapy, 30,* 94-100.

Chisvo, M., Smith, C., Stewart, E., & Thill, D. (2011). *Effectiveness of OT interventions designed for individuals with mild cognitive impairment residing in congregate living facilities.* Unpublished master's thesis, Brenau University, School of Occupational Therapy, Gainesville, GA.

Duncan, E. A. S., Munro, K., & Nicol, M. M. (2009). Research priorities in forensic occupational therapy. *British Journal of Occupational Therapy, 66,* 255-264.

Fidler, G., & Fidler, J. (1963). *Occupational therapy: A communication process in psychiatry.* New York, NY: MacMillan.

Gillen, G. (2013). A fork in the road: An occupational hazard? (Eleanor Clarke Slagle Lecture). *American Journal of Occupational Therapy, 67,* 641-652.

Haglund, H., Ekbladh, E., Thorell, L., & Hallberg, I. (2000). Practice models in Swedish psychiatric occupational therapy. *Scandinavian Journal of Occupational Therapy, 7*(3), 107-113. https://doi.org/10.1080/110381200300006050

Hemphill, B. J. (1980). Mental health evaluations used in occupational therapy. *American Journal of Occupational Therapy, 34,* 721-726.

Kunz, K., & Brayman, S. (1999). The Comprehensive Occupational Therapy Evaluation. In B. J. Hemphill-Pearson (Ed.), *Assessments in occupational therapy mental health: An integrative approach* (pp. 259-274). Thorofare, NJ: SLACK Incorporated.

Li, N., Chen, Y., & Deng, H. (2012). Cross-sectional assessment of the factors associated with occupational functioning in patients with schizophrenia. *Shanghai Archives of Psychiatry, 24,* 222-229.

Margolis, R. L., Harrison, S. A., Robinson, H. J., & Jayaram, G. (1996). Occupational Therapy Task Observation Scale (OTTOS): A rapid method for rating task group function of psychiatric patients. *American Journal of Occupational Therapy, 50,* 380-385.

Mohammed Alotaibi, N., Reed, K., & Shaban Nadar, M. (2009). Assessments used in occupational therapy practice: An exploratory study. *Occupational Therapy in Health Care, 23,* 302-318.

Mosey, A. C. (1970). *Three frames of reference for mental health.* Thorofare, NJ: SLACK Incorporated.

Ralston, L. S., Bell, S. L., Mote, T. B., Rainey, S. B., & Shotwell, M. (2001). Giving up the car keys. *Physical & Occupational Therapy in Geriatrics, 19*(4), 59-70.

Shotwell, M., Alvarado, M. I., & Battle, J. (2001). Comparison of occupational performance measures used in adolescent mental health. Presentation (Short Course) at the American Occupational Therapy Association Conference, Philadelphia, PA.

Wu, M., Wang, T. Y., Chan, F., & Chen, S. P. (2010). Neurocognitive profiles of rehabilitation clients with schizophrenia in Taiwan. *Journal of Rehabilitation, 76,* 10-14.

22

The Independent Living Scales

Nadine Revheim, PhD, OTR/L

There's a big difference between knowing and doing. Knowing is useless without action.
(Vivik, 2015)

I have been impressed with the urgency of doing. Knowing is not enough; we must apply.
Being willing is not enough; we must do.
(da Vinci, n.d.)

Wisdom is knowing what to do next; skill is knowing how to do it, and virtue is doing it.
(Jordan, n.d.)

Every occupational therapist working in an inpatient mental health setting is aware of the importance of a valid and reliable assessment to determine an individual's capacity to function in daily living skills. Results of such an assessment are used for treatment planning, determining discharge readiness, and making recommendations regarding an appropriate fit of the disposition plan for community living. The occupational therapist is frequently the expert on the team when it comes to matching the current functional level of the individual with the expected level of functioning in the future residential context. This matching of skills and capacity for optimal functioning in a given residential setting is also true for the evaluation of outpatients who may be having difficulties maintaining the expected level of functioning and are at risk for failure and rehospitalization. Ideally, assessment within the actual setting where skills are performed is preferred, but many times, an estimate of performance is derived from performance on proxy tasks that are convenient to administer and can produce standardized results. As such, a functional capacity evaluation is the result, rather than a strict functional performance assessment. Therefore, an assessment tool that is reliable and valid, easy to administer in a variety of clinical settings, and has some predictive value for making useful recommendations for community living is essential for an occupational therapist; the Independent Living Scales (ILS) is an excellent example of such a tool.

The ILS is a semistructured interview designed to assess the likelihood of successful independent community living (Loeb, 1996). According to Loeb, the instrument was originally developed for older adults with dementia due to questions and concerns about the

- 383 -

Hemphill, B. J., & Urish, C. K. (Eds.). *Assessments in Occupational Therapy Mental Health: An Integrative Approach, Fourth Edition* (pp. 383-396). © 2020 Taylor & Francis Group.

ability to care for oneself. This assessment has been used to estimate competence of adults diagnosed with psychiatric illness, institutionalized individuals, and those with other disabling conditions and cognitive impairments. The standardization sample included a group of individuals with schizophrenia. As such, the assessment is specifically relevant for individuals diagnosed with severe and persistent mental illness. The ILS is an important assessment tool for occupational therapists to use in mental health settings, not only because of compelling psychometric properties, but because the essential purpose of the ILS is to evaluate functional capacity, which is within the purview of this mental health specialty.

A study by occupational therapists in Canada using an online survey and clinical vignettes was implemented and investigated how adults with mental illness were being assessed (Rouleau, Karyne, & Korner-Bitensky, 2015). The researchers found that the ILS was used with individuals diagnosed with depression and schizophrenia. Canadian occupational therapists reported use of the ILS for approximately 30% of the time vs. 21% of the time with those being treated in the hospital vs. those treated in community-based services, respectively. For hospitalized individuals with depression, occupational therapists reported use of the ILS 7% of the time vs. 1% of the time for depressed individuals treated within community-based services. Results of the study suggested occupational therapists have some familiarity with this standardized instrument and made decisions to use such an assessment in the clinical sample of individuals with schizophrenia who were expected to have more difficulties in community living. Less is known about the use of the ILS by occupational therapists in the United States.

Theoretical Basis

Concepts/Construct

The ILS has five subscales (Memory/Orientation, Managing Money, Managing Home and Transportation, Health and Safety, and Social Adjustment) and two factor-analyzed subscales (Problem Solving and Performance/Information). The Memory/Orientation subscale (8 questions) consisted of items that determined the individual's short-term memory and awareness of his or her surroundings. Items included orientation to time and place, recall of a brief shopping list, hypothetical doctor's appointment, and recognition of a missing object. The Managing Money subscale (17 questions) consisted of calculations, simulations of paying bills, counting change, and awareness of taking precautions with money. The Managing Home and Transportation subscale (15 questions) included items that reflected abilities in the use of telephone and public transportation and engagement in home management skills, such as arranging for household repairs. The Health and Safety subscale (20 questions) includes items that assess the awareness of taking precautions for health problems and responding appropriately to medical emergencies or potential hazards and dangers around the home. The Social Adjustment subscale (10 questions) reflects the individual's concerns and attitudes about relationships with other people.

The Performance/Information and Problem Solving factor subscales were derived from responses to all the items on the five subscales using a principal components analysis. These two-factor subscales were retained because they provide information that was not reflected in the subscales alone but, rather, can reveal patterns of functioning that can differ based on whether someone has the skills to do something (i.e., doing what you know) vs. having the judgment and ability to plan appropriate action (i.e., knowing what to do), which are two distinct contributions to successful community functioning. As such, the ILS provides an opportunity to offer a differential diagnosis of functional deficits related to community living.

The Problem Solving factor subscale is composed of 33 items that utilize information about relevant facts, as well as abstract reasoning and judgment. Items demand an understanding of what the problems might actually be as well as what the likely solutions are. Examples of problem-solving items include figuring out what to do if an unexpected visitor comes to the door late at night, how to react when lights go off in the house or one detects the smell of gas, and what the problem is with directions given to a cab driver.

The Performance/Information subscale is composed of 21 items that test the individual's general knowledge, short-term memory, and actual skills for performing simple daily tasks, such as using a telephone book and a map, making change, remembering a doctor's appointment, and writing a check or money order for the telephone or gas and electric company. This factor reflects actual knowledge or skill used to perform the tasks.

Prior to the formal assessment process and administration of the ILS protocol, there are seven screening questions related to impairments in vision, speech, or hearing that would impede the performance in the functional evaluation. By taking sensory impairment into account, the outcome on the ILS will not be confounded by general issues that could interfere with performance on instrumental activities of daily living (IADLs).

The ILS requires both a semistructured interview and task performance with the identified individual; it does not rely exclusively on self-report or report by family members or staff. It takes approximately 45 to 60 minutes to administer in its entirety and 10 minutes for scoring using easy-to-follow, standardized guidelines. If time is an issue, adaptation of the administration of the ILS is possible by using the Problem Solving factor subscale (33 items) only, which reduces the administration time to 25 minutes. This adaptation is psychometrically valid and can still be useful for its predictive value.

History of Development and Previous Versions/ Important Changes to Note in Current Version

The ILS was developed based on an earlier test, Community Competence Scale, which was also created by Loeb (Anderten, 1979; Loeb, 1983). The refinement of that prototype evaluation led to the development and standardization of the ILS, which ultimately led to its publication by the Psychological Corporation in 1996. Since its original publication, it has not been modified, but it has increasingly been used with psychiatric patients and geriatric populations. It has been cited in the literature 109 times from 1997 through 2015. Citations include studies that used the ILS to measure outcomes related to cognitive remediation intervention (Medalia, Revheim, & Casey, 2001, 2002; Tan & King, 2013); exploration of functionally meaningful measures for clinical trials (Green et al., 2011; Leifker, Patterson, Heaton, & Harvey, 2011; Mausbach, Moore, Bowie, Cardenas, & Patterson, 2009; Patterson & Mausbach, 2010); and the utility of the ILS in civil competency evaluations (Quickel & Demakis, 2013)

Psychometric Properties

Normative Data

The normative sample data was collected during 1994 and 1995. It consisted of a nonclinical group of 590 adults who were older than 65 years, along with a clinical group of 248 adults ages 17 and older, with various diagnoses that could deleteriously affect cognitive functioning.

Reliability

Reliability data for the subscales, including the factor scores and full score, are reported in the test manual for internal consistency, test-retest reliability, and interrater reliability. Alpha coefficients range from 0.72 to 0.92 across the scales, which suggests good internal reliability. The alpha coefficient is 0.86 for the Problem Solving factor and 0.88 for the full scale. Correlations between an initial administration and a second administration of the test range from $r = .81$ to $r = .94$, which suggests very good stability. The Problem Solving factor ($r = .90$) and the full scale ($r = .91$) scores are matched for stability. Interrater reliability is near perfect, with intraclass correlations ranging from 0.95 to 0.99 across all scores; the Problem Solving factor ($r = .98$) and full scale ($r = .99$) scores are equivalent.

Validity

Initial validity studies performed by the test author included content validity using a Q-sort method to ascertain that items measured what they purported to measure and a statistical method using an exploratory principal components analysis to investigate the underlying structure of the test. The results of the factor analysis suggested that items focused on problem solving and complex reasoning were distinct from items that relied on task performance and knowledge of facts. Content validity focused on associations of ILS scores on a geriatric sample with scores on assessments of intelligence (Wechsler Adult Intelligence Scale–Revised), cognition (MicroCog), and ADLs.

Construct validity was performed during test development using clinical populations that involved some form of cognitive impairment. Samples included adults with long-term psychiatric illness, dementia, traumatic brain injury, and mental retardation. For adults with major depression, there were significant differences in ILS classification for several scores (i.e., Managing Money, Health and Safety, Social Adjustment, Problem Solving, and Full Scale). For those with schizophrenia, significant differences also occurred for Managing Money, Health and Safety, Problem Solving, and Full Scale scores. Clinical samples were significantly lower than a group of independent matched controls at the 0.01 level.

Loeb (1996) found that 88% of the normative sample for the schizophrenia group fell below the standardized cut score of 50, which is associated with independent living, with a mean (standard deviation [SD]) score of 34 (12.7). In a convenience sample, Revheim (2015, unpublished data) found that 77.4% of a group of 274 individuals with schizophrenia fell below the cut score of 50 using the Problem Solving factor score only, with a mean (SD) score of 36.7 (12.3), suggesting that, across groups of individuals with schizophrenia, the majority of individuals are in need of moderate or maximum assistance to live independently in the community.

In a study that focused on the use of the Problem Solving subscale with individuals with schizophrenia and schizoaffective disorders (Revheim & Medalia, 2004b), it was found that capacity for problem solving was correlated with severity of deficits on other neuropsychological measures, such as verbal memory ($r = .65$; $p < .01$). However, it was found that daily problem-solving skills, rather than verbal memory, was a significant predictor of living status (inpatient or outpatient) in a sample of 162 persistently ill patients ($R = .34$; $p = .00001$). Therefore, the Problem Solving factor subscale of the ILS may be an important global functional measure.

In addition, it was found that when individuals with persistent mental illness were categorized according to the amount of supervision they actually received in their current living condition (i.e., maximum, moderate, minimum), ILS Problem Solving (ILS-PS) scores were significantly different across the three levels of supervision (maximum vs. moderate, maximum vs. minimum, moderate vs. minimum) when post-hoc comparisons were performed ($F = 35.5$; $df = 2$; $p = .0001$; Revheim & Medalia, 2004a). This suggests that the predictive value using cut scores on the ILS are valid for individuals with schizophrenic spectrum disorders.

Further study suggests that for individuals with serious mental illness, daily problem-solving skills measured with the ILS-PS subscale were significantly associated with negative symptoms, processing speed, verbal memory, and working memory scores. However, working memory and negative symptoms were the only significant predictors of daily problem-solving skills and account for 73.2% of the variance in ILS-PS factor subscale scores (Revheim et al., 2006). Community status (inpatient vs. outpatient) was significantly associated with daily problem-solving skills and negative symptoms. Inpatients were more impaired (lower ILS-PS factor scores and higher negative symptoms), and outpatients were less impaired (higher ILS-PS factor scores and fewer negative symptoms). However, the ILS-PS subscale scores were not related to positive symptoms. The findings provide discriminant validity for the ILS-PS factor subscale when used with this impaired population.

Sensitivity

Criterion-related validity on the ILS established cut scores to compare groups of individuals that were either dependent or independent. Three cut scores were used to determine the sensitivity (i.e., correct identification of the greatest number of individuals who are dependent and classified as moderate and low functioning) and specificity (i.e., correct identification of the greatest number of individuals who are independent and classified as moderate or high functioning).

Assessment Administration

Occupations that are assessed using the ILS include ADLs and IADLs. Client factors entail body functions (e.g., using the senses, especially as they relate to deficits in test-taking ability). Test items involve performance skills related to motor, process, and social interaction skills. Performance patterns that are evaluated include habits and routines. ILS test items presuppose aspects of cultural, personal, and social contexts and environments.

Description of Environment/ Description of Supplies/Materials Required

The ILS is administered in a quiet environment that is free of external distractions. A table and comfortable chair are needed so that the tabletop tasks can be managed with no encumbrance. It is important that the examinee develop rapport with the examiner, as it is important for the examiner to understand the cultural context of the examinee.

Figure 22-1. Sample of an ILS kit.

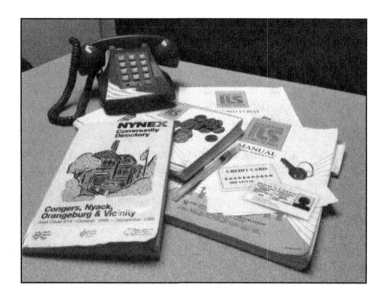

The ILS test kit can be ordered directly from Pearson Education, Inc. at http://www.pearsonclinical.com. Occupational therapists meet the qualification level (B) set by the test publisher. Cost of the complete kit is approximately $350, and replacement record forms can be ordered in packages of 25 for approximately $70. The kit includes a manual; 25 record forms; a stimulus booklet; and a pouch with a facsimile of a driver's license, key, and credit card. Examiners will need to provide a phone, telephone book, envelope, scratch paper, pen, pencil, some money, and a stopwatch (Figure 22-1).

Administration

Guidelines for standardized procedures for test administration are explicitly outlined in the test manual (Loeb, 1996). General directions are given for the order of administration, starting with the screening items. A script to introduce the purpose of the evaluation is provided, and item instructions for all the subscales include detailed information for adaptation of items given the results of the screening, as well as sample answers that are acceptable.

Scoring

Each of the 70 questions on the ILS is assigned a 0-, 1-, or 2-point answer that is delineated in the testing manual with descriptions of acceptable answers. Test protocol booklets provide an easy-to-follow method of scoring so that the sum of all items in each of the five subscales as well as the two-factor subscales are tallied and then transferred to a summary page where these raw scores are converted to standard scores (SS) using tables in the appendices of the manual. SS are obtained for all seven subscales and the full scale. Then the SS are plotted, which creates a graph so that scores are viewed within three categories (i.e., high, moderate, low) for each subscale; factor and full scale scores are separated. High scores for subscales (i.e., SS between 50 and 63) suggest that an individual can live independently in the community; high scores are associated with good functional capacity and predict success in the community without supervision. Moderate scores for subscales (i.e., SS ranging from 40 to 49) suggest that an individual requires moderate levels of supervision to be successful in the community; moderate scores are associated with limitations on independent community functioning. Low scores for subscales (i.e., SS from 20 to 39) suggest than an individual requires maximum levels of supervision to be successful in the community; low scores are associated with severe deficiencies, which interfere with successful community living. The Total Score follows the same rubric in terms of high (i.e., SS ranging from 100 to 121), moderate (i.e., SS ranging from 85 to 99), and low scores (i.e., SS ranging from 55 to 84), with numerical values that are greater because these scores are commensurate with the summed score of the five subscale scores, not including the factor subscales, which are parsed from the actual subscales. The resulting graph within the testing protocol is a pictorial summation of relative strengths and weaknesses, which can be used for interpretation of results and as a guide for treatment planning as per the direction provided in the test manual.

Case Studies

To demonstrate the utility of the ILS for treatment planning for occupational therapists, the 2×2 grid in Figure 22-2 offers an additional perspective of how the scores can be interpreted when the two-factor subscale scores are viewed independently of the five factor subscales or total scores. High/moderate scores vs. low scores on the Performance/ Information subscale can be compared with high/moderate scores vs. low scores on the Problem Solving subscale for any given individual. Essentially, one can use the grid to delineate whether an individual is having more difficulty with skills (i.e., the doing what you know) or with conceptual reasoning (i.e., the knowing what to do). This becomes a helpful template to determine whether someone could benefit from skills training or whether there is a cognitive limitation that might require remediation, compensation, or adaptation of reasoning/problem-solving demands inherent in task performance. The relative strengths and weaknesses using these two subscale dimensions and two levels of performance create four possible subtypes: the capable individual, the unskilled individual, the unaware individual, and the dependent individual (see Figure 22-2).

The capable individual has the skills and the conceptual reasoning to perform IADLs to be successfully integrated into the community. The capable individual may not require occupational therapy intervention to improve performance but might benefit from guidance toward appropriate choices that will optimize or maintain good functioning. For example, the capable individual knows that a budget is essential to tracking information for money management and can implement the budget with appropriate bookkeeping methods, such as checkbook reconciliation, and remembers when to put these skills into action so that bills are paid in a timely manner.

The unskilled individual lacks the necessary skills to optimally perform IADLs in the community. The skill deficiencies may be a result of inexperience and lack of opportunities to practice the skills or could be related to the lack of prior exposure or training. This individual demonstrates the capacity for reasoning and problem solving, which is necessary to learn and to apply the learned skills; therefore, this individual would benefit most from a skills training program. For example, the unskilled individual understands that paying bills on time is the responsible thing to do and that an organizational system would be helpful but cannot add/subtract bills and expenses or fill out money orders because of unfamiliarity with procedures. Skills development and mastery is the focus of skills training treatment.

Figure 22-2. Relationships of two distinct ILS factor subscales.

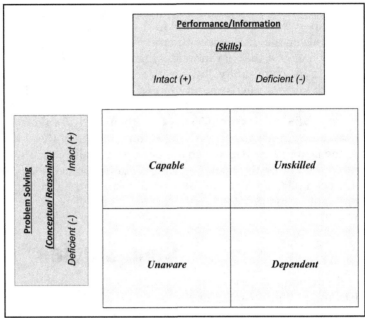

The unaware individual may be able to demonstrate actual skills on demand but lacks the awareness, reasoning capacity, or problem solving in real-life situations that occur within the course of daily living to implement the skills he or she has or understand what is needed if he or she does not have the skills. This individual cannot self-monitor or plan appropriate actions, and as such, it may be harder for this person to learn new skills. In addition, this individual is at risk for accidents or failure in the community if he or she does not have adequate supervision. For example, the unaware individual does not comprehend that there are ways to safeguard money, is careless and unpredictable, and may be ignorant of steps to take for self-protection, but might be able to count change correctly, enumerate prices from a menu, or tell what percentage of his or her spending is for self-care items. Strategies that focus on self-monitoring and self-evaluation, such as checklists or decision trees, can be taught to the individual to compensate for poor planning or lack of anticipation of consequences This will help ensure safety and good judgment when performing expected functional skills in the community.

The dependent individual is limited by deficient reasoning and reduced skills to perform daily living tasks in the community. The individual cannot conceive what is necessary nor can he or she perform what is required. For example, the dependent individual does not understand what monetary resources are accessible or how much money is required for a budget, nor does he or she know how to count money, write out money orders, or perform mathematical operations when shopping. This individual may lack the sufficient amount of awareness to learn the skills and to apply them appropriately without ongoing assistance, which suggests that the individual will require maximum supervision in the community. Please refer to Table 22-1 for information regarding the test subscales and level of functioning

Specific case studies are presented in a manner that displays the differential patterns of performance useful for interpretation and recommendations for occupational therapy treatment planning.

Table 22-1

Intact Skills (Doing), Intact Reasoning (Knowing)

Subscales	High Functioning	Moderate Functioning	Low Functioning
Memory/orientation	61		
Managing money	57		
Managing home and transportation	59		
Health and safety	50		
Social adjustment			22
Problem solving	55		
Performance/information	55		
Full scale standard score	100		

High functioning: subscale SS = 50 to 63, full scale SS = 100 to 121, independent in community; moderate functioning: subscale SS = 40 to 49, full scale SS = 85 to 99, moderate supervision in community; low functioning: subscale SS = 20 to 39, full scale SS = 55 to 84, maximum supervision in community.

Case Study 1: The Capable Individual

Mr. P. is a 49-year-old White man diagnosed with schizophrenia. He was transferred from the county jail after violation of an order of protection with threatening behavior toward a family member. Mr. P. has a history of suicide attempts but is currently stable on medication for psychotic behavior and disorganization.

Mr. P. graduated high school and has worked in a variety of retail stores in the stockroom. Mr. P. stopped working so he could become a caregiver for an ill relative; he currently receives Social Security disability. He likes to rest, relax, sleep, read, draw, and listen to music. Mr. P. has no friends and has conflicted relationships with his family.

According to results on the ILS, Mr. P. demonstrates awareness of safety hazards around the home, anticipates problems in daily living, and plans appropriate and responsible actions. He has good money management and travel skills. Mr. P. has the knowledge and skills necessary to perform tasks commensurate with successful performance in the community; however, his poor social adjustment poses difficulties for his independent living. Mr. P.'s poor interpersonal functioning, isolative behavior, and difficulties with creating and maintaining social support can be addressed in occupational therapy groups, such as Role Playing for Better Communication, Social Cognition, and Exploring Community Resources, where his interests in art and music can be used to help him locate a social network in his neighborhood as part of his discharge planning.

Case Study 2: The Unskilled Individual

Mr. T. is a 25-year-old man who has been diagnosed with schizoaffective disorder, bipolar type. This is his first long-term hospitalization following seven brief inpatient admissions at the county hospital. Mr. T. lives at home with his parents who advocated for this longer hospitalization with the goals of an improved medication regimen, further assessment, and counseling regarding the nature of his illness, which he has denied. He

Table 22-2

Deficient Skills (Doing), Intact Reasoning (Knowing)

Subscales	High Functioning	Moderate Functioning	Low Functioning
Memory/orientation	60		
Managing money	61		
Managing home and transportation		41	
Health and safety		47	
Social adjustment		48	
Problem solving	50		
Performance/information		44	
Full scale standard score	100		

High functioning: subscale SS = 50 to 63, full scale SS = 100 to 121, independent in community; moderate functioning: subscale SS = 40 to 49, full scale SS = 85 to 99, moderate supervision in community; low functioning: subscale SS = 20 to 39, full scale SS = 55 to 84, maximum supervision in community.

does not drive because he has had minor accidents, and the family will not pay for his car insurance. Mr. T. will return to his home after discharge. Please refer to Table 22-2 for an example of the scoring for the unskilled individual.

Mr. T. graduated high school and went directly to a community college. He is an office technology major and has six more credits to take to complete his associate's degree. He has worked with the family in a landscaping business and hopes to continue to do so when he graduates. He has maintained relationships with a few of his high school friends but is starting to think that they do not have much in common anymore, which is stressful. He has never had a girlfriend but does not express interest in romantic pursuits. He spends all his time writing in his journals, some of which are rants against the "powers that be." He does not do any chores around the home because his family does not trust him because he has made errors that have been costly (e.g., leaving water running in a plugged sink, breaking the alarm system, causing a fire in the vent of the clothes dryer). There is a lot of tension and unexpressed anger between the parents and son, and the family has been attending family support groups.

According to the results on the ILS, Mr. T. has intact problem-solving capacity for independent living but lacks many of the skills that would be instrumental in carrying out daily tasks. Mr. T. claims he has not had practice in some of the areas related to money and home management because he has not been responsible for any of them. The occupational therapist has scheduled a family meeting to discuss household chores and responsibilities that Mr. T. can be taught so that he can be share tasks that will give him specific skills that are lacking (e.g., reviewing procedures for operating appliances in the home, budgeting and food shopping, keeping the log of household expenses). Mr. T. will also be referred to the Community Resources group so that he can learn about transportation schedules for traveling on local buses so that he will be less dependent on his parents for car transport to his appointments and classes.

Table 22-3

Intact Skills (Doing), Deficient Reasoning (Knowing)

Subscales	High Functioning	Moderate Functioning	Low Functioning
Memory/orientation	54		
Managing money			37
Managing home and transportation	50		
Health and safety			28
Social adjustment			37
Problem solving			28
Performance/information		47	
Full scale standard score			83

High functioning: subscale SS = 50 to 63, full scale SS = 100 to 121, independent in community; moderate functioning: subscale SS = 40 to 49, full scale SS = 85 to 99, moderate supervision in community; low functioning: subscale SS = 20 to 39, full scale SS = 55 to 84, maximum supervision in community.

Case Study 3: The Unaware Individual

Mr. G. is a 40-year-old Black man with a diagnosis of schizophrenia and polysubstance dependence. He has a history of mental illness since childhood and has served time in prison for sexual violence. After release from prison, he briefly lived in a board and care home, but after threatening another resident, he violated parole and was returned to prison and was ultimately transferred to a state hospital setting for further treatment. Mr. G.'s tenure in the community has been marked by aggression, interpersonal conflict, and noncompliance with medication and after care services. The social worker reports he was recently accepted into an apartment program with minimal supervision. Mr. G's scores are presented graphically in Table 22-3.

Mr. G. had been in special education classes and left school after completing the seventh grade. He reports that he is a hands-on learner. He worked as a housekeeper but was not able to keep his jobs because of confrontation with supervisors and coworkers. He claims he can cook for himself and can perform repetitive household chores. His hobbies include listening to music, dancing, and socializing. He practices good self-care and hygiene. He has contact with his family and a positive relationship with a peer advocate. He frequently gets special privileges and favors from others and becomes argumentative when he does not get what he wants.

According to the results on the ILS, Mr. G. has limited knowledge in the areas of health, safety, and money management while demonstrating strengths in general orientation and matters pertaining to the home and transportation. Notably, Mr. G.'s social adjustment is impaired (as expected by his history), and his problem-solving capacity is fair (which may account for many of his community failures). While Mr. G. demonstrates evidence of some intact skills necessary for independent living, he would benefit from the Life Skills Group, which uses real-life occupations and provides multiple training opportunities so that he could focus specifically on math and money matters. Mr. G. also lacks the judgment and awareness related to appropriate decision making; he would be at risk for failing in a setting unless there were maximum levels of supervision. Therefore, he would benefit from the Have a Problem—Let's Solve It Group for exposure to and practice of compensatory strategies to avoid common risks and dangerous situations because of his poor reasoning. Mr. G. should be counseled about his inability to live independently as he desires because he requires additional skills that can be learned with repetition and practice. More importantly, he requires assistance in areas where he lacks judgment because he is essentially unaware of his potential for error and negative consequences. His ability to accept this level of supervision may hinge on his readiness to reach out to others and to be dependent on their advice, which he does when it is suitable for his needs. Being able to see that his needs may be greater than his limited perception will be critical in his acceptance of a suitable discharge plan, which might be a residential setting with on-site supervision that the apartment program does not provide.

Case Study 4: The Dependent Individual

Ms. M. is a 48-year-old woman diagnosed with schizophrenia who attended school through the 11th grade, when her parents died, and she became psychotic. Her premorbid functioning was marginal since she had difficulty with school and had no friends. After a long hospitalization, she never worked and lived with family. Until recently, she had the support of her five siblings, who, after multiple hospitalizations, felt they could no longer care for her and asked the social worker to place her in a board and care home. While living there for 2 years prior to this hospitalization, she demonstrated poor grooming, isolative behavior, and other negative symptoms of schizophrenia, such as anhedonia and anergia, despite her compliance with medications. She was frequently a victim of her peers, who borrowed money and begged her for cigarettes. She did not attend any psychosocial programming but has maintained relationships with family who frequently take her home for weekend passes.

According to the results on the ILS, Ms. M. demonstrates moderate deficits in memory/orientation and social adjustment but has severe limitations in areas related to instrumental living, which require skill and judgment. She was unable to understand hypothetical situations or predict consequences of actions, and even with concrete tasks, she was unable to perform tasks related to money management, safety, filling out forms, and following directions. Ms. M. may have difficulty learning new skills due to her deficient information processing and inability to monitor her actions. She will require maximum supervision for her safety as she begins to engage in a recovery-oriented program, which will offer her opportunities for GED preparation as requested and socialization with peers while engaging in artistic occupations in the Living Museum. Ms. M's scores are shown in Table 22-4.

Table 22-4

Deficient Skills (Doing), Deficient Reasoning (Knowing)

Subscales	High Functioning	Moderate Functioning	Low Functioning
Memory/orientation		42	
Managing money			34
Managing home and transportation			35
Health and safety			23
Social adjustment		48	
Problem solving			30
Performance/information			34
Full scale standard score			73

High functioning: subscale SS = 50 to 63, full scale SS = 100 to 121, independent in community;
moderate functioning: subscale SS = 40 to 49, full scale SS = 85 to 99, moderate supervision in community;
low functioning: subscale SS = 20 to 39, full scale SS = 55 to 84, maximum supervision in community.

Suggested Future Research

There may be some limitations on the generalizability of some of the items used for performance on some of the subscales. For example, some of the ILS tasks may be dated (e.g., cell phones are replacing landlines, banking may be done online rather than using checkbooks), and knowledge may be influenced by region or cultural group found across the United States (e.g., money orders can be obtained in stores in urban areas, not just at the bank or post office; some individuals believe having a gun in the house ensures personal safety). On the other hand, it may be interesting to develop updated versions of some tasks to perform concurrent validation of new items with the old items (e.g., looking up a phone numbers using a computer search rather than a using a telephone book). Hypothetically, the ability to plan responses and use procedural knowledge and reasoning would be constant, but it could be that experience and exposure to instrumental skills of daily living are more important than the foundational skill set that is assumed by this approach to functional testing.

The ILS may also have limitations regarding its cultural sensitivity or global applicability. Several research studies have explored the relevance of specific functional outcome measures in different countries and cultures and have included the ILS, both from a qualitative perspective when examining modifiability of tests items (Gonzalez, Rubin, Fredrick, & Velligan, 2013) and from a quantitative viewpoint while investigating the adaptability of diverse measures (Velligan et al., 2012). Research that focuses on independent living standards from a global perspective using the ILS could capture the attention of occupational therapists that practice worldwide and have affiliations through the World Federation of Occupational Therapists.

As the ILS did not emerge specifically from an occupational therapy frame of reference, it may be interesting to associate the results of the ILS with other occupational therapy evaluations focusing on IADLs. This type of research would establish construct and criterion-related validity across evaluations and allow for comparisons with additional clinical populations, such as traumatic brain injury.

Summary

The ILS is an important evaluation tool for occupational therapists working in mental health settings because of its utility in assessing performance and reasoning capacity using proxy IADLs and queries about issues and problems that one encounters. It is a standardized and well-designed instrument that assists the clinician in predicting the likelihood of success for community living and in making recommendations for the level of supervision and assistance needed in order to maintain functioning. The ILS has been used in research and findings suggest that it has validity for its intended purpose. Case studies demonstrate how results of the evaluation are helpful in determining patterns of relative strengths and weaknesses and indications for treatment that focuses on skills training, cognitive support, or compensatory strategies to optimize functioning.

References

Anderten, P. (1979). *The elderly, incompetency, and guardianship.* Unpublished master's thesis, St. Louis University, St. Louis, MO.

da Vinci, L. (n.d.). Famous Leonardo da Vinci quotes. Retrieved from http://www.leonardodavinci.net/quotes.jsp

Gonzalez, J. M., Rubin, M., Fredrick, M. M., & Velligan, D. I. (2013). A qualitative assessment of cross-cultural adaptation of intermediate measures for schizophrenia in multisite international studies. *Psychiatry Research, 206,* 166-172.

Green, M. F., Schooler, N. R., Kern, R. S., Frese, F. J., Granberry, W., Harvey, P. D., … Marder, S. R. (2011). Evaluation of functionally meaningful measures for clinical trials of cognition enhancement in schizophrenia. *American Journal of Psychiatry, 168,* 400-407.

Jordan, D. S. (n.d.). David Starr Jordan quotes. Retrieved from https://www.goodreads.com/author/quotes/223714.David_Starr_Jordan

Leifker, F. R., Patterson, T. L., Heaton, R. K., & Harvey, P. D. (2011). Validating measures of real-world outcome: the results of the VALERO expert survey and RAND panel. *Schizophrenia Bulletin, 37,* 334-343.

Loeb, P. A. (1983). *Validity of the community competence scale with the elderly.* Unpublished doctoral dissertation. St. Louis University, St. Louis, MO.

Loeb, P. A. (1996). *ILS: Independent Living Scales manual.* San Antonio, TX: The Psychological Corporation, Harcourt, Brace, Jovanovich, Inc.

Mausbach, B. T., Moore, R., Bowie, C., Cardenas, V., & Patterson, T. L. (2009). A review of instruments for measuring functional recovery in those diagnosed with psychosis. *Schizophrenia Bulletin, 35,* 307-318.

Medalia, A., Revheim, N., & Casey, M. (2001). The remediation of problem-solving skills in schizophrenia. *Schizophrenia Bulletin, 27,* 259-267.

Medalia, A., Revheim, N., & Casey, M. (2002). Remediation of problem-solving skills in schizophrenia: Evidence of a persistent effect. *Schizophrenia Research, 57,* 165-171.

Patterson, T. L., & Mausbach, B. T. (2010). Measurement of functional capacity: A new approach to understanding functional differences and real-world behavioral adaptation in those with mental illness. *Annual Review of Clinical Psychology, 6,* 139-154.

Quickel, E. J., & Demakis, G. J. (2013). The Independent Living Scales in civil competency evaluations: Initial findings and prediction of competency adjudication. *Law and Human Behavior, 37,* 155-162.

Revheim, N., & Medalia, A. (2004a). The Independent Living Scales as a measure of functional outcome for schizophrenia. *Psychiatric Services, 55,* 1052-1054.

Revheim, N., & Medalia, A. (2004b). Verbal memory, problem-solving skills and community status in schizophrenia. *Schizophrenia Research, 68,* 149-158.

Revheim, N., Schechter, I., Kim, D., Silipo, G., Allingham, B., Butler, P., & Javitt, D. C. (2006). Neurocognitive and symptom correlates of daily problem-solving skills in schizophrenia. *Schizophrenia Research, 83,* 237-245.

Rouleau, S., Karyne, D., & Korner-Bitensky, N. (2015). Assessment practices of Canadian occupational therapists working with adults with mental disorders. *Canadian Journal of Occupational Therapy, 82,* 181-193.

Tan, B. L., & King, R. (2013). The effects of cognitive remediation on functional outcomes among people with schizophrenia: A randomised controlled study. *Australian and New Zealand Journal of Psychiatry, 47,* 1068-1080.

Velligan, D. I., Rubin, M., Fredrick, M. M., Mintz, J., Nuechterlein, K. H., Schooler, N. R., … Dube, S. (2012). The cultural adaptability of intermediate measures of functional outcome in schizophrenia. *Schizophrenia Bulletin, 38,* 630-641.

Vivik, R. (2015). Twelve best kept secrets of successful business people. Retrieved from http://fortune.com/2015/03/13/12-best-kept-secrets-of-successful-business-people/

Kohlman Evaluation of Living Skills

Linda Kohlman Thomson, MOT, FAOTA

Authentic and satisfying lives are not built on what someone says are our weaknesses; they do not emerge from fixing what someone decides is wrong with us. We construct a satisfying life when we explore our interests, gravitate toward what we are good at, come to know what settings honor our way of being and which people "get us." When we take a strengths-based approach, we create a tapestry that weaves together the person's interests, skills, and support systems into environments that will support the person's idea of a satisfying life. We foster competence and motivation when the people we serve recognize that we "get them."
(W. Dunn, personal communication, 2015)

The fourth edition of the Kohlman Evaluation of Living Skills (KELS) by Kohlman Thomson (2016), with contributions from Robnett, is an occupational therapy evaluation designed to determine a person's ability to function in basic living skills and to make recommendations for living situations to promote safety, health, and independence. This chapter will provide information on the fourth edition of this assessment from administration to utilization for intervention and discharge planning. A case study is provided for increased understanding of this measure and the utilization within occupational therapy.

The administration of the KELS combines the use of interview and task performance. Assessment administration is easy to learn and can be administered in a short period of time, usually in approximately 45 minutes. The KELS is an appropriate choice for evaluation of basic living skills in settings where time is limited for the development of an intervention and discharge plan. Required equipment for administration of the assessment can be easily assembled and transported. The KELS Score Form was designed to be easy to read and to communicate the results of the assessment effectively. In the KELS fourth edition, 13 living skills are tested in 5 areas: Self-Care, Safety and Health, Money Management, Community Mobility and Telephone, and Employment and Leisure Participation. The KELS provides an occupational therapist with valuable information to be able to make recommendations for living situations that allow clients to function as independently as possible. It provides critical information to match a living environment with a person's strengths, enabling the person to live safely in the least restrictive

Hemphill, B. J., & Urish, C. K. (Eds.). *Assessments in Occupational Therapy Mental Health: An Integrative Approach, Fourth Edition* (pp. 397-405). © 2020 Taylor & Francis Group.

environment possible. The KELS is not a comprehensive evaluation of living skills, but it does provide, in a short amount of time, a significant amount of information about a person's ability to function and perform basic living skills.

Theoretical Basis

Concepts/Construct

When the KELS was first developed in 1978, the assessment did not relate to a specific model of occupational therapy. The KELS was created from an immediate need to have a tool to assess the activities of daily living (ADLs) for clients in a short-term inpatient psychiatric unit. Since that time, various theoretical models have developed in occupational therapy. The KELS is most closely aligned with the Person-Environment-Occupation Model of Occupational Performance (Law, Cooper, Strong, Stewart, Rigby, & Letts, 1996) because the assessment is focused on the interaction of the person, the environment, and the occupation. The interaction of the environment with the person and the occupation affects the success of a person's occupational performance. The KELS helps to identify an environment that supports a person to be safe, healthy, and as independent as possible.

The inability to perform daily living skills is often a factor that may cause an individual to seek treatment. The KELS helps identify a person's areas of strength and those areas in which assistance is needed. In an article about motivation, White (1959) discussed the intrinsic need for individuals to deal with the environment. White (1959) stated that if a person could interact effectively with the environment, his or her sense of competency and satisfaction would be increased. Motivation involves the satisfaction that occurs in successful experiences with the environment. ADLs are all ways in which individuals interact with and control the environment. The KELS helps to match people with environments in which success can be experienced, thereby increasing satisfaction, motivation, and a sense of independence. These are all factors of health for an individual.

History of Development and Previous Versions/ Important Changes to Note in Current Version

The KELS was developed in 1978 at Harborview Medical Center in Seattle, Washington. The chapter author was the only occupational therapist working on a locked inpatient psychiatric unit and needed to evaluate clients in a short period of time to plan discharge. At the time, there were no occupational therapy assessments that addressed this need. Since that time, four editions of the KELS have been published. Each edition had minor changes until the fourth edition was published in 2016.

The following key concepts have driven the development of the KELS:

- The length of time to administer the KELS needed to be no more than 45 minutes for most clients. There are many settings in which an occupational therapist has little time to address the appropriate living environment for a client. This is true for many mental health or behavioral health settings. Therefore, skills such as medication management were never included due to the length of time needed to evaluate this living skill. This does not mean that medication management is not an important skill; rather, it is just not part of the KELS.

- The KELS needed to be easy to learn to administer. The manual was structured so that an occupational therapist can learn to administer the assessment within a short period of time, typically a few sessions. With the limited resources of time and energy, competency needed to be quickly achievable.
- The results of the KELS needed to be easily communicated. Health care professionals have very limited time to review data regarding clients. Therefore, the KELS Score Form is structured so that the information may be processed quickly by a client or any person involved in the care of the client.

The KELS was structured to primarily address the living skill demands present in the culture of the United States; however, the assessment has been used in some foreign countries. Even though the KELS was originally created for use in a short-term inpatient psychiatric unit, with numerous changes in the delivery of health care services and aging of the population, the applicability of the KELS in other intervention settings has grown dramatically. The assessment is an excellent tool for use with the older population. The assessment assists the treatment team, client, and family members in determining the most appropriate living environment for the person to live as independently and safely as possible. Occupational therapists may also use the KELS in acute care hospitals where the therapists are frequently asked to assist in discharge planning and are given very little time to provide the information.

In some states, the KELS has been used within the legal system in court for the determination of commitment and in gravely disabled cases. The KELS is an appropriate assessment for individuals who have cognitively disabling conditions, such Alzheimer's disease, dementia, or brain injury. In settings with a long length of stay, the KELS may not be the best living skills assessment to use, because the individual's financial, transportation, work, and leisure resources have typically dramatically changed due to the long length of stay at the facility.

In the fourth edition, several notable changes were made to update the KELS. The updates were made to more effectively address the many ways people currently access and use different types of telephones, different methods of obtaining telephone information, and the different ways of completing financial transactions. The total number of items was reduced from 17 to 13. An electronic banking option was added to the Money Management section so that a person's ability to perform banking tasks electronically could be evaluated. The Safety pictures were updated. Some items, such as Budgeting, were removed, and other items were modified. Due to significant changes in the fourth edition throughout the manual, it is critical for practitioners to review the new edition closely to ensure each item is administered correctly.

In the fourth edition, a cumulative score is no longer computed. Each individual item is scored. The occupational therapist uses clinical judgment to make recommendations for the most appropriate living situation based on the abilities of the client and the support the client needs to be the most successful in the community. This is a very important change and facilitates the occupational therapist's ability to analyze the strengths of an individual with unique living environments and available support in the community. The KELS Score Form includes the following sections: Areas of Concern and a Summary for making specific living situation recommendations.

Psychometric Properties

A variety of studies were conducted on the first three editions of the KELS. By 2015, three studies were completed on the fourth edition of the KELS. All of these studies further established the reliability and validity of the assessment. Relatively small sample sizes (typically 50 or fewer clients) were used in most of the studies, and many were completed about 30 years ago. Many of the studies were conducted in completion of a master's program. Some of the results were made available to the author; however, many of the studies reside with universities and were not in research publications. As a result, significantly more research needs to be conducted on the KELS, and data need to be made readily available. To assist with this, a website has been created to communicate with interested researchers and occupational therapists (www.kelseval.com).

Reliability

In all of the studies examining the reliability of the KELS (first and second editions), the interrater reliability was in the acceptable to high range from 74% to 98% (Ilika & Hoffman, 1981b; Kohlman McGourty, 1987; Tateichi, 1985).

Validity

Validity studies were conducted comparing the KELS to the Global Assessment Scale (Ilika & Hoffman, 1981a) and to the Bay Area Functional Performance Evaluation (Kaufman, 1982). Results that addressed assessment validity were favorable using the first and second editions. A concurrent validity study was conducted with individuals living in a halfway house and living independently (Tateichi, 1985). These results were viewed as positive because they demonstrated an expected difference in daily living skills between the two groups. The results were significant ($p < .001$), with $U = 47$. Several predictive validity studies were conducted. The results from these studies were mixed, and each study had limitations related to the research design (Kohlman McGourty, 1987; Morrow, 1985).

In one study, researchers found a trend toward false positives. Some clients scoring independently on the KELS item of basic knowledge of the transit system were not able to perform the task independently in the natural environment (Brown, Moore, Hemman, & Yunek, 1996). While this is a concern, the KELS is meant to be administered using all of the items. The KELS was not designed for the individual items to be tested in isolation.

In 2007, Brenau University students completed two master's theses entitled *Kohlman Evaluation of Living Skills Revision: Practitioner and Client Contributions* (Bowra, Joyce, Romeyn, & Todd, 2007) and *Revision of the Kohlman Evaluation of Living Skills: Money Management Section* (Bennett, Shah, Sweigart, & Szczupak, 2007). The results of these studies supported the need to update the KELS and provided the chapter author and Robnett with specific ideas utilized in the creation of the fourth edition. In another Brenau University master's thesis entitled *Concurrent and Predictive Validity of the Revised Kohlman Evaluation of Living Skills* (Cinquemano, Gajjar, & Martin, 2009), the KELS revision created by the students was compared to the Milwaukee Evaluation of Daily Living Skills (MEDLS) and to the third edition of the KELS. This student's version of the KELS and the third edition of the KELS showed a significant correlation with the MEDLS. In addition, research supported that the Mini-Mental State Evaluation (MMSE) score correlated with scores on both versions of the KELS and the MEDLS.

Two additional studies have examined the validity of the KELS in the past. Zimnavoda, Weinblatt, and Katz (2002) administered the KELS to 92 Israelis in various living situations. Concurrent validity was assessed by comparing the KELS scores to the Functional Independence Measure, the Routine Task Inventory–Expanded, and the MMSE (Folstein, Folstein, & McHugh, 1975). Spearman correlations were reported as high. For example, the correlation between the KELS and the MMSE was $r = -.76$ ($p < .001$).

Burnett, Dyer, and Naik (2009) assessed 92 clients referred for *geriatric self-neglect* and 100 community controls to establish convergent validity levels between the KELS and other cognitive measures that were expected to perform similarly. Again, the correlation between the KELS and the MMSE scores was moderate and negative ($r = -.508$; $p < .001$). The researchers concluded that the KELS was a "pragmatic clinical assessment" but also concluded that further research was needed. Robnett et al. (2015) used the KELS as a comparison measure with a home safety screen (Safe at Home) with a small population of adults with acquired brain injuries. As expected, the correlation between the Safe at Home and the KELS was moderate and negative (Spearman's rho = $-.529$; $p = .002$). These studies demonstrated that the KELS has value as a tool to measure basic living skills as it is intended and can be used to supplement information about clients based on scores from other cognitive measures.

In the process of developing the fourth edition, several methods were used to contribute to the content validity. Content validity refers to the opinions of experts (in this case, experienced occupational therapists) with regard to the power of an instrument's test items to operationalize or capture the construct of interest (Kielhofner, 2006). In a session at the 2011 American Occupational Therapy Association annual conference in Philadelphia, Pennsylvania, approximately 40 attendees all agreed that the KELS needed to be updated, but that its structure and overall purpose were still valuable for clinical decision making. Kohlman Thomson and Robnett then developed an online survey focused specifically on the features of the third edition KELS tool and the broad needs of clinicians who assessed independent living skills. The results from 408 occupational therapists indicated that each segment of the KELS was still valued and valid but that a few sections needed significant updating (e.g., safety pictures, phone use, bill paying) and that most sections needed at least minor modifications. Kohlman Thomson and Robnett scrutinized the expert clinician comments when the fourth edition of the KELS was designed.

Content validity was further examined through a beta testing process of the draft of the fourth edition of the KELS in 2014. Thirty-four therapists from 18 different states completed a total of 211 KELS test forms and follow-up surveys. The surveys were used for assessing an aspect of content validity of the draft of the fourth edition of the KELS. Changes were made in the final version of the tool based partially upon expert feedback. The most significant proposed changes were in bill paying (e.g., the addition of optional online banking as requested by survey respondents) and updates to safety photos.

Assessment Administration

The KELS is composed of 13 living skill items in 5 areas of occupations, including Self-Care, Safety and Health, Money Management, Community Mobility and Telephone, and Employment and Leisure Participation. During the administration of the KELS, information is gained about a number of client factors even though they are not specifically tested. Some of these are mental functions, such as higher-level cognitive function, attention, memory perception, thought, and orientation. Information is also obtained about a client's visual and hearing functions and a client's ability to read and write. This information is not scored; however, it is noted on the KELS Score Form.

Interview and task performance are used to assess the living skills of the client. All of the questions, tasks, and supplies are designed to simulate the local environment of the client. The ideal would be to assess clients in their natural living environments; however, in most cases, this is not possible. Therefore, using the simulations in the KELS provides valuable information to be used in discharge, placement, and intervention planning. In the administration section of the manual, information provided includes the method used, necessary equipment, specific administration directions, procedures, and how to score each item. There are separate chapters with specific information on how to assemble the equipment and the necessary forms, labels, and cards. All of the equipment may be assembled in a zippered pouch, box, or notebook to enable it to be easily transported and maintained. Forms may be copied from the manual or from the flash drive included. A telephone (cell or landline) and an electronic device, such as a tablet, notebook, or computer, may be needed. Some forms must be customized to the local area or to the current date when administered. It is critical for the specific administration directions to be followed in order to maintain the reliability and validity of the KELS. The instructions may seem very simple, but they are structured to not lead the client and to be easily understood by clients of varying educational levels. It is important to not provide feedback during the administration process.

Independent and Needs Assistance are the two scoring categories of the KELS. Specific scoring criteria are given for each of the 13 items. The scoring criteria are designed to indicate the minimum standards required to live independently in the community. Independent is defined as the level of competency required to perform the basic living skill in a manner that maintains the safety and health of the individual without direct assistance of other people. For special situations in which the client does not score within the scoring criteria given, the terms "Not Applicable" and "See Note" are used. These terms should be used as infrequently as possible. When they are used, explanations need to be stated on the KELS Score Form.

In the first three editions of the KELS, a composite score was figured and used to decide if a person could live independently or not. In the fourth edition, no composite score is calculated. After the administration of all of the items and detailing any of the client factor areas of concern, the therapist will complete the Summary using clinical judgment. The Summary includes two sections. Section 1 identifies the ability of the client to live alone or the assistance needed, including the specific areas in which assistance is needed and who will provide the assistance. In Section 2 of the Summary, the therapist recommends the best living situation to promote the safety, health, and maximum level of independence for the client. The occupational therapist must use the information gained during the administration of the KELS and any other pertinent information about the client in the process of making the final living situation recommendations.

Intervention Planning
Based on Assessment Results

The KELS is designed to be used in the evaluation process with a client. Depending on the setting and the client's strengths, needs, and wants, information gained from the KELS may be used to design an intervention plan. The KELS is most often used in settings where the client is evaluated and there is limited to no opportunity for further occupational therapy intervention at that site. Even if occupational therapy intervention is not appropriate for the setting where the administration of the KELS occurred, the KELS may identify areas such as occupations, mental functions, and process skills that would be appropriate for intervention in another setting. Financial management, leisure exploration, and participation are some of the occupations that may be identified as appropriate for occupational therapy intervention.

The main purpose of the KELS is to provide information to make recommendations regarding the level of assistance that could be needed by a client and an appropriate living situation to support the client. Because the KELS has only two scoring categories, Independent and Needs Assistance, the assessment does not measure change in the acquisition of living skills. When an intervention plan is implemented, change could be better addressed by assessments that go more in-depth into the evaluation of specific living skills.

Case Study

JR is a 38-year-old man with a diagnosis of bipolar disorder. JR has been living alone in an apartment for the past 3 years and has not been employed for the past 10 years. His family checks in with him via phone or a visit at least every 2 to 3 days. In a call 3 weeks ago, JR's mother noticed that JR's speech appeared to be more pressured with increased speed and loudness in his voice. She then called or visited every day. After a couple of weeks of the family members checking on him frequently, they all had concerns about his ability to care for himself. He was sleeping very little, and during a visit, his family noticed that he had recently purchased many items from a local sporting goods store. JR was very animated in his gestures, was pacing, and his speech was very rapid and loud. JR admitted that he had stopped taking his medications. JR willingly went to the emergency department with his mother and father and was admitted to the inpatient behavioral health unit.

After a week on the unit, JR was stabilized on his medications, and his symptoms of bipolar disorder were significantly decreased. The occupational therapist was asked to administer the KELS to help JR, his family, and his health care providers determine the most appropriate living situation for JR when he would be discharged from the unit. The administration of the KELS took 45 minutes, and the occupational therapist presented the team, client, and family with the results. JR scored Needs Assistance in the following areas (occupations):

- Identification of appropriate action for sickness, accidents, and emergencies
- Payment of bills
- Obtain and maintain source of income
- Leisure activity involvement

In addition, the following Areas of Concern, or client factors and performance skills, were identified for JR:

- JR was able to read and write.
- While completing forms and following directions, he had difficulty staying on task.
- JR was oriented and made no memory errors on the KELS.
- No assistance had been provided for his basic self-care that day.

- In the Summary, the occupational therapist made the assessment that JR appeared to be able to be safe and meet his basic needs while living alone with the following assistance provided during the week or month:
  - At a minimum of once per day, a family member would FaceTime with JR to monitor his mood and behavior more regularly. The call would include a question about his medication compliance.
  - During a weekly visit, JR's mother would pay his bills and monitor his finances.
  - JR would attend a community-based treatment center where he would be assigned a case manager and would attend sessions at least three times a week.

The occupational therapist recommended that JR could return to living in his apartment alone if he had the assistance as described and that he was compliant with the program. JR, his family, and the health care providers were all in agreement of this discharge plan.

Suggested Further Research

Additional research needs to be done on the fourth edition of the KELS to further establish validity and reliability of this edition of the assessment. In addition, a comparison of the results of the KELS to the results of other cognitive and living skill evaluations needs to be completed. Predictive validity studies are needed with a variety of populations to determine how accurately the KELS predicts over time. These can be difficult to design and complete. Isolating living skills as the only changing variable is next to impossible over an extended period of time, especially when the client populations of interest may lead very unstable lives. Studies to investigate the feasibility of adding back a composite score would be helpful in the future development of the KELS. In the future, collaborating and sharing research studies, particularly those done as part of master's and doctoral programs, will be easier via the KELS website (www.kelseval.com).

Summary

The KELS is a valuable assessment tool for occupational therapy practitioners. It is helpful when trying to match a person's strengths with a living environment that will promote safety, health, and maximum independence. Because it requires very little set-up and can be done in a short amount of time, it is extremely useful in settings where there is limited time available to make this type of assessment. The KELS may be used in a variety of settings with many client populations. The KELS has proven to be an essential assessment tool for occupational therapy practitioners and occupational therapy programs.

References

Bennett, B., Shah, V., Sweigart, B., & Szczupak R. (2007). *Revision of the Kohlman Evaluation of Living Skills: Money management section.* Unpublished master's thesis, Brenau University, Gainesville, GA.

Bowra, L. M., Joyce, K. D., Romeyn, J. A., & Todd, A. (2007). *Kohlman Evaluation of Living Skills revision: Practitioner and client contributions.* Unpublished master's thesis, Brenau University, Gainesville, GA.

Brown, C., Moore, W. P., Hemman, D., & Yunek, A. (1996). Influence of instrumental activities of daily living assessment method on judgments of independence. *American Journal of Occupational Therapy, 50,* 202-206.

Burnett, J., Dyer, C. B., & Naik, A. D. (2009). Convergent validation of the Kohlman Evaluation of Living Skills as a screening tool of older adults' ability to live safely and independently in the community. *Archives of Physical Medicine and Rehabilitation, 90,* 1948-1952.

Cinquemano, K., Gajjar, A., & Martin, J. (2009). *Concurrent and predictive validity of the revised Kohlman Evaluation of Living Skills.* Unpublished master's thesis, Brenau University, Gainesville, GA.

Folstein, M., Folstein, S. E., & McHugh, P. R. (1975). "Mini mental state." A practical method for grading the cognitive state of patients for the clinician. *Journal of Psychiatric Research, 12,* 189-198.

Ilika, J., & Hoffman, N. G. (1981a). *Concurrent validity study on the Kohlman Evaluation of Living Skills and the Global Assessment Scale.* Unpublished manuscript.

Ilika, J., & Hoffman, N. G. (1981b). *Reliability study on the Kohlman Evaluation of Living Skills.* Unpublished manuscript.

Kaufman, L. (1982). *Concurrent validity study on the Kohlman Evaluation of Living Skills and the Bay Area Functional Performance Evaluation.* Unpublished master's thesis, University of Florida, Gainesville, FL.

Kielhofner, G. (2006). *Research in occupational therapy: Methods of inquiry for enhancing practice.* Philadelphia, PA: F. A. Davis.

Kohlman McGourty, L. (1987). *Predictive validity of the Kohlman Evaluation of Living Skills.* Unpublished manuscript. Seattle, WA.

Kohlman Thomson, L., & Robnett, R. H. (2016). *The Kohlman Evaluation of Living Skills* (4th ed.). Bethesda, MD: American Occupational Therapy Association, Inc.

Law, M., Cooper, B., Strong, S., Stewart, D., Rigby, P., & Letts, L. (1996). The Person-Environment-Occupation Model: A transactive approach to occupational performance. *Canadian Journal of Occupational Therapy, 63,* 9-23.

Morrow, M. (1985). *A predictive validity study of the Kohlman Evaluation of Living Skills.* Unpublished master's thesis, University of Washington, Seattle, WA.

Robnett, R. H., Bliss, S., Buck, K., Dempsey, J., Gilpatric, H., & Michaud, K. (2015). Validation of the Safe at Home Screening with adults who have acquired brain injury. *Occupational Therapy in Health Care, 30,* 16-28.

Tateichi, S. (1985). *A concurrent validity study of the Kohlman Evaluation of Living Skills.* Unpublished master's thesis, University of Washington, Seattle, WA.

White, R. W. (1959). Motivation reconsidered: The concept of competence. *Psychological Review, 66,* 297-333.

Zimnavoda, T., Weinblatt, N., & Katz, N. (2002). Validity of the Kohlman Evaluation of Living Skills (KELS) with Israeli elderly individuals living in the community. *Occupational Therapy International, 9,* 312-325.

24

Work-Related Assessments
The Worker Role Interview, Work Environment Impact Scale, and Assessment of Work Performance

Brent Braveman, PhD, OTR/L, FAOTA

In order that people may be happy in their work, these three things are needed: they must be fit for it; they must not do too much of it; and they must have a sense of success in it.
(Ruskin, n.d.)

Occupational therapy practitioners help people live life to its fullest by helping them to engage in desired roles, such as the worker role, through the performance of meaningful and purposeful occupations. Work is one of seven areas of occupation identified in the *Occupational Therapy Practice Framework: Domain and Process, Third Edition* (American Occupational Therapy Association [AOTA], 2014). In the *Framework*, areas of work-related occupation are identified and include employment interests and pursuits, employment seeking and acquisition, job performance, retirement preparation and adjustment, and volunteer exploration and participation. Occupational therapy's involvement in work-related practice can be traced back to the roots of the profession and the moral treatment era when harsh treatments, such as regular bleeding and being placed in chains, were replaced by with involvement in occupations including agriculture, tailoring, shoemaking, and sewing (Ross, 2007). Several others have provided detailed descriptions of the evolution of work-related practice in the United States through the 1800s and 1900s (Braveman, 2012; Gordon, 2009; King & Olson, 2009).

Today, occupational therapy practitioners provide work-related interventions in a wide variety of settings across the globe. Examples of such settings include preemployment screening, alternative employment for persons with developmental disabilities, transitional services for adolescents and young adults, supported employment in mental health, employer consultation for job and ergonomic analysis and compliance with the Americans with Disabilities Act, onsite services in the workplace, vocational habilitation settings for people who need to develop work skills, and vocational rehabilitation programs in clinics and in the workplace to help people return to work (Braveman, 2012).

Hemphill, B. J., & Urish, C. K. (Eds.). *Assessments in Occupational Therapy Mental Health: An Integrative Approach, Fourth Edition* (pp. 407-432). © 2020 Taylor & Francis Group.

Occupational therapy practitioners in work-related practice utilize numerous assessments focused on discrete areas that support work performance, such as vision, cognition, physical ability, or person-environment fit. Many of these assessments rely on related knowledge from disciplines such as neurology or psychology rather than knowledge based in the occupational therapy paradigm and are developed from occupational therapy–specific conceptual practice models or theories. Relatively few work-related assessments are explicitly based on occupational therapy knowledge, and the most commonly used are derived from the Model of Human Occupation (MOHO; Kielhofner, 2008). Each of these assessments has been used with a variety of populations, including in areas of mental health practice.

The MOHO has been widely utilized in work programs and has guided research on injured and disabled workers (Bejerholm & Areberg, 2014; Braveman, 2001; Désiron, Donceel, de Rijk, & Van Hoof, 2013; Kielhofner, Braveman, Baron, Fisher, Hammel, & Littleton, 1999; Kielhofner, Braveman, Finlayson, Paul-Ward, Goldbaum, & Goldstein, 2004; Lee & Kielhofner, 2010). Three MOHO assessment tools, the Worker Role Interview (WRI), Work Environment Impact Scale (WEIS), and Assessment of Work Performance (AWP) have been developed for work-related contexts and studied internationally (Braveman et al., 2005; Moore-Corner, Kielhofner, & Olson, 1998; Sandqvist, Lee, & Kielhofner, 2010). The WRI assesses psychosocial factors that influence work performance, the WEIS assesses workplace conditions that impact the worker, and the AWP assesses a worker's observable work-related skills. All three instruments can be used as independent tools but can also be administered simultaneously when therapists and patients want to look more closely at the full range of factors that may be affecting job performance. The purpose of this chapter is to introduce these instruments, including their development and administration, and demonstrate their application through case studies.

Historical Context

In the second half of the 20th century, programs designed for the rehabilitation of injured workers were primarily based on a functional limitations approach. Within this approach, a biomechanical model was widely used in work rehabilitation programs that focused on work capacity or work hardening. These programs simulated the physical demands of a job, building on analyses of work tasks and sites. Patients engaged in tasks designed to enhance their physical capacity to perform a specific job (Bettencourt, Carlstrom, Brown, Lindau, & Long, 1986; Matheson, Ogden, Vilette, & Schultz, 1985).

With time, research indicated that by focusing only on physical limitations for work, the full range of problems faced by persons with disabilities was not addressed (Frederickson, Trief, Van Beveren, Yan, & Baum, 1988; Waddell, 1987). For example, severity of injury in persons with low back pain only partly predicted work disability, while socioeconomic and job-related factors accounted for a larger portion of the variation in outcomes (Waddell, 1987). Interviews at the initiation of work rehabilitation and work prognosis by an experienced team were shown to be better predictors of return to work than biomechanical variables (Frederickson et al., 1988). Consequently, it was recognized that the biomechanical approach overlooked aptitudes, interests, and vocationally relevant skills (Matheson et al., 1985; Waddell, 1987).

The WRI grew out of this context. It was intended to supplement the biomechanical approach by examining psychosocial factors influencing injured or disabled workers. Later, the WEIS was developed to focus more specifically on the work environment of a worker in a specific job, and most recently, the AWP was developed as a complementary assessment focusing on work-related skills.

Table 24-1

The Relationship of Model of Human Occupation Components to Predictive Factors in Return-to-Work Studies

Model Constructs	Model Components	Related Factors Commonly Investigated as Predictive of Return to Work
Volition	Personal causation	• Level of perceived disability • Perceived control over environment • Educational level • Perception of fault for injury • Age
	Values	• Gender • Culture
	Interests	• Job satisfaction prior to injury
Habituation	Roles	• Work status at time of study (light duty vs. nonworking)
	Habits	• Time at job prior to injury • Attendance record at work prior to injury
Performance capacity	Objective	• Nature and severity of injury • Surgery history • Diagnosis
	Subjective	• Perceived level of pain
Environment	Social groups	• Supervisor interaction • Peer interaction • Work environment/stress

The Model of Human Occupation

The WRI, WEIS, and AWP were designed to reflect key concepts from the MOHO, as well as evidence about factors that influence work outcomes in injured or disabled workers. Braveman (1999) reviewed research literature on factors associated with return to work and success at work and organized the factors according to the basic constructs of MOHO. As shown in Table 24-1, most factors that influence return to work can be grouped into the primary theoretical components of MOHO.

MOHO considers the personal and environmental factors that impact a person with a disability. In the context of work, MOHO directs clinicians to consider workers' motivation vis-à-vis work (volition), how workers pattern their everyday lives (habituation), the capacity for work (performance capacity), and how the environment allows and inhibits participation in work (environmental impact).

Volition includes a worker's:

- Values, or the importance and worth one attaches to work
- Interests, or the satisfaction and enjoyment experienced while working
- Personal causation, which is reflected in thoughts and feelings about capacity for work and effectiveness in the workplace

Habituation refers to the semi-autonomous patterning of behavior that structures an individual's life. Habituation is the function of (1) habits, which are tendencies to automatically respond and perform in consistent ways in familiar situations; and (2) roles, which incorporate socially or personally defined status with associated attitudes and expectations for behavior. For the worker, habits regulate how time is spent and how work is done. How a person has internalized the worker role will influence how one engages with others and completes work tasks. Moreover, a person's other life roles can either support or detract from work.

Performance capacity refers to underlying abilities that enable persons to engage in occupation. Performance capacity is not directly assessed in the WRI. Consequently, appropriate work capacity assessments or other functional assessments should be administered along with the WRI when there is any question about work capacity.

The MOHO also considers the impact the environment has on a worker and his or her performance. Impact refers to whether the environment provides resources to support the worker or obstacles that constrain the worker's ability to meet demands. The physical features of an environment include spaces in which the worker acts and objects the worker comes across at work. The social features of an environment include social groups, of which the worker is a part, and occupational forms, which refer to the tasks that the worker must perform.

The MOHO emphasizes that a person's volition and habituation are shaped by culture. This model also emphasizes that the physical and social environments are largely products of culture. Thus, anyone using the MOHO should be aware of how cultural factors influence workers and their context. In order to ensure cultural relevance, MOHO assessments are tested across cultures and languages, and this is also true of the WRI and WEIS.

The Worker Role Interview
Theoretical Basis

The WRI is based on the MOHO and was initially developed by Velozo, Kielhofner, and Fisher (1998). As described earlier, MOHO conceptualizes work behavior as influenced by volition, habituation, performance capacity, and the environment (Kielhofner, 2008). The MOHO's subsystem of performance capacity does not feature as much in the WRI as it focuses more on the worker's perception of his or her capacities rather than actual objective ability.

History of Development and Previous Versions/ Important Changes to Note in Current Version

The WRI was updated in 2005, with a key change being the addition of two new interview formats. Each format is intended for one of three different target groups: (1) injured workers hoping to return to a specific job, (2) patients with longstanding illness or disability who have been out of work for a long time or have limited work history, and (3) patients who may or may not need vocational training. This last interview format combines the WRI with the Occupational Circumstances Assessment Interview and Rating Scale (OCAIRS; Forsyth et al., 2005). The OCAIRS is used to gather general occupational information, and if it emerges that the patient has the possibility of considering work, then the therapist has the opportunity to incorporate necessary WRI questions. If not, then the OCAIRS can be completed alone. This combined format was developed by occupational therapists who were working with patients in a community mental health context and who were charged to identify whether the patient had vocational potential or needs. The OCAIRS is a MOHO-based interview that collects data on 12 major areas: roles, habits, personal causation, values, interests, skills, short-term goals, long-term goals, interpretation of past experiences, physical environment, social environment, and readiness for change.

The questions in all WRI formats are designed to gather information that will provide a holistic picture of the individual's potential as a worker and were developed to broadly represent types of concerns that rehabilitation therapists have about their patients. The content areas of the recommended questions are different for each target group and concern their specific background and experience.

When completing the ratings for the WRI, the therapist can choose one of three different versions of a rating form. The three forms vary in detail and are selected according to the rater's proficiency and knowledge of WRI. The general rating scale form is for the expert WRI rater, because it only contains definitions of the 4-point scale (Figure 24-1). The specific rating scale form is generally for an experienced WRI rater; however, a novice rater who has studied the manual carefully or who uses the manual as a resource when completing the ratings may also use the general rating scale. This scale defines each content area, each item, and has guidelines in the manual on how to score the patient on the items. The criterion-rating guide form presents the scale in detail, with criteria that serve as a guide to making the rating. This form is helpful to use when becoming acquainted with the WRI and with therapeutic reasoning based on the MOHO in a work rehabilitation context. The descriptive criteria provided on this form can serve as a checklist of areas of occupational functioning that the therapist should consider in assessing the patient and beginning treatment planning.

Psychometric Properties

Forsyth et al. (2006) examined the psychometric properties of the WRI scale and determined that the items are valid across ages, diagnoses, and culture and effectively measure a wide range of persons. Data were collected from 21 raters on 440 participants from the United States, Sweden, and Iceland and were analyzed using a many-faceted Rasch model. The authors found that most items of the scale worked effectively to measure the underlying construct for which the WRI was designed. In addition, the items were ordered from least to most of the underlying construct as expected. The scale validly measured 90.23% of the participants, who varied by nationality, culture, age, and diagnostic status. The scale's items distinguished participants into approximately three different strata and were appropriately targeted to the participants. Of the 21 raters, 17 used scale in a valid manner.

Reliability

A series of studies of the WRI indicate that it is a dependable assessment. Biernacki (1993) found it to have high test-retest reliability and high total interrater reliability. Velozo (1993) found initial evidence that the 17 WRI items comprised a unidimensional construct of psychosocial capacity for work. In a subsequent study, Velozo et al. (1999) found that 15/17 items worked together to measure unidimensional construct in a group of 119 workers with low back pain. Two work environment items, boss and work settings, did not

Worker Role Interview Rating Form

Initial Evaluation	Discharge Evaluation
Name of client:	Name of therapist:
Date of birth:	Date of assessment:
☐ Client is rated relative to his/her previous job.	☐ Client is rated relative to return to work in general.

Strongly Supports	Supports	Interferes	Strongly Interferes	Not Applicable
SS	S	I	SI	N/A
Strongly supports client returning to job	Supports client returning to job	Interferes with client returning to job	Strongly interferes with returning to job	Not applicable or not enough information to rate

					Brief comments that support ratings
Personal Causation					
1. Assesses abilities and limitations	SS	S	I	SI	N/A	
2. Expectation of job success	SS	S	I	SI	N/A	
3. Takes responsibility	SS	S	I	SI	N/A	
Values					
4. Commitment to work	SS	S	I	SI	N/A	
5. Work-related goals	SS	S	I	SI	N/A	
Interests					
6. Enjoys work	SS	S	I	SI	N/A	
7. Pursues interests	SS	S	I	SI	N/A	

Figure 24-1. Blank WRI rating form. (Reprinted with permission from the Model of Human Occupation Clearinghouse.)

Worker Role Interview Rating Form (continued)						
Personal Causation						
8. Appraises work expectations	SS	S	I	SI	N/A	
9. Influence of other roles	SS	S	I	SI	N/A	
10. Work habits	SS	S	I	SI	N/A	
11. Daily routines	SS	S	I	SI	N/A	
12. Adapts routine to minimize difficulties	SS	S	I	SI	N/A	
13. Perception of work setting	SS	S	I	SI	N/A	
14. Perception of family and peers	SS	S	I	SI	N/A	
15. Perception of boss	SS	S	I	SI	N/A	
16. Perception of co-workers	SS	S	I	SI	N/A	

Figure 24-1 (continued). Blank WRI rating form. (Reprinted with permission from the Model of Human Occupation Clearinghouse.)

work well with the other items. A later study of a refined WRI scale with environmental items that were reworded to emphasize workers' perceptions showed that all but one item, perception of boss, worked well to constitute a measure of psychosocial capacity for work (Velozo, 1993).

Validity

Ekbladh, Haglund, and Thorell (2004) investigated the predictive validity of the WRI in a 2-year follow-up study of patients attending an insurance medicine investigation center in Sweden. Of the 17 WRI items, 5 predicted return to work and 3 were components of the content personal causation area. These results emphasize the importance of considering the individual's beliefs and expectations of effectiveness at work when assessing patients' work abilities and planning for rehabilitation.

Two studies in Sweden and Iceland examined the psychometric properties of translated versions of the WRI utilizing the Many-Facets Rasch Measurement approach (Fenger & Kramer, 2007; Haglund, Karlsson, Kielhofner, & Lai, 1997). The Swedish study examined patients with psychiatric disabilities, while the Icelandic study included patients with various disabilities. Both studies provided evidence that the translated WRI was valid and culturally relevant. Forsyth et al. (2006) conducted a study of psychometric properties of the WRI rating scale across 3 countries (i.e., Iceland, Sweden, the United States) on 440 participants. The results suggested that 13 items of the scale worked effectively to measure psychosocial capacity for work. The four environmental items appeared to relate more to the environment than to the individual, as might have been expected. The scale validly measured 95% of the participants, who varied by nationality, culture, age, and diagnosis.

More recently, Lohss, Forsyth, and Kottorp (2012) investigated the psychometric properties of the WRI with a psychiatric population in the United Kingdom. Data were collected from 34 psychiatric clients rated by 7 occupational therapists. Rasch analysis was used to examine scale validity, validity of therapists' rating patterns of clients, rater consistency, precision of client measurement, and the scale's aptitude in detecting different ability levels. The authors concluded that all items except one demonstrated acceptable goodness-of-fit to the Rasch model. More than 90% of clients fit the model, and the scale detected five ability levels.

Assessment Administration
Area of Occupation/Performance Skills/ Performance Patterns/Client Factors Assessed

The WRI focuses on the individual's psychosocial/environmental component of work, including paid employment and volunteer work. Performance skills are considered only in general as they influence the client's perception of abilities, limitations, and expectation of success in work. The assessment addresses the performance patterns of habits and routines related to work and the client factors of values and beliefs. Each of these areas is assessed specifically in relation to the context of work. The environment is also considered as it affects the client's perception of the physical work environment, the influence of family and peers, coworkers and bosses, and the organization.

Description of Environment/ Description of Supplies/Materials Required

The WRI is conducted via a semistructured interview process and can be performed in any setting that is quiet and distraction free enough to allow the assessor and the client to engage in the interview. The WRI can typically be completed in 30 to 60 minutes, although it may be conducted over multiple sessions if necessary.

No special materials are needed other than the administration manual, which includes the rating forms and directions. Less experienced practitioners may find that taking limited notes during the interview provides for more accurate scoring, although practitioners are cautioned to not allow note taking to interfere with being totally present during the interview.

Administration

A manual is available that describes, in detail, the background of the WRI, administration procedures, recommended questions, scoring instructions, rating scale, and case studies (Braveman et al., 2005). There are 16 items on the 10.0 version of the WRI rating scale form (see Figure 24-1).

There are five basic steps involved in WRI administration procedures:

1. Preparing for the interview, when the therapist collects preliminary data from the patient's record and decides whether the WRI is appropriate for the patient.
2. Conducting the interview as a conversation, where answers to questions and the patient's emotional responses are monitored along with the inquiries made.
3. Determining or referring to underlying work capacity and/or skill, because the therapist is asked to make a judgment about whether the patient's appraisal of his or her own abilities is realistic. This requires the therapist to have some baseline for comparison. This baseline can come from informal observation, but more typically it is from standardized testing or reports of others on the patient's underlying capacities or skills, such as concentration, strength, endurance, and range of motion.
4. Preparing evaluation scoring and comments by copying the WRI rating form and rating guidelines or the WRI criterion rating guide from the appendix in the manual.
5. Using the WRI for discharge evaluation and to measure change.

Scoring

The 4-point WRI rating scale includes consideration of how each factor represented in the items influences the patient's likelihood of returning to or succeeding at work. The ratings are: strongly supports (SS), supports (S), interferes (I), and strongly interferes (SI). If there is not enough information to rate the item or the item is not applicable, there is an option to indicate the item is not applicable (N/A). A brief comment supporting each rating is recommended as it can help when writing a report. When the ratings are completed, they provide a profile of the patient's strengths and weaknesses. This profile is particularly helpful in clarifying multiple factors that influence the patient's potential for achieving rehabilitation success or succeeding in community adaptation. This information can be important in decisions about providing services, placement, necessary supports, discharge planning, and so on.

Intervention Planning Based on Assessment Results

The WRI can assist in planning intervention to promote occupational performance by helping to identify the relative influence of client factors including personal causation (values and interests) and performance patterns, including roles and habits, and aspects of contexts, and environment. By combining the WRI with other assessments focused on performance skills, the contribution of a client's motor, process, and social interaction skills can be identified. Assessment processes, such as the use of a functional capacity evaluation, may also provide deeper insight.

Case Study

David is a 44-year-old man living in a large urban city. He has been living with HIV/AIDS for 10 years. On the advice of his physician, David left work and applied for private disability through his employer shortly after his first significant HIV-related illness and after being informed that he had progressed to a clinical definition of AIDS. After 6 years of unemployment, David sought counseling from a case manager at a community-based health center and was referred to the occupational therapist who ran a return-to-work program at the center.

The WRI was administered to David to assess his potential for return to work in his field of information technology (IT) or in a new profession. The scores for David are shown in Figure 24-2, and the following qualitative information was gathered in the interview.

David felt as though he barely got through his day-to-day activities and described everything that he did as requiring great effort. He had little energy to complete activities outside of his home and reported becoming socially isolated after having lost contact with most of his friends. He was confident about his work habits but was also positive that his skills were out of date and that the knowledge gap that had evolved during his unemployment would be very difficult to overcome. He had lost confidence in his own capabilities and could not see any solution to his problems.

David was proud of the work he had done in the past and was able to identify many specific accomplishments. He described being embarrassed to be on disability and had very little confidence about his interpersonal skills and his abilities to interact effectively with coworkers, customers, or a boss.

David's habits were ordered, with reasonably satisfying routines, before his major illness. However, he described that after he became ill, his habits and routines began to fall apart and that it become more difficult for him to attend to responsibilities at home. He spent much of his time on his computer playing games and "surfing the internet" with no specific goal. His primary social interactions were with medical and social personnel during his visits to the community health center.

The WRI interview revealed that David had both strengths and weaknesses related to work. His greatest liability was that he had lost control over his situation and confidence in himself and his capabilities. David had loved his job and remembered working with pride when he was employed full time. Without work, David perceived himself as a less valuable person. The occupational therapist thought David's motivation to work might be rekindled through exposure to current innovations and opportunities in his field of IT and began discussions with David about volunteer activities and online communities he might join. David and his occupational therapist also spent time on strategies to more

Worker Role Interview Summary Form

Name of client: DAVID
Name of therapist: BRENT
Client date of birth: ___
Purpose of evaluation   Initial evaluation   Discharge evaluation
Client condition/diagnosis: HIV / AIDS
Date of assessment: 5-15-15
☐ Client is rated relative to his/her previous job
☒ Client is rated relative to return to work in general

	Strongly Supports SS	Supports S	Interferes I	Strongly Interferes SI	Non-Applicable N/A
	Strongly supports client returning to previous employment or finding and keeping work in general	Supports the client returning to previous employment or finishing and keeping work in general	Interferes with the client returning to previous employment or finding and keeping work in general	Strongly interferes with the client returning to previous employment or finding and keeping work in general	Not applicable or not enough information to rate
1. Assess abilities and limitations	SS	(S)	I	SI	N/A
2. Expectation of job success	SS	S	I	(SI)	N/A
3. Takes responsibility	SS	(S)	I	SI	N/A
4. Commitment to work	(SS)	S	I	SI	N/A
5. Work-related goals	SS	(S)	I	SI	N/A
6. Enjoys work	SS	(S)	I	SI	N/A
7. Pursues interests	SS	S	(I)	SI	N/A
8. Appraises work expectations	SS	S	(I)	SI	N/A
9. Influence of other roles	SS	S	(I)	SI	N/A
10. Work habits	SS	(S)	I	SI	N/A
11. Daily routines	SS	(S)	I	SI	N/A
12. Adapts routine to minimize difficulties	SS	S	(I)	SI	N/A
13. Perception of work setting	SS	S	(I)	SI	N/A
14. Perception of family and peers	SS	S	(I)	SI	N/A
15. Perception of boss	SS	S	I	(SI)	N/A
16. Perception of co-workers	SS	S	I	(SI)	N/A

Key comments: PROUD OF PRIOR WORK, STRONG HABITS, SOCIALLY ISOLATED
POOR CONFIDENCE, DOES NOT HAVE HOBBIES OR INTERESTS

Figure 24-2. WRI rating form scores for David. (Reprinted with permission from the Model of Human Occupation Clearinghouse.)

effectively manage his home and to use daily schedules for home management as a way to help David prepare himself for reentry to the workplace. As David began to explore opportunities, he chose to attend a job fair and found that several companies offered full-time training programs and that the only concerns expressed by the recruiters for the programs was that he might be overqualified! David discussed the advantages and disadvantages of disclosing to the recruiters that he had been out of work due to an illness that he now successfully managed and that he saw the training programs as the perfect way to reenter IT.

As this case illustrates, the WRI provides information on volition, habituation, and perception of environment that influences work success and satisfaction. Using performance capacity–oriented assessment alone in this case might have prohibited a revelation of the core problems facing David in reexamination of the worker role.

Suggested Further Research

Further development of the WRI might be indicated, and its usefulness as an outcome measure should be tested with larger samples. While the WRI has been used specifically with populations experiencing mental illness, much of this work has been done outside of the United States, and the influence of health insurance and health care systems on outcomes has not been adequately explored.

The Work Environment Impact Scale
Theoretical Basis

Workers are most productive and satisfied when their motivation (volition), patterns of work habits (habituation), and capacity for doing and interacting at work fit or match the work environment (i.e., physical spaces, objects, social groups, occupational forms). Therefore, the same work environment may affect workers differently. The aim of the WEIS is to determine how a particular work environment impacts a given worker (Moore-Corner et al., 1998).

The WEIS is a semistructured interview accompanied by a therapist-administered, 4-point rating scale. It was designed to gather information on the worker's perception and experience of work settings from workers with physical or psychosocial disabilities. The interview focuses on the impact of work setting on a worker's performance, satisfaction, and well-being from the point of view of the worker. The target groups are (1) people presently working and having difficulties at their job, (2) people who are not presently working but intend to go to a specific job or type of work where the work environment is known, and in unique cases, (3) people out of work who can gain from identifying how past work environments impacted their work productivity and satisfaction.

History of Development and Previous Versions/ Important Changes to Note in Current Version

The WEIS was developed at the University of Illinois at Chicago and published through the MOHO Clearinghouse (http://www.moho.uic.edu) as one of several work-related assessments based on the MOHO. The assessment's construct validity was initially examined through administration to a group of clients with psychiatric disabilities (Corner, Kielhofner, & Lin, 1997). Overall, the items appeared to match the worker's need for performance, satisfaction, and well-being, and the hierarchical order of items measured by the assessment is consistent with literature identifying environmental press and affordance for workers with psychiatric disabilities.

Psychometric Properties

Two studies have been published on the psychometric properties of WEIS. Corner et al. (1997) found that the instrument appears to measure a single construct. However, the scale was not as sensitive as preferred in discriminating between individuals. Based on the results of the previous study, Kielhofner, Lai, and colleagues (1999) revised some scale items to clarify their meaning. Then they scrutinized the psychometric properties of the second American English version and the first Swedish version of the WEIS. Results indicated that the WEIS items worked well together to define a single construct and that the revised instrument had adequate sensitivity and validly measured the participants.

Ekbladh, Fan, Sandqvist, Hemmingsson, and Taylor (2014) examined the psychometric properties of the Swedish version of the WEIS through Rasch analysis of 95 ratings from a sample of clients with experience of sick leave due to different medical conditions. These scholars reported that, overall, the WEIS items together cohered to form a single construct of increasingly challenging work environmental factors. The hierarchical ordering of the items along the continuum followed a logical and expected pattern, and the scale validly measured the participants.

Assessment Administration

Area of Occupation/Performance Skills/ Performance Patterns/Client Factors Assessed

The WEIS focuses on a client's perception of the level of support or interference to working of four environmental factors, including physical space, objects, social groups, and occupational forms (Moore-Corner et al., 1998).

Description of Environment/ Description of Supplies/Materials Required

The WEIS is conducted via a semistructured interview process and can be performed in any setting that is quiet and distraction free enough to allow the assessor and the client to engage in the interview. The WEIS can typically be completed in 30 minutes, although it may be conducted over multiple sessions if necessary.

No special materials are needed other than the administration manual, which includes the rating forms and directions. Less experienced practitioners may find that taking limited notes during the interview provides for more accurate scoring, although practitioners are cautioned to not allow note taking to interfere with being totally present during the interview.

Administration

The WEIS manual introduces and discusses the background of the instrument, the interview process, recommended questions, scoring instructions, and the ratings (Moore-Corner et al., 1998). There are four basic steps involved in WEIS's administration procedures:

1. Obtaining appropriate background data, where the therapist collects preliminary data from the patient's record or interdisciplinary staff to determine whether the WEIS is appropriate for the patient.
2. Conducting the interview, where the therapist carries out the interview like a conversation.
3. Completing the rating scale.
4. Utilizing the information from the interview to improve the work environment.

Scoring

There are 17 items on the WEIS rating scale form, reflecting 17 diverse environmental factors, such as physical space, social contacts and supports, temporal demands, objects utilized, and daily job function. The rating scale indicates the level of support or interference provided to the worker. Two ratings imply environmental support: a 4, in exceptional cases, and a 3, indicating adequate support. Two ratings suggest that the environment interferes: a 2 rating is given when there is some interference, and a 1 rating is given when the interference is perceived to be substantial (Figure 24-3).

The Work Environment Impact Scale

Each item below refers to a feature of the work environment and is scored according to a 4-point scale. Your rating should reflect how each environmental feature impacts (supports or interferes) the worker's needs or preferences for performance, satisfaction, and physical/emotional/social well-being.

General Rating Scale

Rating	Meaning	Description
4	Strongly supports	This environmental factor strongly supports his/her work performance, satisfaction, and physical/emotional/social well-being. (This rating should only be given to items that provide exceptional support.)
3	Supports	This environmental factor supports his/her work performance, satisfaction, and physical/emotional/social well-being (This rating should be given to items that provide adequate support.)
2	Interferes	This environmental factor interferes with his/her work performance, satisfaction, and physical/emotional/social well-being
1	Strongly interferes	This environmental factor strongly interferes with his/her work performance, satisfaction, and physical/emotional/social well-being
N/A	Not applicable	Not enough information to rate the item or item does not apply to the client's particular situation.

Client's Name:	Therapist's Name:
Employer's Name:	Date Administered:

1. **Time Demands:** Time allotted for available/expected amount of work.

1	2	3	4	N/A

Comments:

2. **Task Demands:** The physical, cognitive, and/or emotional demands/opportunities of work tasks.

1	2	3	4	N/A

Comments:

5. **Coworker Interaction:** Interaction/collaboration with coworkers required for job responsibilities.

1	2	3	4	N/A

Comments:

6. **Work Group Membership:** Social involvement with coworkers at work/outside of work.

1	2	3	4	N/A

Comments:

7. **Supervisor Interaction:** Feedback, guidance, and/or other communication/interaction with supervisor(s).

1	2	3	4	N/A

Comments:

8. **Work Role Standards:** Overall climate of work setting expressed in expectations for quality, excellence, commitment, achievement, and/or efficiency.

1	2	3	4	N/A

Comments:

9. **Work Role Style:** Opportunity/expectation for autonomy/compliance when organizing, making requests, negotiating, and choosing how and what work tasks will be done daily.

1	2	3	4	N/A

Comments:

10. **Interaction with Others:** Interaction/communication with subordinates, customers, clients, audiences, students, or others, excluding supervisor or coworkers.

1	2	3	4	N/A

Comments:

11. **Rewards:** Opportunities for job security, recognition/advancement in position, and/or compensation in salary or benefits.

1	2	3	4	N/A

Comments:

3. **Appeal of Work Tasks:** The appeal/enjoyableness or status/value of work tasks.

1	2	3	4	N/A

Comments:

4. **Work Schedule:** The influence of work hours upon other valued roles, activities, transportation, and basic self-care needs.

1	2	3	4	N/A

Comments:

12. **Sensory Qualities:** Properties of the work place such as noise, smell, visual, or tactile properties, temperature/climate, or air quality and ventilation.

1	2	3	4	N/A

Comments:

13. **Architecture/Arrangement:** Architecture or physical arrangement of and between work spaces and environments.

1	2	3	4	N/A

Comments:

14. **Ambience/Mood:** The feeling/mood associated with the degree of privacy, friendliness, morale, excitement, anxiety, frustration in the work place.

1	2	3	4	N/A

Comments:

15. **Properties of Objects:** The physical, cognitive, or emotional demands/opportunities of tools, equipment, materials, and supplies.

1	2	3	4	N/A

Comments:

16. **Physical Amenities:** Non-word-specific facilities necessary to meet personal needs at work such as restrooms, lunchrooms, or break rooms.

1	2	3	4	N/A

Comments:

17. **Meaning of Objects:** What objects signify to a person.

1	2	3	4	N/A

Comments:

General impressions:

_____

_____

_____

_____

_____

Figure 24-3. Blank WEIS rating form. (Reprinted with permission from the Model of Human Occupation Clearinghouse.)

Intervention Planning
Based on Assessment Results

The WEIS gathers information that is useful in establishing the influence of contexts and environments on occupational performance. Assessment of personal, physical, social, and temporal aspects are primary, although some information on cultural and virtual contexts and environments can be gathered if the assessor perceives that these aspects of context and environment might be important. The assessment provides information on how context and performance influence performance with the worker role, and the WEIS can be combined with other assessments to gather additional information on client factors and performance skills.

Case Study

Tamika was a 34-year-old mother of two who was diagnosed with clinical depression. She was referred to occupational therapy for assistance in returning to living independently and for strategies for caring for her home and children as part of outpatient treatment following a short inpatient admission. Tamika was divorced but had good support from family and friends and was on good terms with her ex-husband, who assisted with child care. Tamika worked full time as a medical device salesperson but had only been with her current employer for 9 months when diagnosed.

Tamika was first seen in occupational therapy as an outpatient following a short inpatient hospitalization. During the initial assessment, Tamika complained of moderate-to-severe fatigue, significant feelings of guilt over the impact of her illness on her children, difficulty sleeping that interfered with attendance at work, marked decreased enjoyment during most of her daily activities, and an ongoing sense of restlessness. She denied suicidal ideation but noted that her family was very concerned about her being on her own.

Tamika reported feeling "frustrated and short tempered" because she could not process information as quickly as she used to. At the time of initial assessment, Tamika had returned to work part time but was experiencing some problems. Her supervisor gave her feedback that her pace of work was too slow, that her coworkers had complained about mistakes, and that she did not consistently follow procedures to place orders and to follow up with customers.

The occupational therapist proposed the administration of the WEIS as part of a larger evaluation plan, and Tamika agreed to be interviewed about her work environment. The WEIS was chosen because it would give the therapist and Tamika a better understanding of the fit between her the work environment and Tamika's current work skills and perceptions of the environment. It was expected that insights gained by administration of the WEIS would help Tamika make decisions about her ability to continue in medical sales given her new diagnosis. Results of the WEIS are presented in Figure 24-4.

Tamika reported in the interview that her work tasks had a high level of appeal to her. She appreciated being in different settings in the community and enjoyed interacting with her customers and coworkers, although she felt that some of her coworkers "took their jobs too seriously." She noted that keeping up with the pace of work tasks was not typically difficult, but that at the end of the month, the pace of work became challenging for her given her fatigue and difficulty concentrating. She was aware that she sometimes cut corners, and that this resulted in mistakes that frustrated her coworkers. She also mentioned that at times she was expected to complete work tasks in a prescribed manner and that there

The Work Environment Impact Scale

Each item below refers to a feature of the work environment and is scored according to a 4-point scale. Your rating should reflect how each environmental feature impacts (supports or interferes) the worker's needs or preferences for performance, satisfaction, and physical/emotional/social well-being.

General Rating Scale

Rating	Meaning	Description
4	Strongly supports	This environmental factor strongly supports his/her work performance, satisfaction, and physical/emotional/social well-being. (This rating should only be given to items that provide exceptional support.)
3	Supports	This environmental factor supports his/her work performance, satisfaction, and physical/emotional/social well-being (This rating should be given to items that provide adequate support.)
2	Interferes	This environmental factor interferes with his/her work performance, satisfaction, and physical/emotional/social well-being
1	Strongly interferes	This environmental factor strongly interferes with his/her work performance, satisfaction, and physical/emotional/social well-being
N/A	Not applicable	Not enough information to rate the item or item does not apply to the client's particular situation.

Client's Name: _TAMIKA_   Therapist's Name: _BRENT_

Employer's Name: _JOHNSON SALES_   Date Administered: _5/22/15_

1. **Time Demands:** Time allotted for available/-expected amount of work.

| 1 | (2) | 3 | 4 | N/A |

Comments:

2. **Task Demands:** The physical, cognitive, and/or emotional demands/opportunities of work tasks.

| 1 | (2) | 3 | 4 | N/A |

Comments:

5. **Coworker Interaction:** Interaction/collaboration with coworkers required for job responsibilities.

| (1) | 2 | 3 | 4 | N/A |

Comments:

6. **Work Group Membership:** Social involvement with coworkers at work/outside of work.

| (1) | 2 | 3 | 4 | N/A |

Comments:

7. **Supervisor Interaction:** Feedback, guidance, and/-or other communication/interaction with supervisor(s).

| 1 | (2) | 3 | 4 | N/A |

Comments:

8. **Work Role Standards:** Overall climate of work setting expressed in expectations for quality, excellence, commitment, achievement, and/or efficiency.

| 1 | 2 | (3) | 4 | N/A |

Comments:

9. **Work Role Style:** Opportunity/expectation for autonomy/compliance when organizing, making requests, negotiating, and choosing how and what work tasks will be done daily.

| 1 | 2 | (3) | 4 | N/A |

Comments:

10. **Interaction with Others:** Interaction/communication with subordinates, customers, clients, audiences, students, or others, excluding supervisor or coworkers.

| 1 | 2 | (3) | 4 | N/A |

Comments:

11. **Rewards:** Opportunities for job security, recognition/advancement in position, and/or compensation in salary or benefits.

| 1 | 2 | 3 | (4) | N/A |

Comments:

3. **Appeal of Work Tasks:** The appeal/enjoyableness or status/value of work tasks.

| 1 | 2 | (3) | 4 | N/A |

Comments:

4. **Work Schedule:** The influence of work hours upon other valued roles, activities, transportation, and basic self-care needs.

| 1 | 2 | (3) | 4 | N/A |

Comments:

12. **Sensory Qualities:** Properties of the work place such as noise, smell, visual, or tactile properties, temperature/climate, or air quality and ventilation.

| 1 | 2 | 3 | (4) | N/A |

Comments:

13. **Architecture/Arrangement:** Architecture or physical arrangement of and between work spaces and environments.

| 1 | 2 | 3 | (4) | N/A |

Comments:

14. **Ambience/Mood:** The feeling/mood associated with the degree of privacy, friendliness, morale, excitement, anxiety, frustration in the work place.

| 1 | 2 | 3 | (4) | N/A |

Comments:

15. **Properties of Objects:** The physical, cognitive, or emotional demands/opportunities of tools, equipment, materials, and supplies.

| 1 | 2 | 3 | (4) | N/A |

Comments:

16. **Physical Amenities:** Non-word-specific facilities necessary to meet personal needs at work such as restrooms, lunchrooms, or break rooms.

| 1 | 2 | 3 | (4) | N/A |

Comments:

17. **Meaning of Objects:** What objects signify to a person.

| 1 | 2 | 3 | (4) | N/A |

Comments:

General impressions:

_____

_____

_____

Figure 24-4. WEIS rating form for Tamika. (Reprinted with permission from the Model of Human Occupation Clearinghouse.)

was little room to make decisions on her own, even when she thought her methods of working would be faster. She found this very frustrating.

Through additional discussion, the therapist learned that Tamika found the variability of her work schedule appealing and that she had considerable control over when she completed major parts of her job, such as completing paperwork and orders. While Tamika typically had more energy in the morning, it was also the busiest and most hectic time to work as many of her coworkers used mornings to reach out to coworkers via email and telephone calls.

When asked about the physical setting, Tamika reacted positively, stating that most of the offices and hospitals she visited were very pleasant, that she enjoyed working with different types of people, and that she enjoyed the opportunity to be outdoors between appointments. She was able to complete significant portions of her work at home. She denied any difficulty utilizing the equipment and objects she came across in this job.

Tamika's comments regarding the social environment were notably less positive. Though she stated that she appreciated the diversity she saw in her customers, she did not enjoy the company of her coworkers or of her supervisor. Tamika described herself as "feeling out of place" and said that she preferred to work alone at home rather than at the company's office site. She avoided coworkers outside of the workplace, felt uncomfortable when her supervisor was present, and complained that her office space was too small and noisy for a person to work comfortably. Tamika had chosen not to disclose her disability to her coworkers or supervisor, noting that she was worried about facing discrimination due to her new diagnosis.

Through the assessment, Tamika and the therapist agreed to explore the following in treatment:

- Strategies for managing stress and maintaining attention to work tasks, including scheduling taking more breaks and spreading work across the day
- The advantages and disadvantages of disclosing her illness to her employer and requesting reasonable accommodations, such as continuing to work part time and varying her schedule to accommodate therapy
- Strategies for developing more positive relationships with her coworkers and supervisor
- Strategies for emphasizing her strengths and the parts of the job she found most enjoyable

Suggested Further Research

The WEIS has been utilized with various populations, including those affected by mental illness and various cultures. Continued exploration of the usefulness of the WEIS as part of a comprehensive return to work program in larger populations of persons struggling with mental health issues would be beneficial.

Table 24-2

The Fourteen Skills Assessed by the Assessment of Work Performance, Categorized by Area

Motor Skills					Process Skills						Communication and Interaction Skills			
Posture	Mobility	Coordination	Strength	Physical energy	Mental energy	Knowledge	Temporal organization	Organizational space and objects	Adaptation	Physicality	Language	Relations	Information exchange

The Assessment of Work Performance
Theoretical Basis

As with the WRI and WEIS, the AWP was developed based on concepts from the MOHO (Kielhofner, 2008). Sandqvist et al. (2010) stated that

> The AWP is intended to be used not only by occupational therapists but also by other professionals working with the assessment of work functioning. Because use of the assessment is enhanced by awareness of the theoretical concepts behind it, any user of the AWP should become familiar to concepts of MOHO. Knowledge of MOHO will result in more meaningful and useful interpretation and valuation of the assessment results. (p. 2)

Concepts/Construct

According to Moore-Corner et al. (1998), "the AWP assesses observable, work-related skills of works including information on efficiency and appropriateness of work performance" (p. 2). The AWP assesses three skill domains: motor skills, process skills, and communication and interaction skills. These 3 domains contain 14 skill items categorized in the areas of motor skills, process skills, and communication and interaction skills. These skills are shown in Table 24-2.

The AWP can be used to assess the working skills of individuals with various kinds of work-related problems and who are facing a variety of diagnoses or impairments. The AWP does not target any special tasks or contexts and can be used in various work assessment settings and with work activities performed in actual employment situations/settings, situations where structured work tasks are provided to clients (e.g., work therapy programs, sheltered workshops, work training environments), and in simulated work environments/tasks.

History of Development and Previous Versions/ Important Changes to Note in Current Version

The Swedish National Labour Market Board supported the initial development and evaluation of the AWP financially. The AWP is currently used by many assessors working in a variety of work rehabilitation settings, including the Public Employment Services Office in Sweden, which has chosen the AWP as one of three assessment instruments to be used for all activity-based assessment of their clients (Sandqvist et al., 2010). The AWP has been translated to a Dutch version and other translations, including Danish and Icelandic, and further studies of the psychometric properties are planned or in progress.

Psychometric Properties

Fan, Taylor, Ekbladh, Hemmingsson, and Sandqvist (2013) examined the validity and reliability of the AWP using Rasch analysis. The AWP was administered to 365 clients with a variety of work-related problems. Rasch analysis and principal component analysis were used to examine the appropriateness of the rating scales and unidimensionality of AWP items. The person-response validity, internal consistency, targeting appropriateness, and differential item function were also analyzed. The Rasch analysis confirmed the 4-point rating scale, and the item set met the criteria of unidimensionality. The AWP exhibited satisfactory person-response validity and internal consistency. Among the three subdomains, the targeting of item difficulty was sufficient in the motor skills and process skills subdomains. Differential item functioning was found across genders and diagnoses.

Reliability

Fan et al. (2013) examined reliability via Rasch analysis and found that the item separation reliability was .99, which indicated that the AWP items defined the construct of clients' overall work performance. The person separation reliability was good (.83), and it was considered as the reliability of the person ordering. Therefore, clients' scores in overall work performance were reliably estimated by the Rasch analysis. In addition, the clients in the study could be differentiated into at least three strata.

Validity and Sensitivity

Sandqvist, Björk, Gullberg, Henriksson, and Gerdle (2009) examined the construct validity of the AWP with 364 assessments of clients with a variety of work-related problems assessed by 6 occupational therapists in Sweden between 2004 and 2005. They found that the AWP consisted of two dimensions: one involved motor skills and the other combined process skills with communication and interaction skills. Principal component analysis shows construct validity of the AWP. Moreover, the results indicated that the instrument is sensitive and discriminates between clients, and no gender-related patterns were identified. Evaluation of the psychometric properties of the AWP shows adequate face validity and utility (Sandqvist, Törnquist, & Henriksson, 2006) and acceptable content validity (Sandqvist, Gullberg, Henriksson, & Gerdle, 2008).

Assessment Administration

Area of Occupation/Performance Skills/ Performance Patterns/Client Factors Assessed

The AWP focuses on the work performance of clients and assesses three skill domains: motor skills, process skills, and communication and interaction skills. These 3 domains contain 14 skill items: 5 in the domain of motor skills, 5 in the domain of process skills, and 4 in the domain of communication and interaction skills.

Description of Environment/ Description of Supplies/Materials Required

The AWP does not require observation of any special tasks or contexts (Sandqvist et al., 2010). Rather, the assessment can be applied to any work tasks performed in actual employment situations or in simulated work environments or tasks.

Special materials and supplies are not required beyond the assessment manual and the rating forms for use by an assessor familiar with the AWP. Observation of clients may take place in various settings, and it is useful for the assessor to be able to take specific notes to record observations to assist with completion of the rating.

Administration

The AWP should be utilized as part of a broader assessment methodology that considers the full range of variables that influence work performance. The results can be combined with those obtained through administration of the WRI, WEIS, and other assessments. It is highly recommended that the client takes an active part in the selection of the work tasks used for assessment of the client's performance. This helps the client to feel more involved in the assessment process and facilitates a more meaningful experience for the client when performing the chosen task (Sandqvist et al., 2010).

The assessment authors provide the following recommendations for administration of the AWP (Sandqvist et al., 2010):

- The assessor should inform the client about the purpose of the assessment and where and how the assessment will be carried out as well as the amount of time that the client will need to commit to the assessment process.
- The assessor should discuss the assessment results with the client as soon as possible after the assessment has been carried out.
- The total administration time of the AWP is not predetermined and can vary from a couple hours to much longer, depending on the unique requirements of each client and the complexities and time involved with completing each work task.
- The assessor should rely on his or her competence and experience to determine the appropriate length of observation.

Scoring

Each item on the AWP is scored using a 4-point rating scale, where 1 is the lowest rating (incompetent performance) and 4 is the highest rating (competent performance). A score of 2 indicates limited performance that is inefficient or inappropriate, and a score of 3 indicates not fully competent performance. The AWP uses an ordinal rating scale; therefore, a single summary score cannot be obtained for all items. The assessment authors recommend that, "Instead of calculating a total score of the client's performance, an overview of ratings could be used instead" (Sandqvist et al., 2010, p. 7).

Practitioners use the AWP Assessment Form to assign ratings and to document information to justify rating decisions. Portions of the AWP Assessment Form are provided as examples in Figures 24-5 and 24-6. The full AWP Assessment Form is available as part of the manual when purchased. These ratings then may be transferred to the AWP Summary Form (Figure 24-7). This optional form allows the assessor to record the ratings on a simple form and draw lines between the ratings in order to yield a visual depiction of the strengths and weaknesses of the client's work skills on a specific work task. Rating scores of lack of information (LI) or not relevant (NR) are used when the assessor lacks adequate information or when the item does not apply to the client, respectively. The AWP Summary Form gives details about which skills are strengths or challenges and can be used as a basis for collaborating on the development of treatment goals and strategies. For this reason, it is useful to collaborate with the client in review of the AWP Summary Form and to use it as a tool for intervention planning.

The AWP items are designed to measure the client's work skills (Sandqvist et al., 2006, 2009). Moreover, it recognizes three types of skills (i.e., motor, process, communication and interaction) as proposed in the MOHO (Kielhofner, 2008). Thus, four scores useful for characterizing the client's work skills can be obtained:

- The motor skills subscale score
- The process skills subscale score
- The communication and interaction skills subscale score
- Total work skills score (sum of the 3 subscales)

The subscale scores and total work skills score allow one to compare sections of the AWP and to describe the direction of change in each area upon reevaluation.

Intervention Planning Based on Assessment Results

The AWP helps to gather information focused on the performance skills of motor, process, and communication and interaction skills. The AWP can be combined with other assessments, such as the WRI and WEIS, that aid in the collection of information on client factors, performance patterns, and the context and environment.

Case Study

Xavier is a 28-year-old man who was diagnosed with severe social anxiety disorder at 22 years of age when he dropped out of college for the second time and sought assessment on the recommendation of his primary care physician. He is now employed part time, living with his parents, and taking one college course online. He has experienced

Appendix A: AWP Forms | Assessment Form

AWP (v1.0) Assessment Form

Assessor:____________________ **Assessment number:**________

Client information

Name:____________________

ID number:______________

Sex: Male ☐ Female ☐

Work-related problems:____________________

Assessment situation:____________________

Aids/adaptations:____________________

Dates: Observation:______________

Assessment:______________

Type of observation: Non-participant ☐ Participant ☐

Figure 24-5. Selected portion of AWP Assessment Form. (Reprinted with permission from the Model of Human Occupation Clearinghouse.)

difficulty in maintaining employment and has quit or been fired from his last 3 jobs within 3 months of starting. He recently was hired as a stock clerk in a bookstore but is experiencing difficulty on the job and is concerned about being fired again. He was referred to a vocational program associated with a community-based mental health center and was assessed by the occupational therapist who consults to the center 1 day a week.

Xavier reports feeling severe anxiety in situations where he fears that he will be judged, worries about humiliating himself sometimes to the point of feeling paralyzed, is constantly worried that he has offended coworkers, and can have fear bordering on panic at times when he must interact with strangers. He reports that his symptoms manifest

1	**2**	**3**	**4**
Incompetent performance	**Limited performance**	**Questionable performance**	**Competent performance**
The performance of the work task	The performance of the work task	The performance of the work task is not fully competent with	The performance of the work task
a) is inefficient,	a) is inefficient,	respect to the parameters a-c,	a) is efficient,
b) is inappropriate, and	b) is inappropriate, and/or	but none of them are clearly	b) is appropriate, and
c) gives an unacceptable result. The problems are major and all parameters (a-c) are clearly affected.	c) gives an unacceptable result. One/several (1 or 2) of the parameters (a-c) are clearly affected.	affected. Normally the assessor has a vague feeling that the performance is reduced.	c) gives an acceptable result.

LI = Lack of information, **NR** = Not relevant

Communication and interaction skills

11. Physicality (gesture, gaze, approximate, posture, contact)	LI	NR	1	2	3	4
Comments:						

12. Language (adjust language, adjust speech, focus)	LI	NR	1	2	3	4
Comments:						

13. Relations (engage, relate, respects, collaborate)	LI	NR	1	2	3	4
Comments:						

14. Information exchange (ask, inform)	LI	NR	1	2	3	4
Comments:						

AWP [English Version 1.0]   25

Figure 24-6. Selected portion of AWP Assessment Form (communication and interaction skills). (Reprinted with permission from the Model of Human Occupation Clearinghouse.)

physically through blushing, sweating, trembling, and his voice shaking, which leads him to avoid interactions with others. He has few social contacts outside of his family, although he has recently joined a support group on the recommendation of his psychologist.

The occupational therapist completed the AWP as part of a more comprehensive work-related assessment, and Xavier agreed to allow an observation at work. The therapist completed an observation at the bookstore watching Xavier's direct performance for a little more than 1 hour, during which time Xavier primarily worked alone. However, there were four times that Xavier interacted with two different coworkers and two times that Xavier interacted with customers. The therapist noted the following:

Overview of ratings

Skills	Motor skills					Process skills					Communication and interaction skills			
	Posture	Mobility	Coordination	Strength	Physical Energy	Mental Energy	Knowledge	Temporal Organization	Organizations of Space & Objects	Adaptation	Physicality	Language	Relations	Informations & Exchange
Rating	4	4	4	4	4	4	4	4	4	4	4	4	4	4
	(3)	(3)	3	3	(3)	3	3	(3)	3	3	3	(3)	3	(3)
	2	2	(2)	(2)	2	(2)	(2)	2	2	2	(2)	2	(2)	2
	1	1	1	1	1	1	1	1	(1)	(1)	1	1	1	1
	LI	LI	LI	LI	LI	LI	LI	LI	LI	LI	LI	LI	LI	LI
	NR	NR	NR	NR	NR	NR	NR	NR	NR	NR	NR	NR	NR	NR

Figure 24-7. Selected portion of AWP Summary Form. (Reprinted with permission from the Model of Human Occupation Clearinghouse.)

1. Xavier's motor skills strongly support his performance with competent demonstration of posture, mobility, coordination, strength, and physical energy.
2. Xavier's process skills were generally supportive of performance with competent demonstration of knowledge, temporal organization, and organization of space and objects but with questionable competence in mental energy and adaptation.
3. Communication and interaction skills was the area most problematic to Xavier's performance. The therapist noted limited competence in language and information exchange and noted severe difficulty warranting rating of incompetent in physicality and relations.
4. The therapist assigned a motor skills subscale score of 20, a process skills subscale score of 18, and a communication and interaction subscale score of 6.

The occupational therapist shared his observations with Xavier and provided examples of the strengths and weaknesses observed. The therapist and Xavier began to collaborate on a plan to identify strategies to compensate for weaknesses, to use strategies to manage anxiety recommended by Xavier's psychologist, and to consider adaptations and accommodations that might support Xavier's performance.

Suggested Further Research

The AWP is a newer assessment, and its utilization in practice and in empirical study has been somewhat limited. Inclusion of the AWP in a range of return-to-work programs and in a wider variety of populations, including those with various types of mental health challenges, would be beneficial.

Summary

The WRI, WEIS, and AWP are three work-related assessments based upon the MOHO. The WRI assesses psychosocial factors that influence work performance, whereas the WEIS assesses workplace conditions that impact the worker. The AWP assesses performance of work-related skills through observation. Studies indicate the consistency and dependability of all of these assessments, and they have been used effectively by occupational therapists around the world and in different languages.

References

American Occupational Therapy Association. (2014). Occupational therapy practice framework: Domain and process (3rd ed.). *American Journal of Occupational Therapy, 68*(Suppl. 1), S1-S48.

Bejerholm, U., & Areberg, C. (2014). Factors related to the return to work potential in persons with severe mental illness. *Scandinavian Journal of Occupational Therapy, 21*, 277-286.

Bettencourt, C. M., Carlstrom, P., Brown, S. H., Lindau, K., & Long, C. M. (1986). Using work simulation to treat adults with back injuries. *American Journal of Occupational Therapy, 40*, 12-18.

Biernacki, S. D. (1993). Reliability of the worker role interview. *American Journal of Occupational Therapy, 47*, 797-803.

Braveman, B. (1999). The Model of Human Occupation and prediction of return to work: A review of related empirical research. *Work, 12*, 13-23.

Braveman, B. H. (2001). Development of a community-based return to work program for people with AIDS. *Occupational Therapy in Health Care, 13*, 113-130.

Braveman, B. (2012). An introduction to work and occupational therapy work-related services. In B. Braveman & J. Page (Eds.), *Work: Promoting participation & productivity through occupational therapy*. Philadelphia, PA: F. A. Davis.

Braveman, B., Robson, M., Velozo, C., Kielhofner, G., Fisher, G. S., Forsyth, K., & Kerschbaum, J. (2005). *The Worker Role Interview (Version 10)*. Chicago, IL: Model of Human Occupation Clearinghouse.

Corner, R. A., Kielhofner, G., & Lin, F. L. (1997). Construct validity of a work environment impact scale. *Work, 9*, 21-34.

Désiron, H. A., Donceel, P., de Rijk, A., & Van Hoof, E. (2013). A conceptual-practice model for occupational therapy to facilitate return to work in breast cancer patients. *Journal of Occupational Rehabilitation, 23*, 516-526.

Ekbladh, E., Fan, C. W., Sandqvist, J., Hemmingsson, S., & Taylor, R. (2014). Work environment impact scale: Testing the psychometric properties of the Swedish version. *Work, 47*, 213-219.

Ekbladh, E., Haglund, L., & Thorell, T. H. (2004). The Worker Role Interview—Preliminary data on the predictive validity of return to work of clients after an insurance medicine investigation. *Journal of Occupational Rehabilitation, 14*, 131-141.

Fan, C. W., Taylor, R. R., Ekbladh, E., Hemmingsson, H., & Sandqvist, J. (2013). Evaluating the psychometric properties of a clinical vocational rehabilitation outcome measurement: The Assessment of Work Performance (AWP). *OTJR: Occupation, Participation and Health, 33*, 125-133.

Fenger, K., & Kramer, J. (2007). Worker Role Interview: Testing the psychometric properties of the Icelandic versions. *Scandinavian Journal of Occupational Therapy, 14*, 160-172.

Forsyth, K., Braveman, B., Kielhofner, G., Ekbladh, E., Haglund, L., Fenger, K., & Keller, J. (2006). Psychometric properties of the Worker Role Interview. *Work, 27*, 313-318.

Forsyth, K., Deshpande, S., Kielhofner, G., Henriksson, C., Haglund, L., Olson, L., ... Kulkami, S. (2005). *The Occupational Circumstances Assessment Interview and Rating Scale (OCAIRS)*. (Version 4). Chicago, IL: Department of Occupational Therapy, University of Illinois at Chicago.

Frederickson, B. E., Trief, P. M., Van Beveren, P., Yan, H. A., & Baum, G. (1988). Rehabilitation of the patient with chronic back pain: A search for outcome predictors. *Spine, 13*, 351-353.

Gordon, D. (2009). The history of occupational therapy. In E. B. Crepeau, E. S. Cohn, & B. A. Boyt Schell (Eds.), *Willard and Spackman's occupational therapy* (11th ed., pp. 202-215). Baltimore, MD: Lippincott Williams & Wilkins.

Haglund, L., Karlsson, G., Kielhofner, G., & Lai, J. S. (1997). Validity of the Swedish version of the Worker Role Interview. *Scandinavian Journal of Occupational Therapy, 4*, 23-29.

Kielhofner, G. (2008). *Model of Human Occupation: Theory and application*. Baltimore, MD: Lippincott Williams & Wilkins.

Kielhofner, G., Braveman, B., Baron, K., Fisher, G., Hammel, J., & Littleton, M. (1999). The Model of Human Occupation: Understanding the worker who is injured or disabled. *Work, 12*, 37-45.

Kielhofner, G., Braveman, B., Finlayson, M., Paul-Ward, A., Goldbaum, L., & Goldstein, K. (2004). Outcomes of a vocational program for persons with AIDS. *American Journal of Occupational Therapy, 58*, 64-72.

Kielhofner, G., Lai, J., Olson, L., Haglund, L., Ekbladh, E., & Hedlund, M. (1999). Psychometric properties of the Work Environment Impact Scale: A cross-cultural study. *Work, 12*, 71-77.

King, P. M., & Olson, D. L. (2009). Work. In E. B. Crepeau, E. S. Cohn, & B. A. Boyt Schell (Eds.), *Willard & Spackman's occupational therapy* (11th ed., pp. 615-632). Baltimore, MD: Lippincott Williams & Wilkins.

Lee, J., & Kielhofner, G. (2010). Vocational intervention based on the Model of Human Occupation: A review of evidence. *Scandinavian Journal of Occupational Therapy, 17*, 177-190.

Lohss, I., Forsyth, K., & Kottorp, A. (2012). Psychometric properties of the Worker Role Interview (version 10.0) in mental health. *British Journal of Occupational Therapy, 75*(4), 171-179. https://doi.org/10.4276/030802212X13336366278095

Matheson, L. N., Ogden, L. D., Vilette, K., & Schultz, K. (1985). Work hardening: Occupational therapy in industrial rehabilitation. *American Journal of Occupational Therapy, 39*, 314-321.

Moore-Corner, R. A., Kielhofner, G., & Olson, L. (1998). *A user's guide to Work Environment Impact Scale (WEIS)*. Version 2.0. Chicago, IL: Model of Human Occupation Clearinghouse.

Ross, J. (2007). *Occupational therapy and vocational rehabilitation*. Hoboken, NJ: John Wiley & Sons.

Ruskin, J. (n.d.). Brainy quote. https://www.brainyquote.com/quotes/john_ruskin_132387

Sandqvist, J. L., Björk, M. A., Gullberg, M. T., Henriksson, C. M., & Gerdle, B. U. C. (2009). Construct validity of the Assessment of Work Performance (AWP). *Work, 32*, 211-218. https://doi.org/10.3233/WOR-2009-0807

Sandqvist, J. L., Gullberg, M. T., Henriksson, C. M., & Gerdle, B. U. (2008). Content validity and utility of the Assessment of Work Performance (AWP). *Work, 30*, 441-450.

Sandqvist, J., Lee, J., & Kielhofner, G. (2010). *A user's manual for the Assessment of Work Performance (AWP)*. English Version 1.0. Chicago, IL: Department of Occupational Therapy, University of Illinois at Chicago.

Sandqvist, J. L., Törnquist, K. B., & Henriksson, C. M. (2006). Assessment of Work Performance (AWP)—Development of an instrument. *Work, 26*, 379-387.

Velozo, C. (1993). Work evaluations: Critique of the State of the Art of Functional Assessment of Work. *American Journal of Occupational Therapy, 47*, 203-209. https://doi.org/10.5014/ajot.47.3.203

Velozo, C. A., Kielhofner, G., & Fisher, G. A. (1998). *A user's guide to the Worker Role Interview*. Chicago, IL: Model of Human Occupation Clearinghouse.

Velozo, C., Kielhofner, G., Gern, A., Lin, F. L., Azhar, F, Lai, J. S., & Fisher, G. (1999). Worker Role Interview: Toward validation of a psychosocial work-related measure. *Journal of Occupational Rehabilitation, 9*, 153-168.

Waddell G. (1987). A new clinical model for the treatment of low back pain. *Spine, 12*, 632-644.

25

The Test of Grocery Shopping Skills

Catana Brown, PhD, OTR/L, FAOTA

*The odds of going to the store for a loaf of bread and
coming out with only a loaf of bread are three billion to one.*
(Bombeck, n.d.)

Grocery shopping is an important and challenging instrumental activity of daily living (IADL) that most often occurs in a complex environment. Consider what is involved in locating an item on a grocery list. For example, let us consider finding powdered sugar. When locating an item in the grocery store, one strategy that is helpful is to know the layout of the store. It is also helpful to know how items are categorized, such as knowing what could be found in a section marked "baking goods." Even after the powdered sugar is located, one has to sort through many types of sugar to find the specific item that he or she is looking for and must decide among several brands. Individuals who were efficient and accurate shoppers take much of this information for granted; however, at some point in time, each person had to learn about the grocery store.

The Test of Grocery Shopping Skills (TOGSS), a performance-based assessment, was designed to measure an individual's grocery shopping ability. In addition, the TOGSS allowed the occupational therapist to observe the application of cognitive skills while the individual was engaged in a real-world occupation. An important characteristic of the TOGSS is ecological validity, meaning that the performance of grocery shopping is measured in the real-world environment of a grocery store. The TOGSS was initially developed for use with individuals with serious and persistent mental illness, but it is applicable to other populations with occupational performance issues due to cognitive impairments, such as traumatic brain injury or dementia.

Hemphill, B. J., & Urish, C. K. (Eds.). *Assessments in Occupational Therapy Mental Health: An Integrative Approach, Fourth Edition* (pp. 433-441). © 2020 Taylor & Francis Group.

Theoretical Basis

The Ecology of Human Performance (Dunn, Brown, & McGuigan, 1994) served as a guide to the development of the TOGSS. The Ecology of Human Performance explains that task/occupational performance is based on the interaction between the individual and the environment. Whether an individual can successfully engage in a task depends on the skills and abilities of the individual as well as the environment in which the task was performed. For example, a poor memory (person factor) may make it difficult to remember which items need to be purchased at the grocery store, but a grocery list (environmental factor) can help compensate for memory loss. Conversely, an individual may possess good cognitive skills (person factor), but the grocery store may be so busy (environmental factor) that the individual may decide to come back and shop at a different time. Understanding that the environment plays a major role in performance directed the developers of the assessment toward administration in a natural environment.

Concepts of the Ecology of Human Performance Applied to the Test of Grocery Shopping Skills

According to the Ecology of Human Performance, a person's ability to successfully perform a task is based upon the interaction of the environment (i.e., where the task takes place) and the skills and abilities of the individual. An individual's performance range is increased when his or her skills and abilities match the demands of the environment and the task. In the case of the TOGSS, the task is grocery shopping and, more specifically, finding the correct items at the lowest price.

The environment is the grocery store. This includes the physical environment, which encompasses the building and all of the grocery store items. This aspect of the environment is important due to the massive amount of items and the variability of the items. These are significant considerations in making choices during the task of grocery shopping. The social environment is also a key factor in grocery shopping. During the shopping task, there is social interaction with both the store personnel and other grocery shoppers. Culturally, there are expectations about grocery shopping. Culture affects the items that will be available to the customer in the store. The temporal environment is another consideration. Stores typically have established hours, and it is common that certain times of the day or days of the week will often be busier than others. For example, Friday is payday for many individuals. Friday after work, many people may head to the store to select items for the weekend. This would be a day and time when the store may be busier than at other times during the week.

Many person factors are important for successful performance of grocery shopping. The cognitive skills necessary for grocery shopping are a significant person factor. Other person factors include endurance, sensory processing, and the demand of visual processing requirements. When considering the person, past experience and interest in grocery shopping may impact performance.

The outcomes associated with the TOGSS measure this area of occupation, but because the test is a performance-based measure administered in an actual grocery store, the occupational therapist can use this opportunity to identify person and environmental features that support or interfere with individual performance.

History of Development

The TOGSS was initially developed by an occupational therapist and a nurse. Later in the development of the assessment, a psychologist joined the assessment development team. This individual contributed significantly to the study of the psychometric properties of the instrument. The TOGSS is published by the American Occupational Therapy Association Press (Brown, Rempfer, & Hamera, 2009).

Interest in serious and persistent mental illness and factors that contributed to successful community living facilitated the development of the TOGSS. Although there was a great deal of interest among researchers and clinicians regarding community functioning, few good measures were available to occupational therapy practitioners. Performance-based measures offer advantages over assessment methods, such as self/informant reports (Mausbach, Moore, Bowie, Cardenas, & Patterson, 2009). Performance-based measures, particularly those administered in a natural environment, provide a more direct measure of functioning, offer greater authenticity, and have the potential to capture the complexity of real-world performance. Those involved in the development of the TOGSS chose grocery shopping because this occupation was considered an important IADL. This important occupation requires many different cognitive skills that are known to be impaired in individuals with serious and persistent mental illness, and there were no existing measures of grocery shopping ability.

During the initial development of the TOGSS, it was important to create an assessment that authentically represented grocery shopping for individuals with serious and persistent mental illness (Hamera & Brown, 2000). Assessment developers interviewed individuals with serious and persistent mental illness to identify important characteristics of the grocery shopping experience, including where they shopped, what was typically purchased, and challenges presented by the task. Then the developers accompanied individuals with serious and persistent mental illness during a regular grocery shopping trip to observe performance while engaged in the occupation. Based upon the interviews and observations, the developers concluded that the primary challenges included locating desired items and finding low-cost foods. Efficiency was another important consideration within the grocery shopping task.

As the researchers involved in intervention within the development, it was important to develop two comparable forms of the assessment so that the TOGSS could be used as a pre-test and a post-test. With only one form administered at both time points, one would assume that a second administration would result in improved performance because the test taker would now be familiar with where the items were located and other aspects of the experience. An alternate form provided protection against testing biases associated with already shopping for similar items. The process for developing 2 forms involved initially having individuals with serious and persistent mental illness shop from a long list of 27 items (Hamera & Brown, 2000). The properties of each item were analyzed, and items were dispersed between the two lists so that the two lists were comparable in terms of difficulty and location of the items throughout the store. Originally, the TOGSS was used for research purposes, including assessing the outcomes of a grocery shopping intervention (Brown, Rempfer, & Hamera, 2002). In 2009, the TOGSS was made available to clinicians (Brown et al.).

Psychometric Properties

Reliability

Early development of the TOGSS included a study of reliability (Hamera & Brown, 2002). In a study that examined both test-retest reliability and the comparability of the 2 forms, 26 individuals with schizophrenia or schizoaffective disorder were administered 1 form of the TOGSS. The selection of which form to administer was random. On a subsequent day, the alternate form was administered to the same individual. Because both test-retest and equivalence of the forms were measured simultaneously, it was expected that the reliability coefficient would be lower than if only one form of reliability was studied. The relationship between the two testing times, which also involved the alternate forms, was statistically significant and ranged from 0.64 to 0.83 depending on the specific outcome (i.e., correct item, time, efficiency). The average score for the two forms was almost identical. These results suggest that there is a moderate degree of comparability between the two forms.

Interrater reliability was also examined in this study and was extremely high with correlations of $r = .99$ for Form 1 and $r = 1.00$ for Form 2. The very strong association between the different examiners suggested that different occupational therapists provided similar ratings on the TOGSS.

Validity

Construct validity was examined in studies that reported the relationship between performance on the TOGSS and other cognitive assessments. In one study of individuals with schizophrenia or schizoaffective disorder (Rempfer, Hamera, Brown, & Cromwell, 2003), performance on the TOGSS was associated with verbal learning, attention, and executive functioning. Greenwood, Landau, and Wykes (2005) found similar relationships between TOGSS performance, a measure of working memory, and other executive functions. In another study that used canonical correlations, accuracy and efficiency were distinguished as distinct outcomes (Zayat, Rempfer, Gajewski, & Brown, 2011). This study suggested that working memory was more important for accuracy, whereas problem solving and planning were more important for the efficiency outcomes of time and redundancy.

Other validity studies with the TOGSS have compared the performance of individuals with and without mental illness. An early study compared 26 individuals with schizophrenia, 19 persons with a mental illness diagnosis other than schizophrenia, and 19 individuals without a psychiatric diagnosis but similar in terms of socioeconomic status (Hamera, Brown, Rempfer, & Davis, 2002). All three groups were similar in terms of their performance accuracy, but individuals without mental illness took less time and were less redundant than the two groups with a mental illness. Another study with a slightly modified version of the TOGSS compared individuals with schizophrenia to individuals without schizophrenia (Greenwood et al., 2005). In this study, the researchers further subdivided the group of individuals diagnosed with schizophrenia into individuals with and without negative symptoms. In this study, the group without mental illness performed better on accuracy than the individuals with schizophrenia. Individuals with schizophrenia and negative symptoms were also more impaired in terms of efficiency in time and redundancy. Overall, these studies suggested, as would be expected, that individuals with serious and persistent mental illness performed worse than individuals without mental illness.

The TOGSS has been used as an outcome measure to assess improvement after a grocery shopping intervention (Rempfer, Brown, & Hamera, 2011). This aspect of validity is where the availability of two alternate forms is most important. Although the intervention was not effective in improving performance for the whole group, a measure of learning potential that was administered as part of the study was a predictor of those individuals who received the most benefit from the intervention. In other words, participants with good learning potential benefited from the grocery shopping intervention, whereas individuals who were nonlearners received little to no benefit from the intervention.

Assessment Administration

The primary area of occupation assessed was the IADL of grocery shopping. In addition, through observation of performance, the occupational therapy practitioner was able to assess client performance skills required for grocery shopping, particularly cognitive skills, as well as communication, emotional regulation, and sensory processing.

Description of Environment/
Description of Supplies/Materials Required

A grocery store was selected for administration of the TOGSS. Selection of the grocery store was dependent upon the purpose of administration of the assessment. If the purpose is to determine how well an individual shops at his or her local supermarket, then the TOGSS should be administered in the store where the individual regularly completed grocery shopping. However, in some instances, the occupational therapy practitioner may choose to administer the TOGSS in an unfamiliar store. If the occupational therapist wishes to compare performance of different individuals, all individuals must have the same level of familiarity with the identified store in which the assessment will be administered. Therefore, it may be easiest to select a store where no one shops. Prior to beginning the assessment, it is helpful to notify grocery store personnel that you plan to use the store for the assessment. This is important so that the assessment is not interrupted by curious workers. If possible, there is an advantage to purchasing the grocery items for the participants as this more closely mirrors actual grocery shopping and can also serve as a significant incentive for the participant to locate all of the items on the list.

The supplies needed include two clipboards, two pens, the grocery list, the score sheet, the instructions, a stopwatch, and money if you intend to purchase the groceries. The participant and the tester each receive a clipboard. The score sheets and grocery lists are included with the TOGSS manual (Brown et al., 2009) and can be photocopied from the manual or printed from the compact disc that comes with the manual. The grocery list is placed on the client's clipboard, and the score sheet is placed on the occupational therapist's clipboard. The occupational therapist will need a pen for scoring the assessment. The client is also given a pen and may use it to mark items on the grocery list. The score sheet includes two pages. The first page indicates the 10 items on the list and allows the client to indicate whether the correct item was found. The second sheet is a map of the store, which is used for scoring redundancy. The occupational therapist will need the assessment instructions so they can be read aloud to the client. Once in the grocery store, the occupational therapist should make sure that the client has a cart for placing the items. If items are to be purchased, money will need to be supplied.

Administration

A grocery store should be selected based on the purpose of the assessment. The occupational therapist should determine the store in which the assessment will be conducted. The options may include a store the client shops at on a regular basis or a store the client is less familiar with so that observed performance will occur without prior knowledge of the setting. Before beginning the assessment, notify store personnel so that the assessment process is not interrupted.

Before the TOGSS is administered, the grocery lists provided with the manual (Brown et al., 2009) should be reviewed by the occupational therapist. It is possible that modifications to the list are necessary. All of the items should be available at the designated store. If an item is unavailable, an alternate item can be substituted. The manual describes the features to consider when a new item is substituted for an old item. Most often, only minor modifications to the TOGSS are necessary, such as the changing of item size based on current packaging.

Another preparatory step is the creation of a map of the grocery store. The map of the grocery store is used for scoring redundancy, which serves as an indication of efficiency. Details for creating a store map are included in the TOGSS manual, and a sample is provided (Brown et al., 2009). The grocery store map includes the numbered aisles of the stores and the perimeter of the store labeled according to sections (e.g., produce, dairy).

Administration of the TOGSS takes approximately 30 minutes but may take longer for individuals who find the task more difficult. The time to administer the test does not take into account transportation time to and from the grocery store. Administration begins by reading the instructions to the client. A copy of the instructions is provided to the client, and the client is asked to follow along. The client is then asked to explain what is to be completed while in the store. This ensures that the instructions are understood. If the client misses any of the important points, the occupational therapist shall repeat the specific instructions.

After the instructions are read, the client is asked to start shopping for the items on the list. The occupational therapist follows the client and uses this opportunity to score the assessment and make observations about the process. The occupational therapist should not assist the client with the grocery shopping task, but the client may ask for help from others (e.g., store personnel, shoppers).

Scoring

The TOGSS has three objectively measured subscales, including accuracy, time, and redundancy. The time and redundancy subscales provide measures of efficiency, an aspect of occupational performance that is often neglected. Inefficient performance can be frustrating and tiring and may cause individuals to avoid the task of grocery shopping. Consequently, it is an important aspect of performance to be considered. In addition, because the measure is administered in a natural environment, the grocery store, there are opportunities to observe performance and identify factors that interfere with or support performance.

Accuracy refers to the client's ability to choose the correct item in the correct size and at the lowest price. Each list has 10 items, and because there are 3 possible points for each item, the highest total score for accuracy is 30. Price is the most difficult aspect of the item score. Time is measured with the stopwatch and begins when the client starts shopping and ends when the client reaches the checkout line. Redundancy captures efficiency by identifying how many times the client enters a portion of the store. The occupational therapist uses the store map and places an X each time the client enters a section or aisle of a store. The occupational therapist can determine ahead of time the most efficient path for retrieving the 10 items on the map. Any time the client enters an aisle more than once or goes to sections or aisles where items from the list are not included indicates a redundancy or inefficient shopping. The redundancy score is the actual number of aisles or sections entered minus the minimum number of aisles that are sections required to find all of the items. The redundancy measure is a bit more challenging to score, but the manual provides a detailed explanation (Brown et al., 2009).

In addition, the objective scoring observation of performance provides important information about the process of grocery shopping and performance skill impairments or strengths that affected the outcome of grocery shopping. The scoring form includes some observations, such as "asking for help." Asking for help may be a good strategy if the individual is unable to easily locate an item but becomes inefficient if the individual must continually seek assistance. Asking for help also provides an opportunity to observe communication skills. In developing the measure, a behavior that was frequently noted and observed was "parking the cart." Generally, parking the cart is inefficient because the client must return to the location of the cart after finding an item. When two items are located on the same aisle, it is helpful to identify whether the client finds both items on the same trip, indicating some degree of working memory. Emotional regulation may also be observed in terms of the client's ability to persist or manage frustration.

Observations of the grocery store environment are also helpful, particularly when the TOGSS is administered in a store that the client typically uses. The occupational therapist can identify which aspects of the physical and social environment have the potential to support or interfere with the client's successful performance. For example, perhaps the store includes well-marked overhead signs but the client is unaware of the availability of these cues. The sheer number of items may create additional burdens for someone with decision-making difficulties, or the fluorescent lights may cause difficulty for an individual with visual sensory sensitivity.

Intervention Planning
Based on Assessment Results

The TOGSS provides objective and subjective information that can be used to assist an individual who needs and wants assistance as related to grocery shopping. The inclusion of accuracy and efficiency outcomes help the occupational therapist and client identify the aspects of the task that are most troublesome or challenging. In addition, observing performance in the natural environment provides information about what factors are presenting the greatest barriers to performance in the task of grocery shopping. For example, if the client is taking a long time to complete the task, there could be several reasons. Maybe it takes the client a long time to make a decision. Perhaps the client has trouble locating the item. Or maybe the client is distracted by other shoppers and has difficulty focusing on the task. These observations are crucial for targeting the correct area of focus for intervention.

Case Study

Jerry, a 27-year-old man, is living in an apartment for the first time. Jerry regularly attends a peer-run community program and receives assertive case management, which includes occupational therapy. He is having trouble managing his money, and this includes making his food last for the entire month. Jerry reports that the grocery store is overwhelming and that he tries to get in and out as soon as possible.

The occupational therapist decided to administer the TOGSS in the grocery store where Jerry typically shops. The store is large and full of activity, especially in the early evening hours and on weekends. The employees are friendly and helpful when they are not too busy. Jerry receives 19/30 points for accuracy, with only 4/10 for correctly selecting the lowest-priced item. It takes Jerry 31 minutes to complete the task, which is significantly longer than the average of 19 minutes that it took for individuals with schizophrenia during a validity study (Hamera et al., 2002). In addition, Jerry received a redundancy score of 5, which means he only returned to an aisle or went down an unnecessary aisle or section of the store 5 times.

The occupational therapist made the following observations about Jerry's performance:
- Jerry appears to know the store fairly well and uses the overhead signs or looks down an aisle before entering.
- Once Jerry finds the item on a shelf, this is where he takes a lot of time, as he experiences difficulty figuring out which item is the lowest price. Jerry expresses frustration with the decision-making process by stating, "There are just so many choices."
- In addition, Jerry is reluctant to search within a section in which other shoppers are located and will typically wait until an aisle is clear of all or most shoppers before entering that aisle or section of the store.

Taken together, the objective and subjective outcomes from the TOGSS indicate that Jerry has difficulty locating the lower-priced items in the grocery store. He is able to find the section of the store that contains the items he is looking for but spends a lot of time trying to make a choice among the items. Jerry is also uncomfortable being close to other shoppers, and this can interfere with his efficiency in completing the task.

The occupational therapist and Jerry made a plan to address his challenges with grocery shopping. The plan included learning strategies that will be helpful in finding the lower-priced item through didactic teaching and practice (e.g., how to identify generic items, locating and making sense of the prices on the shelves). Jerry shared that he thinks it will be easier to make decisions once he is more confident that he can locate the lower-priced items on a shelf. To address Jerry's discomfort around other shoppers, they agreed to two strategies: (1) the occupational therapist helped Jerry identify times when the store was less busy, and (2) they decided to practice role playing how Jerry could negotiate the aisle when others are already there.

Suggested Further Research

Normative scores for the TOGSS are not available. Additional research on a large sample to establish norms would be helpful so that scores from a client could be compared to the general population. Although the scores from the reliability and validity studies could be used as guidelines for performance by individuals with mental illness, there is only one small sample of individuals with no mental illness for which results of the TOGSS were published (Hamera et al., 2002). Studies that examined performance of individuals with diagnoses other than schizophrenia or bipolar disorder would also be useful. These studies could provide information about the impact of the diagnosis and related symptoms on the occupation of grocery shopping.

Summary

Few occupational therapy assessments are currently administered in a natural environment. Although there are inconveniences associated with using real-world settings, the benefits often outweigh the disadvantages due to the opportunities for observation as well as the authenticity of the experience. The TOGSS provides occupational therapy practitioners with an assessment of an important IADL that can be used in treatment planning and implementation.

References

Bombeck, E. (n.d.). *Dose of funny*. Retrieved from http://www.doseoffunny.com/erma-bombeck-funny-quote/

Brown, C., Rempfer, M., & Hamera, E. (2002). Teaching grocery shopping skills to people with schizophrenia. *Occupational Therapy Journal of Research, 22*, 90S-91S.

Brown, C., Rempfer, M., & Hamera, E. (2009). *Test of Grocery Shopping Skills manual*. Bethesda, MD: AOTA Press.

Dunn, W., Brown, C., & McGuigan, A. (1994). The Ecology of Human Performance: A framework for considering the effect of context. *American Journal of Occupational Therapy, 48*, 595-607.

Greenwood, K. E., Landau, S., & Wykes, T. (2005). Negative symptoms and specific cognitive impairments as combined targets for improved functional outcome within cognitive remediation therapy. *Schizophrenia Bulletin, 31*, 910-921.

Hamera, E., & Brown, C. E. (2000). Developing a context-based performance measure for persons with schizophrenia: The Test of Grocery Shopping Skills. *American Journal of Occupational Therapy, 54*, 20-25.

Hamera, E., & Brown, C. (2002). *Grocery shopping skills training program*. Retrieved from http://www.ct.gov/dmhas/lib/dmhas/skillbuilding/Test_of_Grocery_Shopping_Skills.pdf

Hamera, E. K., Brown, C., Rempfer, M., & Davis, N. C. (2002). Test of Grocery Shopping Skills: Discrimination of people with and without mental illness. *Psychiatric Rehabilitation Skills, 6*, 296-311.

Mausbach, B. T., Moore, R., Bowie, C., Cardenas, V., & Patterson, T. L. (2009). A review of instruments for measuring functional recovery in those diagnosed with psychosis. *Schizophrenia Bulletin, 35*, 307-318.

Rempfer, M., Brown, C., & Hamera, E. (2011). Learning potential as a predictor of skill acquisition in people with serious mental illness. *Psychiatry Research, 185*, 293-295.

Rempfer, M. V., Hamera, E. K., Brown, C. E., & Cromwell, R. L. (2003). The relations between cognition and the independent living skill of shopping in people with schizophrenia. *Psychiatry Research, 117*, 103-112.

Zayat, E., Rempfer, M., Gajewski, B., & Brown, C. E. (2011). Patterns of association between performance in a natural environment and measures of executive function in people with schizophrenia. *Psychiatry Research, 187*, 1-5.

Part VII
Biological Assessments

Adolescent/Adult Sensory Profile

Catana Brown, PhD, OTR/L, FAOTA

> *In a world where so much happens through computer screens, making a meal by hand,*
> *touching the raw materials, feeling your way through a recipe, tasting, adjusting, engaging all the senses,*
> *can be a soothing relief.*
> (Honore, 2017)

Sensory processing happens automatically as a part of our moment-to-moment existence as living beings. It is through the senses that we perceive, interact with, and understand the world around us. For the most part, we are unaware this is happening; there is no way we can be cognizant of every touch, taste, smell, sight, sound, and motor perception. However, when sensory processing becomes a part of our conscious awareness, many people may have strong reactions and either like or dislike the experience. Consider the following common reactions to a sensory experience: smell can make a person hungry or sick, music can be soothing or annoying, color can make an individual happy or restless, and breezes can be refreshing or bothersome. At times, both reactions occurred even when two different individuals were processing the same sensation.

The Adolescent/Adult Sensory Profile (A/ASP; Brown & Dunn, 2002) was designed to evaluate the behavioral responses that occurred as a reaction to the sensory encounters experienced each day. A self-report assessment intended to capture the traits associated with sensory processing preferences. The assessment does not assess sensory processing at a particular moment in time. Rather, the measure examines how an individual characteristically responds to sensory experiences. The A/ASP assists the occupational therapy practitioner in determining the types of sensory stimuli an individual likes and dislikes.

Hemphill, B. J., & Urish, C. K. (Eds.). *Assessments in Occupational Therapy Mental Health: An Integrative Approach, Fourth Edition* (pp. 445-456). © 2020 Taylor & Francis Group.

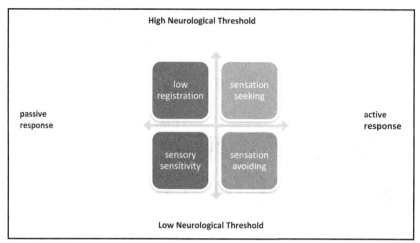

Figure 26-1. Sensory processing differences for individuals with psychiatric conditions.

Theoretical Basis

The theoretical basis for the A/ASP is Dunn's Model of Sensory Processing (Dunn, 1997). The A/ASP was not created as a measure of sensory integration but rather was grounded in sensory processing. This means that the A/ASP does not utilize an impairment model, which would suggest that sensory processing was deficient and needed to be fixed. Instead the theory underlying the A/ASP recognized that all individuals possess sensory processing preferences. Most often, sensory preferences become a problem when they interfere with the client's functional performance and engagement in daily activities. Occupational performance is enhanced when the environment and the occupation match the individual's sensory processing preference. When a mismatch occurs, the individual could demonstrate difficulty with occupational engagement and performance.

According to Dunn's (1997) Model of Sensory Processing, four preferences arise from the intersection of a neurological continuum and a behavioral response continuum, including low registration, sensation seeking, sensory sensitivity, and sensation avoiding (Figure 26-1). The neurological threshold continuum range was from low to high. A low threshold means that it takes very little sensory stimulation for the individual to notice and respond to a sensation. A high sensory threshold means that a more intense stimuli or a longer time period is required for the individual to notice the sensation. The behavioral response continuum range was from passive to active. In a passive response, the individual behaved or responded in a manner that was consistent with the threshold. In an active response, the individual responded in a manner intended to counteract the threshold. All preferences have assets and liabilities depending on the circumstances.

Low Registration (High Threshold, Passive Response in Accordance With the Threshold)

A low registration preference means the individual is slow to notice things that others notice or requires a stronger sensory stimulus to register the sensation. In addition, the individual had a passive response, meaning there was little attempt to find or notice sensations. For example, people with low registration may not hear their names being called or may not see signs directing them to the meeting room. However, individuals with low registration were more likely to be tolerant of a wide range of environments and enjoy a variety of experiences.

Sensation Seeking (High Threshold, Active Response to Counteract the Threshold)

The sensation seeking preference indicated a nervous system with a high threshold, but with this preference, the individual's behavioral response was an active response that counteracted the threshold. Sensation seeking individuals create or place themselves in situations that are loud, colorful, busy, bright, or extreme. The individual may sing to him- or herself, eat spicy foods, touch the items in a store, or engage in intense physical activity. However, sensation seekers may be easily bored and find it difficult to tolerate environments where there is not a lot going on. In extreme situations, these individuals may engage in risk-taking behaviors in an attempt to create a rich sensory experience.

Sensory Sensitivity (Low Threshold, Passive Response to the Threshold)

With a sensory sensitivity preference, the individual was quick to notice sensory stimuli and/or required little stimuli to be aware of the sensation. People with sensory sensitivity were able to identify or notice things quickly. These people distinguished subtle differences and may have been able to detect off-key singers or use their sensitivity for taste testing. However, the sensory sensitive individual can also be easily distracted in sensory-abundant environments and may have trouble staying focused or screening out irrelevant information.

Sensation Avoiding (Low Threshold, Active Response to Counteract the Threshold)

Individuals with sensation avoiding preferences also notice or are easily bothered by sensory stimuli, but they then engage in behaviors to reduce or manage that sensation. For example, sensation avoiders may prefer dimly lit spaces, like to work on only one task at a time, avoid crowded places, and use rituals to promote comfort and familiarity. Sensation avoiders are usually good at adapting environments and creating strategies to manage sensations.

Relationship of the Sensory Processing Preferences

The sensory processing preferences are not mutually exclusive. Individuals may operate in and out of different preferences depending on the particular sensation involved (e.g., an individual may be a movement seeker but an auditory avoider). An individual may also vary his or her preference depending on the occupation at hand. For example, when engaged in a complicated work task, the individual may prefer minimal extraneous stimuli but enjoy sensory-plentiful environments such as ball games or parties when involved in leisure activities. Others may fluctuate from one preference to another for no obvious reason. This is sometimes described as *sensory modulation disorder* and exists when individuals have extreme responses at both ends of a continuum. For example, the same individual may be extremely sensitive in one instance and exhibit low registration in another.

History of Development

The A/ASP benefits from the earlier development of the Sensory Profile by Dunn (1997). The original Sensory Profile was intended for use in children aged 3 to 10 years. The A/ASP was developed somewhat serendipitously after a statistical analysis (specifically a factor analysis) was performed using the data from the Sensory Profile. The assessment author needed a large dataset to analyze as part of a statistics course. Winnie Dunn had such a dataset based on many children's responses to the Sensory Profile. A factor analysis was conducted. The results of the factor analysis spawned Dunn's Model of Sensory Processing (1997). Once the model was developed, the assessment author recognized the salience of this sensory processing theory to occupational therapy practice in mental health. What was discovered was the clear application of the model to individuals with serious and persistent mental illness. As a result, the chapter author began developing an adult version of the Sensory Profile. Eventually, adolescents were included in the development process as the age range for the original Sensory Profile was 3 to 10 years. When considering the applicability of the measure for adolescents and adults, the author decided to design the measure as a self-report rather than an informant report because most adolescents and adults, including those with serious and persistent mental illness, were capable of reporting their behavioral responses to sensory experiences. An important distinction for individuals familiar with the Sensory Profile is that the scores are tabulated such that a higher score indicates more of a particular preference. For example, individuals with high scores on the sensation seeking items were described as sensation seekers.

In creating items for the A/ASP, Dunn's Model of Sensory Processing was taken into account with the idea that an equal number of items would be included to represent each of the four quadrants. In the end, the A/ASP comprised 60 items, including 15 for each quadrant. It was also important to create items that reflected adolescent and adult experiences. Some of the original items could be rewritten so they followed a self-report format, whereas other items were deleted or added. For example, instead of items that related to playground equipment or twirling as found on the Sensory Profile, the A/ASP included items that involved understanding humor and going shopping.

The first set of studies on an earlier version of the measure included a sample of 615 adults ranging in age from 17 to 79 years. They were recruited by students from Midwestern University and from a mailing list of individuals who had expressed interest in the Sensory Profile. These studies were described in greater detail in the original article describing the ASP (at this point, adolescents were not included; Brown, Tollefson, Dunn, Cromwell, & Filion, 2001). Reliability estimates using Cronbach's alpha ranged from 0.66 (sensation avoiding) to 0.82 (low registration). A factor analysis with the same data indicated good separation of the sensation seeking and low registration factors but overlap between sensory sensitivity and sensation avoiding. As a result, items were revised, particularly those in the sensation avoiding quadrant, to better reflect active avoidance of sensory stimuli.

Once it was determined that the measure would include adolescents, a second review of the items was performed. A small pilot group of adolescents reviewed the items to ensure understanding and comprehension of the questions. A few items underwent minor revision to clarify the questions. At this point in its development, it was determined that the A/ASP was ready for in-depth reliability and validity testing.

Psychometric Properties

Studies were undertaken to develop the classification system for the A/ASP and examine the reliability and validity of the measure. Several of these studies are described in the following sections.

Developing the Classification System

The A/ASP is a norm-referenced measure, meaning that an individual's scores can be compared to a standard sample of individuals without disabilities. A standardization sample of 950 adolescents and adults participated in the process of establishing cut scores for the A/ASP (Brown & Dunn, 2002). There were 193 adolescents (ages 11 to 17 years), 496 adults (ages 18 to 64 years), and 261 older adults (ages 65 years and older).

The classification system is used to identify if a particular individual's scores on a particular quadrant are the same as most people, less than most people, or more than most people. Five classification categories were created, and the cut scores were established by applying the percentages to the standardization sample.

- Much less than most people = less than 2% of the standardization sample
- Less than most people = between 2% and less than 16% of the standardization sample
- Similar to most people = between 16% and 84% of the standardization sample
- More than most people = between greater than 84% and 98% of the standardization sample
- Much more than most people = greater than 98% of the standardization sample

The classification system is divided by age group (adolescent, adult, and older adult) and quadrant (low registration, sensation seeking, sensory sensitivity, and sensation avoiding). This means, for example, that there is a separate cut score for low registration for adolescents, adults, and older adults.

Reliability

Item reliability of the A/ASP was analyzed using coefficient alpha as an estimate of internal consistency (Brown et al., 2001). Ninety-three adults with and without psychiatric disability participated in this study. Item reliability was lowest for the sensation seeking subscale ($\alpha=0.60$) but was similar for sensory sensitivity ($\alpha=0.78$), sensation avoiding (α=0.77), and low registration (α=0.78). Item reliability was also examined by comparing the correlation of each item on a subscale with the total score for each A/ASP quadrant subscale. Good reliability was indicated by an item that correlated highest with the intended subscale; this was true of all but two items. One of the items was from the sensation avoiding subscale and one was from the sensation seeking subscale.

An important aspect of reliability that is relevant to the A/ASP is test-retest reliability, but this has yet to be studied.

Validity

Construct validity was examined in a study that compared scores on the A/ASP to a physiological measure of skin conductance (Brown et al., 2001). The skin conductance outcomes included responsiveness and trials to habituation. Five individuals with high scores on one of each of the four quadrants (without high scores on another quadrant) participated in the study, for a total of 20 participants. The results were consistent with the hypothesis. Individuals with sensory sensitivity and sensation avoiding were more responsive (indicative of a low neurological threshold) than were individuals with low registration and sensation seeking. In terms of trials to habituation, the sensory sensitivity and sensation seeking groups took longer to habituate, while the low registration and sensation avoiding groups were quicker to habituate. Being slow to habituate was likely due to different reasons for the sensory sensitivity and sensation seeking groups. The sensitive individuals had trouble adjusting to or ignoring the stimuli, whereas the sensation seeking group desired the stimuli. The low registration group was habituated because they were less likely to notice the continued stimuli, whereas the sensation avoiding group had an active physiological response to disregard the stimuli.

Discriminant validity was supported by studies in which the measure is capable of distinguishing groups of individuals on probable characteristics. Several studies were conducted to examine the scores of individuals with psychiatric disabilities on the A/ASP. Table 26-1 summarizes the results of these studies and indicates distinct patterns of sensory processing for individuals with schizophrenia, bipolar disorder, obsessive compulsive disorder, attention-deficit hyperactivity disorder (ADHD), and autism (Brown et al., 2001; Clince, Connolly, & Nolan, 2016; Rieke & Anderson, 2009). Based on the results of these studies, individuals with autism have the most differences, with scores indicating more than most people for low registration, sensory sensitivity, and sensation avoiding and less than most people on sensation seeking (Clince et al., 2016). When compared to the standardization sample, individuals with schizophrenia were similar to most people on all of the quadrants, except low registration, where they scored more than most people (Brown, Cromwell, Filion, Dunn, & Tollefson, 2002). Their scores in the avoiding area were also close to being more than most people.

Assessment Administration

As a self-reported paper-and-pencil questionnaire, the A/ASP is easy to administer. The questionnaire includes 60 items and summary score sheets.

Table 26-1

Sensory Processing Differences for Individuals With Psychiatric Conditions[a]

Population	Low Registration		Sensation Seeking		Sensory Sensitivity		Sensation Avoiding		Reference
ADHD	40.6	More	44.9	Similar	44.2	More	41.3	Similar	Clince et al., 2016
Autism	42.8	More	40.3	Less	46.7	More	45.6	More	
Obsessive compulsive disorder	36.0	More	46.1	Similar	43.9	More	43.8	More	Reike & Anderson, 2009
Schizophrenia	36.9	More	45.5	Similar	38.9	Similar	40.9	Similar	Brown et al., 2002
Bipolar disorder	34.4	Similar	47.7	Similar	39.7	Similar	43.3	More	

[a]Scores are the reported mean score in the study along with the categorization according to the standardization sample. In all studies, the participants were adults.

Description of Environment/ Description of Supplies/Materials Required

The environment in which the A/ASP is administered can vary with the client. It is possible to provide the questionnaire to the individual for him or her to complete independently and return to the occupational therapist at a later date. In most instances, it is helpful to administer the questionnaire face to face in an interview-type fashion, especially if the client would benefit from assistance with comprehending or understanding the questions. When administering the measure in person, it is useful to have a quiet and comfortable space that is free from unnecessary distractions.

The only required materials are a pencil and the A/ASP Self-Questionnaire. A web-based version of the A/ASP also allows for administration of the measure, automatic scoring, and a summary report. The materials are available from Pearson Education, Inc. and can be ordered at http://www.pearsonclinical.com/therapy/products/100000434/adolescentadult-sensory-profile.html#tab-details.

Administration

The occupational therapist should be familiar with the questionnaire and the underlying theory before administration. The client will likely have a limited background in sensory processing; therefore, it is helpful to explain that the purpose of the A/ASP is to obtain information about how the client responds to everyday sensory experiences.

The responses to each item in the assessment include almost never, seldom, occasionally, frequently, and almost always. The therapist needs to explain to the client that the selected response should indicate how the client responds when presented with the situation described in the item. The occupational therapist should explain that it is important to respond to all of the items because if items are missed or skipped, interpretation and calculation of a final score is difficult.

The A/ASP can be administered in approximately 15 to 20 minutes. If the occupational therapist is administering the measure face-to-face as either the paper-and-pencil questionnaire or the web-based questionnaire, the therapist can clarify questions by further explaining or providing examples but should do so without indicating how the individual should respond. The occupational therapist may choose to read each item aloud to the client if this will help with comprehension. Informant reporting should be avoided; however, some individuals may not be capable of completing the self-report. When using informant reporting, the classification system was found to be much less reliable. The best informants would be those with caretaking responsibilities who have day-to-day interaction with the individual during engagement in activities of daily living.

Scoring

On the A/ASP, a high score indicates a greater amount of that particular sensory processing preference. This is different than the Sensory Profile for children and the Infant/Toddler Sensory Profile; meaning that, for example, an individual with a high score on sensation avoiding tends to engage in behaviors that involve attempting minimize exposure to sensory stimuli. Each item is scored using a 5-point scale:

- 1 = Almost never
- 2 = Seldom
- 3 = Occasionally
- 4 = Frequently
- 5 = Almost always

The four subscales of the A/ASP include low registration, sensation seeking, sensory sensitivity, and sensation avoiding. Each scale has a possible score ranging from 15 to 75. The raw scores are transferred from the Self-Questionnaire to the corresponding number on the Quadrant Grid. This allows the occupational therapist to total the scores for each subscale. The quadrant scores can then be plotted on the classification column to determine if the individual's score is similar to most people or more or less than most people. There is a separate set of classifications for adolescents (ages 11 to 17 years), adults (ages 18 to 64 years), and older adults (65 years and older).

Therapists should also consider extreme scores of items within a sensory category. As mentioned previously, individuals may have extreme scores in one particular sensory category but not in others, and these extreme scores may not be reflected in an overall subscale score. For example, an individual may provide an almost always response to the avoidance items in the auditory processing category. In this case, the occupational therapist would want to further explore situations that involve auditory processing to determine if this is a typical response.

If the web-based version of the A/ASP is used, the scores are tabulated automatically. In addition, a summary report will be provided with the scores.

Intervention Planning
Based on Assessment Results

By identifying an individual's sensory processing preferences, environments can be designed to support engagement and occupational performance. Guidelines regarding how to address the environment for each sensory processing preference follow.

High Scores on Low Registration

For individuals with low registration, it is helpful to increase the salience of the information that is important for the individual to notice. The use of cues, calendars, labels, and lists are useful strategies for individuals with low registration. Increasing the intensity of the stimulus, such as making colors brighter or sounds louder, can also help with noticing. In addition, it is often helpful to slow down the speed at which information is presented and check in often to ensure that the individual has indeed processed the information.

High Scores on Sensation Seeking

The primary intervention strategy for sensation seekers is to provide additional sensory input. This may include providing more opportunities to engage with the environment or increasing the amount or intensity of the sensory stimuli. Providing opportunities to interact with unfamiliar environments as well as frequent changes in the environment are generally desirable for sensation seeking individuals. What may be distracting for others may help increase arousal and attention for the sensation seeker.

High Scores on Sensory Sensitivity

Distractibility is often a concern for individuals with sensory sensitivity, making the removal of distractions a useful intervention strategy for individuals with sensory sensitivity. Supports that help maintain focus can also be useful, such as organizational systems, repetition, and predictability. Tasks may need to be broken down into smaller parts, and new information may need to be introduced gradually.

High Scores on Sensation Avoiding

Reducing the intensity of sensory stimuli in the environment is the primary intervention target for individuals with sensation avoiding preferences. However, sometimes the environment cannot be changed; in these cases, sensation avoiders will benefit from opportunities to remove themselves from environments that are overwhelming by allowing the individual to take breaks. Another beneficial intervention strategy is to provide the individual with control over his or her environment.

Case Study

Sandy, a 47-year-old woman who lives alone in a supported housing apartment, was referred to occupational therapy for personal hygiene issues. She has a diagnosis of schizophrenia and receives aid at a community support services program. Sandy was interested in pursuing an employment search, but her neglect of personal hygiene was a potential barrier.

The occupational therapist administered the A/ASP in addition to an occupational profile. Sandy received a score of 52 on the low registration subscale, indicating that she falls in the classification of much more than most people. This may help explain her inattention to personal hygiene as she may not notice or be bothered by the sensations that most would use as a cue to bathe, brush their teeth, or use deodorant. Other characteristics of schizophrenia seen in Sandy that might be associated with low registration include flat affect (she speaks in a monotone voice and displays very few facial expressions); difficulty with initiating activity; and a general slowness in her thinking, moving, and speaking.

Another feature that stood out on the A/ASP was Sandy's responses to the items in the movement processing category. Sandy uses the "almost always" response to all of the sensory sensitivity and sensation avoiding items related to movement, such as being afraid of heights and easily becoming dizzy. When the therapist further explored movement processing with Sandy, she discovered that she experiences a great deal of postural insecurity. One of the reasons that Sandy avoids bathing is because she is frightened of falling in the tub. She finds it very difficult to get into the tub and is also fearful of slipping once she gets in.

The intervention plan involved addressing the overall high scores in low registration and the specific sensory sensitivity and sensation avoiding issues related to movement, all within the context of the performance of personal hygiene tasks. Sandy was very motivated to participate in the occupational therapy intervention as she understood that improving her self-care was important for success in finding and keeping a job.

First, the occupational therapist used strategies to address Sandy's low registration. The occupational therapist and Sandy created a list of the personal hygiene tasks that should be routinely performed (e.g., tooth brushing, bathing, washing hair, nail care). With this list, they determined the frequency for each task. Based on this list, a weekly color-coded calendar was fashioned that Sandy posted in her bathroom next to the mirror.

Next, the occupational therapist used strategies to address Sandy's sensory sensitivity and sensation avoiding when it came to movement, specifically, her concerns related to bathing. They discussed the option of moving to an apartment with a walk-in shower, but Sandy was not interested in moving. Instead, they decided to adapt the bathroom so that Sandy would feel more secure. Grab bars were added to the tub area, and a tub seat with suction cups was secured to the bathtub. Next, a hand-held shower wand was installed.

In a follow-up visit, it was clear that the strategies were working. Sandy reported that she was delighted with the bathroom modifications. She actually enjoyed showering, and now that she was no longer scared, it was not difficult to carry out the task. In addition, the calendar had been helpful in reminding Sandy about the other personal hygiene tasks.

Suggested Further Research

At this time, no data are available on the test-retest reliability of the A/ASP. It would be useful if studies were carried out in which the measure was administered at two different time points to establish the stability of the scores over time. In addition, it would be interesting for studies to readminister the A/ASP within a short period of time and a long period of time to see if the reliability changed with time. The A/ASP is theorized to measure trait characteristics that do not change dramatically over time. Therefore, a longitudinal study would help determine whether sensory processing is trait-like.

Predictive validity is another area of study that would contribute both to a greater understanding of the measure's usefulness as well as greater understanding of the relationship of sensory processing and occupational performance. These studies would be designed to examine the impact of different sensory processing preference on different aspects of occupational performance. According to Dunn's Model of Sensory Processing (1997), one would hypothesize that each sensory processing preference would have advantages and disadvantages depending on the particular context of occupational performance.

Summary

Although occupational therapists often assess sensory processing to determine its impact on occupational performance, few measures of sensory processing are available for adolescents and adults that include a classification system for comparing results of an individual with others. Individuals with psychiatric conditions often experience sensory processing preferences that are not typical. The A/ASP is a widely used, theory-driven measure that can be useful in better understanding clients with psychiatric conditions and developing intervention plans.

References

Brown, C., Cromwell, R. L., Filion, D., Dunn, W., & Tollefson, N. (2002). Sensory processing in schizophrenia: Missing and avoiding information. *Schizophrenia Research, 55*, 187-195.

Brown, C., & Dunn, W. (2002). *Adolescent/Adult Sensory Profile: User's manual.* San Antonio, TX: The Psychological Corporation.

Brown, C., Tollefson, N., Dunn, W., Cromwell, R., & Filion, D. (2001). The Adult Sensory Profile: Measuring patterns of sensory processing. *American Journal of Occupational Therapy, 55*, 75-82.

Clince, M., Connolly, L., & Nolan, D. (2016). Comparing and exploring the sensory processing patterns of higher education students with attention deficit hyperactivity disorder and autism spectrum disorder. *American Journal of Occupational Therapy, 70*, 7002250010p1-p9.

Dunn, W. (1997). The impact of sensory processing abilities on the daily lives of young children and their families: A conceptual model. *Infants and Young Children, 9*, 23-35.

Honore, C. (2017). Brainy quote. Retrieved from https://www.brainyquote.com/quotes/quotes/c/carlhonore633754.html

Rieke, E. F., & Anderson, D. (2009). Adolescent/Adult Sensory Profile and obsessive-compulsive disorder. *American Journal of Occupational Therapy, 63*, 138-145.

Spiritual Assessments in Mental Health Occupational Therapy

Barbara J. Hemphill, DMin, OTR, FAOTA

Based on the assumption that there is an ontological drive to make sense of life,
particularly in the presence of tragedy, individuals face the task of redefining the meaning of
their existence within the reality of the threat of nonbeing.
(Sorajjakool, 2006, p. 83)

Historically, occupational therapists have been concerned with the care of the whole person—body, mind, and spirit—and have a professional commitment to treat individuals from a holistic perspective. Illness, by its very nature, is a spiritual encounter as well as a physical and emotional experience, but the spiritual is the least visible aspect of the whole. How can occupational therapists effectively address the spirituality of their patients in daily practice?

The term *spirituality* comes from the Latin word *spiritus*, meaning "breath" or "life." The word *spirit* can be a synonym for the living soul. It can mean courage, determination, and energy. Nelson (2011) stated "... spiritual is generally applied to any human essence connecting us to an unseen world that defies scientific measurement but which we nonetheless believe and feel exists, leaving traces here and there" (p. 17). Nelson (2011) further stated that it refers to anything transcendent or anything that can be considered larger than ourselves. It is something beyond the human being. Nelson (2011) defined spiritual as a "direct personal experience, regardless of social context" (p. 26), further quoting from James and Marty (1982) that what makes a personal experience spiritual "is the feelings, acts, and experiences" of individuals who in their solitude understand they have come in contact with "what they may consider to be the divine" (p. 26). This definition is both inclusive and expansive. It means many things to many people and includes concepts such as meaning and purpose, connectedness, peacefulness, personal well-being, and happiness.

Hemphill, B. J., & Urish, C. K. (Eds.). *Assessments in Occupational Therapy Mental Health: An Integrative Approach, Fourth Edition* (pp. 457-468). © 2020 Taylor & Francis Group.

Spirituality, Religion, and Health Care

Spirituality is recognized as an important concept in the study and practice of medicine. Hospitals and health care organizations seem to be listening to what the research says. Since 2000, the Joint Commission has required "that a spiritual history be taken on every patient admitted to an acute care hospital or a nursing home, or seen by a home health agency, and a spiritual history must be documented in the medical record" (Koenig, 2007, p. 4). According to Davis (1997), "We are morally obliged to act in certain ways that reflect what it means to be professional, to respond to fellow human beings who place trust in us because of their vulnerability in time of need" (p. 9). Medical students are educated to understand that taking a patient's spiritual history is as relevant as taking a family history (Spencer, 2004).

In the specific context of occupational therapy, spirituality is viewed as part of the concept of holism and needs to be assessed (American Occupational Therapy Association, 2014). Therapists need to recognize whether their patients relate to spirituality through a traditional religious discipline or through unconventional practices and then assist them in their spiritual process.

To accomplish this, according to Hodge (2001), therapists must distinguish between religion and spirituality. Religion is an institutionalized form of spirit, expressed subjectively through rituals, beliefs, and practices. Spirituality is definitely part of religion, but religion may not be part of spirituality. Spirituality contains the domains of religion, but a person can be spiritual without following religious ideology. Hodge (2001) defined spirituality "as a relationship with God, or whatever is held to be the Ultimate (for example, a set of sacred texts for Buddhists), that fosters a sense of meaning, purpose, and mission in life" (p. 204). This relationship results in concepts such as altruism, love, or forgiveness, which, in turn, affect a person's relationship to the self, nature, others, and the Ultimate Being (Carroll, 1997; Sermabeikian, 1994).

Many clinical assessments of spirituality are limited by their use of terms that are too narrow. These assessments generally assume that the patient is Christian and do not include other traditions. Therapists must take precautions to not use measures that are based on Christian ideology when assessing people who are not of the Christian faith. Further, some people might be offended by the word "God" or find it confusing or meaningless. "Spirituality" is a broader term that can be substituted. Some other examples of alternative words for God could be transcendent being, deity, or higher power.

Thus, the ability of any clinical assessment to capture a patient's spirituality is often limited by the choice of words. Spirituality can be described using words such as higher consciousness, transcendence, self-reliance, love, faith, enlightenment, community, self-actualization, compassion, forgiveness, mysticism, a higher power, and grace. Any of these words can be used to describe the personal meaning someone attaches to human life. Spirituality, although often associated with religion, must be distinct from religion. Occupational therapists need to be careful and use words that are consistent with each individual patient's faith tradition.

A loss of meaning is perhaps the greatest crisis a person might experience when faced with illness or disease. People are able to deal with great physical and emotional trauma, but they might be unable to bear a sense of meaninglessness. People can overcome pain, disease, or hardship, but when they believe they are no longer needed, they can no longer contribute, and their life has no meaning, they are in spiritual crisis (Hay, 1989; Howard & Howard, 1997; Smucker, 1996). Anandarajah and Hight (2001) added to the discussion about spiritual crises and distress when they wrote:

Spiritual distress and spiritual crises occur when individuals are unable to find sources of meaning, hope, love, peace, comfort, strength, and connection in life or when conflict occurs between their beliefs and what is happening in their life. This distress can have a detrimental effect on physical and mental health. Medical illness and impending death can often trigger spiritual distress in patients and family members. (p. 86)

When a patient is in spiritual crisis, as defined by Anandarajah and Hight (2001), it is appropriate for occupational therapists to administer a spiritual assessment, to initiate discussion about spiritual needs, and to refer the patient to appropriate spiritual leaders if necessary. Spiritual crises and spiritual distress are terms "used to describe a pervasive disruption in a person's spiritual life" (Hasselkus, 2011, p. 146). Spiritual crises are the opposite of spiritual health, spiritual well-being, and spiritual integrity.

Spirituality and the Assessment Process

The context for spiritual assessment includes the patient's spiritual locus of control, which includes well-being, personal beliefs, level of spiritual maturity, and religious traditions and values. Richards and Bergin (1997) proposed five reasons why spiritual assessment is essential in a therapeutic relationship: (1) to understand a patient's worldview so the therapist can become more empathetic and sensitive; (2) to increase the therapist's understanding of how healthy or unhealthy a patient's spiritual orientation is and to what extent it affects the presenting problem; (3) to see whether the patient's beliefs and the community can be used as resources for coping methods and growth; (4) to find out which spiritual interventions may be beneficial for the patient; and (5) to determine whether the patient has unresolved spiritual issues.

Further, Richards and Bergin (1997) proposed the following eight dimensions that should be included in a spiritual assessment:

1. Metaphysical worldview
2. Religious affiliation or denomination
3. Religious problem-solving style (self-directing involves only the self; deferring is giving it to God; collaborating involves others, such as medical healers)
4. Spiritual identity and tradition
5. God image
6. Value and lifestyle congruence
7. Doctrinal knowledge (i.e., the patient's knowledge of the sacred texts of his or her faith)
8. Religious and spiritual health and maturity

Gathering data does not constitute an assessment in itself; the information must be interpreted, organized, integrated with theory, and made meaningful.

Spiritual assessments can sometimes raise concerns. Occupational therapists must try to keep a balance between using and developing patients' spiritual strengths and remaining focused on treatment goals. Therapy should always be the primary focus. Occupational therapists need to avoid assuming the role of spiritual expert, instead referring their patients to their own spiritual or religious healer (Hodge, 2001).

When practitioners have firmly held values, they risk imposing their own positions on patients. In this case, they should not conduct spiritual assessments with people who hold values different from theirs. Also, some people consider spirituality a private matter and may object to exploring this area in a rehabilitative setting. Still others do not believe in a higher power, and therapists should respect this. In short, therapists should never administer a spiritual assessment without obtaining consent.

Therapist's Spiritual Self

Anandarajah and Hight (2001) indicated that two factors can increase the likelihood of a successful discussion of spiritual needs: spiritual self-understanding and spiritual self-care. They asserted that therapists must understand their own spiritual beliefs, values, and biases to remain patient-centered and nonjudgmental when dealing with patients' spiritual concerns. This concept is compatible with the relationship-centered care concept, and it is especially relevant when the therapist's and patient's beliefs differ.

Anandarajah and Hight (2001) further stated, "Spiritual self-care is integral to serving the multiple needs and demands of patients in the current health care system" (p. 6). Later, Koenig (2004) described some of the barriers therapists might encounter in obtaining spiritual histories. They included lack of time on the part of the therapist, lack of training, discomfort with the subject, worries about imposing religious beliefs on patients, and lack of interest or awareness. Ultimately, it is important that therapists first look at their spiritual selves.

Spiritual Assessment Process

Koenig (2004) suggested four questions that occupational therapists can use when gathering information from patients about their spiritual histories:

1. Are they drawing on religion or spirituality as a method of coping with their illness?
2. Do they have a supporting spiritual community?
3. Do they have spiritual questions of concern?
4. Do they hold spiritual beliefs that may affect their medical care?

Similarly, Gorsuch and Miller (1999) proposed that therapists integrate three questions into the clinical setting during therapy:

1. Do you currently practice your religion?
2. Do you believe in God or a higher power?
3. Are there certain practices that you engage in on a regular basis?

To assess a sense of meaning, therapists also might ask, "What is important to you, and what gives you meaning and purpose in life?" All of these questions are helpful to consider when conducting a spiritual assessment.

Another spiritual history tool, referred to as the *FICA* (faith or beliefs; importance or influence; community; address in care), asks a series of questions about patients' faith, the importance of their beliefs, if they belong to a spiritual community, and if there are spiritual practices they wish to develop. Through these questions, the FICA examines four concepts: faith or beliefs, importance, community, and address. Puchalski and Romer (2000) suggested that therapists use the FICA to explore their own personal spiritual histories.

A spiritual history assessment should be administered during the admission process and during the initial occupational therapy evaluation process. Care should be taken that the same questions are not repeated. If a spiritual history is not taken at the time of admission, it is appropriate for the occupational therapist to administer a spiritual history evaluation. Koenig (2007) suggested the best times to conduct an initial spiritual history are the following:

- When taking the medical history during a new patient evaluation. The spiritual history is taken during the initial evaluation process and integrated into the interview; it is part of obtaining the patient's occupational profile.
- When taking the medical history while admitting a patient to a health facility.
- When doing a health maintenance visit as part of a well-person evaluation. This includes obtaining information about the patient's environment and support system, such as family, job, and sources of stress.

The spiritual history assessment can be repeated after several months or years if appropriate. It needs to be reviewed and updated to reflect the patient's current condition and medical, social, and physical environment. It is important to distinguish between a spiritual history assessment and a spiritual assessment that is intended to reflect the patient's current spirituality and relates to clinical goals and objectives. An example of a question in a spiritual history assessment would be, "What was your faith tradition growing up?" A spiritual assessment would ask, "What faith tradition do you currently follow?"

Other Spiritual Assessments

Illness and disability raise fundamental questions about spiritual well-being. Why me? Why do I suffer? Does my suffering have meaning? Maugans (1996) created an assessment examining concepts of meaning and purpose. Maugans (1996) drew from the work of Frankl (1984) for the development of a framework for taking a spiritual interview and answering these questions based on the concept of spiritual suffering. Frankl (1984) stated that physical discomfort and deprivation, no matter how extreme or brutal, do not cause suffering. The cause of suffering is the loss of meaning and purpose in life. Maugans's (1996) assessment examined the concepts of meaning and purpose.

An assessment rooted in the theory of logotherapy is the Engleside Skilled Nursing and Rehabilitation Center Assessment Tool developed by Frankl (1984). The underlying premise of this assessment is that people search for meaning in life up until the moment of death. This tool can be used to assess the meaning of a higher power.

An example of a questionnaire form of assessment is the Spiritual Assessment Guidelines by Schnorr (1999). This assessment was initially designed for persons of the Quaker faith. The questions ask about source of spiritual strength, meaning and purpose, love and relatedness, forgiveness, hope, effects of illness, and religious affiliation.

The Multidimensional Spiritual/Religiousness measure is a researched instrument that can be obtained free of charge from the Fetzer Institute and the National Institute on Aging Working Group (1999). A presentation regarding administration and scoring is available online. This assessment is reported from Fetzer to be valid with various populations when compared to other spiritual assessments. The constructs examined that relate to health care are as follows: daily activities, spiritual experiences, meaning, values, beliefs, forgiveness, private religious practices, religious/spiritual history, commitment, organizational religiousness, and religious preference. The assessment is available in a short or long form. The entire assessment does not have to be administered to obtain results.

Another spiritual assessment tool that addresses this specifically is the HOPE concept:

- H stands for the patient's sources of hope, strength, comfort, meaning, peace, love, and connection.

- O is the role of organized religion for the patient.
- P represents the patient's personal spirituality and practices.
- E stands for effects on medical care and end-of-life decisions.

The HOPE questions serve to introduce spiritual content into the interviewing process. The questions have not yet been validated by research, but they allow open-ended inquiry into the patient's spiritual resources and concerns. For example, in the interview process, a therapist can ask, "For some people, their religious or spiritual beliefs act as a source of comfort and strength in dealing with life's ups and downs; is this true for you?" If the answer is "yes," the assessment can proceed. If the answer is "no," the clinician can ask, "Was it ever important to you?" If the answer is "yes," the clinician can follow up by asking, "What changed?" This can lead to further inquiry, or the therapist can cease asking questions about spiritual matters.

As this brief survey of possible tools indicates, spiritual assessments come in a variety of formats. There are questionnaires, observational scales, and interview guides. Plus, other types of assessments can be used to reevaluate patients in addition to gathering a spiritual history. Appendix H offers a list of recommended assessments.

Guidelines for Selecting Spiritual Assessments

Fitchett (2002) suggested seven issues to consider when selecting a spiritual assessment process or tool:
1. "Is the model's concept of spirituality explicit or implicit?" (p. 90). The assessments in this area of occupation are objective and therefore implicit.
2. "Is it substantive or functional?" (p. 91). Substantive means that the assessment focuses on the patient's beliefs and values. Functional assessments focus on the practice of beliefs and values.
3. "Does it include one or more dimensions of spiritual life?" (p. 91). An assessment that asks only one question is one-dimensional (e.g., "What religion do you practice?"). An assessment that asks multiple questions is one that looks at spiritual life from a number of perspectives.
4. "Is it static or developmental?" (p. 92). Is change expected, and does the assessment measure change? A developmental assessment expects change, such as Fowler's (1981) five stages of spiritual development.
5. "Does it have a dynamic perspective?" The therapist needs to "know what people say what they believe and feel as well as observations of unconscious attitudes and emotions that might or might not be consistent with those that are consciously held" (p. 93).
6. "Is the context for spiritual assessment holistic?" (p. 93). The patient's religious practices, culture, personality, family, and health should be interrelated. The therapist should be aware of patients' behaviors that may be caused by an infarct on the brain, such as brain injury, medication reaction, or stress.
7. "Is the spiritual dimension distinct from the psychosocial one?" (p. 94). Be sure the assessment tests spirituality and not psychosocial aspects. Do not substitute a psychological test for a spiritual one.

The FICA is an example of an assessment that meets all of these criteria and is brief. However, other assessments also meet some of these guidelines. In considering the occupational therapy process and conducting a spiritual assessment, occupational therapists must first select a spiritual assessment that is most appropriate for use with an individual patient. Because there are many spiritual assessments available, therapists must choose the assessment(s) they feel will best illuminate their patients' needs and concerns. Next, therapists must clearly and competently understand how to administer and interpret the assessment(s), seeking outside guidance from a colleague or supervisor if there are areas of uncertainty or a lack of understanding. Lastly, therapists must consider how to interpret the data gathered during a spiritual assessment. Consider the case of Lauren and George as an example of the process of conducting a spiritual assessment.

Case Study

Lauren was an occupational therapist in an outpatient substance abuse treatment clinic and psychosocial clubhouse. George was a 32-year-old, first-generation Mexican-American who was living with his parents. He was caught between the values, beliefs, and religion of his parents, who were Catholic, and his emerging Buddhist beliefs.

When Lauren met him, George had been recently discharged following 5 years of incarceration for the manufacturing and sale of methamphetamine. This was George's third incarceration, and he now had a felony on his record. While in prison, George received treatment for his addiction and began learning about Buddhism. However, he began using methamphetamine 1 hour after discharge from prison. He went to the outpatient clinic where Lauren was employed after his parole officer required a random urine screen to ensure he was not using methamphetamine. George, referred to outpatient addictions treatment, had not been able to see his 3 children for the past 5 years because his ex-wife had a restraining order against him.

After entering the outpatient treatment environment, George began to question his Catholic upbringing and the beliefs and values his parents appeared to be trying to impose upon him. He felt lost, overwhelmed, and did not know what to believe. George's primary motivations for treatment were to be able to see his children and remain out of prison. His parole officer indicated that his primary responsibility was to stay off drugs and get a job and that this would help him stay out of prison.

Lauren considered herself to be a holistic therapist. Her assessments included reviewing George's medical record, including his family history, personal narrative, life turning points, physical health, nutrition, and social relationships. She administered the HOPE assessment during the interviewing process. She found that George's beliefs from Buddhism helped him cope with the ups and downs of being away from his family. Lauren examined carefully George's spiritual environment because this provided a framework through which he was attempting to accept, make sense of, and find meaning within his life; resolve loss and grief issues; solve problems related to employment and life outside prison; make major life decisions; cope with daily living challenges; embrace joys; adjust to change; find inner strength; face his fears; and learn how to take appropriate risks.

In the process of her comprehensive assessment, Lauren discovered that many of the issues George was struggling with pertained to Buddhism and his desire to practice this spiritual tradition in all aspects of his life, while his parents insisted that he return to the Catholic church. Lauren shared with George, "I think I can assist you in the things you struggle with, but I have limited knowledge of the Buddhist religion. With your permission, I would like to consult with a colleague who is a Buddhist. I also may recommend a Buddhist teacher to you to help you clarify some specific beliefs you mentioned earlier. Is this acceptable to you?" George agreed.

In the case of Lauren and George, Lauren needed to understand her own spiritual grounding and then step beyond it. She both reassured George and acknowledged her limitations when she said, "I think I can assist you in the things you struggle with, but I have limited knowledge of the Buddhist religion." She then offered two additional resources/approaches for assistance and asked for his permission.

In addition, Lauren knew enough about Buddhism to understand that she needed to approach George in a mindful way. This approach—a means for interacting with patients from the Buddhist tradition—is, according to Bien (2006), a keen awareness of a calm presence. It entails experiencing and accepting reality fully. It is a method of listening reflectively; allowing silence in interactions with patients; and using metaphor, storytelling, and other methods.

This case study involves someone with interests in Buddhism, but the same approach can be used whenever the occupational therapist and patient have different spiritual or religious beliefs and/or practices. Successful work with a diverse population necessitates that therapists view spiritual practices as a reciprocal process. Therapists must meet their patients on the patient's own playing field. In the case of this Buddhist patient, the playing field was a therapeutic relationship wrapped in compassion, acceptance, mindfulness, ethical conduct, and wisdom, which might result in the lessening of suffering and thereby contribute to effective habilitation and rehabilitation.

As this case study shows, occupational therapists can contribute to patients' change, growth, and development by supporting the patient within his or her preferred spiritual environment. By listening to the unique needs and issues shared by the patient, and by critical examination of their own knowledge, ideas, feelings, and beliefs so they are not barriers to understanding the patient's current or previous experiences, therapists can work closely with patients to identify the beliefs and practices that will promote, support, and encourage recovery (Egan & Phillips, 2011).

Treatment Planning and Intervention

During a spiritual assessment, occupational therapists can learn about the uniqueness of each person and the contexts that support or hinder his or her occupational performance. Barriers may need to be examined and addressed, as the case of Lauren and George demonstrates. However, by gathering this information, therapists can develop a treatment plan based on the experiences a person most values and wishes to retain.

General Intervention Planning

Galanti (2008) has offered some suggestions that are culturally and spirituality sensitive when developing treatment plans and interventions:

- "Honor patient requests for same-sex providers whenever possible.
- Respect … patient's religious beliefs, even when they conflict with your own.
- Allow patients privacy for prayer.
- Be aware that different religions have different holy days. It is Friday for Muslims, Saturday for Jewish people, and Sunday for Christians.
- Allow patients to make informed choices regarding risks when medical procedures conflict with their religious beliefs.
- Learn what symbols are sacred to those who are treated, and respect them" (p. 78).

Koenig (2007) suggested that a spiritual director should be made available, if possible, although medical centers are cutting budgets and clergy may not be available. Pastoral services may be combined with social services to meet budgetary needs.

Specific Intervention Planning

Ideally, occupational therapists and patients should collaborate, based upon information gathered in the assessment, to develop treatment plans and interventions that value and honor the patients' individual needs (Egan & Phillips, 2011). Just as each spiritual assessment is unique to each patient, each intervention should be planned to address their unique needs, values, and goals.

Through examination of spiritual assessments, occupational therapists can develop interventions to help their patients accept, make sense of, and find meaning in life (Egan & Phillips, 2011). Further, interventions can address grief and loss issues patients may be dealing with that could be hindering their engagement in valued occupations. By examining a patient's spiritual focus, therapists can structure interventions to foster improved problem-solving, coping, and decision-making skills. Interventions designed to assist patients in facing fears; adjusting to uncertainty; and addressing change from a physical, mental, or emotional perspective can be addressed (Egan & Phillips, 2011).

Of utmost importance in intervention planning and spiritual assessment is the occupational therapist's role in fostering independence with each patient. Therapists need to plan interventions that promote and enable occupational participation rather than dependency on the therapist or the therapy process (Egan & Phillips, 2011).

At times, a patient may look to the occupational therapist as the keeper of the knowledge when, in fact, the patient is the one who knows him- or herself better than anyone. Patients should be directly, consistently, and regularly consulted regarding their insights about therapeutic interventions and any perceived benefits, concerns, and outcomes. By engaging in ongoing conversations with their patients, occupational therapists can ascertain if the therapeutic interventions selected are valuing the individual's spiritual being and providing a meaningful connection to their world (Schulz, 2011).

In considering intervention planning, implementation, and modification from a spiritual perspective, occupational therapists need to be ever mindful that individuals' spirituality can evolve, change, and grow as they adapt to life and that changes may occur related to acute illness, chronic illness, or disability (Schulz, 2011). An occupational therapist who provides an intervention to a patient for a hand injury in 2015 and who then sees the same person 2 years later cannot rely on previous spiritual assessment data. The individual may have made minor or significant changes from a spiritual perspective. However, that person may not willingly offer this information or perspective to the therapist; this leads to the importance of conducting ongoing spiritual assessments (Schulz, 2011).

Using a valued occupation that patients find meaningful on a daily basis as an orienting force may significantly influence the therapy process in a positive manner. For example, incorporating time in the morning and before bedtime for quiet reflection or meditation may help individuals critically examine goals for the day (AM reflection) and progress that has transpired during the day (PM reflection). Encouraging patients to engage in meaningful, valued occupations in a consistent fashion also can help them feel a sense of empowerment, stability, and calmness, especially for individuals who may be encountering many areas of their lives in which they feel they have little to no control (e.g., certain medical procedures).

Finally, occupational therapists need to make sure that intervention plans include spiritually meaningful occupations that can help individuals celebrate the joys of change, skill development, and adaptation as they cope with daily challenges.

Ethical Considerations

Incorporating spirituality into the assessment and treatment process can create ethical concerns for occupational therapists. Possible concerns might be imposing one's own religious beliefs on the patient and/or the need to address a spiritual crisis the patient may be experiencing. To avoid such ethical difficulties, therapists must assess their own spiritualities and where they are on their spiritual journeys. As previously mentioned, they need to understand how to incorporate their own spiritualities into their practices. In addition, therapists need to understand how patients' values and religious beliefs influence their decision making. Some people base their identity (i.e., idiosyncrasies that make a person unique) on what is perceived as right and wrong, and some draw on the spiritual aspect of life, following specific beliefs that have meaning to them.

The following is a set of universal ethics to guide clinicians' thinking as they interact with patients who are experiencing a spiritual crisis:

- Be human, be real, be honest.
- Be present and listen, with an emphasis on being with the patient, not doing.
- Include spiritual concerns in treatment planning.
- Respect the patient's belief system, regardless of your own feelings about religion and spirituality.
- Provide access to spiritual resources by referring to spiritual healers, such as chaplains, priests, ministers, rabbis, and imams.
- Be a caring professional; encourage patients and their family members to give voice.
- Explore, but do not probe; help people to feel heard.
- Avoid judging beliefs, practices, or emotional responses; refrain from proselytizing or imposing your own beliefs.
- Be aware of your beliefs and the influence they have on the health care process.
- Be careful if you and a patient share the same religious traditions; beliefs and practices vary widely.
- Avoid discussions of doctrine, dogma, and complicated theological questions. Patients usually do not want or need intellectual discussions; they need comfort and reassurance.
- Avoid clichés such as "It is God's will" or "God never gives you more than you can bear." Do not use this language unless the patient and family members have used these phrases themselves.
- Respect the patient's and family's spiritual traditions and practices, as well as their privacy in this area.
- Do not initiate participation in the patient's religious observances. Let the family do the inviting.
- Follow the plan for spiritual care agreed upon by the patient, family, and health team.

Summary

Spiritual history assessments are an integral part of occupational therapists' holistic practice with their patients. Such assessments generally take the form of interviews, questionnaires, and inventories. Although there are no published articles to date demonstrating the benefits of conducting a spiritual assessment, there is indirect evidence to support this practice. First, spiritual practices are ways in which patients cope with medical illnesses. Second, spiritual beliefs have been found to influence medical decisions. Third, the patient's faith community is a source of support and can be associated with adherence to medical therapy. Finally, patient satisfaction with the emotional aspects of care is high when their spiritual needs are recognized and faith traditions are respected (Koenig, 2004).

Spiritual assessments usually focus on health care and end-of-life issues (e.g., HOPE). Occupational therapists should consider administering a spiritual assessment at the beginning of the evaluation process and again at reevaluation. Prior to the start of clinical practice and on a regular basis (perhaps annually), occupational therapists also should complete a spiritual assessment of themselves to ensure their own values and spiritual ideas do not influence their patient care in clinical practice or research. Ultimately, spiritual issues can be approached as an aspect of diversity and treated with the same respect as any other personal issue.

Acknowledgments

I wish to thank those who contributed to this chapter. Christine K. Urish, PhD, OTR/L, BCMH, FAOTA, contributed information about the case study. Nancy Powell, PhD, FAOTA, OTR, contributed information about Buddhism in relation to occupational therapy.

References

American Occupational Therapy Association. (2014). Occupational therapy practice framework: Domain and process (3rd ed.). *American Journal of Occupational Therapy, 68*(Suppl. 1), S1-S48.

Anandarajah, G., & Hight, E. (2001). Spirituality and medical practice: Using the HOPE questions as a practical tool for spiritual assessment. *American Family Physician, 63*, 81-89.

Bien, T. (2006). *Mindful therapy: A guide for therapists and helping professionals.* Boston, MA: Wisdom Publications.

Carroll, M. (1997). Spirituality and clinical social work: Implications of past and current perspectives. *Arete, 22*, 25-34.

Davis, C. (1997). Psychoneuroimmunology: The bridge to the coexistence of two paradigms. In C. Davis (Ed.), *Complementary therapies in rehabilitation.* (pp. 1-16). Thorofare, NJ: SLACK Incorporated.

Egan, M., & Phillips, S. (2011). The spiritual environment. In C. Brown & V. C. Stoffel (Eds.), *Occupational therapy in mental health* (pp. 453-461). Philadelphia, PA: F. A. Davis.

Fetzer Institute and the National Institute on Aging Working Group. (1999). *Multidimensional measurement of religious/spirituality for use in health research.* Retrieved from: http://www.fetzer.org/resources/multidimensional-measurement-religiousnessspirituality-use-health-research

Fitchett, G. (2002). *Assess spiritual needs: A guide for caregivers.* Lima, OH: Academic Renewal Press.

Fowler, J. (1981). *Stages of faith.* San Francisco, CA: HarperOne.

Frankl, V. (1984). *Man's search for meaning.* New York, NY: Washington Square Press.

Galanti, G. A. (2008). *Caring for patients from different cultures.* Philadelphia, PA: University of Pennsylvania Press.

Gorsuch, R., & Miller, W. (1999). Assessing spirituality. In W. Miller (Ed.), *Integrating spirituality into treatment: Resources for practitioners.* Washington, DC: American Psychological Association.

Hasselkus, B. (2011). *The meaning of everyday occupation.* (2nd ed.). Thorofare, NJ: SLACK Incorporated.

Hay, M. (1989). Principles in building spiritual assessments tools. *American Journal of Hospital Care, 6*, 25-31.

Hodge, D. (2001). Spiritual assessment: A review of major qualitative methods and a new framework for assessing spirituality. *Social Work, 46*, 203-213.

Howard, B. S., & Howard, J. R. (1997). Occupation as spiritual activity. *American Journal of Occupational Therapy, 51*, 181-185.

James, W., & Marty, M. (1982). *Varieties of religious experience: A study in human nature.* New York, NY: Penguin Books.

Koenig, H. G. (2004). Taking a spiritual history. *Journal of the American Medical Association, 291*, 2881.

Koenig, H. (2007). *Spirituality in patient care: Why, how, when, and what.* West Conshohocken, PA: Templeton Press.

Maugans, T. (1996). The SPIRITual history. *Archives of Family Medicine, 5*, 11-16.

Nelson, K. (2011). *The spiritual doorway in the brain: A neurologist's search for the God experience.* New York, NY: Plume.

Puchalski, C., & Romer, A. L. (2000). Taking a spiritual history allows clinicians to understand patients more fully. *Journal of Palliative Medicine, 3*, 129-137.

Richards, S., & Bergin, A. (1997). *A spiritual strategy for counseling and psychotherapy.* Washington, DC: American Psychological Association.

Schnorr, M. (1999). Spiritual caregiving. In P. Solari-Twadell & M. A. McDermott (Eds.), *Parish nursing: Promoting whole person health within faith communities* (pp. 43-53). Thousand Oaks, CA: Sage Publications.

Schulz, E. (2011). Spiritual occupation. In C. Brown & V. C. Stoffel (Eds.), *Occupational therapy in mental health* (pp. 755-763). Philadelphia, PA: F. A. Davis.

Sermabeikian, P. (1994). Our clients, ourselves: The spiritual perspective and social work practice. *Social Work, 39*, 178-183.

Smucker, C. (1996). A phenomenological description of the experiences of spiritual distress. *Nurses Diagnosis, 7*, 81-91.

Sorajjakool, S. (2006). *When sickness heals: The place of religious belief in healthcare.* West Conshohocken, PA: Templeton Press.

Spencer, P. (2004, December 7). The healing power of prayer. *Woman's Day.*

List of Spiritual Assessments

Anandarajah, G., & Hight, E. (2001). Spirituality and medical practice: Using the HOPE questions as a practical tool for spiritual assessment. *American Family Physician, 63*, 81-89.

Fetzer Institute and the National Institute on Aging Working Group. (1999). *Multidimensional measurement of religious/spirituality for use in health research.* Retrieved from: http://www.fetzer.org/resources/multidimensional-measurement-religiousnessspirituality-use-health-research

Fitchett, G. (2002). 7 X 7 model for spiritual assessment. In G. Fitchett, *Assessing spiritual needs* (p. 39). Lima, OH: Academic Renewal Press.

Koenig, H. G. (2004). Taking a spiritual history. *Journal of the American Medical Association, 291*, 2881.

Kravitz, Y. J. (2007). Spiritual intelligence assessment. Retrieved from http://www.spiritualintelligence.com

Maugans, T. (1996). The SPIRITual history. *Archives of Family Medicine, 5*, 11-16.

Puchalski, C., & Romer, A. L. (2000). Taking a spiritual history allows clinicians to understand patients more fully. *Journal of Palliative Medicine, 3*, 129-137.

Schnorr, M. (1999). Spiritual caregiving. In P. Solari-Twadell & M. A. McDermott (Eds.), *Parish nursing: Promoting whole person health within faith communities* (pp. 43-53). Thousand Oaks, CA: Sage Publications.

Schulz, E. (2008). OT-QUEST assessment. In B. Hemphill (Ed.), *Assessments in occupational therapy mental health* (p. 263). Thorofare, NJ: SLACK Incorporated.

Underwood, L., & Teresi, J. A. (2000). The daily spiritual experience scale: Development, theoretical description, reliability, exploratory factor analysis, and preliminary construct validity using health-related data. *Annals of Behavioral Medicine, 24*, 22-33.

28

The OT-QUEST
The Occupational Therapy Quality of Experience and Spirituality Assessment Tool

Emily Schulz, PhD, OTR/L, CFLE, ACUE

In the meantime, you live here on Earth and you have tasks to fulfill, both physical and spiritual. Come down to Earth and develop love; this is something tangible. It is something you can feel, you can give and you can receive. Since love is connected with bliss, it is connected with all that lies further and beyond. Catch this substance—which is within your grasp—with humility. For the time being, forget all that is not within your reach. Bliss is within your heart to experience: knowing, growing, bringing fulfillment to your physical body, your emotional aspect and the deepening of your soul.

(Purna, 2014, p. 21)

This chapter will offer a definition of spirituality for occupational therapy, offer a three-dimensional model of spirituality based on a review of the literature, and explore the role of spirituality in occupational therapy intervention. A spirituality assessment tool for occupational therapy practice, the OT-QUEST (Occupational Therapy Quality of Experience and Spirituality Assessment Tool) will be presented, including the history of its development, its reliability and validity, rationale for use, and its administration and scoring, along with two case studies illustrating its use. Finally, a discussion of the tool's strengths and limitations, as well as suggestions for future research, will be provided.

Literature Review

General interest in spirituality and its use in health care have been increasing (Congdon & Magilvy, 2001; Farrar, 2001; MacKinlay & Burns, 2017; Miller & Thoresen, 2003; Puchalski, 1998; Ross, 1995; Ziegler, 1998). Studies have been conducted demonstrating the positive impact of spirituality, faith, and religion on the physical, mental, and emotional health issues of individuals with a variety of conditions (Chibnall, Videen, Duckro, & Miller, 2002; Ferrell, Smith, Juarez, & Melancon, 2003; Kirby, Coleman, & Daley, 2004; Lowry & Conco, 2002; MacKinlay & Burns, 2017; Touhy, 2001; Zimmer, Jagger, Chiu, Ofstedal, Rojo, & Saito, 2016).

Hemphill, B. J., & Urish, C. K. (Eds.). *Assessments in Occupational Therapy Mental Health: An Integrative Approach, Fourth Edition* (pp. 469-513). © 2020 Taylor & Francis Group.

In the occupational therapy literature addressing spirituality, the focus has primarily been on exploring the term as it relates to occupation (Algado, Gregori, & Egan, 1997; Champagne, Ryan, Saccomando, & Lazzarini, 2007; Christiansen, 1997; Egan & DeLaat, 1997; Frank et al., 1997; Howard & Howard, 1997; Kirsh, 1996; Levack, 2003; Low, 1997; Luboshitzky & Bennett-Gaber, 2001; Neuhaus, 1997; Peloquin, 1997; Toomey, 1999; Unruh, 1997) or investigating its role in practice (J. S. Collins, Paul, & West-Frasier, 2001; M. Collins, 2016; Csontó, 2009; Engquist, Short-DeGraff, Gliner, & Oltenbruns, 1997; Farrar, 2001; Jones, Topping, Wattis, & Smith, 2016; Morris, Stecher, Briggs-Peppler, Chittenden, Rubira, & Wismer, 2014; Mthembu, Wegner, & Roman, 2017; Prochnau, Liu, & Boman, 2003; Rose, 1999; Taylor, Mitchell, Kenan, & Tacker, 2000; Udell & Chandler, 2000). The next section of this chapter first offers a definition of spirituality for occupational therapy along with a three-dimensional model, which is then followed by a discussion of the role of spirituality in occupational therapy.

Definition of Spirituality

The way the term *spirituality* has been defined in the profession of occupational therapy has evolved over time. For example, in its first edition, the *Occupational Therapy Practice Framework: Domain and Process* (American Occupational Therapy Association [AOTA], 2002) placed the term spirituality under the contextual category of Spiritual Context. In its second edition, the term was moved to the Client Factors section, under Values, Beliefs, and Spirituality, and the following definition was provided:

[T]he personal quest for understanding answers to ultimate questions about life, about meaning, and about relationship with the sacred or transcendent, which may (or may not) lead to or arise from the development of religious rituals and the formation of community. (Moreira-Almeida & Koenig, 2006, p. 844)

The third edition of the *Framework* retains the term spirituality under Client Factors and provides the following definition of spirituality:

The aspect of humanity that refers to the way individuals seek and express meaning and purpose and the way they experience their connectedness to the moment, to self, to others, to nature, and to the significant or sacred. (AOTA, 2014, p. S22)

Definition of Spirituality and Three-Dimensional Model of Spirituality Based on a Review of Literature

Through a review of the literature, it becomes apparent that spirituality is a multidimensional construct (Meraviglia, 1999; Puchalski et al., 2009; Ross, 1995). First, to clarify an issue that is often raised, spirituality and religion are not the same thing, although they can overlap for some people, as is clear from the definition provided previously (Zinnbauer et al., 1997). Koenig, McCollough, and Larson (2001), who have researched religion and health extensively, differentiate between spirituality and religion. They explain that spirituality, when compared to religion, is "individualistic, less visible and measurable, less formal, less orthodox, less systematic, emotionally oriented, inward directed, not authoritarian, [as having] little accountability, and … [being] unifying, not doctrine oriented" (Koenig et al., 2001, p. 18). In contrast, they describe religion as "community focused, observable, measurable, objective, formal, orthodox, organized, behavior oriented, [having] outward practices, [being] authoritarian in terms of behaviors, and [having] a doctrine separating good from evil" (Koenig et al., 2001, p. 18). In summary, religion appears to be more concerned with rules and rituals, whereas spirituality focuses more on personal meaning and the experience of unity (Koenig et al., 2001; Zinnbauer et al., 1997). When describing spirituality in the literature, most health care professions seem to focus on the quality of unity or connectedness as a main characteristic of the term (Bellingham, Cohen, Jones, & Spaniol, 1989; Bosacki & Ota, 2000; Burkhardt, 1994; Dossey, 1998; Dyson, Cobb, & Forman, 1997; Hodge, 2001; Hodge, Cardenas, & Montoya, 2001; Hungelmann, Kenkel-Rossi, Klassen, & Stollenwerk, 1985; Kessler, 1999; Piedmont, 2001; Pike, 2000; Ross, 1995).

Connectedness, according to the literature (Puchalski et al., 2009), is multifaceted. Connectedness can be to the self (Bellingham et al., 1989); others, (Bellingham et al., 1989; Burkhardt, 1994; Dyson et al., 1997; Hungelmann et al., 1985; Pike, 2000), the world (Burkhardt, 1994; Dyson et al., 1997; Pike, 2000), and the divine (Burkhardt, 1994; Hungelmann et al., 1985; Pike, 2000).

Because of the profession's unique attention to meaningful occupation, the occupational therapy literature seems to concentrate on the expressive aspect of spirituality when discussing its nature (Algado et al., 1997; Champagne et al., 2007; Christiansen, 1997; Do Rozario, 1994; Egan & DeLaat, 1997; Frank et al., 1997; Howard & Howard, 1997; Kirsh, 1996; Levack, 2003; Low, 1997; Luboshitzky & Bennett-Gaber, 2001; Neuhaus, 1997; Peloquin, 1997; Spencer, Davidson, & White, 1997; Toomey, 1999; Unruh, 1997). According to the occupational therapy literature, the expression of one's of spirituality can manifest through a person's reflections (Low, 1997; Neuhaus, 1997; Spencer et al., 1997; Unruh, 1997), narratives (Kirsh, 1996; Toomey, 1999), and actions (Christiansen, 1997; Do Rozario, 1994; Egan & DeLaat, 1997; Frank et al., 1997; Howard & Howard, 1997; Peloquin, 1997).

Finally, because human beings are embodied on a physical plane of existence (rather than on some ethereal realm, for instance), the natural laws of physics apply to us, including those of linear time (Smith, 1978). While there are some theories in quantum physics (Greene, 2005; Wolf, 2004) and metaphysics (Nager, 2005; Purna, 2012) in which time and physical matter are viewed as illusions (e.g., for those rare individuals in an enlightened state), in general, most human beings, including most occupational therapy clients, have not achieved such a state and therefore are still subject to the laws of physics and linear time.

The definition of spirituality offered in this chapter is for the majority of human beings rather than those who are enlightened, as the enlightened most likely will not require occupational therapy services. *Enlightenment* is having conscious awareness of our true spiritual nature and is a by-product of the process of *liberation*, which happens when we free ourselves of all of our self-imposed limitations (Purna, 2012). For the majority of humanity, it is through the act of existing on the physical plane, with its confines of linear and historical/cultural time and physical/societal Barriers and Facilitators (AOTA, 2014), that a demand for mastery (Schkade & Schultz, 1992; Schultz & Schkade, 1992) and an opportunity for the human spirit to shine forth and evolve (Schulz, 2002, 2005) are created.

Indeed, Meyer (1922) stated that it is humankind's ability to remember the past, recognize and use the present moment, and realize that there is a future to plan for that separates it as a species from the rest of the animal kingdom. In fact, it is during the present moment that a state of flow can occur for a person engaged in a meaningful creative occupation (Csikszentmihalyi, 1998; Csikszentmihalyi & Csikszentmihalyi, 1998).

Therefore, taking into consideration the literature, the following can be used as the definition of spirituality within occupational therapy: experiencing a meaningful connection to our core selves, other beings, the world, and/or a Greater Power, as expressed through our reflections, narratives, and actions, within the context of space and time. This definition is illustrated in a three-dimensional model in Figure 28-1.

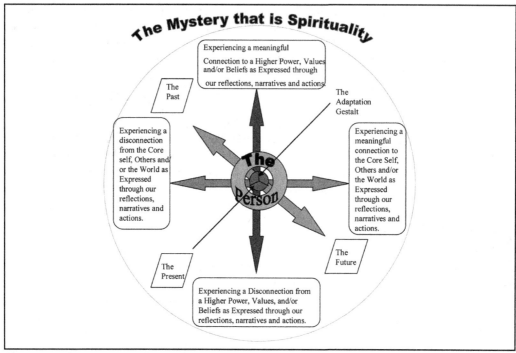

Figure 28-1. Three-Dimensional Spirituality Model.

In the model depicted in Figure 28-1, spirituality as a whole is viewed as a mystery. The model can be used to portray a person's spirituality in a snapshot in time or a person's spiritual evolutionary process across linear time. The three dimensions of spirituality illuminated in the model are the vertical element (on a continuum from connectedness to disconnectedness to a Greater Power, which includes the divine, values, and beliefs), the horizontal element (on a continuum from connectedness to disconnectedness to self, others, and the world), and the temporal element (past, present, and future). The individual person is in the center of the model and holistically adapts to challenges in life (Schkade & Schultz, 1992; Schultz & Schkade, 1992) across linear time; as this occurs, he or she may change in levels of connectedness/disconnectedness to the vertical and horizontal aspects of spirituality. The model is fluid and dynamic (Schulz, 2002).

Figures 28-2 through 28-5 illustrate examples of the types of people at the extremes of the four quadrants of the model in a snapshot of time for the purpose of clarifying how the model works:

- High connectedness to both vertical and horizontal elements (see Figure 28-2)
- High connectedness to the horizontal element with high disconnectedness to the vertical element (see Figure 28-3)
- High disconnectedness to both the vertical and horizontal elements (see Figure 28-4)
- High disconnectedness to the horizontal element with high connectedness to the vertical element (see Figure 28-5)

These are merely examples, as most likely the majority of humans do not fall into the extremes nor do people necessarily stay in one quadrant due to the dynamic nature of the model across linear time, as previously mentioned.

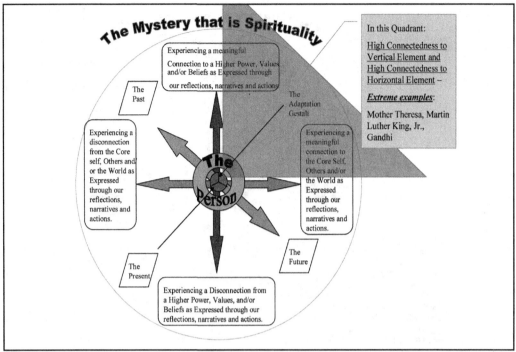

Figure 28-2. Quadrant 1—High connectedness to vertical element and high connectedness to horizontal element.

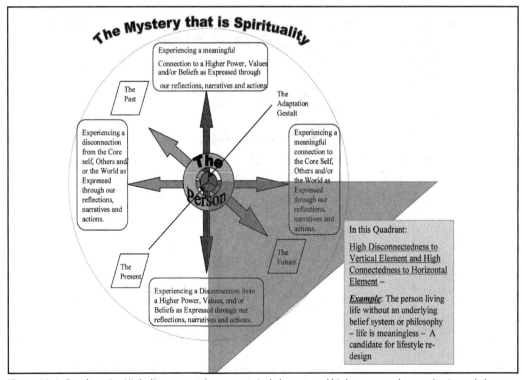

Figure 28-3. Quadrant 2—High disconnectedness to vertical element and high connectedness to horizontal element.

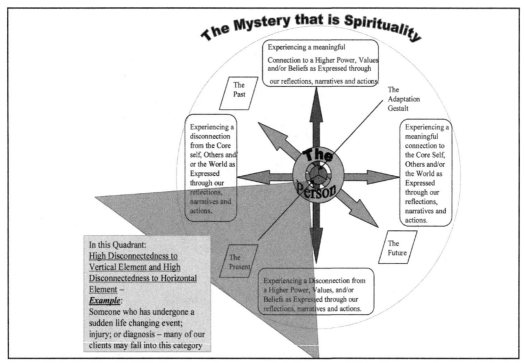

Figure 28-4. Quadrant 3—High disconnectedness to vertical element and high disconnectedness to horizontal element.

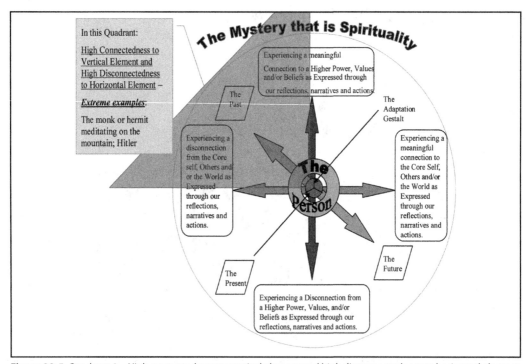

Figure 28-5. Quadrant 4—High connectedness to vertical element and high disconnectedness to horizontal element.

Role of Spirituality in Occupational Therapy

Many occupational therapy scholars have questioned the role of spirituality in the profession (J. S. Collins et al., 2001; M. Collins, 2016; Csontó, 2009; Engquist et al., 1997; Farrar, 2001; Morris et al., 2014; Prochnau et al., 2003; Rose, 1999; Taylor et al., 2000; Udell & Chandler, 2000). After all, occupational therapists are not clergy nor are they trained to be clergy. In fact, even though most occupational therapists value highly their own spirituality, many occupational therapists have not been trained on how to address spirituality in practice (J. S. Collins et al., 2001; M. Collins, 2016; Mthembu et al., 2017). It is definitely not the role of the occupational therapist to proselytize, attempt to convert, or otherwise coerce a client into embracing the therapist's own spiritual or religious beliefs. In the case of a client being in a spiritual crisis or needing spiritual counseling, after actively listening to him or her, it is appropriate for the occupational therapist to refer the client to a chaplain or clergy member of that client's faith rather than trying to counsel the client personally (M. Collins, 2016). That being said, what are suitable boundaries to adhere to when approaching the issue of spirituality in practice? This is a legitimate question and is best addressed by therapists remembering our profession's domain of concern: facilitating the engagement of people in their meaningful occupations for optimum participation in their environments (AOTA, 2014).

According to the *Framework*, spirituality is, at its most basic level, about the essential underlying foundation that provides meaning in life for human beings (AOTA, 2014). Therefore, if we tap into our clients' spirituality, we can discover what is meaningful to them, and thus collaboratively create treatment goals, plans, and interventions that are client centered and have the potential to be truly powerful, healing, and transformative (Nosek, 1995; Schulz, 2002). By facilitating the engagement of clients in the occupations or outward manifestations of their spirituality or faith (or their values or beliefs, for nonreligious people), occupational therapists can address spirituality in a way that is ethically sound and within the domain of the profession.

Using the Definition of Spirituality and Spirituality Model to Guide Clinical Reasoning

Perhaps this point can best be illustrated through using Figure 28-6 and Table 28-1. Figure 28-6 is the now-familiar three-dimensional model of spirituality with the addition of numbers on a continuum from -3 to +3 for both the vertical elements and the horizontal elements. Table 28-1 is a grid-like structure that can be used to guide the therapist's thinking when using the model in practice with a client. The grid in Table 28-1 has not been tested in practice nor has it been researched for validity and reliability—it is simply a tool to help readers more fully understand the definition of spirituality and the three-dimensional model presented in this chapter.

A therapist wanting to broach the topic of spirituality with a client for the first time can begin by saying something like the following: "Sometimes it helps people receiving services if we include spirituality in our interventions. I know spirituality is a personal topic, and I was wondering if I could ask you some questions about yours to help me to better help you." If the person gives consent, then the therapist can ask a client to reflect on and rate how connected he or she felt to the self before receiving services (on a scale from -3 to +3); how he or she feels regarding connectedness to the self now; and how he or she wants to feel in terms of connectedness to the self in the future. The therapist can ask the following questions:

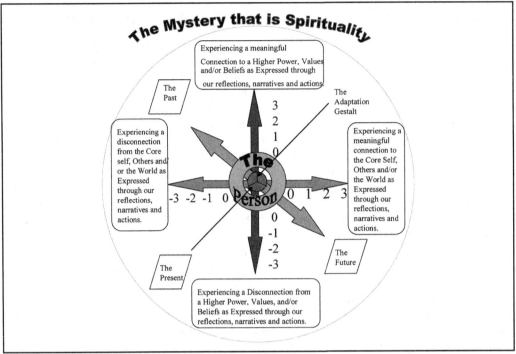

Figure 28-6. Three-Dimensional Spirituality Model with numbers included to qualify levels of connectedness and disconnectedness to vertical and horizontal elements.

- Why do you think you felt (feel) that way?
- How did you connect to yourself in the past?
- How do you want to connect to yourself in the future?

From this type of discussion with the person, client-centered collaborative goals and treatment plans can be written for the aspect of spirituality related to connectedness to the self. This same process can be repeated for the other aspects of connectedness to others, the world, and a Greater Power across linear time.

Important Considerations

There are some issues that may arise for people as they explore their spirituality deeply. People who are very devout or who focus a great deal of attention on their spiritual life can sometimes experience what is termed a *dark night of the soul*, *spiritual crisis*, or even a *spiritual emergency*. It is important for clinicians working in mental health to be aware of these possibilities and be able to differentiate between what is a spiritual process and therefore not pathological, just challenging and usually temporary, vs. a psychological condition, which may be more long lasting and may involve pathology. In the case of the former, spiritual guidance and support are suggested; in the case of the latter, clinical psychological intervention is helpful and often required, depending on the severity of the issue. Definitions of the three terms follow.

Table 28-1

Spirituality Model Assessment Grid

Spirituality Concept	Past	Present	Future	How?	Why?	Goals?
Level of connectedness to self • High connectedness = 3 • Moderate connectedness = 2 • Low connectedness = 1 • Neutral = 0 • Low disconnectedness = -1 • Moderate disconnectedness = -2 • High disconnectedness = -3	Level ____	Level ____	Level ____			
Level of connectedness to others • High connectedness = 3 • Moderate connectedness = 2 • Low connectedness = 1 • Neutral = 0 • Low disconnectedness = -1 • Moderate disconnectedness = -2 • High disconnectedness = -3	Level ____	Level ____	Level ____			
Level of connectedness to the world • High connectedness = 3 • Moderate connectedness = 2 • Low connectedness = 1 • Neutral = 0 • Low disconnectedness = -1 • Moderate disconnectedness = -2 • High disconnectedness = -3	Level ____	Level ____	Level ____			

(continued)

Table 28-1 (continued)

Spirituality Model Assessment Grid

Spirituality Concept	Past	Present	Future	How?	Why?	Goals?
Level of connectedness to a greater power • High connectedness = 3 • Moderate connectedness = 2 • Low connectedness = 1 • Neutral = 0 • Low disconnectedness = -1 • Moderate disconnectedness = -2 • High disconnectedness = -3	Level ____	Level ____	Level ____			
Total Scores						
Horizontal Element (add self, others, and world scores and divide by 3)	Horizontal element:	Horizontal element:	Horizontal element:			
Vertical Element (greater power score)	Vertical element:	Vertical element:	Vertical element:			

The term *dark night of the soul* comes from the Christian tradition, out of the written work and life experiences of Saint John the Divine and Saint Teresa of Avila, who were devout mystics living in Spain in the 1500s (May, 2009). May (2009) explains that the dark night of the soul is a spiritual process through which we become freed from behaviors and circumstances in our lives that no longer serve us so we can become more loving and free to live a more fulfilled life. However, the dark night of the soul can be a painful process if we fight it. The process is mysterious and happens on a subtle level, which is why it is called dark. We cannot control the process, which is why it feels frightening, yet the outcome is always beneficial.

A spiritual crisis occurs when one experiences a test of faith. Agrimson and Taft (2009) define *spiritual crisis* as:

A unique form of grieving or loss, marked by a profound questioning of or lack of meaning in life, in which an individual or community reaches a turning point, leading to a significant alteration in the way life is viewed. Possible antecedents include sudden acute illness and loss of important relationships. Potential consequences may include physical and emotional responses. (p. 454)

A *spiritual emergency* (Grof, 1989) is a process that can mimic psychosis (M. Collins, 2014). As Collins (2007) explains:

People can experience a transformational crisis through engaging in spiritual growth and development, a phenomenon that has been termed a "spiritual emergency." A spiritual emergency manifests itself as a crisis within ego-identity and can include experiences of disorientation and de-adaptation, which affect a person's ability to function in daily life. Consequently, a person may be diagnosed and treated for a mental health problem; however, a spiritual emergency may present a person with opportunities to engage in a process of self-renewal rather than being considered ill. (p. 504)

Spiritual emergency and the dark night of the soul experiences typically come about through a process of spiritual purification and are brought on by sincere and devout spiritual effort. As one Himalayan Master explains:

Purification of mind and body is essential for one who seeks enlightenment … The way to liberation is an arduous path which requires total dedication and faultless preparation … Communion with God is the highest; such powerful energies are not perceived if one is not attuned to the higher wave-length, nor if one's motives are impure. (Purna, 2012, p. 22)

In another discourse, Purna (2014) explains:

One of the conditions of Enlightenment is that you have to be strong: it is not the way of one who is feeble or scared. It is the Path of one who is courageous. It is a mystical journey where you must overcome those things you dislike the most—or those that frighten you the most. All must be approached in the spirit of humility and trust. You will be put in to a difficult situation where you must find a way out. (pp. 18-19)

It is clear that these three processes are different yet may be related. For example, we can go through a dark night of the soul process that we cannot control, which can lead to a loss of circumstances that no longer serve us, even though we wish to hold on to them. During that process, we might experience a spiritual crisis or loss of faith due to those losses. If the purification process is intense, it may lead to a spiritual emergency. However, the underlying purposes of these processes are actually for spiritual growth and are usually in response to a spiritual need. The purification process occurs in response to that profound need for spiritual growth. Occupational therapists need to be aware of these nuances and be able to identify them whenever possible so that the correct professionals can be brought in to address them on the treatment team.

As it is frequently the case that both a spiritual issue and a psychological issue can arise together, it is recommended that practitioners from both areas of expertise work together for the benefit of the client. A practitioner with a background in transpersonal psychology also has the knowledge base to work with both spiritual and psychological arenas together. Transpersonal psychology addresses positive human potential. Rather than focusing on psychological pathology and its causes and cures, it instead involves holding an understanding of the positive and sacred that exists within everyday existence, as well as those expansive aspects of human experience that occur beyond mundane life (Hartelius, Caplan, & Rardin, 2007). Therefore, it embraces the spiritual dimension of human experience as an authentic and necessary aspect of what it means to be a human being. Other helpful practitioners to refer clients to would be clergy from their specific faith tradition, a spiritual director, or a spiritual guide, depending on the clients' backgrounds and comfort levels.

Rationale

Now that spirituality has been defined, and some spiritual growth processes have been explained, the next section of this chapter will focus on the OT-QUEST itself. The OT-QUEST was developed to meet a perceived need of the profession that was a structured way to address spirituality in clinical practice. Individuals with disabilities have stated that they would like their spirituality to be included when receiving rehabilitation services (Nosek, 1995). The *Framework* includes the spiritual context in the scope of practice for the profession (AOTA, 2014). However, before intervention can be provided, assessment must be done. Assessment tools have been needed to be developed to appropriately measure and address spirituality in health care (Lowry & Conco, 2002). While there are spirituality assessments available for other professions, such as the Spiritual Health in Four Domains Index (Fisher, Francis, & Johnson, 2000), the Spiritual Well-Being Scale (SWBS; Paloutzian & Ellison, 1982), and the Spiritual Experience Index–Revised (Genia, 1991, 1997), the OT-QUEST is a spirituality assessment tool that offers therapists a way to assess spirituality that is specifically designed by an occupational therapist and for occupational therapy practice.

History and Development

The first edition of the OT-QUEST was developed by the author as an assignment in an assessment course in the doctoral program at Texas Woman's University. It is based on Collins's (1998) model, as well as the Occupational Adaptation Frame of Reference (Schkade & Schultz, 1992; Schultz & Schkade, 1992). The questions in the instrument were developed based upon those models and modified after receiving feedback from an expert in the field. The first edition comprised 11 visual analog questions to gather quantitative data and 12 sentence completion questions to retrieve qualitative information from the participants. It was pilot tested as an anonymous survey in 1999 with a nonclinical population ($n = 41$). Participants were primarily White women aged 18 to 55 years. With one item removed, the OT-QUEST scored a Cronbach's alpha of 0.71 and factor analysis revealed four noncorrelated factors.

Psychometric Properties

The OT-QUEST was modified for the second edition to make the instrument more specific in its wording. The resulting revised OT-QUEST includes 14 Likert scale questions and 15 open-ended questions. A Likert scale was used instead of a visual analog scale in the second edition to ease administration and scoring. A study was conducted in 2005, the purpose of which was to determine the test-retest reliability, concurrent validity, and internal consistency of the second edition of the OT-QUEST with older adults with low vision. Patients with low vision who were aged 50 years and older were recruited from a clinic for this study (Tables 28-2 and 28-3).

The intended design for this study was to recruit 120 participants; however, due to time constraints and a drop-in clientele at the clinic, doing so was problematic. The study design called for two telephone interviews to be conducted prior to the participants' first visit to the clinic to avoid bias. The second interview occurred 1 to 2 weeks after the first interview. However, some participants only responded to the first survey and others changed appointment dates and could not be interviewed for the follow-up, resulting in a small study group ($n = 45$). In the first interview, eight surveys were given—a demographic survey, the OT-QUEST, the Spiritual Health in Four Domains Index, the SWBS, and the Spiritual Experience Index–Revised—to ascertain the OT-QUEST's concurrent validity. Those surveys were followed by several others: the Center for Epidemiologic Studies Depression Scale (Schein & Koenig, 1997), which measured participants' depressive symptoms; the National Eye Institute Visual Function Questionnaire (Cole, Beck, Moke, Gal, & Long, 2000), which addressed participants' visual functioning; and the Short Portable Mental Status Questionnaire (Roccaforte, Burke, Bayer, & Wengel, 1994), which measured participants' cognitive status. For the second interview, participants only responded to the OT-QUEST to determine its test-retest reliability. A chart audit was done after the participants attended the low vision clinic for the first time as new patients.

Results of the study indicated that the OT-QUEST had strong, significant test-retest reliability (Spearman's correlation = 0.57; $p < .0001$) for items on the Likert scale and moderate concurrence in the themes from the sentence completion questions (50% to 72%). It had significant moderate concurrent validity with the SWBS (Spearman's Correlation = 0.35; $p = .0178$) and with the Spiritual Health in Four Domains Index (Spearman's correlation = 0.34; $p = .0206$). Concurrent validity was nonsignificant and weak with the Spiritual Experience Index–Revised (Spearman's correlation = -.22; $p = .1566$). Internal consistency was also weak (overall Cronbach's alpha = 0.68); Cronbach's alpha ranged from 0.59 to 0.70 for the six factors (Spiritual = 0.70; Being = 0.65; Meaning = 0.59; Expression = 0.65; Intention = 0.64; and Adaptation = 0.62).

Table 28-2

Study Participants' Demographics

Gender			Race		
Category	N	%	Category	N	%
Male	14	31%	White	35	78%
Female	31	69%	Black	10	22%
Gender			Race		
Mean	SD		Category	N	%
73.86	15.71		Christianity	45	100%
Marital Status			Education		
Category	N	%	Category	N	%
Married	18	40%	< 12th grade	16	35%
Single	5	11%	Graduated 12th grade	9	20%
Divorced	7	16%	Some college	10	22%
Widowed	15	33%	College degree	7	16%
			Graduate degree	3	7%
Employment Status			Income		
Category	N	%	Category	N	%
Retired	39	87%	<$20,000	25	60%
Working	2	4%	$20,000-$39,000	11	26%
Disability	4	9%	≥$40,000	6	14%

Assessment Administration

The next part of this chapter will describe the administration and scoring of the OT-QUEST. A case study will be presented also to illustrate how to score the instrument.

How the Tool Is Administered

The OT-QUEST can be administered as a paper-and-pencil survey or as a 15- to 20-minute interview.

Concepts Being Measured

The concepts measured by the OT-QUEST are the Five Key Factors within the person that relate to spirituality and quality of experience—Spiritual, Being, Meaning, Intention, and Expression, as found in Collins's (1998) model—and Adaptation, as found in the Occupational Adaptation Frame of Reference (Schkade & Schultz, 1992; Schultz & Schkade, 1992). Collins's (1998) model states that if people are having a good

Table 28-3

Study Participants' Conditions and Areas for Treatment

Medical Conditions[a]			Ocular Conditions[a]		
Category	N	%	Category	N	%
Arthritis	16	36%	Cataract	35	78%
Hypertension	15	33%	Age-related macular degeneration	27	60%
Cardiovascular disease	11	24%	Glaucoma	10	22%
Diabetes	8	18%	Scotoma	10	22%
Hearing problems	6	13%	Diabetic retinopathy	6	13%
Balance problems	3	7%	Hemianopsia	3	7%
Stroke/transient ischemic attack	3	7%	Stargardt's disease	1	2%

Depressive Symptoms (CESD)[b]		Cognitive Status (SPMSQ)[c]	
Mean Score	SD	Mean Score	SD
17.56	7.98	0.84	0.60

Visual Functioning (NEI-VFQ)[d]			Expectations and Goals: Areas for Treatment[a]
Category	Mean Score	SD	Activities of Daily Living
General health	36.67	27.49	Communication device use
General vision	30.67	17.37	Community mobility
Ocular pain	75.56	23.07	Financial management
Near vision	30.28	23.74	Functional mobility
Distance vision	37.41	26.06	Home establishment and management
Social functioning	54.72	29.83	Improve vision/visual perception
Mental health	44.72	25.56	Leisure
Role difficulties	31.94	26.99	Meal preparation
Well-being/distress	43.33	34.75	Personal hygiene
Driving[e]	95.83	36.71	Shopping
Color vision	69.44	33.24	Social participation
Peripheral vision	46.02	29.99	

[a]From chart audit.

[b]Score of 16 to 18+=Possible depression.

[c]Participants had intact cognition.

[d]Higher score (1 to 100)=Better functioning.

[e]Only driving participants responded to this item.

Abbreviations: CESD=Center for Epidemiologic Studies Depression Scale; NEI-VFQ=National Eye Institute Visual Function Questionnaire; SPMSQ=Short Portable Mental Status Questionnaire.

quality of experience in their lives, then their spiritual selves are also well. According to Collins (1998), evidence of clients having healthy spirituality becomes apparent to therapists if those clients exhibit the following qualities:

- Positive renewal and acceptance (Spiritual Factor)
- Awareness and understanding (Being Factor)
- Purpose and discovery (Meaning Factor)
- Motivation and will (Intention Factor)
- Exploration and causation (Expression Factor)

Collins (1998) developed questions for each of the Five Key Factors and their subcomponents. Those questions were modified slightly in wording for the first edition of the OT-QUEST, and some were expanded in the second edition for clarity. A question about adaptation and spirituality was included in the tool to measure whether spirituality was a factor when adapting to challenges for persons responding to the tool.

How Concepts Are Measured

As stated previously, the second edition of the OT-QUEST is comprised of 14 Likert scale questions (on a 5-point scale) and 15 open-ended questions.

How to Score the OT-QUEST

There are two to three Likert scale questions for each of the Five Key Factors (Collins, 1998) and one item for the Adaptation reference (Schkade & Schultz, 1992; Schultz & Schkade, 1992). The mean score for the items for each Key Factor and the one score for the Adaptation item are used in scoring the Likert scale section; a range is set for low, medium, and high mean scores. An overall mean score is also calculated. A low overall score or a low score for one of the Five Key Factors indicates that the person may be struggling with spirituality and quality of experience in general (in the case of the overall score) or with that particular issue (in the case of the factor). Further information about the Five Key Factors and Adaptation comes to light through the sentence completion section of the instrument because those items closely relate to the Likert scale questions. The sentence completion questions are not scored in a traditional sense; however, general themes can be written down to summarize issues the client is having. Those themes are divided under two categories on the score sheet: Facilitators and Barriers.

Goal Writing

Goal writing should be collaborative and client centered and flow naturally from the findings of the assessment. It should be done in a collaborative conversation with the client.

Case Studies

T.L.

T.L. is a woman in her 40s with three grown children who live out of state. She is currently living in the Midwest after having recently moved from another part of the United States. She is going through a second divorce. She is recovering from a hairline hip fracture after a fall down the stairs and has Crohn's disease. She is having difficulty adjusting to her new living situation and is experiencing reactionary depression. She does not consider herself religious but does consider herself to be spiritual and feels a strong connection to angelic beings. She enjoys doing crafts, volunteering to take care of babies with AIDS, and participating in the Society for Creative Anachronism; however, because of a series of traumatic events in her life over the past 4 years (e.g., death of family member, loss of two homes, divorce, bankruptcy, recent relocation to another state, stressful job), she no longer does these things. She completed the OT-QUEST as a survey. Her responses on the tool and scoring are shown in Table 28-4. Goal writing was completed in collaboration with her.

In looking at T.L.'s mean overall score, she is on the low-end cusp of the high range. However, when looking at her mean scores for the Five Key Factors, her lowest score is a medium score for the Being Factor (when averaging her responses to the two questions "Do you usually feel good about yourself?" and "Do you regularly take the time to meet your own needs?"). The themes for Facilitators and Barriers that came up for her in the sentence completion questions related to the Likert scale Being Factor items ("I feel most positive about myself when …" "I am best able to pay attention to my own needs when …") clarified why she scored lower on Being, and goals were written to help her address this factor. This process continued for all of the factors.

D.S.

D.S. is a 43-year-old, divorced, White woman who lives alone. She works two part-time jobs as a consultant in the natural health supplement industry. She has been married and divorced twice. She has two teenaged children whom she co-parents with her first ex-husband in a nearby town. Her son has graduated from high school, and her daughter is close to finishing high school. Her parents and brother and his family live in another state. She has a history of depression and is struggling with the residual symptoms of Lyme disease. She has painful sciatica in her back, which leads to numbness in her lower extremities, and at times has difficulty with walking. She is a sincere spiritual seeker.

D.S. is seeking assistance because she wants clarity and guidance and needs help with overcoming low self-esteem and compulsiveness. She completed the OT-QUEST on her own, and then together she and her therapist went over her responses and created some goals. She stated that she gained some new insights from the process. Her responses and score sheet are shown in Table 28-5.

Table 28-4

T.L.'s Responses to the OT-QUEST

Instructions: Circle or state your response to each question. (Note: T.L.'s responses are in brackets.)

1. How important is an experience of inner peace to you?

1	2	3	4	[5]
Not at all important	Not very important	Somewhat important	Very important	Extremely important

2. Do you usually feel good about yourself?

1	2	[3]	4	5
Never	Rarely	Sometimes	Most of the time	Always

3. Do you regularly take the time to meet your own needs?

1	2	[3]	4	5
Never	Rarely	Sometimes	Most of the time	Always

4. How do you usually feel about the actions you have taken?

1	2	[3]	4	5
Not at all positive	Not very positive	Somewhat positive	Very positive	Extremely positive

5. How do you usually feel about the decisions you have made?

1	2	[3]	4	5
Not at all positive	Not very positive	Somewhat positive	Very positive	Extremely positive

6. Do you value being engaged in doing something?

1	2	3	4	[5]
Never	Rarely	Sometimes	Most of the time	Always

7. Is it important to you to express yourself in a manner that is uniquely you?

1	2	3	4	[5]
Not at all important	Not very important	Somewhat important	Very important	Extremely important

8. Does the physical environment around you have an impact on your ability to express yourself to the fullest degree possible?

1	2	3	[4]	5
No impact at all	Not a very strong impact	Somewhat of an impact	Very strong impact	Extremely strong impact

(continued)

Table 28-4 (continued)

T.L.'s Responses to the OT-QUEST

9. Do the people around you have an impact on your ability to express yourself to the fullest degree possible?

1	2	3	[4]	5
No impact at all	Not a very strong impact	Somewhat of an impact	Very strong impact	Extremely strong impact

10. Is it important to you to plan ahead what you will do in life?

1	2	[3]	4	5
Not at all important	Not very important	Somewhat important	Very important	Extremely important

11. How easy is it for you to follow through with plans?

1	2	3	[4]	5
Not at all easy	Not very easy	Somewhat easy	Very easy	Extremely easy

12. How easy is it for you to stay interested in an activity?

1	2	3	4	[5]
Not at all easy	Not very easy	Somewhat easy	Very easy	Extremely easy

13. Does spirituality have an important role in how you adapt to change?

1	2	3	4	[5]
Not at all important	Not very important	Somewhat important	Very important	Extremely important

14. How valuable is spirituality to you?

1	2	3	4	[5]
Not at all valuable	Not very valuable	Somewhat valuable	Very valuable	Extremely valuable

Instructions: Please finish the following sentences as briefly or as thoroughly as you wish.
(Note: T.L.'s responses are in all caps.)

15. Spirituality to me is A PART OF MY LIFE.
16. I experience inner peace when I'M LISTENING TO MUSIC.
17. I feel most positive about myself when I CREATE SOMETHING.
18. I am best able to pay attention to my own needs when EVERYTHING IS QUIET.
19. I feel best about what I do when I'M THINKING POSITIVELY.
20. I feel best about my decisions when I GET POSITIVE FEEDBACK.
21. I am most engaged in an activity when MY MIND IS INVOLVED.
22. I am most able to express myself in my own unique way when COMMUNICATION IS EASY.
23. I am most able to express myself when the physical environment ALLOWS ME TO USE MY HANDS.
24. When I plan for the future I—THAT'S NOT SOMETHING I DO.
25. I am able to follow through with plans when I WRITE THEM DOWN.
26. I am able to stay interested in an activity when MY MIND IS ENGAGED.
27. When going through a difficult change or transition in my life, I usually adapt by GOING TO MY SPIRITUALITY.
28. I would define spirituality as THE WHOLE OF MY BEING AND MY ANGELS AROUND ME.

(continued)

Table 28-4 (continued)

T.L.'s Responses to the OT-QUEST

Factor	Likert Scale Questions	Add Scores	Divide By	Factor Score (Average)	Low (Score of 1.0-2.3)	Medium (Score of 2.4-3.7)	High (Score of 3.8-5.0)
1. Spiritual (Renewal and Acceptance)	1 & 14 1. How important is an experience of inner peace to you? 14. How valuable is spirituality to you?	Q1: 5 + Q14: 5	2	Factor 1 Score: 5			X
2. Being (Awareness and Understanding)	2 & 3 2. Do you usually feel good about yourself? 3. Do you regularly take the time to meet your own needs?	Q2: 3 + Q3: 3	2	Factor 2 Score: 3		X	
3. Meaning (Purpose and Discovery)	4, 5, & 6 4. How do you usually feel about the actions you have taken? 5. How do you usually feel about the decisions you have made? 6. Do you value being engaged in doing something?	Q4: 3 + Q5: 3 + Q6: 5	3	Factor 3 Score: 3.66		X	

(continued)

Table 28-4 (continued)

T.L.'s Responses to the OT-QUEST

Factor	Likert Scale Questions	Add Scores	Divide By	Factor Score (Average)	Low (Score of 1.0-2.3)	Medium (Score of 2.4-3.7)	High (Score of 3.8-5.0)
4. Expression (Exploration and Causation)	7, 8, & 9 7. Is it important to you to express yourself in a manner that is uniquely you? 8. Does the physical environment around you have an impact on your ability to express yourself to the fullest degree possible? 9. Do the people around you have an impact on your ability to express yourself to the fullest degree possible?	Q7: 5 + Q8: 4 + Q9: 4	3	Factor 4 Score: 4.33			X
5. Intention (Motivation and Will)	10, 11, & 12 10. Is it important to you to plan ahead what you will do in life? 11. How easy is it for you to follow through with plans? 12. How easy is it for you to stay interested in an activity?	Q10: 3 + Q11: 4 + Q12: 5	3	Factor 5 Score: 4			X
6. Adaptation (Spirituality and Adaptation)	13 13. Does spirituality have an important role in how you adapt to change?	Q13: 5	1	Factor 6 Score: 5			X
Total				Total factor score: 24.99	Low (6-13.3)	Medium (13.4-21.8)	High (21.9-30) X

(continued)

Table 28-4 (continued)

T.L.'s Responses to the OT-QUEST

Instructions: Using the themes found in the OT-QUEST sentence completion questions (15-28), and collaborating with your client, fill in the spaces below. (Note: T.L.'s responses are bolded in the first two columns.)

Factor Scores From Likert Scale and Ratings	Sentence Completion Questions	Facilitators of Client's Quality of Experience/ Spirituality	Barriers to Client's Quality of Experience/ Spirituality	Goals to Address
Factor 1: Spiritual 5 Lo Med **Hi**	15, 16, & 28 15. Spirituality to me is **a part of my life.** 16. I experience inner peace when I'm **listening to music.** 28. I would define spirituality as **the whole of my being and my angels around me.**	• Music and whole self, angels	• Making time for music and self	• Put aside 30 min/ day to write out daily schedule • At the end of day write if she did it or not in her journal
Factor 2: Being 3 Lo Med Hi	17 & 18 17. I feel most positive about myself when I **create something.** 18. I am best able to pay attention to my own needs when **everything is quiet.**	• Quiet environment • Creative expression (e.g., painting, writing, sewing)	• Not having a place of quiet solitude and privacy • Not having a place to work • Not creating time	• Put aside 15 min/day for creativity • Clear a space for basket of craft materials
Factor 3: Meaning 3.66 Lo Med Hi	19, 20, & 21 19. I feel best about what I do when I'm **thinking positively.** 20. I feel best about my decisions when **I get positive feedback.** 21. I am most engaged in an activity when **my mind is involved.**	• Thinking positively • Positive feedback from others • Mind is involved in activity	• Getting negative feedback from peers or someone important • Being put down by others unjustly • Being intimidated when trying to complete a thought or activity	• Practice taking a deep breath when conflict is happening for 5 min/ day in front of a mirror • Also with a trusted other person 1x/week

(continued)

Table 28-4 (continued)

T.L.'s Responses to the OT-QUEST

Factor Scores From Likert Scale and Ratings	Sentence Completion Questions	Facilitators of Client's Quality of Experience/ Spirituality	Barriers to Client's Quality of Experience/ Spirituality	Goals to Address
Factor 4: Expression 4.33 Lo Med **Hi**	22 & 23 22. I am most able to express myself in my own unique way when **communication is easy.** 23. I am most able to express myself when the physical environment **allows me to use my hands.**	• Easy communication • Expression with hands (gestures)	• Having people who want to have their own opinions heard rather than hearing mine • If environment is too small	• Practice asking people to listen all the way through • 1x/week find a spacious environment to express self • Volunteer helping with babies and holding them 1x/month
Factor 5: Intention 4 Lo Med **Hi**	24, 25, & 26 24. When I plan for the future I—**that's not something I do.** 25. I am able to follow through with plans when **I write them down.** 26. I am able to stay interested in an activity when **my mind is engaged.**	• Planning day and journaling • Mind engaged— learning new things or more about old things • Society for Creative Anachronism engages her mind and learning	• Does not plan because of major stress and grief in a 4-year period	• Daily use of journal • Plan an activity with new society group
Factor 6: Adaptation 5 Lo Med **Hi**	27 27. When going through a difficult change or transition in my life, I usually adapt by **going to my spirituality.**	• Spirituality • Angel altar • Prayer at altar	• Not making time for it	• Put aside 10 min/day to make time for prayer at her angel altar

Table 28-5

D.S.'s Responses to the OT-QUEST

Instructions: Circle or state your response to each question. (Note: D.S.'s responses are in brackets.)

1. How important is an experience of inner peace to you?

1	2	3	4	[5]
Not at all important	Not very important	Somewhat important	Very important	Extremely important

2. Do you usually feel good about yourself?

1	2	[3]	4	5
Never	Rarely	Sometimes	Most of the time	Always

3. Do you regularly take the time to meet your own needs?

1	2	3	[4]	5
Never	Rarely	Sometimes	Most of the time	Always

4. How do you usually feel about the actions you have taken?

1	2	[3]	4	5
Not at all positive	Not very positive	Somewhat positive	Very positive	Extremely positive

5. How do you usually feel about the decisions you have made?

1	2	[3]	4	5
Not at all positive	Not very positive	Somewhat positive	Very positive	Extremely positive

6. Do you value being engaged in doing something?

1	2	3	[4]	5
Never	Rarely	Sometimes	Most of the time	Always

7. Is it important to you to express yourself in a manner that is uniquely you?

1	2	[3]	4	5
Not at all important	Not very important	Somewhat important	Very important	Extremely important

8. Does the physical environment around you have an impact on your ability to express yourself to the fullest degree possible?

1	2	3	4	[5]
No impact at all	Not a very strong impact	Somewhat of an impact	Very strong impact	Extremely strong impact

9. Do the people around you have an impact on your ability to express yourself to the fullest degree possible?

1	2	3	[4]	5
No impact at all	Not a very strong impact	Somewhat of an impact	Very strong impact	Extremely strong impact

(continued)

Table 28-5 (continued)

D.S.'s Responses to the OT-QUEST

10. Is it important to you to plan ahead what you will do in life?

1	2	3	[4]	5
Not at all important	Not very important	Somewhat important	Very important	Extremely important

11. How easy is it for you to follow through with plans?

1	[2]	3	4	5
Not at all easy	Not very easy	Somewhat easy	Very easy	Extremely easy

12. How easy is it for you to stay interested in an activity?

1	[2]	3	4	5
Not at all easy	Not very easy	Somewhat easy	Very easy	Extremely easy

13. Does spirituality have an important role in how you adapt to change?

1	2	3	4	[5]
Not at all important	Not very important	Somewhat important	Very important	Extremely important

14. How valuable is spirituality to you?

1	2	3	4	[5]
Not at all valuable	Not very valuable	Somewhat valuable	Very valuable	Extremely valuable

Instructions: Please finish the following sentences as briefly or as thoroughly as you wish. (Note: D.S.'s responses are in all caps.)

15. Spirituality to me is THE UMBRELLA UNDER WHICH ALL OF LIFE FALLS.
16. I experience inner peace when I AM IN MEDITATION.
17. I feel most positive about myself when I AM COMPETENTLY EXECUTING MY ROLE AND LIFE SEEMS BALANCED.
18. I am best able to pay attention to my own needs when THERE AREN'T OUTER DISTRACTIONS.
19. I feel best about what I do when I AM ENRICHING OTHERS' LIVES.
20. I feel best about my decisions when THERE APPEARS TO BE A HIGHER OUTCOME.
21. I am most engaged in an activity when IT IS ALIGNED WITH A DIVINE PURPOSE.
22. I am most able to express myself in my own unique way when I HAVE TIME AWAY FROM WORK.
23. I am most able to express myself when the physical environment IS POSITIVE.
24. When I plan for the future I BECOME ANXIOUS AND UNCERTAIN.
25. I am able to follow through with plans when THEY ARE CONCRETE.
26. I am able to stay interested in an activity when IT HAS MEANING AND PURPOSE AND IS ALIGNED WITH THE GREATER GOOD.
27. When going through a difficult change or transition in my life, I usually adapt by GETTING HELP FROM FAMILY, FRIENDS, AND PRACTITIONERS.
28. I would define spirituality as ONE'S PERSONAL JOURNEY TOWARD WHOLENESS.

(continued)

Table 28-5 (continued)

D.S.'s Responses to the OT-QUEST

Factor	Likert Scale Questions	Add Scores	Divide By	Factor Score (Average)	Low (Score of 1.0-2.3)	Medium (Score of 2.4-3.7)	High (Score of 3.8-5.0)
1. Spiritual (Renewal and Acceptance)	1 & 14 1. How important is an experience of inner peace to you? 14. How valuable is spirituality to you?	Q1: 5 + Q14: 5	2	Factor 1 Score: 5			X
2. Being (Awareness and Understanding)	2 & 3 2. Do you usually feel good about yourself? 3. Do you regularly take the time to meet your own needs?	Q2: 3 + Q3: 4	2	Factor 2 Score: 3.5		X	
3. Meaning (Purpose and Discovery)	4, 5, & 6 4. How do you usually feel about the actions you have taken? 5. How do you usually feel about the decisions you have made? 6. Do you value being engaged in doing something?	Q4: 3 + Q5: 3 + Q6: 4	3	Factor 3 Score: 3.3		X	

(continued)

Table 28-5 (continued)

D.S.'s Responses to the OT-QUEST

Factor	Likert Scale Questions	Add Scores	Divide By	Factor Score (Average)	Low (Score of 1.0-2.3)	Medium (Score of 2.4-3.7)	High (Score of 3.8-5.0)
4. Expression (Exploration and Causation)	7, 8, & 9 7. Is it important to you to express yourself in a manner that is uniquely you? 8. Does the physical environment around you have an impact on your ability to express yourself to the fullest degree possible? 9. Do the people around you have an impact on your ability to express yourself to the fullest degree possible?	Q7: 3 + Q8: 5 + Q9: 4	3	Factor 4 Score: 4			X
5. Intention (Motivation and Will)	10, 11, & 12 10. Is it important to you to plan ahead what you will do in life? 11. How easy is it for you to follow through with plans? 12. How easy is it for you to stay interested in an activity?	Q10: 4 + Q11: 2 + Q12: 2	3	Factor 5 Score: 2.67		X	
6. Adaptation (Spirituality and Adaptation)	13 13. Does spirituality have an important role in how you adapt to change?	Q13: 5	1	Factor 6 Score: 5			X
Total				Total factor score: 23.47	Low (6-13.3)	Medium (13.4-21.8)	High (21.9-30) X

(continued)

Table 28-5 (continued)

D.S.'s Responses to the OT-QUEST

Instructions: Using the themes found in the OT-QUEST sentence completion questions (15-28), and collaborating with your client, fill in the spaces below. (Note: D.S.'s responses are bolded in the first two columns.)

Factor Scores From Likert Scale and Ratings	Sentence Completion Questions	Facilitators of Client's Quality of Experience/ Spirituality	Barriers to Client's Quality of Experience/ Spirituality	Goals to Address
Factor 1: Spiritual 5 Lo Med **Hi**	15, 16, & 28 15. Spirituality to me is **the umbrella under which all of life falls.** 16. I experience inner peace when I **am in meditation.** 28. I would define spirituality as **one's personal journey toward wholeness.**	• Giving herself regular time to meditate, reflect on goals and refocus on guru's teachings at least 1x/day	• Compulsivity around work • Getting into a frenzy because there is always more to do • Can't stop workaholic behavior • Not taking time for self • Not taking time to rest	• Schedule regular breaks on calendar and stick to them • Make taking breaks part of daily routine: 1.5 hrs in a.m. for meditation/yoga; 1.5 hrs meditation/ relaxation during day; 1 hr for home/self-maintenance daily
Factor 2: Being 3.5 Lo **Med** Hi	17 & 18 17. I feel most positive about myself when I **am competently executing my role and life seems balanced.** 18. I am best able to pay attention to my own needs when **there aren't outer distractions.**	• Having reflection time during meditation to review life areas for more balance • Having the phone/ computer off	• Constant texts, emails, and phone calls • No goal list	• Turn off phone and computer after 10 p.m. and during meditation time • Write a daily goal list for self every morning and stick to it

(continued)

Table 28-5 (continued)

D.S.'s Responses to the OT-QUEST

Factor Scores From Likert Scale and Ratings	Sentence Completion Questions	Facilitators of Client's Quality of Experience/ Spirituality	Barriers to Client's Quality of Experience/ Spirituality	Goals to Address
Factor 3: Meaning 3.3 Lo **Med** Hi	19, 20, & 21 19. I feel best about what I do when **I am enriching others' lives.** 20. I feel best about my decisions when **there appears to be a higher outcome.** 21. I am most engaged in an activity when **it is aligned with a divine purpose.**	• Having clients • Giving classes • Friends and family • Inner intuition	• Lack of knowledge about what to do to promote work she wants to do, which is to educate people about health and disseminate her guru's spiritual teachings • Lack of an audience	• Daily prayer for guidance • At least 2x/week do something to educate self about how to market oneself (e.g., talk to someone who is successful, do an internet search, take a workshop, read a book)
Factor 4: Expression 4 Lo Med **Hi**	22 & 23 22. I am most able to express myself in my own unique way when **I have time away from work.** 23. I am most able to express myself when the physical environment **is positive.**	• Setting boundaries • Living alone in a quiet space	• Compulsivity • Fear of lack of money • Feeling irresponsible due to debt • Phone calls/texts • Children dropping in unannounced	• Include in budget money to pay off debt every month • Do not accumulate more debt and keep track by writing down daily expenses

(continued)

Table 28-5 (continued)

D.S.'s Responses to the OT-QUEST

Factor Scores From Likert Scale and Ratings	Sentence Completion Questions	Facilitators of Client's Quality of Experience/ Spirituality	Barriers to Client's Quality of Experience/ Spirituality	Goals to Address
Factor 5: Intention 2.67 Lo **Med** Hi	24, 25, & 26 24. When I plan for the future I **become anxious and uncertain.** 25. I am able to follow through with plans when **they are concrete.** 26. I am able to stay interested in an activity when **it has meaning and purpose and is aligned with the greater good.**	• Having a plan that is working • Relaxation time • Connecting to spiritual path	• Lack of finances • Uncertainty about future • Children are grown/ leaving • Time management challenges • Distractions	• Take continuing education classes or study something every other week to increase skills • Investigate new places to live/move every other week
Factor 6: Adaptation 5 Lo Med **Hi**	27 27. When going through a difficult change or transition in my life, I usually adapt by **getting help from family, friends, and practitioners.**	• Listening to inner voice guidance when it suggests it is time to reach out for help • Recognizing more and more when help is needed	• Not wanting to burden others • Financial lack • Feeling indebted to others	• Keep a list of how she helps others and review it 1x/week • Make a list of people to whom she feels indebted (to make it seem more manageable) and pray for them daily

E.W.

E.W. is a 75-year-old, retired, divorced, White woman who lives alone. She was married for 28 years and divorced in 1987; her ex-husband passed away last year. She explained that much of who she is today is directly related to who she became working through the ramifications of her relationship with her ex-husband. She had never been by herself or had experienced a broken relationship before that. Accepting something like that was required for her to live and move through it. She has 2 adult children and 4 grandchildren who live about 5 hours away. She has two sisters and two brothers with whom she has a close relationship but who do not live locally. She was the sole caretaker for her elderly father for 10 years before he passed away 4.5 years ago. She is a sincere spiritual seeker.

E.W. is seeking assistance because she was feeling stuck in her spiritual progress and thought that a session might help her be able to see herself more clearly. She has some residual issues and feelings about her ex-husband coming up to be released after his recent death. She also has rheumatoid arthritis, which roams around the body. The rheumatoid arthritis affects her neck, hands, arms, and feet. It began around the same time she began working as an engineer in 1974. It is not as severe as it used to be.

E.W. has an aversion to goals because they feel coercive to her, so the score sheet was modified to make the suggestions/plans for the future into *intentions* rather than definite goals. We worked on the intentions collaboratively after she completed the OT-QUEST on her own. E.W.'s responses to the OT-QUEST and her score sheet are shown in Table 28-6.

Appropriate Populations for Use

Appropriate populations for use of the OT-QUEST are adults who are able to answer abstract questions.

Strengths and Limitations

The OT-QUEST has yet to be trialed with clients receiving occupational therapy services, so how it translates to practice is unknown. The weak internal consistency finding in the previous study is of concern; however, it may partly be a result of the small number of participants and the small number of items per subscale. Results of the previous study also indicate that the OT-QUEST is a tool with good concurrent validity, which means that it appears to measure what it sets out to measure. It also has and strong test-retest reliability, which means that over time, it elicits consistent responses from people. It also offers therapists useful quantitative and qualitative information about the spiritual aspect of the person, which has the potential to lead to meaningful treatment goals, plans, and interventions for clients.

Table 28-6

E.W.'s Responses to the OT-QUEST

Instructions: Circle or state your response to each question. (Note: E.W.'s responses are in brackets.)

1. How important is an experience of inner peace to you?

1	2	3	4	[5]
Not at all important	Not very important	Somewhat important	Very important	Extremely important

2. Do you usually feel good about yourself?

1	2	[3]	4	5
Never	Rarely	Sometimes	Most of the time	Always

3. Do you regularly take the time to meet your own needs?

1	2	[3]	4	5
Never	Rarely	Sometimes	Most of the time	Always

4. How do you usually feel about the actions you have taken?

1	2	3	[4]	5
Not at all positive	Not very positive	Somewhat positive	Very positive	Extremely positive

5. How do you usually feel about the decisions you have made?

1	2	[3]	4	5
Not at all positive	Not very positive	Somewhat positive	Very positive	Extremely positive

6. Do you value being engaged in doing something?

1	2	3	[4]	5
Never	Rarely	Sometimes	Most of the time	Always

7. Is it important to you to express yourself in a manner that is uniquely you?

1	2	3	4	[5]
Not at all important	Not very important	Somewhat important	Very important	Extremely important

8. Does the physical environment around you have an impact on your ability to express yourself to the fullest degree possible?

1	2	[3]	4	5
No impact at all	Not a very strong impact	Somewhat of an impact	Very strong impact	Extremely strong impact

9. Do the people around you have an impact on your ability to express yourself to the fullest degree possible?

1	2	3	[4]	5
No impact at all	Not a very strong impact	Somewhat of an impact	Very strong impact	Extremely strong impact

(continued)

Table 28-6 (continued)

E.W.'s Responses to the OT-QUEST

10. Is it important to you to plan ahead what you will do in life?

1	2	[3]	4	5
Not at all important	Not very important	Somewhat important	Very important	Extremely important

11. How easy is it for you to follow through with plans?
DEPENDS ON WHAT I'M PLANNING AND IF $$ ARE INVOLVED.

1	2	3	[4]	5
Not at all easy	Not very easy	Somewhat easy	Very easy	Extremely easy

12. How easy is it for you to stay interested in an activity?
DEPENDS. CLEAR INSTRUCTION? DEPENDING ON OTHERS? DEPTH OF INTEREST?

1	2	[3]	4	5
Not at all easy	Not very easy	Somewhat easy	Very easy	Extremely easy

13. Does spirituality have an important role in how you adapt to change?

1	2	3	4	[5]
Not at all important	Not very important	Somewhat important	Very important	Extremely important

14. How valuable is spirituality to you?

1	2	3	4	[5]
Not at all valuable	Not very valuable	Somewhat valuable	Very valuable	Extremely valuable

Instructions: Please finish the following sentences as briefly or as thoroughly as you wish.
(Note: E.W.'s responses are in all caps.)

15. Spirituality to me is PRIORITY IN LIFE.
16. I experience inner peace when I'M IN ACCEPTANCE OF SELF AND OTHERS.
17. I feel most positive about myself when RHEUMATOID ARTHRITIS IS NOT HIGH AND WHEN I ACCEPT MYSELF AS I AM.
18. I am best able to pay attention to my own needs when I'M BY MYSELF AND NOTHING IS PUSHING ME … INTERNALLY OR EXTERNALLY.
19. I feel best about what I do when I CAN HELP ANOTHER OR A SOLUTION TO A PROBLEM IS GENERATED/CREATED.
20. I feel best about my decisions when THEY DON'T IMPACT OTHERS NEGATIVELY.
21. I am most engaged in an activity when IT INTERESTS ME, OR SOMETHING I'M ENGAGED IN HAS A COMPLETION REQUIREMENT.
22. I am most able to express myself in my own unique way when … I GUESS ALWAYS, BUT DEPTH OF COMMUNICATION DEPENDS ON RECEPTION RESPONSE OF OTHERS.
23. I am most able to express myself when the physical environment MATCHES MY INTENT.
24. When I plan for the future I KNOW THAT FLEXIBILITY IS REQUIRED.
25. I am able to follow through with plans when FINANCIAL AND THE UNIVERSE SUPPORT THE PLAN … AND I DON'T CHANGE THE ORIGINAL PLAN …
26. I am able to stay interested in an activity when IT DOESN'T CONCERN A LOT OF OTHERS AND DOESN'T REQUIRE A LOT OF WORDS WITHOUT PRODUCT. AND IT'S EASIER IF I'M INTERESTED.
27. When going through a difficult change or transition in my life, I usually adapt by GOING THROUGH IT TO GET TO IT.
28. I would define spirituality as LIVING LIFE HEART CENTERED AND REACHING FOR SOURCE/GOD/ONE.

(continued)

Table 28-6 (continued)

E.W.'s Responses to the OT-QUEST

Factor	Likert Scale Questions	Add Scores	Divide By	Factor Score (Average)	Low (Score of 1.0-2.3)	Medium (Score of 2.4-3.7)	High (Score of 3.8-5.0)
1. Spiritual (Renewal and Acceptance)	1 & 14 1. How important is an experience of inner peace to you? 14. How valuable is spirituality to you?	Q1: 5 + Q14: 5	2	Factor 1 Score: 5			X
2. Being (Awareness and Understanding)	2 & 3 2. Do you usually feel good about yourself? 3. Do you regularly take the time to meet your own needs?	Q2: 3 + Q3: 3	2	Factor 2 Score: 3		X	
3. Meaning (Purpose and Discovery)	4, 5, & 6 4. How do you usually feel about the actions you have taken? 5. How do you usually feel about the decisions you have made? 6. Do you value being engaged in doing something?	Q4: 4 + Q5: 3 + Q6: 4	3	Factor 3 Score: 3.67		X	

(continued)

Table 28-6 (continued)

E.W.'s Responses to the OT-QUEST

Factor	Likert Scale Questions	Add Scores	Divide By	Factor Score (Average)	Low (Score of 1.0-2.3)	Medium (Score of 2.4-3.7)	High (Score of 3.8-5.0)
4. Expression (Exploration and Causation)	7, 8, & 9 7. Is it important to you to express yourself in a manner that is uniquely you? 8. Does the physical environment around you have an impact on your ability to express yourself to the fullest degree possible? 9. Do the people around you have an impact on your ability to express yourself to the fullest degree possible?	Q7: 5 + Q8: 3 + Q9: 4	3	Factor 4 Score: 4			X
5. Intention (Motivation and Will)	10, 11, & 12 10. Is it important to you to plan ahead what you will do in life? 11. How easy is it for you to follow through with plans? 12. How easy is it for you to stay interested in an activity?	Q10: 3 + Q11: 4 + Q12: 3	3	Factor 5 Score: 3.33		X	
6. Adaptation (Spirituality and Adaptation)	13 13. Does spirituality have an important role in how you adapt to change?	Q13: 5	1	Factor 6 Score: 5			X
Total				Total score: 24	Low (6-13.3)	Medium (13.4-21.8)	High (21.9-30) X

(continued)

Table 28-6 (continued)

E.W.'s Responses to the OT-QUEST

Instructions: Using the themes found in the OT-QUEST sentence completion questions (15-28), and collaborating with your client, fill in the spaces below. (Note: E.W.'s responses are bolded in the first two columns.)

Factor Scores From Likert Scale and Ratings	Sentence Completion Questions	Facilitators of Client's Quality of Experience/ Spirituality	Barriers to Client's Quality of Experience/ Spirituality	Goals to Address
Factor 1: Spiritual 5 Lo Med **Hi**	15, 16, & 28 15. Spirituality to me is **priority in life.** 16. I experience inner peace when **I'm in acceptance of self and others.** 28. I would define spirituality as **living life heart centered and reaching for source/God/One.**	• Trying to do contemplation and a lot of mantra work • Reading her guru's books (*Life: A Mysterious Journey*) and other related books (*Call of the Sun; Towards a Solar Civilization*) • Attending retreats • Prayer for self, prayer for others • Developing a practice gathering 1x/week for anyone who wants to come • Moving through each day with calmness	• Laziness • Lack of discipline • Hate doing something I have to do • Feel like have to meditate but may not want to today • Goals are bothersome	• Substitute out a practice that is related to her spiritual path that she doesn't want to do for a different practice that is also related to her spiritual path that she does want to do

(continued)

Table 28-6 (continued)

E.W.'s Responses to the OT-QUEST

Factor Scores From Likert Scale and Ratings	Sentence Completion Questions	Facilitators of Client's Quality of Experience/Spirituality	Barriers to Client's Quality of Experience/Spirituality	Goals to Address
Factor 2: Being 3 Lo **Med** Hi	17 & 18 17. I feel most positive about myself when **rheumatoid arthritis is not high and when I accept myself as I am.** 18. I am best able to pay attention to my own needs when **I'm by myself and nothing is pushing me … internally or externally.**	• Walking and staying away from processed foods • Results of prayer or meditation prayer are helpful with self-acceptance • Solitude • Treating goals as intentions without deadlines	• Rheumatoid arthritis flare-ups • Poor self-image; body image, age • Harsh self-judgment • Not feeling good enough • Feeling alone—not feeling the oneness with anything (e.g., with nature, the birds outside the window) • Missing deceased loved ones	• Continue with walking, not eating processed foods, doing prayer and meditation • Reframing to see age as wisdom and strength and share that with others • Remembering "I am not my body" • Talking to deceased loved ones to feel connected to them

(continued)

Table 28-6 (continued)

E.W.'s Responses to the OT-QUEST

Factor Scores From Likert Scale and Ratings	Sentence Completion Questions	Facilitators of Client's Quality of Experience/ Spirituality	Barriers to Client's Quality of Experience/ Spirituality	Goals to Address
Factor 3: Meaning 3.67 Lo **Med** Hi	19, 20, & 21 19. I feel best about what I do when I **can help another or a solution to a problem is generated/created.** 20. I feel best about my decisions when **they don't impact others negatively.** 21. I am most engaged in an activity when **it interests me, or something I'm engaged in has a completion requirement.**	• Intuition • Using wisdom gained from years • Good communication skills • Ability to intuitively read others for best words to use in communication • Dealing with issues with others directly • Activity being done is pleasurable, fun, or challenging	• The other person trying to help is unreachable or closed off • Solution costs money • Physical pain in hands from rheumatoid arthritis • Feeling compelled to speak and/or act for truth and justice, which may negatively impact others • Choosing to lose interest in an activity • Don't like it, don't want to do it, not interested in it, don't want to do it any more, withdrawing from activity	• Acceptance of what is • Take a second look at the activity, find something enjoyable about it, and redirect the self to do it in a positive way

(continued)

Table 28-6 (continued)

E.W.'s Responses to the OT-QUEST

Factor Scores From Likert Scale and Ratings	Sentence Completion Questions	Facilitators of Client's Quality of Experience/ Spirituality	Barriers to Client's Quality of Experience/ Spirituality	Goals to Address
Factor 4: Expression 4 Lo Med **Hi**	22 & 23 22. I am most able to express myself in my own unique way when … **I guess always, but depth of communication depends on reception response of others.** 23. I am most able to express myself when the physical environment **matches my intent.**	• Humor • Speaking with gentleness • Avoidance of harm • Flexibility in changing intent • Acceptance of the physical environment	• People not wanting to hear • Impatience • Not asking for help	• Practicing patience when communicating with others • Asking for help when the physical environment does not match intent
Factor 5: Intention 3.33 Lo **Med** Hi	24, 25, & 26 24. When I plan for the future I know that **flexibility is required.** 25. I am able to follow through with plans when **financial and the universe support the plan … and I don't change the original plan …** 26. I am able to stay interested in an activity when **it doesn't concern a lot of others and doesn't require a lot of words without product. And it's easier if I'm interested.**	• The world is a great teacher of flexibility • Tailoring plans to finances • Leave the universe freedom to support whatever the plan is; not trying to control the outcome • Life at the moment does not involve a lot of people • Interest in getting the project done • Project involves serving others • Project is a worthwhile project	• Stubbornness—wanting it my way • Too many cooks spoil the broth • Too many people creates overwhelming energy • The unknown, unforeseen occurrences (e.g., catch-22, Murphy's law) • Project is unworthy of time, attention, interest	• Acceptance, letting it go, working through it • Divide larger groups into smaller groups • Prayer to navigate through the unexpected • Hunkering down and getting it done anyway • Reframing or finding an element of worth in the completion of the project

(continued)

Table 28-6 (continued)

E.W.'s Responses to the OT-QUEST

Factor Scores From Likert Scale and Ratings	Sentence Completion Questions	Facilitators of Client's Quality of Experience/ Spirituality	Barriers to Client's Quality of Experience/ Spirituality	Goals to Address
Factor 6: Adaptation 5 Lo Med **Hi**	27 27. When going through a difficult change or transition in my life, I usually adapt by **going through it to get to it.**	• Prayer • Acceptance • Contemplation • Patience • Flexibility • Knowing what is happening around me is going to change	• Stubbornness, wanting it my way • It is unfair • Why is this happening to me? • Low self-image • Low self-worth	• Reframing the situation • Practicing acceptance • Forgiveness of others • Forgiveness of self

Suggested Further Research

The low number of participants in the reliability and validity study decreased the power of the results. Therefore, more research with a larger set of participants is suggested. Further research is also needed to ascertain which clinical populations it is best suited for and how outcomes of occupational therapy intervention would be affected by using it in clinical practice.

To date, two more completed studies have been attempted to validate the OT-QUEST. The first study, a faculty-led research process, was conducted with 10 entry-level master's occupational therapy students as researchers using electronic surveys comparing the concurrent validity of the OT-QUEST (Humpherys, Pomeranz, Roschkowsky, Swope, & Tartaglia, 2011) using the SWBS (Paloutzian & Ellison, 1982), the Spiritual Health and Life-Orientation Measure (Fisher, 2010), and the Spiritual Experience Index–Revised (Genia, 1991, 1997) as comparison measures. The study also examined how health professional faculty and students view spirituality (Coup, Rowe, Smith, Whitewood-Zaslavsky, & Hastings, 2011). Results were inconclusive due to a limited sample size ($N = 49$).

A second faculty-led study was conducted with 8 entry-level master's occupational therapy students as researchers using electronic surveys looking at the concurrent validity of the OT-QUEST (Brass, Campbell, Clark, & Demick, 2012) against the SWBS only to make the study less cumbersome for participants. The study also examined how nursing and occupational therapy faculty and students view spirituality (Hepworth, Jones, Macziewski, & Murphy, 2012). Results were inconclusive due to limited sample size ($N = 151$). However, another potential model of spirituality (instead of Collins's 1998 model) was suggested from the data. From these two attempts, it became evident that more testing of the OT-QUEST with a larger sample size is needed.

To that end, another study is in progress with a revised third edition of the OT-QUEST, which has 38 Likert scale items. Concurrent validity in this study is being measured against the SWBS and the Mindful Awareness Attention Scale. The data collection process, now completed, occurred using an online survey format (Schulz, Thomas, Rollins, & Booher, 2017). Data analysis has begun, but at the writing of this chapter is not yet completed. However, with the larger sample size obtained from this attempt, it is hoped that the most salient items to include in accordance with the best model will be determined and the concurrent validity of the OT-QUEST may be finally established.

Acknowledgments

The author would like to thank the following people:
- Kathlyn L. Reed, PhD, OTR, FAOTA, MLIS, AHIP, Visiting Professor, Texas Woman's University—Houston Center, Houston, Texas, for inspiration, mentoring, and guidance provided to the author in developing the OT-QUEST
- Cynthia Owsley, PhD, Professor of Ophthalmology at the University of Alabama at Birmingham
- Gerald McGwin Jr., PhD, Associate Professor in the School of Public Health/Trauma/Ophthalmology at the University of Alabama at Birmingham
- Donald Fletcher, MD, Director of Low Vision Clinic in the Department of Ophthalmology at the University of Alabama at Birmingham, for mentoring and collaboration provided to the author in the reliability and validity research on the second edition of the OT-QUEST

- Mary Voytek, OTD, MC, OTR/L, Assistant Professor, Occupational Therapy Program, Arizona School of Health Sciences, A. T. Still University in Mesa, Arizona, for collaborating and co-leading with the author the research groups of the entry-level master's students studying the OT-QUEST
- R. Curtis Bay, PhD, Professor, Biostatistics, Department of Interdisciplinary Health Sciences, and Chair, Institutional Review Board, Arizona School of Health Sciences, A.T. Still University in Mesa, Arizona, for his statistical support
- The MSOT students involved in the research groups studying the OT-QUEST:
  - 2010-2011 Group: Kim Coup, OTS; Katelyn Rowe, OTS; Shelby Smith, OTS; Alison Whitewood-Zaslavsky, OTS; Meagan Hastings, OTS; Kay Humpherys, OTS; Marla Pomeranz, OTS; Kathy Roschkowsky, OTS; Jackie Swope, OTS; Marietta Tartaglia, OTS
  - 2011-2012 Group: Brandon Hepworth, OTS; Brandon Jones, OTS; Tabitha Macziewski, OTS; Nicole Murphy, OTS; Julie Brass, OTS; Cari Campbell, OTS; Jacquelyn Clark, OTS; Laura Demick, OTS
- Frank N. Thomas, PhD, LMFT-S, Professor of Counseling and Counselor Education at the College of Education, Texas Christian University, Fort Worth, Texas, for his collaboration in leading his doctoral students through the current research study process
- Kimberly Grigg, MEd in Counseling, doctoral student at Texas Christian University, for her assistance with research design for the current study
- Erin Acker Booher, MEd, LPC, doctoral student at Texas Christian University, for her ongoing assistance with the current study
- (Lisa) Michelle Rollins, MEd in Counseling, doctoral student at Texas Christian University, for her ongoing assistance with the current study

Funding

The validity and reliability study conducted in 2005 on the second edition of the OT-QUEST was funded by a Research to Prevent Blindness grant from the University of Alabama at Birmingham, Department of Ophthalmology—Clinical Research Unit, and a matching grant from the University of Alabama at Birmingham, School of Health-Related Professions, Department of Occupational Therapy.

The funding to purchase use of the SWBS was provided by the Occupational Therapy Department at A.T. Still University, Arizona School of Health Sciences, for the research conducted from 2010 to 2017.

References

Agrimson, L. B., & Taft, L. B. (2009). Spiritual crisis: A concept analysis. *Journal of Advanced Nursing, 65,* 454-461.

Algado, S. S., Gregori, J. M. R., & Egan, M. (1997). Spirituality in a refugee camp. *Canadian Journal of Occupational Therapy, 64,* 138-145.

American Occupational Therapy Association. (2002). Occupational therapy practice framework: Domain and process. *American Journal of Occupational Therapy, 56,* 609-639.

American Occupational Therapy Association. (2014). Occupational therapy practice framework: Domain and process (3rd ed.). *American Journal of Occupational Therapy, 68*(Suppl. 1), S1-S48.

Bellingham, R., Cohen, B., Jones, T., & Spaniol, L. (1989). Connectedness: Some skills for spiritual health. *American Journal of Health Promotion, 4,* 18-31.

Bosacki, S., & Ota, C. (2000). Preadolescents' voices: A consideration of British and Canadian children's reflections on religion, spirituality, and their sense of self. *International Journal of Children's Spirituality, 5*, 203-219.

Brass, J., Campbell, C., Clark, J., & Demick, L. (2012). *Concurrent validity of the OT-QUEST: Assessing spirituality in occupational therapy*. Unpublished manuscript, A.T. Still University, Mesa, AZ.

Burkhardt, M. A. (1994). Becoming and connecting: Elements of spirituality for women. *Holistic Nursing Practice, 8*, 12-21.

Champagne, T. T., Ryan, J. K., Saccomando, H. M., & Lazzarini, I. (2007). A nonlinear dynamics approach to exploring the spiritual dimensions of occupation. *Emergence: Complexity and Organization, 9*(4), 29-43.

Chibnall, J. T., Videen, S. D., Duckro, P. N., & Miller, D. K. (2002). Psychosocial-spiritual correlates of death distress in patients with life-threatening medical conditions. *Palliative Medicine, 16*, 331-338.

Christiansen, C. (1997). Nationally speaking: Acknowledging a spiritual dimension in occupational therapy practice. *American Journal of Occupational Therapy, 51*, 169-172.

Cole, S. R., Beck, R. W., Moke, P. S., Gal, R. L., & Long, D. T. (2000). The National Eye Institute Visual Function Questionnaire: Experience of the ONTT. Optic Neuritis Treatment Trial. *Investigative Ophthalmology & Visual Science, 41*, 1017-1021.

Collins, J. S., Paul, S., & West-Frasier, J. (2001). The utilization of spirituality in occupational therapy: Beliefs, practices, and perceived barriers. *Occupational Therapy in Health Care, 14*(3/4), 73-92.

Collins, M. (1998). Occupational therapy and spirituality: Reflecting on quality of experience in therapeutic interventions. *British Journal of Occupational Therapy, 61*(6), 280-284.

Collins, M. (2007). Spiritual emergency and occupational identity: A transpersonal perspective. *British Journal of Occupational Therapy, 70*, 504-512.

Collins, M. (2014). *The unselfish spirit: Human evolution in a time of global crisis*. London, United Kingdom: Permanent Publications.

Collins, M. (2016). Spirituality and occupational therapy: Reflections on professional practice and future possibilities. In M. de Souza, J. Bone, & J. Watson (Eds.), *Spirituality across disciplines: Research and practice* (pp. 203-216). New York, NY: Springer International Publishing.

Congdon, J. G., & Magilvy, J. K. (2001). Themes of rural health and aging from a program of research. *Geriatric Nursing, 22*, 234-238.

Coup, K., Rowe, K., Smith, S., Whitewood-Zaslavsky, A., & Hastings, M. (2011). *Comparing attitudes toward and experience of spirituality among health care students and professionals*. Unpublished manuscript, A.T. Still University, Mesa, AZ.

Csikszentmihalyi, M. (1998). The flow experience and its significance for human psychology. In M. Csikszentmihalyi & I. S. Csikszentmihalyi (Eds.), *Optimal experience: Psychological studies of flow in consciousness* (pp. 15-35). Cambridge, United Kingdom: Cambridge University Press.

Csikszentmihalyi, M., & Csikszentmihalyi, I. S. (Eds.). (1998). *Optimal experience: Psychological studies of flow in consciousness*. Cambridge, United Kingdom: Cambridge University Press.

Csontó, S. (2009). Occupational therapy students' consideration of clients' spirituality in practice placement education. *British Journal of Occupational Therapy, 72*, 442-449.

Do Rozario, L. (1994). Ritual, meaning and transcendence: The role of occupation in modern life. *Journal of Occupational Science, 1*, 46-53.

Dossey, B. M. (1998). Florence Nightingale. *Journal of Holistic Nursing, 16*, 111-163.

Dyson, J., Cobb, M., & Forman, D. (1997). The meaning of spirituality: A literature review. *Journal of Advanced Nursing, 26*, 1183-1188.

Egan, M., & DeLaat, M.D. (1997). The implicit spirituality of occupational therapy practice. *Canadian Journal of Occupational Therapy, 64*, 115-121.

Engquist, D. E., Short-DeGraff, M., Gliner, J., & Oltenbruns, K. (1997). Occupational therapists' beliefs and practices with regard to spirituality and therapy. *American Journal of Occupational Therapy, 51*, 173-180.

Farrar, J. E. (2001). Addressing spirituality and religious life in occupational therapy practice. *Physical & Occupational Therapy in Geriatrics, 18*(4), 65-85.

Ferrell, B. R., Smith, S. L., Juarez, G., & Melancon, C. (2003). Meaning of illness and spirituality in ovarian cancer survivors. *Oncology Nursing Forum, 30*, 249-257.

Fisher, J. (2010). Development and application of a spiritual well-being questionnaire called SHALOM. *Religions, 1*, 105-121.

Fisher, J. W., Francis, L. J., & Johnson, P. (2000). Assessing spiritual health via four domains of spiritual wellbeing: The SH4DI. *Pastoral Psychology, 49*, 133-145.

Frank, G., Bernardo, C. S., Tropper, S., Noguchi, F., Lipman, C., Maulhardt, B., & Weitze, L. (1997). Jewish spirituality through actions in time: Daily occupations of young orthodox Jewish couples in Los Angeles. *American Journal of Occupational Therapy, 51*, 199-206.

Genia, V. (1991). The Spiritual Experience Index: A measure of spiritual identity. *Journal of Religion and Health, 30*, 337-347.

Genia, V. (1997). The Spiritual Experience Index: Revision and reformulation. *Review of Religious Research, 38,* 344-381.

Greene, B. (2005). *The fabric of the cosmos: Space, time, and the texture of reality.* New York, NY: Vintage.

Grof, S. (1989). *Spiritual emergency: When personal transformation becomes a crisis.* New York, NY: TarcherPerigree.

Hartelius, G., Caplan, M., & Rardin, M. A. (2007). Transpersonal psychology: Defining the past, divining the future. *The Humanistic Psychologist, 35*(2), 135-160.

Hepworth, B., Jones, B., Macziewski, T., & Murphy, N. (2012). *Comparing spirituality: Nursing vs. occupational therapy.* Unpublished manuscript, A.T. Still University, Mesa, AZ.

Hodge, D. R. (2001). Spiritual assessment: A review of major qualitative methods and a new framework for assessing spirituality. *Social Work, 46,* 203-214.

Hodge, D. R., Cardenas, P., & Montoya, H. (2001). Substance use: Spirituality and religious participation as protective factors among rural youths. *Social Work Research, 25,* 153-161.

Howard, B. S., & Howard, J. R. (1997). Occupation as spiritual activity. *American Journal of Occupational Therapy, 51,* 181-185.

Humpherys, K., Pomeranz, M., Roschkowsky, K., Swope, J., & Tartaglia, M. (2011). *Concurrent validity of the OT-QUEST: A comparison between four measures of spirituality.* Unpublished manuscript, A.T. Still University, Mesa, AZ.

Hungelmann, J., Kenkel-Rossi, E., Klassen, L., & Stollenwerk, R. M. (1985). Spiritual well-being in older adults: Harmonious interconnectedness. *Journal of Religion and Health, 24,* 147-153.

Jones, J., Topping, A., Wattis, J., & Smith, J. (2016). A concept analysis of spirituality in occupational therapy practice. *Journal for the Study of Spirituality, 6*(1), 38-57.

Kessler, R. (1999). Nourishing students in secular schools. *Educational Leadership, 56*(4), 49-52.

Kirby, S. E., Coleman, P. G., & Daley, D. (2004). Spirituality and well-being in frail and nonfrail older adults. The *Journals of Gerontology Series B: Psychological Sciences and Social Sciences, 59,* 123-129.

Kirsh, B. (1996). A narrative approach to addressing spirituality: Exploring personal meaning and purpose. *Canadian Journal of Occupational Therapy, 63,* 55-61.

Koenig, H. G., McCullough, M. E., & Larson, D. B. (2001). *Handbook of religion and health.* London, United Kingdom: Oxford University Press.

Levack, H. (2003). Adventure therapy in occupational therapy: Can we call it spiritual occupation? *New Zealand Journal of Occupational Therapy, 50*(1), 22-28.

Low, J. F. (1997). Religious orientation and pain management. *American Journal of Occupational Therapy, 51,* 215-219.

Lowry, L. W., & Conco, D. (2002). Exploring the meaning of spirituality with aging adults in Appalachia. *Journal of Holistic Nursing, 20,* 388-402.

Luboshitzky, D., & Bennett-Gaber, L. (2001). Holidays and celebrations as a spiritual occupation. *Australian Occupational Therapy Journal, 48,* 66-74.

MacKinlay, E., & Burns, R. (2017). Spirituality promotes better health outcomes and lowers anxiety about aging: The importance of spiritual dimensions for baby boomers as they enter older adulthood. *Journal of Religion, Spirituality & Aging,* 1-18.

May, G. G. (2009). *The dark night of the soul.* New York, NY: Harper Collins.

Meraviglia, M. G. (1999). Critical analysis of spirituality and its empirical indicators. *Journal of Holistic Nursing, 17,* 18-33.

Meyer, A. (1922). The philosophy of occupational therapy. *Archives of Occupational Therapy, 1*(1), 1-10.

Miller, W. R., & Thoresen, C. E. (2003). Spirituality, religion, and health: An emerging research field. *American Psychologist, 58,* 24-35.

Moreira-Almeida, A., & Koenig, H. G. (2006). Retaining the meaning of the words religiousness and spirituality: A commentary on the WHOQOL SRPB group's "A cross-cultural study of spirituality, religion, and personal beliefs as components of quality of life." *Social Science & Medicine, 63,* 843-845.

Morris, D. N., Stecher, J., Briggs-Peppler, K. M., Chittenden, C. M., Rubira, J., & Wismer, L. K. (2014). Spirituality in occupational therapy: Do we practice what we teach? *Journal of Religion and Health, 53,* 27-36.

Mthembu, T. G., Wegner, L., & Roman, N. V. (2017). Exploring occupational therapy students' perceptions of spirituality in occupational therapy groups: A qualitative study. *Occupational Therapy in Mental Health,* 1-27.

Nager, B. (2005). *The ego identity crisis: Handbook for enlightenment.* Orlando, FL: RTN Publishing.

Neuhaus, B. E. (1997). Brief or new: Including hope in occupational therapy practice: A pilot study. *American Journal of Occupational Therapy, 51,* 228-234.

Nosek, M. A. (1995). The defining light of Vedanta: Personal reflections on spirituality and disability. *Rehabilitation Education, 9,* 171-182.

Paloutzian, R. F., & Ellison, C. W. (1982). Loneliness, spiritual well-being and the quality of life. In L. A. Peplau & D. Perlman (Eds.), *Loneliness: A sourcebook of current theory, research, and therapy* (pp. 224-237). New York, NY: Wiley-Interscience.

Peloquin, S. M. (1997). Nationally speaking: The spiritual depth of occupation: Making worlds and making lives. *American Journal of Occupational Therapy, 51*, 167-168.

Piedmont, R. L. (2001). Spiritual transcendence and the scientific study of spirituality. *Journal of Rehabilitation, 67*(1), 4-14.

Pike, M. (2000). Spirituality, morality, and poetry. *International Journal of Children's Spirituality, 5*, 177-191.

Prochnau, C., Liu, L., & Boman, J. (2003). Personal-professional connections in palliative care occupational therapy. *American Journal of Occupational Therapy, 57*, 196-204.

Puchalski, C. M. (1998). Spirituality and medicine. *World & I, 13*, 180-185.

Puchalski, C., Ferrell, B., Virani, R., Otis-Green, S., Baird, P., Bull, J., ... & Pugliese, K. (2009). Improving the quality of spiritual care as a dimension of palliative care: The report of the Consensus Conference. *Journal of Palliative Medicine, 12*(10), 885-904.

Purna, S. (2012). *The truth will set you free.* New Delhi, India: New Age Books.

Purna, S. (2014). *Life: A mysterious journey.* New Delhi, India: New Age Books.

Roccaforte, W. H., Burke, W. J., Bayer, B. L., & Wengel, S. P. (1994). Reliability and validity of the Short Portable Mental Status Questionnaire administered by telephone. *Journal of Geriatric Psychiatry & Neurology, 7*(1), 33-38.

Rose, A. (1999). Spirituality and palliative care: The attitudes of occupational therapists. *British Journal of Occupational Therapy, 62*, 307-312.

Ross, L. (1995). The spiritual dimension: Its importance to patients' health, well-being and quality of life and its implications for nursing practice. *International Journal of Nursing Studies, 32*, 457-468.

Schein, R. L., & Koenig, H. G. (1997). The Center for Epidemiological Studies Depression (CES-D) Scale: Assessment of depression in the medically ill elderly. *International Journal of Geriatric Psychiatry, 12*, 436-446.

Schkade, J. K., & Schultz, S. (1992). Occupational adaptation: Toward a holistic approach for contemporary practice, part 1. *American Journal of Occupational Therapy, 46*, 829-838.

Schultz, S., & Schkade, J. K. (1992). Occupational adaptation: Toward a holistic approach for contemporary practice, part 2. *American Journal of Occupational Therapy, 46*, 917-926.

Schulz, E. K. (2002). *The meaning of spirituality in the lives and adaptation processes of individuals with disabilities.* Unpublished doctoral dissertation, Texas Woman's University, Denton, TX.

Schulz, E. K. (2005). The meaning of spirituality for individuals with disabilities. *Disability and Rehabilitation, 27*, 1283-1295.

Schulz, E., Thomas, F., Rollins, M., & Booher, E. (2017). *The role of spirituality in family resiliency.* Unpublished raw data, A.T. Still University, Mesa, AZ and Texas Christian University, Fort Worth, TX.

Smith, H. (1978). *The world's religions: Our great wisdom traditions.* New York, NY: HarperCollins.

Spencer, J., Davidson, H., & White, V. (1997). Helping clients develop hopes for the future. *American Journal of Occupational Therapy, 51*, 191-198.

Taylor, E., Mitchell, J. E., Kenan, S., & Tacker, R. (2000). Attitudes of occupational therapists toward spirituality in practice. *American Journal of Occupational Therapy, 54*, 421-426.

Toomey, M. (1999). Reflections on...the art of observation: Reflecting on a spiritual moment. *Canadian Journal of Occupational Therapy, 66*, 197-199.

Touhy, T. A. (2001). Nurturing hope and spirituality in the nursing home. *Holistic Nursing Practice, 15*, 45-56.

Udell, L., & Chandler, C. (2000). The role of the occupational therapist in addressing the spiritual needs of clients. *British Journal of Occupational Therapy, 63*, 489-494.

Unruh, A. M. (1997). Spirituality and occupation: Garden musings and the Himalayan blue poppy. *Canadian Journal of Occupational Therapy, 64*, 156-159.

Wolf, F. A. (2004). *Yoga of time travel: How the mind can defeat time.* New York, NY: Quest Books.

Ziegler, J. (1998). Spirituality returns to the fold in medical practice. *Journal of the National Cancer Institute, 90*, 1255-1257.

Zimmer, Z., Jagger, C., Chiu, C. T., Ofstedal, M. B., Rojo, F., & Saito, Y. (2016). Spirituality, religiosity, aging and health in global perspective: A review. *SSM-Population Health, 2*, 373-381.

Zinnbauer, B. J., Pargament, K. I., Cole, B., Rye, M. S., Butter, E. M., Belavich, T. G., ... Kadar, J. L. (1997). Religion and spirituality: Unfuzzying the fuzzy. *Journal for the Scientific Study of Religion, 36*, 549-564.

Part VIII
Additional Assessments

29

Measuring Life Balance

Kathleen Matuska, PhD, OTR/L, FAOTA

Balance is not something you find, it's something you create.
(Kingsford, 2015)

Occupational therapy was founded on the idea that practicing a kind of balanced rhythm between work, play, rest, and sleep leads to wholesome living (Meyer, 1977). Life balance should be a consideration in any occupational therapy intervention, and the desired outcome is life satisfaction and improved quality of life. Until recently, there were no assessment tools available to measure life balance. This chapter will describe the Life Balance Inventory (LBI), which can be used to identify unhealthy patterns of occupation and help people create new, more satisfactory and healthy patterns.

Occupational therapy is an important profession for addressing lifestyles in preventative and restorative ways because of the expertise and understanding of occupational patterns. Lifestyles are unique patterns of everyday occupations, including roles, habits, routines, and rituals, and can lead to an overall life balance or imbalance with long-term consequences on health, well-being, and quality of life. *Life balance* refers to a perception that one's patterns of everyday occupations are satisfactory and include a range of meaningful occupations. Life balance is defined as "a satisfying pattern of daily activity that was healthful, meaningful, and sustainable to an individual within the context of his or her current life circumstances" (Matuska & Christiansen, 2008, p. 11).

Hemphill, B. J., & Urish, C. K. (Eds.). *Assessments in Occupational Therapy Mental Health: An Integrative Approach, Fourth Edition* (pp. 517-525). © 2020 Taylor & Francis Group.

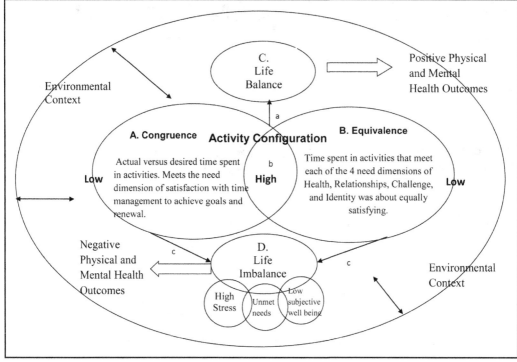

Figure 29-1. The Life Balance Model.

Theoretical Basis

The LBI is a tool that measures the constructs from the Life Balance Model (LBM; Matuska, 2012a, 2012b). The LBM depicts the relationships between occupational patterns (i.e., habits, routines, rituals), life outcomes, and the environment. Occupational patterns should enable people to meet four important needs:

1. Support biological health and physical safety (i.e., exercise, rest, medication management)
2. Contribute to positive relationships (i.e., friends and family)
3. Feeling engaged and challenged (i.e., hobbies, stimulating work)
4. Create a positive personal identity (i.e., caregiving, volunteering; Matuska & Christiansen, 2008)

To the extent that people are able to engage in patterns of occupations that addressed all of these needs, they will perceive their lives as more satisfying, less stressful, and more meaningful, or *balanced*. People also need to have the skill to organize their time and energy in ways that enable them to meet their important personal goals and renewal (Matuska, 2012a).

In other words, life balance requires having the skill to create a match between how much time one desires to engage in activities and how much time one actually engages in the activities that meet important needs.

Figure 29-1 displays the theoretical LBM. The two large ovals in the center (ovals A and B) represent the activity configurations people engage in. It was expected that activity configurations would vary across people because individuals have different personalities, values, and interests. It was also expected that activity configurations would vary for individuals across situations and time because people have different roles and role requirements in different situations. The LBM proposed that life balance was best understood by knowing how people live their lives and that life balance could be conceptualized through actual configurations of activities that people engage in on a regular basis. In other words, what people actually do (activity configurations) was a representation of their lives, and certain configurations were considered balanced or imbalanced depending on whether their needs were met (Matuska, 2009).

To address the balance part of the LBM, two components were considered: activity configuration congruence and activity configuration equivalence. Oval A in Figure 29-1 represents congruence of activity configurations, which means that one's actual activity configuration in everyday life matches one's desired activity configuration in everyday life. If people report the amount of time spent in most activities was about right—not too much or too little—then they would have high congruence. This represents the skill dimension in the LBM about organizing time and energy to meet goals and renewal and was reflected by a person's reported congruence in activity configurations. In balanced lives, need-based activities were engaged in through time in a manner that, at the end of the day, week, month, or year, people felt satisfied that their needs and important goals were achieved.

It was conceivable that an individual might regularly spend a large amount of time in one activity with very little time in other activities. For example, zero hours desired and zero hours actually spent on a given activity shows congruence, and 15 hours desired and 15 hours actually spent on a given activity also shows congruence. Thus, for example, a person who works 15 hours a day (as desired) and spends no time in relationships (as desired) would be considered balanced. The LBM addresses the potential limitations by proposing another component to life balance: activity configuration equivalence.

Oval B represents equivalence of activity configurations. The LBM proposes that the second component of a balanced life includes activity configurations that allow people to meet the four need dimensions identified in the LBM. High equivalence means that there was an approximate equal apportion of satisfaction with time use across various activities that met the need-based dimensions in the LBM. Low equivalence means that people did not perceive equal levels of satisfaction with time use across various activities that met the need dimensions of the LBM (e.g., being satisfied in all relationship- and health-related activities but feeling dissatisfied with the level of challenge in activities or in activities that contribute to a satisfactory identity). An important distinction of the LBM was that it does not prescribe certain activities as important for life balance. Rather, it suggests that the activities engaged in meet the needs of physiological health, satisfactory relationships, positive identity, and challenge (Matuska, 2012a).

The LBM depicted an overlap (area B) between equivalence and congruence because both were proposed as necessary for a balanced life (Matuska 2012a). Figure 29-1 suggests that both high congruence and high equivalence lead to a balanced life (line a), and low congruence or low equivalence (or both) lead to an imbalanced life (line c).

Life balance, represented by oval C in Figure 29-1, relates to lower stress, higher need satisfaction, and higher personal well-being (Matuska, 2012a). Life imbalance was represented by oval D. Low congruence and/or low equivalence in activity configurations were expected to relate to life imbalance and to reports of high stress, low need satisfaction, and low personal well-being. Life imbalance was characterized by configurations of daily activities that were perceived to be unsatisfactory to the individual and which:

- Increase the risk for physical and mental health problems
- Limit participation in valued relationships

- Were incongruent with a satisfactory identity
- Were felt to be mundane, uninteresting, or unchallenging
- Were not sufficiently organized or comprehensible to enable self-renewal or goal achievement (Matuska, 2009; Matuska & Christiansen, 2009)

The entire figure was surrounded by a large oval representing the supports and barriers of the environmental context (physical, social, cultural, political, economic, and temporal). The interaction between the person and the environment was dynamic; one's presence and actions influence the environment, and alternatively, the characteristics of the environment influence the emotions and actions of the individual (Shaw, 2003). The LBM suggests that choosing activity patterns that were optimal for one's overall perception of a balanced life was not entirely within one's personal control. The forces of the environment may make it difficult to engage in the kinds of activities desired. Matuska (2012a) found that life balance was lower for people of a racial minority and was negatively affected by employment and having children at home. A highly supportive environment could improve life balance. For example, having enough financial security to create a satisfactory life was also viewed as important for life balance among Swedish men and women (Wagman, Håkansson, Matuska, Björklund, & Falkmer, 2011).

History of Development and Previous Versions/ Important Changes to Note in Current Version

The author used the basic categories of activities of daily living, instrumental activities of daily living, work, rest, play, education, leisure, and social participation as a beginning framework for creating the activity categories. Each activity category includes several possible activities. For example, the activity category of "getting regular exercise" could be expressed through various activities (e.g., swimming, walking, tennis). "Doing things with friends" could vary greatly (e.g., hanging out, going for walks, sharing a meal).

The items were meant to be broad to encompass the various ways people engage in the activity categories. The items were shared with 6 experts in occupational science and 52 colleagues, friends, relatives, or graduate students for feedback. As a result of this combined feedback, the LBI was created with 53 items thought to represent broad categories of activities that people in Western cultures engage in (Matuska, 2012b).

Rating and Scoring

The following three important principles guided the development of the LBI rating and scoring methods: (1) configurations of daily activities will be unique for each person, (2) imbalance could result from spending too little or too much time in an activity, and (3) the activity categories in the scale should reflect the four need-based dimensions in the LBM (i.e., health, relationships, challenge, identity).

First, to allow unique configurations of daily activities, respondents first indicate on a dichotomous scale of yes/no whether they want to do the activity. This individualizes the results to reflect the unique activity configuration of each individual by ignoring activities the person does not do or does not want to do (Matuska, 2012b).

Second, to measure the congruence construct, for each of the items that they do or want to do, they rate their perceived satisfaction with the amount of time they spent doing that activity in the past month compared to the amount of time they wanted to do the activity. The rating scale was created where the center score, "about right for me," represents perceived congruence in that activity, and was scored the highest (3). Ratings of either "too little" or "too much" on any item represent imbalance, and were scored (2) if rated "sometimes" and (1) if rated "always." Scoring of the LBI generates a total average score across all items respondents do or want to do (sum of ratings divided by number of items rated) and reflects the congruence component of the LBM (Matuska, 2012b).

Finally, the LBI contains four subscales, each containing clusters of items intended to reflect one of the four need-based dimensions in the LBM (Matuska, 2012b). For example, items such as relaxing and getting regular exercise were in the health subscale and were intended to reflect activities that met the need-based LBM dimension of maintaining health. Items such as doing things with friends and having an intimate sexual relationship were in the relationships subscale and intended to reflect activities that met the need-based dimension of having satisfactory relationships. Items such as taking care of your appearance and participating in religious events were in the identity subscale and intended to reflect activities that met the need-based dimension of creating a satisfactory identity. Items such as working for pay, making music, and gardening were in the challenge/interest subscale and intended to reflect activities that met the need-based dimension of being challenged.

The four subscales were scored by taking an average satisfaction score across all items respondents do or want to do within the subscale items (sum of ratings divided by number of items rated in the subscale). The relative equivalence of scores in each of the subscales reflects the equivalence construct.

Psychometric Properties

The LBI was tested with Rasch analysis in 2 studies with 118 and 458 participants, respectively, and in both studies, every item had a mean square value between 1.82 and 0.82 and also demonstrated good internal consistency (Cronbach's alpha 0.89 and 0.97; Matuska, 2012b). Recent research on the LBM has provided validity evidence for each of the constructs of the LBM. In a study of 458 demographically mixed participants, overall life balance and balance among the four need-based dimensions was associated with lower stress, higher subjective well-being, and need satisfaction. In addition, the influence of environmental factors was supported when certain demographic characteristics, such as working, having children at home, and being non-White, moderated life balance (Matuska, 2012a; Matuska, Bass, & Schmitt, 2013).

The validity of the need-based dimensions in the LBM (i.e., health, relationships, identity, challenge) was also supported in several phenomenological studies. Women who had multiple sclerosis (Matuska & Erickson, 2008) or stress-related disorders (Håkansson & Matuska, 2010) expressed life balance or imbalance in terms of whether they were able to meet their needs in each dimension through their everyday activities. Similarly, working adults in Sweden who did not have a chronic health condition also expressed their perceptions of life balance in terms of the need-based dimensions in the life balance (Wagman et al., 2011).

Assessment Administration

Life balance is a performance pattern because it reflects satisfaction with time spent in a variety of activities that meet essential needs. One's habits, routines, rituals, and roles will definitely influence that satisfaction. The LBI is a self-report instrument that can be taken by anyone at any time and can be found in Appendix I. The LBI can be accessed online at http://minerva.stkate.edu/LBI.nsf, and the output consists of an overall life balance score and balance scores in each subscale. The range of possible scores is 1.0 to 3.0, with the following interpretations:

- 1.0 to 1.5 = Very unbalanced
- 1.5 to 2.0 = Unbalanced
- 2.0 to 2.5 = Moderately balanced
- 2.5 to 3.0 = Very balanced

It is recommended that you print out the output page for your records.

Intervention Planning Based on Assessment Results: Utilizing the *Occupational Therapy Practice Framework* Language

LBI scores can be used for research questions related to life balance. The LBI can also be used as a starting point for life coaching or occupational therapy intervention. Life balance is important to everyone, not just the clients seen in current occupational therapy practice. The LBI is useful for individuals who simply want to live a more balanced and satisfying life and do not have any medical conditions or illnesses. Examples include individuals who feel their lives are too stressful or busy or who want more meaningful activities in their lives. The LBI may be useful for individuals who are "at risk" for eventual disability and need to prevent physical or mental decline by living a more balanced life. An example is an individual who is obese and unsuccessful following diet and exercise regimes. The LBI will identify other activities that this individual wants to do and could lead to goal setting to increase overall activity patterns. Individuals who have activity limitations or participation restrictions may feel their lives are not balanced and could use the LBI to identify activity categories where they were least and most satisfied. When a client shows a lower balance score in one or more of the subscales, this could be a good starting point for discussion and goal setting. For example, if the scores in the relationship subscale were low, the focus could be on creating positive relationships. Similarly, if scores in the health subscale were low, the focus could be on increasing healthy behaviors. Because life balance was about creating satisfactory patterns of occupation and because it was highly influenced by the environmental context, it was not enough to simply get a score and create a goal. The LBI was a starting point to identify areas of dissatisfaction and imbalance and could be followed with interview (refer to Chapter 3). The occupational therapist needs to examine critically the supports and barriers of the environment and the routines and habits related to the areas of dissatisfaction.

Case Studies

Robin

Robin was an unmarried woman, 27 years old, and was working as an administrative assistant for a law firm. She had been fatigued and depressed most of the time for the past 2 years. It was difficult for her to get moving in the morning, and she was frequently late for work, causing her boss to be dissatisfied. She was about 80 pounds overweight and had many complaints about abdominal discomfort. She felt that she was sleeping too much, but her sleep was often fitful, and she frequently woke up feeling tired. Her doctor prescribed medication for depression, and the dietician counseled her on diet and suggested she stay away from glucose to rule out glucose intolerance. After several visits to the doctor and dietician with moderate results, she was referred to an occupational therapist to help her create healthier patterns of living. As part of the team, the occupational therapist supported the goals for diet and depression and broadened the intervention to include healthy occupational patterns.

Robin's total score on the LBI was 1.7, or unbalanced. Her lowest subscale score was the health subscale, where she scored 1.2, or very unbalanced, followed by the challenge subscale, where she scored 1.7, or unbalanced. She had better scores in the identity and relationship subscales. These scores helped the occupational therapist focus discussion on areas of dissatisfaction. Robin was unhappy with her diet, exercise, and sleep patterns. She also had low scores in the challenge subscale because she was bored with her job and had quit doing several hobbies she used to love, like playing the piano and needlecraft. She wanted more intellectual stimulation and was interested in enrolling in some art classes.

The most important area for Robin was to increase her activity level and lose some weight. As an intervention based upon the LBI results, the occupational therapist had Robin create a time diary to examine how she used her time and prioritized her activities. Robin and the occupational therapist also identified the environmental barriers that made exercising difficult and found that she was too embarrassed to join a fitness club and that the winter weather often limited her ability to walk outside. Robin eventually started walking with a friend either outside or in a nearby shopping mall 4 evenings per week because mornings were not her best time. The occupational therapist assisted the client in establishing goals to add more challenge to her life. As a result, Robin signed up for an art class based upon the goals she collaborated on with the occupational therapist. Robin appreciated the social and physical benefits of her walking with a friend and the uplift to her spirit when she engaged in art. This led to new goals and new strategies to address other areas where she felt unbalanced.

Robert

Robert was 77 years old and recently lost his wife to whom he was married for 49 years. Robert and his wife enjoyed working in their large suburban yard and always had a large vegetable garden and canned/preserved the vegetables. They were friends with two neighbors and enjoyed monthly card games and dinner. They spent time with their three adult children and five grandchildren who lived within a 1-hour drive. Robert loved to do the maintenance on his car and other mechanical work in the garage. After Robert's wife was diagnosed with Alzheimer's disease, the family home was sold, and they moved into a senior apartment that provided various levels of care. For 2 years prior to his wife's death, Robert spent most of his time taking care of her. The caretaking role was very stressful at times, and he gave up doing things that he enjoyed. The new apartment had a woodworking and hobby room and an underground garage. The senior apartment complex offered occasional social gatherings, but none of these opportunities appealed to Robert.

After his wife's death, Robert became more and more isolated. His children were concerned he might be depressed and that he did not have anything to keep him busy during the day. The senior apartment services included an occupational therapist who consulted for 1 day per month. Robert's children asked the occupational therapist for some advice regarding their concerns for their father.

The occupational therapist met with Robert and shared his children's concerns. He admitted to "having nothing to do" because he did not have a yard or garage to work in and stated he missed his old neighborhood friends. Without the caretaking role, Robert felt lost and without value. The occupational therapist administered the LBI to Robert by asking him each item verbally and entering his answers in the online form. Robert's overall score was "very imbalanced," which meant he was not satisfied with the time spent doing activities. He expressed feeling as if he was spending too much time on activities like watching TV and sleeping and not enough time in social activities and his hobbies of repairing things and gardening. The occupational therapist used the results of the LBI and began the process of goal setting. After reviewing each item with Robert, he wanted to make changes in the items he rated the lowest: TV watching (1, always too much), gardening (1, always too little), and socializing with friends (1, always too little). The occupational therapist coached him to identify opportunities and barriers in these areas and together problem solved strategies to achieve his goals. The occupational therapist reinforced the importance of engagement in activities he enjoyed as health promoting and emphasized people's need for activities to build relationships, maintain physical health, provide challenge, and contribute to a positive identity. With coaching, the first thing Robert did was gather information about local community gardens and talked to the gardener for the apartment complex about possible gardening opportunities at the complex. He identified a goal to play a game of cards with his old neighbors, so his first step was to call and invite them over. He felt that TV watching would be reduced if he did these things. He admitted when the goals were accomplished that he might be motivated help his children with car maintenance, which he missed.

Suggested Further Research

The concept of life balance may be completely inappropriate for individuals in environments where personal choices are constrained by poverty or limited resources. For example, Matuska et al. (2013) found that people in lower income and education groups had lower life balance scores than individuals of higher income and education groups. In addition, the life balance concept reflects a Western value of individualism and may not resonate with cultures with collectivist values that prioritize group goals over individual goals. Research is needed about the concept of life balance with other, more diverse and non-Western groups. The LBM asserted that life balance was associated with positive health and well-being outcomes. The LBI was used to test personal well-being and need satisfaction, but other outcomes such as happiness, life satisfaction, and other physical and mental health indicators should be tested.

Summary

Participation patterns (i.e., habits, routines, rituals) create the framework of people's lives and, together, make up lifestyles that are unique to each person. Living a balanced life is one component that contributes to health and well-being. People who are stressed or have other participation restrictions would benefit from the LBI as it identifies the activity categories where the time spent doing these activities does not match what they desire. This leads to goal setting for the improvement in the balance in activities important to individuals. Occupational therapy practitioners could use the LBI described in this chapter to identify unhealthy patterns of occupation and help their clients create new patterns that are more satisfactory and healthy. The desired outcome for any occupational therapy intervention is life satisfaction and improved quality of life. The LBI instrument is available in Appendix I in the text.

References

Håkansson, C., & Matuska, K. M. (2010). How life balance was perceived by Swedish women recovering from a stress-related disorder: A validation of the life balance model. *Journal of Occupational Science, 17,* 112-119.

Kingsford, J. (2015). Balance. Retrieved from http://www.bigdreamsbootcamp.com/

Matuska, K. (2009). *Life balance: Multidisciplinary theories and research.* Bethesda, MD: AOTA Press.

Matuska, K. (2012a). Validity evidence for a model and measure of life balance. *OTJR: Occupation, Participation and Health, 32,* 229-237.

Matuska, K. (2012b). Description and development of the Life Balance Inventory. *OTJR: Occupation, Participation and Health, 32,* 220-228.

Matuska, K., Bass, J., & Schmitt, J. S. (2013). Life balance and perceived stress: Predictors and demographic profile. *OTJR: Occupation, Participation and Health, 33,* 146-158.

Matuska, K. M., & Christiansen, C. H. (2008). A proposed model of lifestyle balance. *Journal of Occupational Science, 15,* 9-19.

Matuska, K., & Christiansen, C. (2009). *Life balance: Multidisciplinary theories and research.* Bethesda, MD: SLACK Incorporated and AOTA Press.

Matuska, K., & Erickson, B. (2008). Lifestyle balance: How it is described and experienced by women with multiple sclerosis. *Journal of Occupational Science, 15,* 20-26.

Meyer, A. (1977). The philosophy of occupational therapy. Reprinted from the Archives of Occupational Therapy, Volume 1, pp. 1-10, 1922. *American Journal of Occupational Therapy, 31,* 639-642.

Shaw, R. (2003). The agent-environment interface: Simon's indirect or Gibson's direct coupling? *Ecological Psychology, 15,* 37-106.

Wagman, P., Håkansson, C., Matuska, K., Björklund, A., & Falkmer, T. (2011). Validating the model of lifestyle balance on a working Swedish population. *Journal of Occupational Science, 4,* 1-9.

30

Goal Attainment Scaling

Ann Chapleau, DHS, OTR/L

The only man who behaves sensibly is my tailor; he takes my measurements anew every time he sees me,
while all the rest go on with their old measurements and expect me to fit them.
(Shaw, 1903)

Traditionally, occupational therapists have utilized an individualized approach to assessment by considering the unique attributes of each client, such as client factors and performance skills and patterns. However, in the current health care arena, there is increasing pressure for the occupational therapist to demonstrate client improvement. Passage of the Affordable Care Act of 2010 has expanded initiatives such as pay-for-performance, which has been implemented by Medicaid, Medicare, and private insurers in clinical settings, such as ambulatory care facilities, hospitals, nursing homes, and home health care agencies (Robert Wood Johnson Foundation, 2014).

The pay-for-performance, or value-based payment, initiatives provide monetary incentives for improvements in health care delivery systems and increased patient outcomes. The Hospital Readmissions Reduction Program reduces payments to hospitals that have a high rate of readmissions within 30 days of discharge. These pay-for-performance initiatives are designed to reward improvements in health care by focusing on measurement, transparency, and accountability (O'Kane, 2007). In the education setting, legislative reform, including the No Child Left Behind Act of 2001 and the Individuals with Disabilities Education Act of 2004, has also mandated greater accountability through the use of outcome measures (U.S. Department of Education, 2014).

To meet these accountability demands, occupational therapists must ensure that each client's evaluation process includes documentation of functional goal outcomes. In a typical mental health setting in which diverse clients of varied ages and backgrounds present with a wide range of disabling conditions, occupational therapists rely on an

Hemphill, B. J., & Urish, C. K. (Eds.). *Assessments in Occupational Therapy Mental Health: An Integrative Approach, Fourth Edition* (pp. 527-536). © 2020 Taylor & Francis Group.

Table 30-1	
The Goal Scaling Template	
Goal Attainment Levels	*Goal*
Much less than expected outcome (-2)	
Somewhat less than expected outcome (-1)	
Projected level of performance (0)	
Somewhat more than expected outcome (+1)	
Much more than expected outcome (+2)	

individualized approach for assessment of each client. Despite the variety of mental health assessment tools reviewed in this text, there is no one-size-fits-all clinical assessment tool to measure meaningful, functional changes in clients' daily living skills.

One option that can address this need to quantify and compare outcomes among diverse groups is Goal Attainment Scaling (GAS), a method for measuring individual goal attainment. GAS provides a structured framework for identifying specific, measurable, and objective goals using a 5-point scale, typically ranging from +2 to -2 (Table 30-1).

Development of Goal Attainment Scaling

GAS was originally developed for practitioners in mental health to measure the efficacy of community mental health programs (Kiresuk & Sherman, 1968). GAS has been used for more than 40 years for the measurement of both individual and program goal achievements. It allows for a comparison of scores among multiple participants with different goals, making it useful for program evaluation (Jones, Walley, Leech, Paterson, Common, & Metcalfe, 2006; Kolip & Schaefer, 2013; Ottenbacher & Cusick, 1990). GAS has been found to be a useful and simple outcome measure when used for clients with complex, multiple needs (Lannin, 2003; Miller, Coll, & Schoen, 2007; Stolee et al., 2012) and when used in conjunction with the Canadian Occupational Performance Measure (Chapleau, Seroczynski, Meyers, Lamb, & Buchino, 2012; Doig, Fleming, Kuipers, & Cornwell, 2010). It has also been used in school-based research, as its scaling method can be used to operationalize Individualized Education Plan objectives (Oren & Ogletree, 2000). It has also been studied as an outcome measure of student learning during occupational therapy field experience (Chapleau & Harrison, 2015; Koski & Richards, 2015). A review of the literature (Schlosser, 2004) reveals support for GAS as a versatile method of evaluating individualized longitudinal change, adaptable to any *International Classification of Functioning, Disability and Health* levels and domains (World Health Organization, 2001).

Psychometric Properties

When examining the psychometric properties of GAS, it is important to differentiate the original Kiresuk and Sherman (1968) 5-point scale from the modified versions that can be found in the literature. Due to the variability in how the GAS scores are obtained, it is difficult to assess the psychometric properties. Content validity is dependent on the

Table 30-2

Comparison of Goal Scaling Methods
Used by Various Researchers

Level	Scaling Method			
	Ottenbacher & Cusick (1990)	King et al. (1999)	Miller et al. (2007)	Kiresuk, Smith, & Cardillo (1994)
-2	Most unfavorable outcome likely	Baseline	Regression from current level	Much less than expected outcome
-1	Less than expected outcome	Less than expected outcome	Current level of performance	Somewhat less than expected outcome
0	Expected level	Expected level	Expected level	Projected level of performance
+1	Greater than expected outcome	Greater than expected outcome	Greater than expected outcome	Somewhat more than expected outcome
+2	Most favorable outcome likely	Much greater than expected outcome	Much greater than expected outcome	Much more than expected outcome

Reprinted with permission from Mailloux, Z., May-Benson, T. A., Summer, C. A., Miller, L. J., Brett-Green, B., Burke, J., … Schoen, S. A. (2007). The issue is—Goal attainment scaling as a measure of meaningful outcomes for children with sensory integration disorders. *American Journal of Occupational Therapy, 61*, 254-259.

expertise of the goal writer in both predicting outcomes and creating an equally distributed scale of performance of a single dimension of change (Palisano, 1993).

GAS is a criterion-referenced (rather than norm-referenced) outcome measure, which makes it highly sensitive to even minimal changes in client performance. The original use of GAS by Kiresuk and Sherman (1968) was based on the premise that the scale levels were equally distributed above and below the expected outcome level (0). There have been a number of scaling variations found in the literature. Table 30-2 provides a comparison of scaling methods, as reported by Mailloux et al. (2007). When using GAS for research purposes, it is best to set the client's initial baseline level at -2, the lowest scale level, even when decompensation is possible, in order to obtain comparable scores (Krasny-Pacini, Hiebel, Pauly, Godon, & Chevignard, 2013). More recently, some researchers have changed the numbers within the 5-point scale to eliminate negative numbers. For example, a 0 to 4 scale to reflect progress may provide a more positive perspective for clients and family/caregivers.

In a study of interrater reliability of GAS in rehabilitation, Steenbeck, Ketelaar, Lindeman, Galama, and Gorter (2010) reported interrater reliability ranging from 0.49 to 0.91, with some variation between primary therapist raters and independent raters. The authors concluded that interrater reliability was good, particularly for scales constructed by the child's own therapist. In a study of psychometric properties of GAS in psychotherapy (Shefler, Canetti, & Wiseman, 2001), mean interrater reliability was $r = .88$, and moderate to high correlations with the Health-Sickness Rating Scale, the Target Complaints Scale, and the Brief Symptom Inventory were found. Conversely, as reported by Krasny-Pacini et al. (2013), GAS scores are poorly correlated with a number of standard scales that are commonly used in health care. However, GAS was found to be highly sensitive to change when used with varied populations and settings. Other scaled assessments that are not as sensitive to change may not detect meaningful functional improvements or decline. Mailloux et al. (2007) found GAS to be an effective method of capturing diverse and highly individualized outcomes for children with sensory integration disorders, and parents valued the focus on individualized and functional goals.

Assessment Administration

GAS is a method of identifying and scaling goals; it is not an assessment tool itself. The occupational therapist should first complete an individualized evaluation, incorporating standardized and/or nonstandardized assessment tools, interviews, and review of the client's history to obtain a comprehensive understanding of the client's needs and preferences. Any of the assessment tools identified in this text can be used to complete this evaluation process. Goal scaling is the technique by which the occupational therapist translates the evaluation data into a full range of measurable goal outcomes. In a typical clinical setting, the occupational therapist will record a number of treatment goals for each client. Each goal is either met or unmet; the client either succeeds or fails in meeting each goal. Using GAS, the occupational therapist guides the client and/or the client's family/caregiver in envisioning a full range of potential outcomes for each goal.

In a client-centered approach to treatment, it is ideal for the client to be involved in the goal scaling selection and scaling process. When working with young children or those with significant cognitive limitations, the therapist may select and scale goals, consulting with family/caregivers when possible. Typically, three to five goals are selected; more than five goals would be difficult for any individual to achieve simultaneously. The GAS template can be modified to fit the number of goal columns needed.

The GAS methodology is as follows (Krasny-Pacini et al., 2013):

1. Define the occupational performance goal.
2. Choose an observable behavior that can be measured.
3. Determine baseline/preintervention level of performance.
4. Complete the 5-point scaling process.
5. Establish a time interval for reevaluation.
6. Complete the reevaluation, determining the level of goal attainment.
7. Calculate the GAS score for all goal scales.

In the first step, the occupational therapist and client and/or client's caregiver meet to discuss the expectations for functional improvement. Client factors, performance skills and patterns, and the client's context and environment should all be considered. The second step ensures that the target behavior is measurable and consistent with the overall occupational performance goal. It is imperative that each scale only measure one element of change. The third step entails an assessment of the level and type of assistance currently needed to perform the activity. The fourth step involves determining the time, quantity, and frequency of the target behavior. Levels of performance are scaled based on the level of assistance required or the quality of the performance.

After all goals have been scaled, the occupational therapist and client may choose to differentially weight each goal by rank ordering in order of importance. For example, if you have scaled four treatment goals for your client, you will assign a weight of 1, 2, 3, or 4 to each of the goals, depending on their level of importance. This weighting step is for statistical purposes. For clinicians who are using GAS raw scores only, weighting is not needed.

Evaluation and intervention are a dynamic process, and goals are adjusted based on the client's response to treatment. The goal scale can be revised at each reevaluation interval after determining any changes in goal behavior. GAS is also a measure of one's ability to predict outcomes; therefore, when using GAS for research purposes, do not make any changes to the scaled goals before the scheduled reevaluation.

Effectively using GAS requires skill both in accurately predicting outcomes and in scaling goals that are measurable and objective, with equidistant difficulty between the scale levels. Predicting outcomes involves the selection of outcome behaviors that match the goal scales. For example, +2 should be very difficult to achieve. If the therapist finds that the clients are attaining all goals at the +2 level, this would indicate that the goals are too easy to attain. Conversely, if the therapist finds that the clients are consistently unable to move beyond the -2 or -1 level, this would indicate a need to reassess what is realistic for the clients within the particular treatment setting. This process of reflecting on the ability to predict outcomes may help enable the therapist to improve his or her goal-setting ability, which is a potential benefit of this tool. Scaling goals requires practice. Ensure adequate opportunities to practice goal scaling prior to clinical use. When you are first learning to scale goals, it can be helpful to engage the assistance of a supervisor, colleague, or, in the case of research, a member of the research team.

There are also online training resources to provide additional instruction and guidance in goal scaling (Chapleau, 2017; Chapleau & Evans, 2019a, 2019b). A mobile and web-based application for GAS is now available to simplify the data entry and scoring process with additional features for increased communication/support between client and therapist beyond in-person treatment sessions. Readers can contact the author for additional information.

Scoring

There are several options for scoring, each with its own advantages and disadvantages. The original T-score calculation (Kiresuk & Sherman, 1968; Kiresuk, Smith, & Cardillo, 1994) is often used for research purposes to create a standardized value. The T-score can be weighted by rank ordering the goals in order of importance. In a review of the GAS literature, Krasny-Pacini et al. (2013) concluded that use of rank tests and nonparametric statistics to analyze the median of the raw scores was the most appropriate method of statistical analysis given the ordinal nature of GAS. However, for therapists using GAS for clinical purposes, it might be more relevant to just use the raw scores of the scale. This method is most easily understood by clients and caregivers.

Therapists can choose to simply document the change in performance levels or, to provide an average of overall level of goal attainment for all scaled goals for all clients on a caseload, the therapist can add up the total scale numbers and divide by the number of goals. For example, if a therapist is working with eight clients who each have three scaled goals, and for each goal scale, clients achieved a 0, 0, and a +1, the calculation would be: $0+0+1=1$; 1×8 (number of clients) $=8$; $8 \div 24$ (the total number of goal scales) $=0.33$. This final number reflects the average level of performance between 0 and +1, or between projected and somewhat more than expected level of goal attainment for the caseload.

Case Studies

Grace

Grace is a 42-year-old client at the mental health drop-in center at the local homeless center. She received a diagnosis of bipolar disorder when she was 25 years old and was diagnosed with diabetes mellitus 1 year ago. She has been participating in case management services for over 15 years, with a history of unstable housing with frequent episodes of shelter housing and a history of medication (both psychotropic and medical) noncompliance, resulting in four hospitalizations over the past year for medical conditions related to diabetes mellitus. She currently has daily contact with her case manager due to an inability to manage her daily living needs without assistance. Case management services include a weekly grocery shopping group outing, one-on-one assistance with money management, and a daily activity group provided at the drop-in center.

Prior to the GAS intervention, Grace was 30 pounds overweight and was unable to maintain her blood glucose levels. The occupational therapy case manager met with Grace to assess her daily living skills and functional cognition and to talk with her about her occupational performance needs and goals. The occupational therapist administered the Allen Cognitive Level Screen (ACLS-5; Allen, Austin, David, Earhart, McCraith, & Riska-Williams, 2007) and the Canadian Occupational Performance Measure (Law, Baptiste, Carswell, McColl, Polatajko, & Pollock, 2014). Grace identified a primary goal of learning how to manage her diabetes mellitus. Other goals were to learn to take the bus independently from her apartment to the downtown location of her medical doctor's office and to learn to cook healthier foods. Her performance on the ACLS-5 indicated a potential to learn and apply new strategies for instrumental activities of daily living. All three goals were scaled, with a reevaluation date of 1 month (Table 30-3). Grace's baseline level of functioning for diabetes management was scaled at the -1 level, or somewhat less than expected outcome. As she was at risk of medical complications and hospitalization related to her diabetes mellitus, the -2 level (or much less than expected outcome) reflects a potential for decompensation. Grace's baseline level of performance in both her community mobility and cooking goals were noted to be at the -2 level, or much less than expected outcome. Her overall baseline performance was -1 + -2 + -2 = -5; -5 ÷ 3 = -1.67, indicating a baseline average between -1 and -2.

At the 1-month reevaluation session, the occupational therapist and client determined current level of functioning to assess functional improvement. For the diabetes management goal, Grace's level of performance changed from a -1 to a 0. Community mobility also improved from a -2 to 0. Although Grace did not meet her projected level of performance (0) for her cooking goal, she did improve from her baseline of -2 to the -1 level, or somewhat less than expected outcome. The occupational therapist talked with Grace about her progress on this goal; although she did not meet the projected goal, Grace was able to visually see her progress from -2 to -1 on the GAS template. Scoring was as follows: 0 + 0 + -1 = -1; -1 ÷ 3 = .33. A score of .33 indicates an overall average performance between projected (0) and somewhat more than expected outcome (+1).

Table 30-3

Goal Attainment Scaling for Three Goals—Grace

*Place * next to scale level that indicates baseline performance*

Goal Attainment Levels	Goal: Diabetes Management	Goal: Community Mobility	Goal: Cooking
Much less than expected outcome (-2)	Requires hospitalization for a medical condition related to diabetes	*Does not ride bus to/from downtown	*Does not identify any new healthy recipes
Somewhat less than expected outcome (-1)	*Is noncompliant with diabetes management and precautions in her diet	Will ride bus to/from downtown with assist of family/friend to accompany her and ensure correct bus selection, by 1 month	Identifies 1 or 2 healthy recipes of her choice
Projected level of performance (0)	With prompting, can list ways in which she can make healthy nutritional choices	Will independently ride the bus to/from downtown, by 1 month	Prepares 1 or 2 healthy recipes
Somewhat more than expected outcome (+1)	With prompting, adheres to diet when making purchases during shopping outing	Will independently ride bus to/from downtown, by 3 weeks	Prepares 3 or 4 healthy recipes
Much more than expected outcome (+2)	Independently adheres to diet needs when shopping	Will independently ride bus to/from downtown by 2 weeks	Prepares 3 or 4 healthy recipes for 2 consecutive weeks

Joseph

Joseph is an 8-year-old student who attends a psychosocial after-school program. He is diagnosed with attention-deficit/hyperactivity disorder and has a history of poor peer interactions due to impulsivity. He has also had academic difficulties due to limited sustained attention in the classroom. The occupational therapist met with both Joseph and his mom, who is a single parent working two part-time jobs while attending community college. Joseph was observed in both structured and unstructured play environments. The occupational therapist completed the Sensory Profile (Dunn, 1999) to identify any underlying sensory processing patterns that might be affecting occupational performance. In addition, she utilized the Social Skills Improvement System (Gresham & Elliott, 2008) to assess social and academic abilities. His mother was interviewed and asked to complete the parent rating scale of the Social Skills Improvement System, and Joseph's elementary school teacher completed the teacher form to provide information about his social and academic competence compared to other children in his grade.

Results of the evaluation indicated that Joseph's sensory seeking behaviors were negatively impacting his occupational performance at school and home. Joseph's above average scores in the problem behaviors subscale, specifically the hyperactivity/inattention and externalizing subscales, also reflected significant occupational performance deficits, which were contributing to below average math and reading skills.

Table 30-4		
Goal Attainment Scaling for Two Goals—Joseph		
Place * next to scale level that indicates baseline performance		
Goal Attainment Levels	*Goal: Sustained Attention*	*Goal: Sensory Regulation*
Much less than expected outcome (-2)	Consistently demonstrates less than 2 minutes of sustained attention to task	*Is unable to identify or utilize any sensory strategies to help self-regulate sensory seeking behaviors
Somewhat less than expected outcome (-1)	*Consistently demonstrates 2 minutes of sustained attention to task	Is able to identify one sensory strategy but does not utilize during group activities
Projected level of performance (0)	Consistently demonstrates 3 to 5 minutes of sustained attention to task	Is able to identify one sensory strategy and is able to implement it during after-school time, with minimal verbal cues
Somewhat more than expected outcome (+1)	Consistently demonstrates 6 to 8 minutes of sustained attention to task	Is able to identify one sensory strategy and is able to independently initiate implementation during after-school time
Much more than expected outcome (+2)	Consistently demonstrates 9 or more minutes of sustained attention to task	Is able to identify 2 or more sensory strategies and is able to independently implement strategies as needed during after-school time

In working with Joseph, his mother, and the after-school staff, two mutually agreed-upon goals were identified: increase sustained attention to task and improve sensory self-regulation. All parties believed that improvement in these areas was necessary in order to address other social and academic issues. Both goals were scaled, with a reevaluation date of 3 months (Table 30-4). With an initial measurement of 2 minutes of sustained attention to task, there was potential for a decrease in length of attention; therefore, Joseph's baseline level of functioning for sustained attention was scaled at the -1 level, or somewhat less than expected outcome. Joseph's baseline level of functioning in sensory self-regulation was noted to be at the -2, or much less than expected outcome, as he had not yet participated in any learning activities related to sensory strategies.

At the 3-month reevaluation session, the occupational therapist and Joseph's mother determined his current level of performance. Joseph was able to consistently engage in tasks for 3 to 4 minutes before becoming distracted (his projected level of performance), in contrast to his baseline of 2 minutes. Joseph also demonstrated improvement in his sensory regulation goal. By the second week of intervention, Joseph had tried out several sensory items and identified a preferred sensory strategy of sitting on a balance cushion during tasks. By the ninth week of intervention, Joseph had developed a routine of independently retrieving the balance cushion from the shelving in the activity room and being able to remain seated for up to 4 minutes at a time. This use of the sensory strategy facilitated his successful goal attainment of increasing sustained attention, which was his other goal. The occupational therapist documented Joseph's progress, noting that sustained attention had improved from -1 (somewhat less than expected outcome) to 0 (projected level of performance), and that the sensory regulation goal had been met at a much more than expected level of attainment, improving from -2 to +1.

Summary

GAS has been shown to be an effective outcome measure for both individual and program goal attainment. Although GAS has challenges related to reliability and validity, due to its highly individualized methodology, GAS is responsive to changes in client functioning. Moreover, GAS can be an empowering process because the client can visualize a full range of potential outcomes rather than a single measurement of success or failure to attain a goal. The use of GAS may be useful in meeting the health care mandates for accountability and evidence-based practice while maintaining a highly individualized evaluation process.

References

Allen, C. K., Austin, S. L., David, S. K., Earhart, C. A., McCraith, D. B., & Riska-Williams, L. (2007). *Manual for the Allen Cognitive Level Screen-5 (ACLS-5) and Large Allen Cognitive Level Screen-5 (LACLS-5)*. Camarillo, CA: ACLS and LACLS Committee.

Chapleau, A. (2017). Goal attainment scaling: An outcome measure for clinicians, educators, and researchers. Online continuing education course. Seattle, WA: Medbridge. Available at medbridgeeducation.com

Chapleau, A., & Evans, D. (2019a) Goal attainment scaling: An academic example. Instructional video. [DVD]. Available at: https://youtu.be/OrdoJUH2ICY

Chapleau, A., & Evans, D. (2019b). Goal attainment scaling: How to scale goals for clinical practice. Instructional video. [DVD]. Available at: https://youtu.be/LOW8bGXCRh4

Chapleau, A., & Harrison, J. (2015). Fieldwork I program evaluation of student learning using goal attainment scaling. *American Journal of Occupational Therapy, 69*(Suppl. 2), 6912185060. http://dxdoi.org/10.5014/ajot.2015.018325

Chapleau, A., Seroczynski, A. D., Meyers, S., Lamb, K., & Buchino, S. (2012). The effectiveness of a consultation model in community mental health. *Occupational Therapy in Mental Health, 28*, 379-395.

Doig, E., Fleming, J., Kuipers, P., & Cornwell, P. L. (2010). Comparison of rehabilitation outcomes in day hospital and home settings for people with acquired brain injury—A systematic review. *Disability and Rehabilitation, 32*, 2061-2077.

Dunn, W. (1999). *Sensory Profile: User's manual*. San Antonio, TX: The Psychological Corporation.

Gresham, F. M., & Elliott, S. N. (2008). *Social Skills Improvement System (SSIS) rating scales*. San Antonio, TX: Pearson Education Inc.

Jones, M. C., Walley, R. M., Leech, A., Paterson, M., Common, S., & Metcalfe, C. (2006). Use of goal attainment scaling to evaluate a needs-led exercise programme for people with severe and profound intellectual disabilities. *Journal of Intellectual Disabilities, 10*, 317-335.

King, G. A., McDougall, J., Tucker, M. A., Gritzan, J., Malloy-Miller, T., Alambets, P., ... Gregory, K. (1999). An evaluation of functional, school-based therapy services for children with special needs. *Physical and Occupational Therapy in Pediatrics, 19*, 5-29.

Kiresuk, T. J., & Sherman, R. E. (1968). Goal attainment scaling: A general method for evaluating comprehensive community mental health programs. *Community Mental Health Journal, 4*, 443-453.

Kiresuk, T. J., Smith, A., & Cardillo, J. E. (1994). *Goal attainment scaling: Applications, theory and measurement*. Mahwah, NJ: Lawrence-Erlbaum.

Kolip, P., & Schaefer, I. (2013). Goal attainment scaling as a tool to enhance quality in community-based health promotion. *International Journal of Public Health, 58*, 633-636.

Koski, J., & Richards, L. G. (2015). Brief report—Reliability and sensitivity to change of Goal Attainment Scaling in occupational therapy nonclassroom educational experiences. *American Journal of Occupational Therapy, 69*(Suppl. 2), 6912350030. http://dx.doi.org/10.5014/ajot.2015.016535

Krasny-Pacini, A., Hiebel, J., Pauly, F., Godon, S., & Chevignard, M. (2013). Goal attainment scaling in rehabilitation: A literature-based update. *Annals of Physical and Rehabilitation Medicine, 56*, 212-230.

Lannin, N. (2003). Goal attainment scaling allows for program evaluation of a home-based occupational therapy program. *Occupational Therapy in Healthcare, 17*, 43-54.

Law, M., Baptiste, S., Carswell, A., McColl, M. A., Polatajko, H., & Pollock, N. (2014). *Canadian Occupational Performance Measure* (5th ed.). Ottawa, Ontario, Canada: CAOT Publications ACE.

Mailloux, Z., May-Benson, T. A., Summer, C. A., Miller, L. J., Brett-Green, B., Burke, J., ... Schoen, S. A. (2007). The issue is—Goal attainment scaling as a measure of meaningful outcomes for children with sensory integration disorders. *American Journal of Occupational Therapy, 61*, 254-259.

Miller, L. J., Coll, J. R., & Schoen, S. A. (2007). A randomized controlled pilot study of the effectiveness of occupational therapy for children with sensory modulation disorder. *American Journal of Occupational Therapy, 61*, 228-238.

O'Kane, M. E. (2007). Performance-based measures: The early results are in. *Journal of Managed Care Pharmacy, 13*(Suppl. B), S3-S6.

Oren, T., & Ogletree, B. T. (2000). Program evaluation in classrooms for students with autism: Student outcomes and program processes. *Focus on Autism and Other Developmental Disabilities, 15*, 170-175.

Ottenbacher, K. J., & Cusick, A. (1990). Goal attainment scaling as a method of clinical service evaluation. *American Journal of Occupational Therapy, 44*, 519-525.

Palisano, R. J. (1993). Validity of goal attainment scaling in infants with motor delays. *Physical Therapy, 73*, 651-658.

Robert Wood Johnson Foundation. (2014). Pay-for-performance. Retrieved from www.rwjf.org/ed/topics/search-topics/P/pay-for-peformance.html

Schlosser, R. W. (2004). Goal attainment scaling as a clinical measurement technique in communication disorders: A critical review. *Journal of Communication Disorders, 37*, 217-239.

Shaw, G. B. (1903). *Man and superman*. London, United Kingdom: Penguin Books.

Shefler, G., Canetti, L., & Wiseman, H. (2001). Psychometric properties of goal-attainment scaling in the assessment of Mann's time-limited psychotherapy. *Journal of Clinical Psychology, 57*, 971-979.

Steenbeck, D., Ketelaar, M., Lindeman, E., Galama, K., & Gorter, J. (2010). Interrater reliability of goal attainment saling in rehabilitation of children with cerebral palsy. *Archives of Physical Medicine and Rehabilitation, 91*, 429-435.

Stolee, P., Awad, M., Byrne, K., DeForge, R., Clements, S., & Glenny, C. (2012). A multi-site study of the feasibility and clinical utility of Goal Attainment Scaling in geriatric day hospitals. *Disability and Rehabilitation, 34*, 1716-1726.

U. S. Department of Education (2020, March 16). No child left behind. https://www2.ed.gov/nclb/landing.jhtml

World Health Organization. (2001). *International Classification of Functioning, Disability and Health*. Geneva, Switzerland: Author.

Stress Management Questionnaire

Franklin Stein, PhD, OTR/L, FAOTA

> *It is not stress that kills us, but our reaction to it.*
> (Selye, n.d.)

A report by the American Psychological Association released in 2015 stated the following:

> The number of Americans saying that stress has a very strong or strong impact on their physical (25 percent in 2014 vs. 37 percent in 2011) or mental health (28 percent in 2014 vs. 35 percent in 2011) appears to be declining. However, 75 percent of Americans report experiencing at least one symptom of stress in the past month. The most commonly reported symptoms of stress in the past month include feeling irritable/angry (37 percent), being nervous/anxious (35 percent), having a lack of interest/motivation (34 percent), feeling fatigued (32 percent), feeling overwhelmed (32 percent) and being depressed/sad (32 percent).

Definition of Stress

In this chapter, stress is defined as a cause of symptoms, as well as the body's reaction to everyday events. Stress reactions are a result of the body's attempt to self-regulate physiological and psychological responses. The Stress Management Questionnaire (SMQ) is consistent with the definition that follows.

Stress is a term used for certain types of experiences, as well as the body's response to such experiences. The term generally refers to challenges, real or implied, to the homeostatic regulatory processes of the organism. Thus, heat and cold, as well as physical

Hemphill, B. J., & Urish, C. K. (Eds.). *Assessments in Occupational Therapy Mental Health: An Integrative Approach, Fourth Edition* (pp. 537-546). © 2020 Taylor & Francis Group.

trauma, are direct assaults on homeostasis, whereas fear, joy, surprise, and other emotions represent internal states that threaten the internal stability of the body. Of particular interest have been the factors that determine whether the body's response to stress leads to adaptation or to maladaptation and disease. Both outcomes involve changes in brain and behavior arising from the ability of the brain to control body functions through neural and hormonal output (McEwen & Mendelson, 1993, p. 101).

The SMQ (Stein & Cutler, 2002) was devised to enable occupational therapists to evaluate the effects of stress on their patients' physical or psychological disabilities and to devise an intervention plan based upon the results. There are currently three versions of the SMQ: the group version, self-scored computer version, and individual card version (Sorting Out Stress [SOS]). This chapter includes the history of stress research as it relates to the SMQ; a discussion of stress and its relationship to precipitating disease symptoms; a review of the theoretical basis of the SMQ; a discussion of the psychometric properties of the three versions of the SMQ; and information on the strategies that can be used to implement an individual stress management program based on the findings from the SMQ.

Research on the Concept of Stress

The SMQ is based on the assumption that stress comes from the everyday experiences in living. What is stress and its relationship to everyday living? Stress can precipitate symptoms, as well as a positive and motivating force. As a cause, stress can be categorized as good stress (eustress), bad stress (distress), overstress (hyperstress), and understress (hypostress; Selye, 1974). Eustress, defined by Selye (1974) as pleasant or curative stress, can be a mobilizing force in an individual's life, such as when performing in a competitive sport or playing a musical instrument at a public concert. In these situations, the individual is motivated to perform at his or her best effort. Conversely, distress, defined by Selye (1974) as unpleasant or disease-producing stress, can be debilitating and precipitate symptoms of an illness, such as headaches, gastrointestinal pain, back pain, and depression. Distress is like a trigger to symptoms and can cause relapse in individuals with existing diseases, such as in arthritis or clinical depression. For example, it is known that stress can trigger a relapse in individuals with a diagnosis of multiple sclerosis (Brown, Tennant, Sharrock, Hodgkinson, Dunn, & Pollard, 2006).

Hyperstress, defined by Selye (1979) as chronic or prolonged stress, is unremitting without resolution and can produce damage to the internal organs of the body, such as the heart, kidneys, and blood vessels. Physically, the body reacts to extreme pressure or prolonged stress in a variety of ways that can precipitate a disease or an illness in an individual (e.g., stroke). Physical damage from stress will occur if external causes are intense and long-lasting. Research has presented overwhelming evidence that severe stress over prolonged periods has a detrimental effect on an individual's life (Prather et al., 2015). For example, among patients with coronary heart disease, acute psychological stress has been shown to induce transient myocardial ischemia, and long-term stress can increase the risk of recurrent heart attacks and mortality (Steptoe & Kivimäki, 2012). Work stress can also increase the risk of coronary heart disease (Li, Zhang, Loerbroks, Angerer, & Siegrist, 2014). Hypostress, or understress, can be conceptualized as lack of motivation or hopelessness in the face of danger or threat (Selye, 1974). In hypostress, the individual has given up and is passive to the demands of life.

In general, stress is a complex concept that is dynamic and affects the everyday events in a person's life. The intensity of the stress reaction and its consequences will depend on the individual's inner ability to cope and the external resources available to reduce stress, such as friends, music, and exercise. When a person is able to use available resources for coping, the response to stress lessens. Some examples of everyday stressful situations are the pressure to do well on an examination, the fear of being rejected by a friend, the reaction to a loss of a job, or an anxious thought about the future. These situations are referred to as stressors that can trigger a reaction in the individual. The body reacts to these stressors by increasing the response rate, such as increasing heart rate, blood pressure, and metabolism. When an individual perceives that he or she is under pressure, the body mobilizes as if it is under attack. If the response is intense or prolonged, it can lead to symptoms such as headaches, heartburn, blurring of vision, anxiety, or numerous other common problems. Stress also refers to the everyday pressures in living that are the result of daily or occasional situations or hassles that make life difficult and/or create discomfort.

Stressors are specific to the individual. There are external stressors that are generated by the environment, including crowds, noise, poor lighting, inadequate ventilation, and environmental pollutants. Internal stressors are generated by the individual and are caused by feelings of insecurity and fearfulness. Social stressors include major life changes, such as divorce, job loss, major illness, financial problems, family death, car breakdown, and accidents. These stressors may compromise the immune system, leading to a psychneuroimmune reaction (Holmes, Plichta, Gamelli, & Radek, 2015). Coping skills are everyday activities or behavioral efforts to master, reduce, or tolerate the demands created by a stressful situation. *Coping* refers to an individual's efforts to manage demands, regardless of the success of those efforts (Folkman, Lazarus, Pinley, & Novacek, 1987). When successful, coping skills manage or reduce stress by bringing about a feeling of relaxation, reduced anxiety, and an increased sense of well-being. Meng and D'Arcy (2015) found that positive coping indicated a higher level of personal well-being, whereas negative coping was associated with a lower level of personal well-being and related to distress.

Chronic Stress

In general, recent evidence shows that stress can trigger a number of symptoms in individuals who have a chronic disease, such as in stroke (Zhang et al., 2015), multiple sclerosis (Artemiadis, Vervainioti, Alexopoulos, Rombos, Anagnostouli, & Darviri, 2012), low back pain (Christensen et al., 2015), and schizophrenia (Corcoran, Mujjca-Parodi, Yale, Leitman, & Malaspina, 2002).

> Chronic stress may lead to psychotic symptoms (hallucinations, delusions), either in the context of post-traumatic stress disorder or depression. In these conditions, when psychosis is present, there are abnormalities in the hypothalamic-pituitary-adrenal (HPA) "stress" axis. As for schizophrenia, stress (life events) seems to be associated with the worsening or relapse of psychotic symptoms. This is like all kinds of medical conditions, where stress often seems to make symptoms worse. (Corcoran et al., 2002)

Theoretical Basis

The underlining theoretical model for the development of the SMQ was derived from the concept of self-regulation. This is based on the work of Walter Cannon (1939) in his classic work, *The Wisdom of the Body*, who as a physiologist identified homeostasis as the body's maintenance of a steady state that is controlled by the autonomic nervous system

(ANS). For example, through neurological and hormonal mechanisms, the ANS tries to maintain steady states in heart rate, blood pressure, respiratory rate, temperature, salt concentration, blood sugar, oxygen, and carbon dioxide levels in the blood, as well as other physiological and emotional reactions. When an individual experiences stress, the ANS responds. The ANS, which is composed of the sympathetic system, activates the organism to fight or flight, and the parasympathetic system that slows down the organism tries to maintain stable functions.

The SMQ is based on the physiological principle that the body reacts by increasing cardiac and respiratory functions when an individual is under stress and that the parasympathetic system slows down the physiological responses when the organism is resting or relaxed, such as in meditation. If the stressful state is prolonged or intense, it can lead to cognitive symptoms, such as impaired thinking, remembering, and concentrating; physiological symptoms, such as headaches, rapid heart rate, and stomach pain; emotional symptoms, such as anxiety, anger, and panic; and behavioral symptoms, such as insomnia, smoking, and problems relating to others. These four areas (i.e., cognitive, emotional, physiological, behavioral) were used as the basis of the initial research on the SMQ, with open questions such as, "What symptoms do you have when you are stressed?" The researcher found that these symptoms were unique to the individual and could be mild, moderate, or severe. One way for the individual to quantify the symptoms was to have the individual rank the symptoms from 1 (the most severe) to 10 (the most mild).

The next part of the SMQ was to identify the stressors in the individual's daily life. These can be considered the hassles of daily life. Holmes and Rahe (1967) developed the Social Readjustment Rating Scale, which listed 43 life events that cause stressful reactions, including major stressors (e.g., the death of a spouse, divorce, imprisonment, health problems) to minor stresses (e.g., holidays, vacation). Each stressor was given a weighted score, wherein death of a spouse was assigned 100 points and moving residence was assigned 20 points. Holmes and Rahe (1967) made the assumption that these stressors were fixed and that individuals who had a high number of points would be experiencing severe stress.

The limitation of the SMQ is that stressors could affect individuals differently, so a high stressor for one person may not have an equal weight to another individual. The SMQ is based on the assumption that stressors are experienced uniquely, and only the individual can weigh the impact of a stressor on one's life. Dohrenwend and Dohrenwend (1974), expanding upon the work of Holmes and Rahe (1967), found that major life events could cause major stress reactions and prolonged physical and psychological symptoms. The debate among researchers in measuring stress regarding critical life events vs. daily hassles as the major precipitators of stressful reactions was analyzed by Kanner, Coyne, Schaefer, and Lazarus (1981). Researchers compared two modes of stress measurement: daily hassles and uplifts vs. major life events. The SMQ follows in the tradition of measuring the daily stressors of life rather than examining major life events, such as divorce, death of a spouse, and changes in work, finances, and living situations. The SMQ measures stressors such as everyday events involving arguments with spouses or coworkers, driving in traffic, or being late for an appointment. These daily stressors were compiled by asking a large group of people what everyday situations or thoughts cause them stress. There have been a number of stress assessments developed for specific populations. Sheras, Abidin, and Konold (1998) developed and researched the Stress Index for Parents of Adolescents, which can provide valuable information regarding stressful areas of parent-adolescent interactions, as observed by an adolescent's parent or guardian.

History of Development

The SMQ is a tool that occupational therapists can use in the assessment, evaluation, and treatment of stress disorders. The SMQ is the result of the author's research on stress over the past 40 years. The author's clinical experiences as an occupational therapist at New York State Psychiatric Institute and the Brooklyn Day Hospital demonstrated how stress could precipitate episodes of mental illness in individuals diagnosed with schizophrenia and deepening the symptoms of depression in people who had been hospitalized. At that time (in the 1960s), stress was not identified as a precipitator or trigger of psychiatric symptoms.

The SMQ was first developed from unstructured questions and later as a self-administered paper-and-pencil questionnaire. The major purposes of the SMQ are to help the individual to gain insight into one's stress, to determine how stress triggers symptoms, and to discuss the activities or occupations that can be used in managing stress. The 3 versions of the SMQ were developed over a 20-year period with the help of undergraduate and graduate occupational therapy students at the University of Wisconsin—Milwaukee and the University of South Dakota. The SMQ can be administered in a group or individually. The original paper-and-pencil questionnaire consists of 158 items and takes about 30 to 45 minutes to complete. The questionnaire uses a forced choice format for each item and a section for ranking the top 10 symptoms, stressors, or coping skills covered in each section.

The purpose of the SMQ is to help the client identify the symptoms and problems precipitated by stress, the stressors in the individual's life that cause a stress response, and coping activities that the individual currently uses to manage or alleviate stress. From these results, the client, with guidance from the occupational therapist, would be able to incorporate the coping skills into his or her daily schedule as a means of alleviating stress or to apply newly learned coping skills, such as prescriptive exercise, tai chi, meditation, or music.

The first set of descriptors in the SMQ describes the symptoms that individuals experience while under stress. From the original research, the specific symptoms and problems resulting from stress were organized into the following four factors:

1. Physiological, such as headaches, tremors, and neck/low back pain

2. Cognitive, such as difficulty concentrating, remembering, and decision making

3. Emotional, such as feeling angry, hopeless, tense, and sad

4. Behavioral, such as difficulty sleeping, eating, and speaking

In total, 72 descriptors were listed: 27 are physiological symptoms, 8 are cognitive, 18 are emotional, and 19 are behavioral.

The second set of descriptor choices on the SMQ identifies situations that cause the stress response. These stressors include arguments, criticism, encountering red tape, and driving in heavy traffic. Stressors are those aspects of the environment that increase demands on the individual and tend to increase stress. The stress-inducing occurrences of daily events parallel major life changes in their potential to produce stress. The SMQ is similar to the Survey of Recent Life Experiences (SRLE; Kohn & Macdonald, 1992), a measure that comprises a list of experiences to measure how much everyday stressors affect physical and mental health, in identifying stressors. The 51-item scale of the SRLE incorporates 4 levels of intensity of the stress experience: not at all, only slightly, moderately, and very much. The SMQ includes a range of daily hassles under the stressors heading that is related to the SRLE. Everyday stressors precipitating stress reactions were grouped under nine factors:

1. Interpersonal, such as arguments with family members

2. Intrapersonal, such as low self-esteem

3. Time demands, such as meeting a deadline at work

4. Mechanical breakdown, such as dealing with a broken household appliance

5. Performance, such as taking a test

6. Financial pressures, such as loss of income

7. Illness, such as having the flu

8. Environmental disturbance, such as excessive noise

9. Complex situations, such as raising a child alone

Thirty-six items are included under the question, "What are the everyday situations or thoughts that cause stress for you?"

The third section of the SMQ lists coping responses, such as exercise, listening to music, and talking to a friend. Interactional theories emphasize the mediating role of coping and adaptive mechanisms in determining overall levels of stress. A related scale, the Health Promotion Lifestyle Profile, incorporates six areas as indicators of positive coping: health responsibility, physical activity, nutrition, spiritual growth, interpersonal relations, and stress management (Walker, Sechrist, & Pender, 1987). Everyday activities that manage or reduce stress, coping skills were organized in the SMQ into nine factors:

1. Creative, such as writing a poem

2. Construction, such as knitting a sweater

3. Exercise, such as walking

4. Appreciation, such as listening to music

5. Self-care, such as taking a bath

6. Social, such as talking to friends

7. Plant and animal care, such as having a pet

8. Performance, such as singing in a choir

9. Sports, such as swimming

Forty-eight items are included under the statement, "List the following activities that help you relieve stress."

A final section of the questionnaire asks for demographic information and poses questions concerning the experience of completing the questionnaire itself, such as:

- Was the questionnaire too long?

- Were the directions clear?

- Did the questionnaire accurately reflect your feelings?

- Did the questionnaire help you to become more aware of the stressors in your everyday life?

- Did you identify from the questionnaire any new methods to manage stress?

- Do you feel you would benefit from an individualized stress management program?

Natz (1995) developed a computer version of the SMQ. This included a printout of the client's stress profile. The latest computer version of the SMQ allows the client to complete the questionnaire in a clinic, work environment, or the privacy of one's own home or office. Stein, Grueschow, Hoffman, Taylor, and Tronback (2003) published the SOS cards, which is the individual version of the SMQ. The SOS cards can be used by a variety of clinical populations to identify activities that promote healthy adjustment, lower anxiety, and increase quality of life. A reliability study of the SOS was published by Stein et al. (2003). The forced-choice format of the SOS cards provides an opportunity for self-monitoring of symptoms, stressors, and coping skills. The format is somewhat similar to the principle of the Q-sort technique developed by Stephenson (1953), who used a deck of cards with printed statements, such as energetic, active, or organized, that the participant read and then placed into piles of personality categories that applied to him- or herself. Its game-like presentation is innovative, and it is an appealing alternative to paper-and-pencil tests.

Psychometric Properties

In the initial development of the SMQ, Stein (1986) conducted 2 descriptive studies collecting data from 113 participants in the first pilot study and 639 participants in the second study. These studies identified the most common symptoms, stressors, and coping skills that were listed by 752 participants. The SMQ was developed from the results of these studies (Stein, 1986). The results from the normative and reliability studies have been published previously by (Stein, 2003). In summarizing the results, it was found that the concurrence of agreement in a test-retest reliability study of 34 normal participants showed that reliability ranges from .85 to .89.

The instrument was later applied in three clinical research studies (Stein & Neville, 1987; Stein & Nikolic, 1989; Stein & Smith, 1989). In these studies, the SMQ was used to establish the extent and nature of improved stress responses and lowered stress levels following relaxation and biofeedback therapy. In general, the SMQ provides a personal stress profile that helps the individual identify stressors and reduce resultant symptoms by incorporating individual coping skills into one's everyday life. It is envisaged that the SMQ has wide potential for self-monitoring symptoms, stressors, and coping skills as part of holistic stress management programs. It can serve as a comprehensive interactive measuring instrument for guided self-understanding and healthy lifestyle planning, such as in health promotion and disease prevention programs in school and work environments.

In the first test of validity of the SMQ, Stein, Bentley, and Natz (1999) involved comparing scores with the Health Promotion Lifestyle Profile (Walker et al., 1987), which incorporates six factor areas as indicators of positive coping. The SMQ was also compared to the SRLE, which comprises a list of experiences to measure how much everyday stressors affect physical and mental health (Kohn & Macdonald, 1992). This is considered to be a decontaminated form of the Hassles Scale by retaining an indirect relationship to the stress-appraisal process, which Lazarus, DeLongis, Folkman, and Gruen (1985) maintained was a critical determinant of the adverse consequences of stress. This 51-item scale of the SRLE incorporates four levels of intensity of the experience: not at all, only slightly, moderately, and very much. The SMQ includes a range of daily hassles under the stressor's heading. From this, it was evident that the SMQ, in its questionnaire form, matched stressors, stress experiences, and coping behavior (as identified in Health Promotion Lifestyle Profile and the SRLE lifestyle measures) with a statistically significant positive correlation.

The second test of validity used independent t test–based comparisons of the SMQ between normal and clinical samples of participants (Stein, 1986). In general, the SMQ is able to distinguish between individuals in clinical groups and those who are healthy. Reliability was later measured by examining the internal consistency of the SMQ subscales and by comparing scores over 2 administrations of the questionnaire to provide test-retest data, separated by approximately 1 month (Stein, 2003).

Can the SMQ be generalized? Feedback from respondents indicated satisfaction with the SMQ in length, clarity, and diversity of items concerning stress and with learning new ways to manage stress. Using the SMQ in conjunction with the change process could potentially deter maladaptive behavior from being established by having the individual identify appropriate coping activities. Coping activities need to fit the daily routine of the individual.

Strategies to Implement a Stress Management Program

The results of the SMQ can be used to develop an intervention program that uses the client's identification of symptoms, stressors, and coping skills. For example, if a client lists headaches as the primary symptom of stress, then the occupational therapist can use this symptom as a baseline measure of progress. The goal would be to help the client to identify and try to eliminate or lessen those situations that are stressors, such as arguments with spouses. The identified coping skills can be used to self-regulate the stress encountered. For example, if the client has found that classical music is calming, then the individual can schedule a time each day to listen to relaxing music. The occupational therapist and client can identify new activities, such as tai chi and aerobic exercise, that can be used to self-regulate stress. The management of stress by an occupational therapist includes relaxation therapy, prescriptive exercise, creative arts, biofeedback, meditation and visualization, and social skills training. The therapist helps the client to incorporate the stress management technique into his or her everyday life.

Learning to cope more effectively with stressors in the environment is the basis for changing the stressful behavior. By changing thought processes and regulating situations that have previously been labeled stressful, one can relearn behaviors. For example, the anxiety of driving can be changed by using relaxation techniques before and after driving. The greater the desire to change, the more willing the individual is to assume responsibility for his or her behavior. The more active the involvement in instigating changes, the greater the probability that the necessary changes will occur. Generally, three types of solutions exist for any problem or stressor. First, it can be tolerated, often leading to continued stress. Second, taking charge of the stressful situation by adapting to it can change the situation. Third, the solution is to avoid the stressor, such as in arguments with spouses. Through stress management, the client is taught to recognize, record, and monitor the stressors, symptoms, and coping skills on a daily basis. The occupational therapist and the client can jointly monitor the effectiveness of the coping skills to reduce symptoms. Because the occupational therapist's focus is on purposeful and meaningful occupation, it is important to educate clients to be aware of their activity levels and the implications of changes in level of activity. It is important to develop strategies that can be used on an everyday basis to be better able to manage the everyday stress. A sense of self-efficacy is thought to be an essential coping resource. Findings indicate that both personal factors (age) and the type of stressor influence the choice of specific coping responses. Flexibility in the choice of a coping skill helps an individual to deal effectively with everyday stress.

The general principles of stress management for a client to self-regulate stress are the following:

- Incorporate the coping skill into your everyday schedule as a personal habit, such as brushing your teeth.
- Try to engage in the coping activity on a daily basis at a convenient time, such as right before breakfast, during an afternoon break, or before dinner.

- Keep a daily log of stress management activities and coping skills and how they affect your symptoms, mood, energy level, and productivity.
- Be realistic in setting up a schedule that is relevant, appropriate, and attainable.
- Do the stress management techniques in increments starting out for 5 or 10 minutes and working up to 30 minutes. For example, in walking, which is an excellent coping skill for many individuals, start out with a 15-minute relaxing walk and increase the walk to 30 minutes.
- Monitor the impact of each coping skill in reducing anxiety, depressive feelings, and self-esteem.
- Try to establish a quiet, unobtrusive environment for carrying out relaxation exercises or meditation.

A stress management program can help clients understand that by addressing everyday hassles with a healthy outlook, hardiness will be developed and resistance to stress-related health problems will be better attained. Incorporation of daily activities that reduce tension, enhance self-esteem, and increase coping are facilitated by using a stress management program as part of a holistic approach in rehabilitation.

Summary

Distress and post-traumatic stress disorders are pervasive problems in our society. Stress is a major cause of personal symptoms and a trigger in chronic diseases. In this chapter, the author demonstrates how occupational therapists can use the SMQ as a clinical tool in helping clients identify the symptoms, stressors, and coping skills in designing an individual program for stress management.

Specifically, a stress management program based on any of the three formats of the SMQ (i.e., group, individual, computerized) can help the client to identify and monitor everyday hassles and identify coping activities to self-regulate the symptoms of distress. The incorporation of daily activities that reduce distress, such as exercise, music, meditation, and meaningful arts and crafts, have been shown to be effective as part of a holistic approach to treatment. Occupational therapists can facilitate stress management through teaching relaxation therapy exercises, setting up a prescriptive exercise program, and using creative arts that the client has shown interest in, as well as the traditional therapeutic programs of social skills training, visualization, and meditation.

References

American Psychological Association. (2015). *Stress in America: Paying with our health*. Retrieved from http://www.apa.org/news/press/releases/stress/2014/stress-report.pdf

Artemiadis, A. K., Vervainioti, A. A., Alexopoulos, E. C., Rombos, A., Anagnostouli, M. C., & Darviri, C. (2012). Stress management and multiple sclerosis: A randomized controlled trial. *Archives of Clinical Neuropsychology, 27*, 406-416.

Brown, R. F., Tennant, C. C., Sharrock, M., Hodgkinson, S., Dunn, S. M., & Pollard, J. D. (2006). Relationship between stress and relapse in multiple sclerosis: Part I. Important features. *Multiple Sclerosis, 12*, 453-464.

Cannon, W. B. (1939). *The wisdom of the body*. New York, NY: W. W. Norton & Company.

Christensen, J., Fisker, A., Mortensen, E. L., Olsen, L. R., Mortensen, O. S., Hartvigsen, J., & Langberg, H. (2015). Comparison of mental distress in patients with low back pain and a population-based control group measured by Symptoms Check List: A case-referent study. *Scandinavian Journal of Public Health, 43*, 638-647.

Corcoran, C., Mujjca-Parodi, L., Yale, S., Leitman, D., & Malaspina, D. (2002). Could stress cause psychosis in individuals vulnerable to schizophrenia? *CNS Spectrums, 7*(1), 33-42.

Dohrenwend, B. S., & Dohrenwend, B. F. (1974). *Stressful life events: The nature and effects.* New York, NY: John Wiley & Sons.

Folkman, S., Lazarus, R. S., Pinely, S., & Novacek, J. (1987). Age differences in stress and coping processes. *Psychology and Aging, 2,* 171-184.

Holmes, C. J., Plichta, J. K., Gamelli, R. L., & Radek, K. A. (2015). Dynamic role of host stress responses in modulating the cutaneous microbiome: Implications for wound healing and infection. *Advances in Wound Care, 4*(1), 24-37.

Holmes, T. H., & Rahe, R. H. (1967). The Social Readjustment Scale. *Journal of Psychosomatic Research, 11,* 213-218.

Kanner, A. D., Coyne, J. C., Schaefer, C., & Lazarus, R. S. (1981). Comparison of two modes of stress measurement: Daily hassles and uplifts versus major life events. *Journal of Behavioral Medicine, 4,* 1-39.

Kohn, P. M., & Macdonald, J. E. (1992). The survey of recent life experiences: A decontaminated Hassles Scale for adults. *Journal of Behavioral Medicine, 15,* 221-236.

Lazarus, R. S., DeLongis, A., Folkman, S., & Gruen, R. (1985). Stress and adaptational outcomes: The problem of confounded measures. *American Psychologist, 40,* 770-779.

Li, J., Zhang, M., Loerbroks, A., Angerer, P., & Siegrist, J. (2014). Work stress and the risk of recurrent coronary heart disease events: A systematic review and meta-analysis. *International Journal of Occupational Medical and Environmental Health, 27,* 1-12.

McEwen, B. S., & Mendelson, S. (1993). Effects of stress on the neurochemistry and morphology of the brain: Counter-regulation versus damage. In L. Goldberger & S. Breznitz (Eds.), *Handbook of stress theoretical and clinical aspects* (pp. 101-126). New York, NY: The Free Press.

Meng, X., & D'Arcy, C. (2015). Coping strategies and distress reduction in psychological well-being? A structural equation modelling analysis using a national population sample. *Epidemiology and Psychiatric Science, 16,* 1-14.

Natz, M. (1995). *Comparing computer based and traditional versions of the Stress Management Questionnaire in a general population.* Unpublished manuscript. University of South Dakota, Vermillion, SD.

Prather, A. A., Epel, E. S., Arenander, J., Broestl, L., Garay, B. I., Wang, D., & Dubal, D. B. (2015). Longevity factor klotho and chronic psychological stress. *Translational Psychiatry, 5,* e585.

Selye, H. (n.d.). Brainy quote. Retrieved from https://www.brainyquote.com/authors/hans_selye

Selye, H. (1974). *Stress without distress.* Philadelphia, PA: Springer.

Selye, H. (1979). Stress, cancer and the mind. In J. Tache, H. Selye, & S. B. Day (Eds.), *Cancer, stress and death* (pp. 11-19). New York, NY: Plenum Medical Book Co.

Sheras, P. L. Abidin, R. R., & Konold, T. R. (1998). *The Stress Index for Parents of Adolescents (SIPA): Professional manual.* Odessa, FL: Psychological Assessment.

Stein, F. (1986). *Reliability and validity of the Stress Management Questionnaire.* Unpublished manuscript. University of Wisconsin—Milwaukee, Milwaukee, WI.

Stein, F. (2003). *Stress Management Questionnaire: An instrument for self-regulating stress.* Clifton Park, NY: Thomson Delmar Learning.

Stein, F., Bentley, D., & Natz, M. (1999). Computerized assessment: The Stress Management Questionnaire. In B. Hemphill-Pearson (Ed.), *Assessment in occupational therapy mental health: An integrative approach* (pp. 301-317). Thorofare, NJ: SLACK Incorporated.

Stein, F., & Cutler, S. (2002). *Psychosocial occupational therapy: A holistic approach* (2nd ed.). Clifton Park, NY: Thomson Delmar Learning.

Stein, F., Grueschow, D., Hoffman, M., Taylor, S., & Tronback R. (2003). The Sorting Out Stress Cards—A version of the SMQ: A reliability study. *Occupational Therapy in Mental Health, 19,* 41-59.

Stein, F., & Neville, S. A. (1987). *Biofeedback, locus of control and reduction of anxiety in alcohol dependent adults.* Unpublished manuscript. University of Wisconsin–Milwaukee, Milwaukee, WI.

Stein, F., & Nikolic, S. (1989). Teaching stress management techniques to a schizophrenic patient. *American Journal of Occupational Therapy, 43,* 162-169.

Stein, F., & Smith, J. (1989). Short-term stress management program with acutely depressed in-patients. *Canadian Journal of Occupational Therapy, 56,* 185-192.

Stephenson, W. (1953). *The study of behavior: Q-technique and its methodology.* Chicago, IL: University of Chicago Press.

Steptoe, A., & Kivimäki, M. (2012). Stress and cardiovascular disease. *National Review of Cardiology, 34,* 360-370.

Walker, S. N., Sechrist, K. R., & Pender, N. J. (1987). The health-promoting lifestyle profile: Development and psychometric characteristics. *Nursing Research, 36,* 76-81.

Zhang, H., Qian, H. Z., Meng, S. Q., Shu, M., Gao, Y. Z., Xu, Y., … Xiong, R. H. (2015). Psychological distress, social support and medication adherence in patients with ischemic stroke in the mainland of China. *Journal Huazhong University Science Technology Medical Sciences, 35,* 405-410.

Appendices

Writing as an Assessment Tool in Mental Health
Resources

The following are just a small sample of available resources.

Adams, K. (1990). *Journal to the self: Twenty-two paths to personal growth*. New York, NY: Warner Books.

Kathleen Adams is cited by other authors as contributing much to the application of the journal process both in personal and professional/therapist venues. This book is written from the perspective of a therapist regarding the transformative powers of a journal. The writing and format are easy to read. Several suggestions and tools are given related to the art of journal writing. Special note: Much of this book refers to and builds upon the works of Progoff.

Adams, K. (1994). *Mightier than the sword: The journal as a path to men's self-discovery*. New York, NY: Warner Books.

Adams discusses how journal writing may be used by men to work through issues caused by role models who may have taught emotional restriction. The author cites the book as "practical, immediately useful ways to use a journal for personal growth, problem solving, stress management, creative expression, and a whole host of other applications."

Adams, K. (1998). *The way of the journal: A journal therapy workbook for healing* (2nd ed.). Baltimore, MD: Sidran Institute Press.

A series of exercises are presented that are designed to help the reader come to self-understanding, deal with personal conflicts, and work toward personal growth. The book may be helpful to use in conjunction with Adams's (1990) *Journal to the Self: Twenty-Two Paths to Personal Growth*.

Hemphill, B. J., & Urish, C. K. (Eds.). *Assessments in Occupational Therapy Mental Health: An Integrative Approach, Fourth Edition* (pp. 549-552). © 2020 Taylor & Francis Group.

Baldwin, C. (1991). *Life's companion: Journal writing as a spiritual quest.* New York, NY: Bantam Books.

Christina Baldwin discusses the inner process and spiritual journey of journal writing as it contributes to the development of the self in life's journey. Baldwin uses a split format for the book, writing the actual text on the right-hand side of the book and offering quotes, journal excerpts, and providing exercises on the left-hand side of the book. The book itself is written as a journey through life and a journey through writing.

Baldwin, C. (1991). *One to one: A new and updated edition of the classic self-understanding through journal writing.* New York, NY: M. Evans and Company.

This book is a revision of a previous book written by Christina Baldwin. It provides a general overview of journal writing, as well as exercises and discussions of how to promote self-awareness and personal growth through the use of the journal.

Bender, S. (2000). *A year in the life: Journaling for self-discovery.* Cincinnati, OH: Walking Stick Press.

This book provides a basic overview of journaling in the first three chapters, followed by a series of chapters that include multiple exercises designed to take the journal writer through a year of structured writing. Each exercise includes additional suggestions for variations on the central theme.

Bolton, G., Howlett, S., Lago, C., & Wright, J. K. (Eds.). (2004). *Writing cures: An introductory handbook of writing in counseling and therapy.* New York, NY: Brunner-Routledge.

A compilation of authors present the therapeutic benefits of writing in a variety of venues, including poetry, journal writing, expressive techniques, and reflective writing. The theoretical background and research findings are presented, along with writing applications within theoretical frameworks. This book is well suited to health care practitioners who wish to utilize writing in the healing process.

Borkin, S. (2014). *The healing power of writing: A therapist's guide to using journaling with clients.* New York, NY: W. W. Norton.

This book is written by a psychotherapist and presents a comprehensive overview of therapeutic journaling and how it may be used with clients who have a variety of mental health diagnoses.

Bouton, E. E. (2000). *Journaling from the heart: A writing workshop in three parts.* San Luis Obispo, CA: Whole Heart Publications.

This book is set up as a three-part workshop designed to take the journal writer through a series of exercises for personal use and reflection. The exercises range from light to fairly heavy and deep and are focused quite heavily on introspection.

Capacchione, L. (1989). *The creative journal: The art of finding yourself.* Tarzana, CA: New Castle Publications.

This book presents ideas for personal creativity designed to teach the journal writer about the self through drawing and writing.

Chavis, G. (2011). *Poetry and story therapy: The healing power of creative expression.* Philadelphia, PA: Jessica Kingsley Publishers.

This book presents an overview of the use of narrative, writing, and poetry in the therapeutic relationship.

Heart, R. D., & Strickland A. (1999). *Harvesting your journals: Writing tools to enhance your growth and creativity.* Santa Fe, NM: Blessingway Books.

The authors provide various exercises and ideas for personal learning through the use of the journal. The focus is often on rereading and learning from past journal writing.

Jacobs, B. (2004). *Writing for emotional balance.* Oakland, CA: New Harbinger Publications.

This book provides guided journal exercises, many of which come out of techniques similar to cognitive behavioral therapy to facilitate self-understanding and self-control over emotions. The book provides a background of each concept presented followed by exercises designed to help emotional regulation.

Mallon, T. (1995). *A book of one's own: People and their diaries.* St. Paul, MN: Hungry Mind Press.

Mallon presents an interesting book on the importance of diaries. This book is often cited by others and offers information from published diaries.

Neubauer, J. N. (2001). *The complete idiot's guide to journaling.* Indianapolis, IN: Alpha Books.

Neubauer's book is a general elementary overview of principles for journaling. The book does not go into great detail or depth and therefore is best suited for the beginning diarist who has little to no experience with journal/diary writing. For those most serious with journaling, I would recommend consideration of other books.

Phifer, N. (2012). *Memoirs of the soul: Writing your spiritual autobiography.* Cincinnati, OH: Walking Stick Press.

This book takes a powerful look at writing one's memoirs. The content differs some from reflections on journals and diaries in that the writing of memoirs may involve sharing with others and/or the production of a lasting product and therefore the development of memoirs involve more drafts and editing than may otherwise be used within a personal journal or diary.

Progoff, I. (1992). *At a journal workshop: Writing to access the power of the unconscious and evoke creative ability.* New York, NY: Penguin Putnam Books.

Progoff is often considered one of the key contemporary writers on the journal process. He combines psychological roots with an intensive prescriptive process for journal writing. Progoff spends a fair amount of time discussing how each phase/section of the journal relates to life and the development of the self. This book is a compilation of his previous classic works on journal writing.

Rainer, T. (1978). *The new diary: How to use a journal for self-guidance and expanded creativity.* Los Angeles, CA: Jeremy P. Tarcher Inc.

Although Rainer's book is dated, much of the information presented holds true for present day journaling and diary techniques. Rainer uses the term *diary* interchangeably with *journal* and provides extensive insights into the history, techniques, and practical suggestions for diary writing. At times, she indicates favor of maintaining a diary in chronological order and cites concerns about Progoff's numerous sections; she contends that the use of numerous sections can be difficult to use when rereading and reflecting on the diary contents within the continuity of the individual's life.

Ramsland, K. (2000). *Writing to find your true self: Bliss.* Cincinnati, OH: Walking Stick Press.

This book takes a look at the role of writing and self-reflection in finding one's direction in life. The concept of flow is discussed, as is the pursuit of bliss, which is identified as coming to know what is meant to be for one's life. Ramsland offers several exercises for individual and group reflection.

Woodward, P. (1996). *Journal jumpstarts: Quick topics and tips for journal writing.* Fort Collins, CO: Cottonwood Press.

This book is fairly small and simplistic and compiles a series of questions the journal writer may use as jumpstarts to journal writing.

Zimmerman, S. (2010). *Writing to heal the soul: Transforming grief and loss through writing.* New York, NY: Harmony Publications.

This book presents a series of writing exercises that may be used to cope with grief and loss. The author gives a self-account of her own journey and provides suggestions for helping the self and clients through grief/loss.

Zukav, G. (2003). *The mind of the soul: Responsible choice.* New York, NY: Free Press.

Zukav's book is a *New York Times* best seller. The book has information and exercises focused on personal choices, personal control, and means to facilitate responsible choice. The book may be used alone or in conjunction with Zukav and Francis's (2003) *Self-Empowerment Journal.*

Zukav, G., & Francis, L. (2003). *Self-empowerment journal: A companion guide to the mind of the soul: Responsible choice.* New York, NY: Free Press.

This journal workbook provides a series of exercises designed to go along with Zukav's (2003) book. The exercises are easy to read and provide clear directions for use.

B

Creative Participation Assessment

Hemphill, B. J., & Urish, C. K. (Eds.). *Assessments in Occupational Therapy Mental Health: An Integrative Approach, Fourth Edition* (pp. 553-557). © 2020 Taylor & Francis Group.

Levels of Creative Ability

	Tone	Self-Differentiation	Self-Presentation	Passive Participation	Imitative Participation	Active Participation	Competitive Participation
Action	Undirected and unplanned	Incidentally constructive or destructive (1- to 2-step task)	Explorative (3- to 4-step task)	Fairly product centered (5- to 7-step task); experimental	Product centered (7- to 10-step task)	With originality; transcends norm/expectations	Product centered
Volition	Egocentric; to maintain existence	Egocentric; to differentiate self from others	Seems willing to try to present self, unsure	Robust; directed to attainment of skill	Directed to produce a good product Acceptable behavior	Directed to improvement of product/procedures	Directed to participation with others, to compare and evaluate self in relation to others
Handle Tools and Materials	Not evident	Only simple everyday tools (e.g., spoon); poor handling	Basic tools for activity participation; poor handling	Appropriate → skill	Good	With initiative	Very good
Relate to People	No awareness	Fleeting awareness	Identification selection; makes contact; tries to communicate; superficial interpersonal relationship	Communicate	Communicate/interact	Close interpersonal relationship; intimacy; can assist others	Adapts, makes allowances shows consideration

(continued)

Levels of Creative Ability (continued)

	Tone	Self-Differentiation	Self-Presentation	Passive Participation	Imitative Participation	Active Participation	Competitive Participation
Handle Situations	No awareness of different situations	No awareness or ability shown	Stereotype handling; makes effort, but unsure/timid	Follower; will manage fairly in a variety of situations; participates in a passive way	Manages variety of situations; appropriate behavior	Can evaluate, adapt, adjust, according to need; can deal with problems	↑
Task Concept (T/C)	No T/C; basic concepts	No T/C; basic and elementary concepts	Partial T/C; compound concepts	Total T/C; extended compound concepts (abstract element)	Comprehensive T/C; integrated abstract concepts	Abstract reasoning	↑
Product	None	None	Simple, familiar activities; poor quality product	Product fair quality (aware of expectations)	Product good quality (according to expectations)	Open labor market quality; can adapt, modify, evaluate, upgrade; exceeds expectations	↑
Assistance/ Supervision Needed	Total assistance and supervision assistance and (24-hour) constant supervision; requires nursing care	↑	Constant supervision needed for task completion	Regular supervision	Guidance; supervision— regular: for new activities/tasks; occasionally: for known activities	Guidance needed with formal training; own responsibility; help to supervise others	↑

(continued)

Levels of Creative Ability (continued)

	Tone	Self-Differentiation	Self-Presentation	Passive Participation	Imitative Participation	Active Participation	Competitive Participation
Behavior	Bizarre; disorientation	Bizarre; little reaction; disorientation	At times strange behavior; hesitant/unsure/ unwilling to try out	Follower, but will participate passively; occasionally strange	Socially acceptable behavior; symptoms generally controlled	Acceptable; shows originality; may decide to act contrary to norm	Socially acceptable/ correct; adaptable to a variety of situations. Plan action behavior
Norm Awareness	None noted	None noted	Starts to be aware of norms	Norm awareness (aware of expectations [e.g., related to appearance])	Norm compliance (do as expected/ required/ standard)	Norm transcendence (e.g., do better, more than norm, adapt) Graded from activities to situations to variety of situations ⟶	
Anxiety and Emotional Responses	Limited responses; +ve/-ve	Limited uncontrolled basic emotions; +ve/-ve; comfort/ discomfort shown	Varied responses, usually low self-esteem and anxiety; poor control	Varied and anxiety; poor control	Full range of emotions, mostly controlled; makes effort	Subtle differences; compassion; ↑ self-awareness; anxiety used +ve	New situations → anxiety normal emotional responses (anxiety motivator)

(continued)

Levels of Creative Ability (continued)

	Tone	Self-Differentiation	Self-Presentation	Passive Participation	Imitative Participation	Active Participation	Competitive Participation
Initiative and Effort	None noted	No initiative; fleeting/minimal; effort not sustained	Effort inconsistent/not maintained; ↓ frustration tolerance	Varies; needs guidance to sustain effort	As expected/require; sustained	Consistent and originality	
Totals							

Level of creative ability:

Phase within level:	Therapist directed
	Patient directed
	Transition

Patient: Date:

Instructions:
Mark each appropriate block with an X/color.
Add up. The highest total(s) indicate on which level the patient is functioning.

Important notes:
1. Familiar/repetitive learnt activity will seem to increase a level.
2. At least three activities/situations are needed to make adequate evaluations. Always include unfamiliar/novel tasks.

Abbreviations: +ve = positive; -ve = negative.

Reprinted with permission from van der Reyden, D. (2017). *Creative participation assessment.* Unpublished assessment.

C

Routine Task Inventory– Expanded

Scoring Sheet			
Physical Scale-ADL (score range 1-5)	S	C	T
Grooming			
Dressing			
Bathing			
Walking/Exercising			
Feeding			
Toileting			
Taking Medications (1-6)			
Using Adaptive Equipment (1-6)			
Mean scale (sum/8)			
Community Scale-IADL (score range 2-6)	S	C	T
Housekeeping			
Preparing/Obtaining Food			
Spending Money			
Doing Laundry			
Traveling			
Shopping			
Telephoning			
Child Care			
Mean scale (sum/8)			
			(continued)

Hemphill, B. J., & Urish, C. K. (Eds.). *Assessments in Occupational Therapy Mental Health: An Integrative Approach, Fourth Edition* (pp. 559-560). © 2020 Taylor & Francis Group.

Scoring Sheet (continued)

Communication Scale (score range 1-6)	S	C	T
Listening/Comprehension			
Talking/Expression			
Reading/Comprehension			
Writing/Expression			
Mean scale (sum/4)			
Work Readiness Scale (score range 3-6)	S	C	T
Maintaining Pace/Schedule			
Following Instruction			
Performing Simple/Complex Tasks			
Getting Along With Co-Workers			
Following Safety Precautions/Responding to Emergencies			
Planning Work/Supervising Others			
Mean scale (sum/6)			

Summary of scores: S = self-report of the patient; C = caregiver report of behavior prior to admission; T = therapist observation of behavior while in hospital; NA = not applicable; NT = not tested.

The number recorded is the cognitive level (1-6); it parallels to the Medicare assistance code:
6 = independent; 5 = standby assistance/supervision; 4 = minimum assistance; 3 = moderate assistance; 2 = maximum assistance; 1 = total assistance.

Reprinted with permission from Katz, N. (2006). *Routine Task Inventory–Expanded (RTI-E)*. Retrieved from http://www.allen-cognitive-network.org/pdf_files/RTIManual2006.pdf, based on Allen, 1989.

Role Assessments Used in Mental Health

Task Skills		
Client: _____ Date: _____ Practitioner: _____		
Task Behavior	**Rating**	**Comments**
1. *Willingness to engage in doing tasks.* Is the level of readiness, eagerness, or enthusiasm to engage in tasks compatible with what would be the typical expectation for the tasks? Is the level of prompting or encouragement needed compatible with what would be the typical expectation for the tasks?		
2. *Physical capacity.* Is posture, strength, gross and fine motor coordination, and endurance compatible with what would be the typical expectation for the tasks?		
3. *Ability to maintain concentration on task.* Is the level of attention to tasks and number of breaks satisfactory so that the tasks are completed within time periods compatible with the typical expectation for the tasks?		
4. *Ability to organize task in a logical manner.* Is the level of organization satisfactory so that there is evidence of planning for tasks prior to beginning, including having all the items needed for task completion close at hand, and considering what should be done first, second, and so forth?		
		(continued)

Hemphill, B. J., & Urish, C. K. (Eds.). *Assessments in Occupational Therapy Mental Health: An Integrative Approach, Fourth Edition* (pp. 561-574). © 2020 Taylor & Francis Group.

Task Skills (continued)

Client: _____ Date: _____ Practitioner: _____

Task Behavior	Rating	Comments
5. *Ability to follow directions.* Is the level of following directions compatible with the typical expectation for the tasks regarding comprehension of directions, following directions without assistance, and returning to directions to check whether tasks are being done correctly?		
6. *Rate of performance.* Is the rate of performance compatible with the typical expectation for the tasks regarding working at a steady pace so as not to be excessively slow in performing a task so that little is accomplished in comparison to others, or excessively fast so that quality is sacrificed? Is the rate of performance compatible with the typical expectation for the tasks being completed correctly and on time?		
7. *Attention to detail.* Is the level of attention to detail compatible with the typical expectation for the tasks so that there is the required amount of detail without too little or excessive detail and is considerate of aspects of a task that are more or less important?		
8. *Tolerates frustration.* Is the level of frustration tolerance reflective of an ability to emotionally and socially address frustration with tasks when confronted with a problem, mistake, delay, or setback?		

1 = Significantly below essential performance standards = Significantly fails to achieve standards defined for the group (e.g., does not work on the task, may show deviant or abusive behaviors toward the task).
2 = Below essential performance standards = Fails to meet standards defined for the group (e.g., needs assistance to productively engage in the task).
3 = Meets essential performance standards = Meets, but does not exceed, standards defined for the group (e.g., engages in the task as required or appropriate for the activity).
4 = Above essential performance standards = Exceeds standards defined for the group (e.g., readily and independently engages in task and exceeds level of performance required for task).
5 = Significantly above essential performance standards = Significantly exceeds standards defined for the group (e.g., can teach and supervise others in task completion, assistant to the group leader).

Additional Comments:

Adapted with permission from Mosey, A. C. (1986). *Psychosocial components of occupational therapy.* New York, NY: Raven Press.

Interpersonal Skills

Client: _____   Date: _____   Practitioner: _____

Interpersonal Behavior	Rating	Comments
1. *Ability to initiate, respond to, and sustain verbal interactions.* Does the level of interaction reflect the expectation for spontaneously initiating a conversation with another person, spontaneously responding to others, carrying on a conversation, and participating in the normal give-and-take of conversation?		
2. *Keeps all statements appropriate to context.* Does the level of interaction reflect the expectation for following the thread of discussion, making statements that are appropriate and relevant to the subject matter?		
3. *Communicates accurately and expresses self clearly.* Does the level of interaction reflect the expectation for communicating in a way that is sensible to the listener, communicating accurate statements, and expressing ideas in a straightforward manner?		
4. *Interacts comfortably with staff.* Does the level of interaction reflect the expectation for requesting or receiving attention or assistance, and interacting in a way that is friendly and respectful?		
5. *Interacts comfortably with peers.* Does the level of interaction reflect the expectation for the appropriate amount of interaction, friendliness and respectfulness, consideration of the needs of others, collaboration with peers, and acceptance of help from peers?		
6. *Uses appropriate nonverbal behavior and tone of voice.* Does the level of interaction reflect the expectation for maintaining space between others, tone of voice, and the level in which nonverbal gestures are consistent or appropriate to verbal content or context of the situation?		
7. *Cooperates as a member of a group.* Does the level of interaction reflect the expectation for group interaction including acting independently and collaboratively where cooperation is required, and appropriately accepting being the winner or the loser in a competitive group situation?		

(continued)

Interpersonal Skills (continued)

Client: _____ Date: _____ Practitioner: _____

Interpersonal Behavior	*Rating*	*Comments*
8. *Controls impulsive, offensive, or annoying behavior.* Does the level of interaction reflect the expectation for regulating and managing emotions and behaviors so as not to act out toward self or others in a negative or harmful manner, intentionally irritate, torment, tease, or cause anguish to others, or be verbally degrading or abusive to others?		

1 = Significantly below essential performance standards = Significantly fails to achieve standards defined for the group (e.g., does not interact with others, may show deviant or abusive behaviors toward others).

2 = Below essential performance standards = Fails to meet standards defined for the group (e.g., needs assistance for productive interaction with others).

3 = Meets essential performance standards = Meets, but does not exceed, standards defined for the group (e.g., engages in interaction as required or appropriate for the activity; is not disruptive to the group process).

4 = Above essential performance standards = Exceeds standards defined for the group (e.g., readily engages others in interactions, is helpful to others).

5 = Significantly above essential performance standards = Significantly exceeds standards defined for the group (e.g., assumes appropriate group leadership role, assistant to the group leader).

Additional Comments:

Adapted with permission from Mosey, A. C. (1986). *Psychosocial components of occupational therapy.* New York, NY: Raven Press and Rogers, E. S., Sciarappa, K., & Anthony, W. A. (1991). Development and evaluation of situational assessment instruments and procedures for persons with psychiatric disabilities. *Vocational Evaluation and Work Adjustment Bulletin, 24,* 61-67.

School		
Client: _____ Date: _____ Practitioner: _____		

School Behavior	Rating	Comments
1. *Class attendance.* Does the school behavior reflect the expectation for class attendance, arrival to class, and remaining in class for the duration of class periods?		
2. *Group behavior.* Does the school behavior reflect the expectation for paying attention, and participating in tasks, discussions, and interactions?		
3. *Relationship with teachers.* Does the school behavior reflect the expectation for following the teacher's instructions, approaching the teacher for guidelines or assistance when needed, adapting to the style of the teacher, and acting independently as appropriate?		
4. *Relationship with classmates.* Does the school behavior reflect the expectation for the level and quality of interaction with classmates, including being friendly and respectful, considerate of the needs of others, working collaboratively with peers, and accepting help from peers?		
5. *Academic performance.* Does the school behavior reflect the expectation for grades that are at or above the level one would expect given the individual's apparent abilities, that are consistent across subjects and/or grading periods, that demonstrate the amount of effort required, and demonstrate responsibility for one's own academic performance?		
6. *Participation in academic evaluations.* Does the school behavior reflect the expectation for studying for tests, giving appropriate attention to each item, and managing test anxiety and preoccupation with grades?		

1 = Significantly below essential performance standards = Significantly fails to achieve standards defined for school (e.g., does not work on the task, may show deviant or abusive behaviors toward the task).

2 = Below essential performance standards = Fails to meet standards defined for school (e.g., needs assistance to productively engage in the task).

3 = Meets essential performance standards = Meets, but does not exceed, standards defined for school (e.g., engages in the task as required or appropriate for the assignment).

4 = Above essential performance standards = Exceeds standards defined for school (e.g., readily and independently engages in the task and exceeds level of performance required for the task).

5 = Significantly above essential performance standards = Significantly exceeds standards defined for school (e.g., can teach and supervise others in task completion, assistant to the teacher).

Additional Comments:

Adapted with permission from Mosey, A. C. (1986). *Psychosocial components of occupational therapy.* New York, NY: Raven Press.

Work

Client: _____ Date: _____ Practitioner: _____

Work Behavior	Rating	Comments
1. *Attendance.* Does the work behavior reflect the expectation for work attendance, arrival to work, and remaining at work for the duration of the work session?		
2. *General attitude.* Does the work behavior reflect the expectation for the role of worker as an important social role, viewing the self as a worker, and a positive attitude at work?		
3. *Performance.* Does the work behavior reflect the expectation for productivity, including organizing tasks relative to priority, working at increased speeds when required, returning to work after interruptions, planning work periods so that required amount of work is accomplished, assuming responsibility, completing assigned tasks in an acceptable manner, and completing assigned tasks on time?		
4. *Take direction from work supervisor.* Does the work behavior reflect the expectation for accepting direction, accepting constructive criticism, and working independent of the supervisor as required?		
5. *Relationship to coworkers.* Does the work behavior reflect the expectation for the level and quality of interaction with coworkers, including giving and receiving assistance, carrying on a conversation, and working collaboratively?		
6. *Response to norms of the work setting.* Does the work behavior reflect the expectation for appropriate dress, topics of conversation, and other rules of the setting?		

1 = Significantly below essential performance standards = Significantly fails to achieve standards defined for work (e.g., does not work on the task, may show deviant or abusive behaviors toward the task).

2 = Below essential performance standards = Fails to meet standards defined for work (e.g., needs assistance for to productively engage in the task).

3 = Meets essential performance standards = Meets, but does not exceed, standards defined for work (e.g., engages in the task as required or appropriate for the activity).

4 = Above essential performance standards = Exceeds standards defined for work (e.g., readily and independently engages in task and exceeds level of performance required for the task).

5 = Significantly above essential performance standards = Significantly exceeds standards defined for the group (e.g., can teach and supervise others in task completion, assistant to the group leader).

Additional Comments:

Adapted with permission from Mosey, A. C. (1986). *Psychosocial components of occupational therapy.* New York, NY: Raven Press.

Group Membership

Client: _____   Date: _____   Practitioner: _____

Group Membership Behavior	Rating	Comments
1. *Group attendance.* Does the group behavior reflect the expectation for group attendance, arrival to the group sessions, and remaining in the group for the duration of the sessions?		
2. *Group behavior.* Does the group behavior reflect the expectation for paying attention and participating in tasks, discussions, and interactions?		
3. *Relationship with group leaders.* Does the group behavior reflect the expectation for following the leader's instructions, approaching the leader for guidelines or assistance when needed, adapting to the style of the leader, and acting independently as appropriate?		
4. *Relationship with group members.* Does the group behavior reflect the expectation for the level and quality of interaction with group members, including conversing, giving and receiving assistance, and working collaboratively?		
5. *Performance.* Does the group behavior reflect the expectation for the demand to be productive, to organize tasks relative to priority, to complete tasks at increased speeds when required, to return to tasks after interruptions, to plan tasks so that the required amount of work is accomplished, to assume responsibility, to complete assigned tasks in an acceptable manner, and to be an active participant in discussions?		
6. *Response to norms of the setting.* Does the group behavior reflect the expectation for appropriate dress, topics of conversation, and other rules of the setting?		

1 = Significantly below essential performance standards = Significantly fails to achieve standards defined for the group (e.g., does not work on the task, may show deviant or abusive behaviors toward the task).

2 = Below essential performance standards = Fails to meet standards defined for the group (e.g., needs assistance to productively engage in the task).

3 = Meets essential performance standards = Meets, but does not exceed, standards defined for the group (e.g., engages in the task as required or appropriate for the activity).

4 = Above essential performance standards = Exceeds standards defined for the group (e.g., readily and independently engages in the task and exceeds level of performance required for the task).

5 = Significantly above essential performance standards = Significantly exceeds standards defined for the group (e.g., can teach and supervise others in task completion, assistant to the group leader).

Additional Comments:

Adapted with permission from Mosey, A. C. (1986). *Psychosocial components of occupational therapy.* New York, NY: Raven Press.

Family Member—Parent Role

Client: _____ Date: _____ Practitioner: _____

Family Member Behavior—Parent Role	Rating	Comments
1. *Child's physical needs.* Does behavior reflect the expectation for providing adequate food, clothing, and shelter; securing periodic physical, dental, and eye examinations; maintaining a safe home; and securing adequate childcare assistance (e.g., baby sitter, childcare centers)?		
2. *Child's emotional needs.* Does behavior reflect the expectation for demonstrating affection, being aware of the child's emotional needs, interacting with the child, and expressing positive feelings toward the child?		
3. *Play/recreational activities with child.* Does behavior reflect the expectation for seeing play/recreation as part of a parental role, providing appropriate toys, and showing appropriate concern about the child's recreational activities?		
4. *Communication.* Does behavior reflect the expectation for communicating in a clear manner, and at the child's level of understanding and interests, giving the child the opportunity to discuss matters of concern, and using an appropriate level of one's own expression of thoughts and feelings?		
5. *Discipline.* Does behavior reflect the expectation for setting specific behavioral expectations, showing consistency in disciplining the child relative to expectations, maintaining adequate balance between giving the child freedom and imposing limits, and maintaining self-control when the child does not meet behavioral expectations?		
6. *Education.* Does behavior reflect the expectation for demonstrating concern for the child's education, knowing about the child's academic performance or behavior in school, assisting in or providing guidelines for the child's completion of homework assignments, maintaining contact with the school, and encouraging the child to attend school on a regular basis?		
7. *Responsibilities.* Does behavior reflect the expectation for giving the child appropriate self-care and household responsibilities, giving the child responsibilities at his or her capacity, and adequately rewarding the child for taking appropriate responsibilities?		

(continued)

Family Member—Parent Role (continued)

Family Member Behavior—Parent Role	Rating	Comments
8. *Encourage appropriate independence.* Does behavior reflect the expectation for encouraging the child's independence, and rewarding independent behavior that is appropriate to a parent-child relationship?		

1 = Significantly below essential performance standards = Significantly fails to achieve standards defined for work (e.g., does not work on the task, may show deviant or abusive behaviors toward the task).

2 = Below essential performance standards = Fails to meet standards defined for work (e.g., needs assistance to productively engage in the task).

3 = Meets essential performance standards = Meets, but does not exceed, standards defined for work (e.g., engages in the task as required or appropriate for the activity).

4 = Above essential performance standards = Exceeds standards defined for work (e.g., readily and independently engages in task and exceeds level of performance required for the task).

5 = Significantly above essential performance standards = Significantly exceeds standards defined for the group (e.g., can teach and supervise others in task completion, assistant to the group leader).

Additional Comments:

Adapted with permission from Mosey, A. C. (1986). *Psychosocial components of occupational therapy.* New York, NY: Raven Press.

Family Member—General Family Interaction

Client: _____ Date: _____ Practitioner: _____

Family Member Behavior—General Family Interaction	Rating	Comments
1. *Quantity of roles.* Does behavior reflect the expectation for a satisfying number of roles appropriate to one's age, gender, and family situation?		
2. *Quality of family roles.* Does behavior reflect the expectation for viewing the family member roles as important social roles, seeing the self as a family member or in family roles, and experiencing satisfaction in family member roles?		
3. *Communication with family members.* Does behavior reflect the expectation for communicating ideas and feelings in an appropriate manner and giving and receiving emotional support?		
4. *Relationship to partner.* Does behavior reflect the expectation for an acceptable degree of responsibility for the relationship, appropriate independence, treatment of partner in a positive supportive manner, and mutual satisfaction of sexual needs?		
5. *Relationship to family members.* Does behavior reflect the expectation for an acceptable degree of responsibility for the relationship, appropriate independence, treatment of family members in a positive supportive manner, and engagement in activities of daily living that are appropriate to the relationship?		

1 = Significantly below essential performance standards = Significantly fails to achieve standards defined for work (e.g., does not work on the task, may show deviant or abusive behaviors toward the task).

2 = Below essential performance standards = Fails to meet standards defined for work (e.g., needs assistance to productively engage in the task).

3 = Meets essential performance standards = Meets, but does not exceed, standards defined for work (e.g., engages in the task as required or appropriate for the activity).

4 = Above essential performance standards = Exceeds standards defined for work (e.g., readily and independently engages in task and exceeds level of performance required for the task).

5 = Significantly above essential performance standards = Significantly exceeds standards defined for the group (e.g., can teach and supervise others in task completion, assistant to the group leader).

Additional Comments:

Adapted with permission from Mosey, A. C. (1986). *Psychosocial components of occupational therapy.* New York, NY: Raven Press.

Friendships

Client: _____   Date: _____   Practitioner: _____

Friendship Behavior	Rating	Comments
1. *Initiates friendships.* Does behavior reflect an appropriate quantity and quality of friendships, and knowledge and skill of how to find a friend and start a friendship?		
2. *Maintains friendships.* Does behavior reflect an appropriate amount of time spent with a friend or friends and the overall length of friendships?		

1 = Significantly below essential performance standards = Significantly fails to achieve standards defined for the group (e.g., does not interact with others, may show deviant or abusive behaviors toward others).

2 = Below essential performance standards = Fails to meet standards defined for the group (e.g., needs assistance for productive interaction with others).

3 = Meets essential performance standards = Meets, but does not exceed, standards defined for the group (e.g., engages in interaction as required or appropriate for the activity; is not disruptive to the group process).

4 = Above essential performance standards = Exceeds standards defined for the group (e.g., readily engages others in interactions, is helpful to others).

5 = Significantly above essential performance standards = Significantly exceeds standards defined for the group (e.g., assumes appropriate group leadership role, assistant to the group leader).

Additional Comments:

Adapted with permission from Mosey, A. C. (1986). *Psychosocial components of occupational therapy.* New York, NY: Raven Press.

Community Member

Client: _____ Date: _____ Practitioner: _____

Community Member Behavior	Rating	Comments
1. *Leisure/recreation.* Does behavior reflect the appropriate amount of time spent in leisure/recreational activities, a variety in leisure/recreational activities, and satisfaction with leisure/recreation activities? Are leisure/recreational activities within the bounds considered acceptable by one's cultural group?		
2. *Community activities.* Does behavior reflect the appropriate amount of community activities? Does behavior reflect acceptance by the community, and are the community activities within the bounds considered acceptable by one's cultural group?		

1 = Significantly below essential performance standards = Significantly fails to achieve standards defined for work (e.g., does not work on the task, may show deviant or abusive behaviors toward the task).

2 = Below essential performance standards = Fails to meet standards defined for work (e.g., needs assistance to productively engage in the task).

3 = Meets essential performance standards = Meets, but does not exceed, standards defined for work (e.g., engages in the task as required or appropriate for the activity).

4 = Above essential performance standards = Exceeds standards defined for work (e.g., readily and independently engages in task and exceeds level of performance required for the task).

5 = Significantly above essential performance standards = Significantly exceeds standards defined for the group (e.g., can teach and supervise others in task completion, assistant to the group leader).

Additional Comments:

Adapted with permission from Mosey, A. C. (1986). *Psychosocial components of occupational therapy.* New York, NY: Raven Press.

Health Maintenance

Client: _____   Date: _____   Practitioner: _____

Health Maintenance Behavior	Rating	Comments
1. *Ability to understand what health is and what is required to maintain health.* Does behavior reflect the appropriate amount of knowledge regarding healthy living and the components of healthy living? Does behavior reflect a healthy lifestyle in the areas of diet and exercise? Does behavior reflect the appropriate amount of knowledge regarding illnesses and diseases?		
2. *Ability to understand and implement medication management.* Does behavior reflect the appropriate amount of knowledge regarding medications currently prescribed, as well as the dosing requirements, effects, side effects, and precautions? Does behavior reflect the appropriate amount of knowledge regarding how to locate information about medications?		
3. *Ability to understand and implement a healthy, well-balanced diet.* Does behavior reflect a healthy diet that includes the recommended amounts of fruits, vegetables, proteins, fat, sugar, and calories?		
4. *Ability to understand how to maintain an appropriate exercise program.* Does behavior reflect an exercise or fitness routine that contributes to an appropriate exercise program? Does behavior reflect the recommended amount or type of fitness or exercise activity?		

1 = Significantly below essential performance standards = Significantly fails to achieve standards defined for work (e.g., does not work on the task, may show deviant or abusive behaviors toward the task).

2 = Below essential performance standards = Fails to meet standards defined for work (e.g., needs assistance to productively engage in the task).

3 = Meets essential performance standards = Meets, but does not exceed, standards defined for work (e.g., engages in the task as required or appropriate for the activity).

4 = Above essential performance standards = Exceeds standards defined for work (e.g., readily and independently engages in task and exceeds level of performance required for the task).

5 = Significantly above essential performance standards = Significantly exceeds standards defined for the group (e.g., can teach and supervise others in task completion, assistant to the group leader).

Additional Comments:

Adapted with permission from Mosey, A. C. (1986). *Psychosocial components of occupational therapy*. New York, NY: Raven Press.

Home Maintenance

Client: _____   Date: _____   Practitioner: _____

Home Maintenance Behavior	Rating	Comments
1. *Meal planning, preparation, and cleanup.* Does behavior reflect an ability to plan, prepare, and serve well-balanced, nutritional meals and clean up food and equipment after meals?		
2. *Shopping.* Does behavior reflect an ability to prepare a shopping list, select and purchase items, select method of payment, and complete money transaction?		
3. *Home establishment and management.* Does behavior reflect an ability to develop and maintain personal and household possessions and environment (e.g., home, yard, garden, appliances, vehicles), including maintaining and repairing personal possessions (e.g., clothing, household items) and knowing how to seek help or whom to contact?		
4. *Safety.* Does behavior reflect an ability to know and perform preventive procedures to maintain a safe environment as well as recognizing sudden, unexpected hazardous situations and initiating emergency action to reduce the threat to health and safety?		

1 = Significantly below essential performance standards = Significantly fails to achieve standards defined for work (e.g., does not work on the task, may show deviant or abusive behaviors toward the task).

2 = Below essential performance standards = Fails to meet standards defined for work (e.g., needs assistance for to productively engage in the task).

3 = Meets essential performance standards = Meets, but does not exceed, standards defined for work (e.g., engages in the task as required or appropriate for the activity).

4 = Above essential performance standards = Exceeds standards defined for work (e.g., readily and independently engages in task and exceeds level of performance required for the task).

5 = Significantly above essential performance standards = Significantly exceeds standards defined for the group (e.g., can teach and supervise others in task completion, assistant to the group leader).

Additional Comments:

Adapted from American Occupational Therapy Association. (2014). Occupational therapy practice framework: Domain and process (3rd ed.). *American Journal of Occupational Therapy, 68*(Suppl. 1), S1-S48.

E

The Performance Assessment of Self-Care Skills

Hemphill, B. J., & Urish, C. K. (Eds.). *Assessments in Occupational Therapy Mental Health: An Integrative Approach, Fourth Edition* (pp. 575-578). © 2020 Taylor & Francis Group.

Performance Assessment of Self-Care Skills
Tasks Categorized by Functional Domains

Domain	Tasks
FM	• Bed mobility • Stair use • Toilet mobility and management • Bathtub and shower mobility • Indoor walking
BADLs	• Oral hygiene • Trimming toenails • Dressing
CIADLs	• Shopping (money management) • Bill paying by check (money management) • Checkbook balancing (money management) • Mailing (money management) • Telephone use • Medication management • Obtaining critical information from the media (auditory current events) • Obtaining critical information from the media (visual current events) • Small repairs (home maintenance) • Home safety (environmental awareness) • Playing Bingo (leisure) • Oven use (meal preparation) • Stovetop use (meal preparation) • Use of sharp utensils (meal preparation)
PIADLs	• Clean-up after meal preparation (light housework) • Changing bed linens (heavy housework) • Sweeping (home maintenance) • Bending, lifting, and carrying out the garbage (heavy housework)

Abbreviations: BADLs = basic activities of daily living; CIADLs = IADLs with a cognitive emphasis; FM = functional mobility; IADLs = instrumental activities of daily living; PIADLs = IADLs with a physical emphasis.

Rating Scales for PASS Independence, Safety, and Adequacy

Score	Independence	Safety	Adequacy	
			Process	*Quality*
3	No assists given for task initiation, continuation, or completion	Safe practices were observed	Subtasks performed with precision and economy of effort and action	Optimal (performance matches the quality standards listed in each subtask)
2	No Level 7 to 9 assists given, but occasional Level 1 to 6 assists given	Minor risks were evident but no assistance provided	Subtasks generally performed with precision and economy of effort and action; occasional lack of efficiency, redundant or extraneous action; no missing steps	Acceptable (performance, for the most part, matches or nearly matches the quality standards listed in each subtask)
1	No Level 9 assists given; occasional Level 7 or 8 assists given OR Continuous Level 1 to 6 assists given	Risks to safety were observed and assistance given to prevent potential harm	Subtasks generally performed with lack of precision and/or economy of effort and action; consistent extraneous or redundant actions; steps may be missing	Marginal (performance, for the most part, does not match the quality standards listed in each subtask)
0	Level 9 assists given OR Continuous Level 7 or 8 assists given OR Unable to initiate, continue, or complete subtask or task	Risks to safety of such severity were observed that task was stopped or taken over to prevent harm	Subtasks are consistently performed with lack of precision and/or economy of effort and action so that task progress is unattainable	Unacceptable (performance does not match the quality standards listed in each subtask, perhaps with a few exceptions)

Sample PASS Data Collection and Scoring Form: Medication Management

Task # C14: CIADL: Medication Management

Assistive Technology Devices (ATDs) used during task:

1.
2.
3.

Total # of ATDs used: _____

Subtasks	MOBILITY/ADL/IADL SUBTASKS	No Assistance (0)	Verbal Supportive (Encouragement) (1)	Verbal Non-Directive (2)	Verbal Directive (3)	Gestures (4)	Task or Environment Rearrangement (5)	Demonstration (6)	Physical Guidance (7)	Physical Support (8)	Total Assist (9)	Independence scores for subtasks	Unsafe Observations (SAFETY DATA)	PROCESS: Imprecision, lack of economy, missing steps	QUALITY: Standards not met / improvement needed
1 Med 1 C-P*	Reports next time first medication is to be taken correctly (based on testing time, matches direction on label)														
2 Med 1 C-P	Opens first pill bottle with ease (by second try)														
3 Med 1 C-P	Distributes pills from first pill bottle into correct time slots for the next 2 days (all pills & all slots indicated; days indicated)														
4 Med2 N-C-P*	Reports next time second medication is to be taken correctly (based on testing time, matches direction on label)														
5 Med2 N-C-P	Opens second pill bottle with ease (by second try)														
6 Med2 N-C-P	Distributes pills from second pill bottle into correct time slots for the next 2 days (all pills and all slots indicated; days indicated)														

SUMMARY SCORES

ADEQUACY SCORE →   SAFETY SCORE →   INDEPENDENCE MEAN SCORE →

Definitions of Terms for the Comprehensive Occupational Therapy Evaluation Scale

Definitions of Terms for the COTE Scale

I. General Behaviors

Provide for an overall impression of the patient's general level of performance patterns. These performance patterns include behaviors that influence function.

A. Appearance	
Reflects how the client is doing at self-care. The factors selected to assess appearance are considered to be within the client's control within a clinical or community setting. These include neatness, cleanliness, and appropriate attire. Appearance is rated according to the number of factors involved. The following six factors are involved: 1. Clean skin 2. Clean hair 3. Hair combed 4. Clean clothes 5. Clothes neat 6. Clothing suitable for the occasion	0 No problems in any area 1 Problem in 1 area 2 Problem in 2 areas 3 Problem in 3 or 4 areas 4 Problem in 5 or 6 areas

(continued)

Hemphill, B. J., & Urish, C. K. (Eds.). *Assessments in Occupational Therapy Mental Health: An Integrative Approach, Fourth Edition* (pp. 579-587). © 2020 Taylor & Francis Group.

Definitions of Terms for the COTE Scale (continued)

B. Nonproductive Behavior Includes such behaviors as rocking, playing with hands, or talking to self. When clients engage in nonproductive behaviors, their opportunities for successful performance in areas of occupation become compromised. Nonproductive behavior may be an indicator of a dominating habit resulting in a dysfunctional performance pattern (e.g., rocking, playing with hands, repetitive statements, appears to be talking to self, preoccupied with own thoughts).	0 No nonproductive behavior during session 1 Nonproductive behavior occasionally during session 2 Nonproductive behavior for half of the session 3 Nonproductive behavior for three-fourths of the session 4 Nonproductive behavior the entire session	

| *C. Activity Level*
A. Hypoactive
B. Hyperactive
A level of activity is problematic when it is so high or low that is attracts the attention of others, disrupts performance, or prevents participation. Activity level is rated according to its effects on participation. | **A. Hypoactive**
0 No hypoactivity
1 Occasional hypoactivity
2 Hypoactivity level attracts the attention of other clients/staff, but can participate
3 Hypoactivity level such that client can only participate with great difficulty
4 So hypoactive that client cannot participate | **B. Hyperactive**
0 No hyperactivity
1 Occasional hyperactivity
2 Hyperactivity level attracts the attention of other clients/staff, but can participate
3 Hyperactivity level such that client can only participate with great difficulty
4 So hyperactive that client cannot participate |

| *D. Expression*
Includes the many elements that can provide indications of a client's feelings. Some of these elements are body language, volume and tone of voice, facial expression, posture and bearing, and the degree of animation displayed. Expression is rated according to its appropriateness to the situation. | 0 Expression consistent with situation and setting
1 Communicates with expression, occasionally inappropriate
2 Shows inappropriate expression several times during session
3 Show of expression but inconsistent with situation
4 Extremes of expression (e.g., bizarre, uncontrolled, or no expression) | |

| *E. Responsibility*
A measure of the client's personal accountability. This behavior is reflected by attendance patterns, adherence to known rules, care of equipment and supplies, and adherence to behavioral contracts. Responsibility is measured according to the degree it is assumed. | 0 Takes responsibility for own actions
1 Denies responsibility for 1 or 2 actions
2 Denies responsibility for several actions
3 Denies responsibility for most actions
4 Denial of all responsibility (i.e., messes up project and blames others) | |

(continued)

Definitions of Terms for the COTE Scale (continued)

F. Attendance/Punctuality Attendance is a behavior that reflects an individual's commitment and motivation to participate. The amount of encouragement needed for attendance/participation is the basis for rating this behavior.	0 Consistently ready for therapy 1 Needs encouragement 20% of the time 2 Needs encouragement 50% of the time 3 Refuses up to 50% of the time 4 Refuses more than 50% of the time
G. Reality Orientation Addresses the client's awareness of person, time, place, and situation. The behavior rating is based on the number of factors of which the client is aware.	0 Complete awareness of person, place, time, and situation 1 General awareness but inconsistency in 1 area 2 Awareness of only 2 areas 3 Awareness in 1 area 4 Lack of awareness of person, place, time, and situation
H. Conceptualization A higher-level cognitive function that represents the client's level of learning and response to situations. It is rated on a continuum that reflects responses that range from concrete to abstract.	0 Demonstrates abstract thinking 1 Responds abstractly 1+ times 2 Relevant concrete responses 3 Responds concretely 1+ times 4 Responses unrelated to situation

II. Interpersonal Behaviors

Interpersonal relationships affect performance in all social activities. Effective performance in areas of occupation often depends upon effective social interactions. Occupational therapy provides both structured and nonstructured opportunities for these interactions to occur.

I. Independence Shows how independently the client can function in occupational therapy. While occupational therapy may include structured activity, opportunities exist in each session for a client to be independent. Independence is rated according to the number of independent actions observed.	0 Independent functioning 1 Only 1 or 2 dependent actions 2 50% independent and 50% dependent actions 3 Only 1 or 2 independent actions 4 No independent actions
J. Cooperation Indicates how well the client cooperates with the intervention program. Indicators used for rating this behavior are compliance and opposition to the program and the therapist as demonstrated by the client's ability to follow directions.	0 Cooperates with program 1 Follows most directions, opposes less than 50% 2 Follows 50%, opposes 50% 3 Opposes 75% of the session 4 Opposes all directions/suggestions

(continued)

Definitions of Terms for the COTE Scale (continued)

K. Self-Assertion **A. Passive** **B. Aggressive** Behaviors can vacillate between passivity and dominance with self-assertion lying midway.	**A. Passive** 0 Assertive when appropriate 1 Passive less than 50% of the session 2 Passive 50% of the session 3 Passive more than 50% of the session 4 Passive the entire session	**B. Aggressive** 0 Assertive when appropriate 1 Dominant less than 50% of the session 2 Dominant 50% of the session 3 Dominant more than 50% of the session 4 Dominates aggressively
L. Sociability **A. Withdrawn** **B. Overly Social** Refers to a performance skill related to communication and interaction. This behavior is demonstrated by how well the client socializes with the staff and other clients during the therapy session. This behavior is rated by whether the client can participate, initiate, and respond to social interactions.	**A. Tends to be withdrawn** 0 Socializes appropriately with staff and other clients 1 Socializes with staff and occasionally with other clients or vice versa 2 Socializes only with staff or only with other clients 3 Socializes only if approached 4 Does not join others in activities, unable to carry on casual conversation even if approached	**B. Tends to oversocialize** 0 Socializes appropriately with staff and other clients 1 Socializes with staff/clients and occasionally needs cueing to stop talking with others during group activity 2 Socializes with staff/clients and frequently needs cueing to stop talking with others during group activity 3 Socializes with only staff or only with other clients and frequently needs cueing to stop talking with others during group activity 4 Oversocialization is so extreme it is disruptive to the group

(continued)

Definitions of Terms for the COTE Scale (continued)

M. Attention-Getting Behavior Reflects the amount of time that the client spends seeking attention. Examples include recreated questions, frequent requests for assistance, and overt requests for approval or merely doing nothing in order to get attention.	0 1 2 3 4	No reasonable attention-getting behavior Less than 50% of the time spent in attention-getting behavior 50% of the time spent in attention-getting behavior 75% of the time spent in attention-getting behavior Verbally or nonverbally demands constant attention
N. Negative Response From Others Is an indicator of the client's effect on the therapist and other clients. Examples of this behavior include asking or demanding special privileges or interactions with fellow clients that result in negative responses. This behavior is rated according to the number of negative responses evoked from other persons during the session.	0 1 2 3 4	Evokes no negative responses Evokes 1 negative response Evokes 2 negative responses Evokes 3 or more negative responses during the session Evokes numerous negative responses from others, and therapist must take some action

III. Occupational Behaviors

Occupational therapy provides a unique opportunity to observe a patient's behavior during occupations that reflect the challenges of daily life. The occupational therapist can select numerous types of tasks/activities/occupations that require performance skills that are not readily observable in group or individual talk therapy.

O. Engagement Reflects the commitment made to performance in occupations or activities as a result of self-choice motivation and meaning. This is a significant behavior as no task can be accomplished unless it is begun.	0 1 2 3 4	Needs no encouragement to begin task Encourage once to begin activity Encourage 2 or 3 times to engage in activity Engages in activity only after much encouragement Does not engage in activity
P. Concentration/Attention An important patient factor and can be measured by the client's ability to sustain engagement in activities and occupations. This mental function is measured by the amount of time spent attending to the activity at hand.	0 1 2 3 4	No difficulty concentrating during session Off task less than 25% of the time Off task 50% of the time Off task 75% of the time Inability to maintain concentration on task for more than 1 minute
Q. Coordination A performance skill that relates to using more than one body part to interact with task objects in a manner that supports task performance. This skill is an indicator of a motor skill that demonstrates how well the body and brain function together. Coordination can serve as a measurable indicator of the client's response to medication or other treatments.	0 1 2 3 4	No problems with coordination Occasionally has trouble with fine detail, manipulating tools and materials Occasionally has trouble manipulating tools and materials but has frequent trouble with fine detail Some difficulty in gross movement, unable to manipulate some tools and materials Has great difficulty in movement (gross motor), virtually unable to manipulate tools and materials

(continued)

Definitions of Terms for the COTE Scale (continued)

R. Follow Directions Reflects the ability to respond to an activity demand in order to carry out the desired activity.	0 Carries out directions without problems 1 Carries out simple 1- to 2-step directions, has trouble with 2- to 3-step directions 2 Carries out 1 direction, has trouble with 2 3 Can only carry out very simple 1-step directions (demonstrated, written, or verbal) 4 Unable to carry out any directions	
S. Activity Neatness/Attention to Detail **A. Lack of Attention to Detail** **B. Over-Focused/Detailed** Reflects opposite ends of a continuum related to how well a client can accomplish a task and to the quality of that task.	**A. Lack of attention to detail** 0 Activity neatly done 1 Occasionally ignores fine detail 2 Often ignores fine detail and materials are scattered 3 Ignores fine detail and work habits disturbing to those around 4 Unaware of fine detail; so sloppy that therapist has to intervene	**B. Over-focused/detailed** 0 Pays attention to detail appropriately 1 Occasionally too detailed/precise 2 More attention to several details than is required 3 So detailed/precise that project will take twice as long as expected 4 So concerned (obsessed with details) that project will never get finished
T. Problem Solving A client factor that represents a higher level of cognitive functioning. It requires the client to plan and carry out actions in response to a challenge.	0 Solves problems without assistance 1 Solves problems after assistance is given once 2 Can solve only after repeated instruction 3 Recognizes a problem but cannot solve it 4 Unable to recognize or solve a problem	
U. Complexity and Organization of Task Can be rated using multilevel activities.	0 Organizes and performs tasks given 1 Occasionally has trouble with organization of complex activities that client should be able to do 2 Can organize simple but not complex activities 3 Can do only very simple activities with organization imposed by therapist 4 Unable to organize or carry out an activity when all tools, materials, and directions are available	

(continued)

Definitions of Terms for the COTE Scale (continued)

V. Initial Learning Evaluated when the client is performing an activity that is unfamiliar and requires instruction.	0 Learns a new activity quickly and without difficulty 1 Occasionally has difficulty learning a complex activity 2 Has frequent difficulty learning a complex activity 3 Unable to learn complex activities, occasionally has difficulty learning simple activities 4 Unable to learn a new activity
W. Interest in Activities Illustrates the client's willingness to try new or different activities.	0 Interested in a variety of activities 1 Occasionally not interested in a new activity 2 Shows occasional interest in a part of an activity 3 Engages in activity but shows no interest 4 Does not participate
X. Interest in Accomplishment Indicates whether the client can set goals and work toward them by taking the steps needed to complete the activity. This behavior requires the expenditure of physical and mental energy.	0 Interested in finishing activities 1 Occasional lack of interest or pleasure in finishing a long-term activity 2 Interest or pleasure in accomplishment of a short-term activity, lack of interest in a long-term activity 3 Only occasional interest in finishing an activity 4 No interest or pleasure in finishing an activity
Y. Decision Making This higher-level cognitive function refers to an individual's ability to process knowledge in order to select a course of action. Decision making is dependent on the number and kinds of choices and degree of support available.	0 Makes own decisions 1 Makes own decisions but occasionally seeks therapist's approval 2 Makes own decisions but often seeks therapist's approval 3 Makes decisions when given only 2 alternatives 4 Cannot make or refuses to make any decisions
Z. Frustration Tolerance An indicator of the client's ability to persevere in activities when each phase does not come easily. The ability to tolerate frustration reflects the ability to adapt and make accommodations or adjustments.	0 Handles all tasks without becoming overly frustrated 1 Occasionally becomes frustrated with 1 or more complex tasks; can handle simple tasks 2 Often becomes frustrated with more complex tasks but is able to handle simple tasks 3 Often becomes frustrated with any task but attempts to continue 4 Becomes so frustrated with simple tasks that refuses or is unable to function

COTE Recording Form

Client: _____ Observer: _____ Date: _____

Type of Behavior	Score	Comments
I. General Behaviors		
A. Appearance		
B. Nonproductive Behavior		
C. Activity Level ☐ A. Hypoactive ☐ B. Hyperactive		
D. Expression		
E. Responsibility		
F. Attendance/Punctuality		
G. Reality Orientation		
H. Conceptualization		
General Behaviors Subtotal		
II. Interpersonal Behaviors		
I. Independence		
J. Cooperation		
K. Self-Assertion ☐ A. Passive ☐ B. Aggressive		
L. Sociability ☐ A. Withdrawn ☐ B. Overly Social		
M. Attention-Getting Behavior		
N. Negative Response From Others		
Interpersonal Behaviors Subtotal		
		(continued)

COTE Recording Form (continued)

Type of Behavior	Score	Comments
III. Occupational Behaviors		
O. Engagement		
P. Concentration/Attention		
Q. Coordination		
R. Follow Directions		
S. Activity Neatness/Attention to Detail ☐ A. Lack of Attention to Detail ☐ B. Over-Focused/Detailed		
T. Problem Solving		
U. Complexity and Organization of Task		
V. Initial Learning		
W. Interest in Activities		
X. Interest in Accomplishment		
Y. Decision Making		
Z. Frustration Tolerance		
Occupational Behaviors Subtotal		
Total		

Scale (Observed Impairment): 0 = Typical, 1 = Minimal, 2 = Mild, 3 = Moderate, 4 = Severe.

KidCOTE

Demographic _____

Patient Goal _____

Evaluation Procedures Administered:

__Chart Review	__Task Evaluation	__Clinical Observation
__Piers Harris	__Bruininks-Oseretsky	__Test of Visual Perceptual Skills
__Test of Visual-Motor Skills	__Gessell	__Other: _____

General Behavior	ADM	D/C	Cognitive Behavior	ADM	D/C
Activities of Daily Living			Attention Span/Concentration		
Responsibility			Memory		
Reality Orientation			Sequencing and Categorization		
Attendance/Punctuality			Concept Formation		
			Problem Solving/Judgment		
Psychosocial Behaviors			Follows Directions		
Self-Concept			Organizational Skills		
Social Conduct			Decision Making		
Self-Expression			Initial Learning		
Coping Skills			Interest in Activity		
Time Management			Interest in Accomplishment		
Insight			Frustration Tolerance		

Scale:
0 = WNL: Functions to satisfaction of self and environment; independent
1 = MIN: Requires assist/cueing 1 to 2 times per session; occasional difficulties
2 = MOD: Frequently needs assist 3+ times per session; requires supervision; frequent difficulties
3 = SEVERE: Requires constant supervision or is completely unable to perform

Assets:_____   **Problems:**_____
     _____   _____
     _____   _____

Hemphill, B. J., & Urish, C. K. (Eds.). *Assessments in Occupational Therapy Mental Health: An Integrative Approach, Fourth Edition* (pp. 589-591). © 2020 Taylor & Francis Group.

Sensorimotor Performance:

Sensory Awareness/Processing _____

Neuromuscular

　Fine Motor _____

　Gross Motor _____

Expected Outcomes:

_____

_____

Short-Term Objectives:

_____

_____

Treatment Plan:

_____

_____

_____ Therapist　　_____ Date

Evaluation Results/Standardized Tests
Bruininks-Oseretsky Tests/Complete Battery

Gross Motor Composite	Sum	Standard Score	Percentile Rank	Stanine	Age Equivalent	Standard Deviation
Upper Limb Coordination Fine Motor Composite Battery Composite						

Short Form:　　Point Score ____　　Standard Score ____ Percentile Rank ____　　Stanine ____

Test of Visual Perceptual Skills:　　Sum of Scaled Scores ____　　Percentile Rank ____
　　　　　　　　　　　　　　　　　　Perceptual Quotient ____　　Median Perceptual Age ____

Test of Visual-Motor Skills:　Total Raw Scores ____　　Motor Age ____
　　　　　　　　　　　　　　Standard Scores ____　　Percentile Rank ____　　Stanine ____

Piers Harris Self-Concept Scale:　　Raw Score ____　　Percentile Rank ____　　Stanine ____

Clusters:　　Behavior ____　　Intellectual ____　　Physical Appearance ____
　　　　　　Anxiety ____　　Popularity ____　　Happiness and Satisfaction ____

Other: _____

Report: _____

_____

_____

_____

_____

_____

_____

_____

_____

_____

_____

_____

Recommendations:

Consult outpatient occupational therapy appointments for the following:

____ Social Skills Training

____ Developmental Assessment/Treatment

____ Sensory Motor

_____ Therapist   _____ Date

H

List of Spiritual Assessments

Anandarajah, G., & Hight, E. (2001). Spirituality and medical practice: Using the HOPE questions as a practical tool for spiritual assessment. *American Family Physician, 63,* 81-89.

Fetzer Institute and the National Institute on Aging Working Group. (1999). *Multidimensional measurement of religious/spirituality for use in health research.* Kalamazoo, MI: Fetzer Institute. Retrieved from http://www.fetzer.org/resources/ multidimensional-measurement-religiousnessspirituality-use-health-research

Fitchett, G. (2002). 7 X 7 model for spiritual assessment. In G. Fitchett, *Assessing spiritual needs: A guide for caregivers* (p. 39). Lima, OH: Academic Renewal Press.

Koenig, H. (2004). Taking a spiritual history. *Journal of the American Medical Association, 291,* 2881-2882.

Kravitz, Y. J. (2007). *Spiritual Intelligence Assessment.* Melrose Park, CA: Center for Spiritual Intelligence. Retrieved from http://www.spiritualintelligence.com

Maugans, T. (1997). The spiritual history. *Archives of Family Medicine, 5,* 11-16.

Puchalski, C., & Romer, A. L. (2000). Taking a spiritual history allows clinicians to understand patients more fully. *Journal of Palliative Medicine, 3,* 129-137.

Schnorr, M. A. (2005). Spiritual Assessment Guidelines. Friends General Conference of the Religious Society of Friends. Retrieved from https://www.fgcquaker.org/ resources/resources-fostering-vital-friends-meetings

Underwood, L., & Teresi, J. (2000). The daily spiritual experience scale: Development, theoretical description, reliability, exploratory factor analysis and preliminary construct validity using health-related data. *Annals of Behavioral Medicine, 24*(1), 22-33.

Hemphill, B. J., & Urish, C. K. (Eds.). *Assessments in Occupational Therapy Mental Health: An Integrative Approach, Fourth Edition* (p. 593). © 2020 Taylor & Francis Group.

Life Balance Inventory

To rate the following items, Step 1, indicate if you do the activity or want to do the activity by circling "Yes" or "No."

Then, Step 2, for the activities you circled "Yes," think about yourself doing each activity in the past month, and rate how much time you actually spend in each activity compared to the amount of time you want to spend in each activity.

Step 1: I Do This Activity or Want to Do This Activity		Step 2: For the Activities You Circled Yes, the Amount of Time I Spend Doing This Activity Is:				
Yes/No		Activity	Always Less Than I Want	Sometimes Less Than I Want	About Right for Me	Sometimes More Than I Want	Always More Than I Want
Yes	No	Taking care of personal hygiene and bathing	1	2	3	2	1
Yes	No	Taking care of your appearance	1	2	3	2	1
Yes	No	Getting adequate sleep	1	2	3	2	1
Yes	No	Relaxing	1	2	3	2	1
Yes	No	Getting regular exercise	1	2	3	2	1
Yes	No	Eating nutritiously	1	2	3	2	1

(continued)

Hemphill, B. J., & Urish, C. K. (Eds.). *Assessments in Occupational Therapy Mental Health: An Integrative Approach, Fourth Edition* (pp. 595-598). © 2020 Taylor & Francis Group.

Step 1: I Do This Activity or Want to Do This Activity		Step 2: For the Activities You Circled Yes, the Amount of Time I Spend Doing This Activity Is:				
Yes/No		Activity	Always Less Than I Want	Sometimes Less Than I Want	About Right for Me	Sometimes More Than I Want	Always More Than I Want
Yes	No	Managing your health needs	1	2	3	2	1
Yes	No	Managing money (bills/budget/ investments)	1	2	3	2	1
Yes	No	Driving	1	2	3	2	1
Yes	No	Taking the bus	1	2	3	2	1
Yes	No	Doing things with family members	1	2	3	2	1
Yes	No	Doing things with spouse/significant other	1	2	3	2	1
Yes	No	Doing things with friends	1	2	3	2	1
Yes	No	Taking care of children or family members	1	2	3	2	1
Yes	No	Having an intimate sexual relationship	1	2	3	2	1
Yes	No	Participating in groups (clubs, classes, etc.)	1	2	3	2	1
Yes	No	Meeting new people	1	2	3	2	1
Yes	No	Working for pay	1	2	3	2	1
Yes	No	Gaining competence in your job	1	2	3	2	1
Yes	No	Socializing at work	1	2	3	2	1
Yes	No	Participating in formal religious activities	1	2	3	2	1
Yes	No	Participating in traditional rituals, holidays	1	2	3	2	1

(continued)

Step 1: I Do This Activity or Want to Do This Activity			Step 2: For the Activities You Circled Yes, the Amount of Time I Spend Doing This Activity Is:				
Yes/No		Activity	Always Less Than I Want	Sometimes Less Than I Want	About Right for Me	Sometimes More Than I Want	Always More Than I Want
Yes	No	Participating in educational opportunities	1	2	3	2	1
Yes	No	Participating in professional organizations	1	2	3	2	1
Yes	No	Volunteering in the community	1	2	3	2	1
Yes	No	Participating in organized sports	1	2	3	2	1
Yes	No	Doing outdoor activities (hunting, fishing)	1	2	3	2	1
Yes	No	Gardening	1	2	3	2	1
Yes	No	Communing with nature	1	2	3	2	1
Yes	No	Planning and coordinating events	1	2	3	2	1
Yes	No	Decorating or organizing spaces	1	2	3	2	1
Yes	No	Cooking	1	2	3	2	1
Yes	No	Doing housework	1	2	3	2	1
Yes	No	Shopping	1	2	3	2	1
Yes	No	Taking care of pets	1	2	3	2	1
Yes	No	Going to restaurants/bars	1	2	3	2	1
Yes	No	Going to plays, movies, sporting events	1	2	3	2	1
Yes	No	Doing crafts, hobbies	1	2	3	2	1
Yes	No	Making music	1	2	3	2	1
Yes	No	Making art	1	2	3	2	1

(continued)

Step 1: I Do This Activity or Want to Do This Activity			Step 2: For the Activities You Circled Yes, the Amount of Time I Spend Doing This Activity Is:				
Yes/No		Activity	Always Less Than I Want	Sometimes Less Than I Want	About Right for Me	Sometimes More Than I Want	Always More Than I Want
Yes	No	Maintaining or repairing equipment	1	2	3	2	1
Yes	No	Sewing/ needlework	1	2	3	2	1
Yes	No	Reading	1	2	3	2	1
Yes	No	Using computers (text, internet, blogs)	1	2	3	2	1
Yes	No	Reflecting or meditating	1	2	3	2	1
Yes	No	Journaling	1	2	3	2	1
Yes	No	Composing, writing (music, poetry, etc.)	1	2	3	2	1
Yes	No	Dancing, yoga, etc.	1	2	3	2	1
Yes	No	Playing games of skill (cards, electronic, etc.)	1	2	3	2	1
Yes	No	Watching TV	1	2	3	2	1
Yes	No	Mentoring (teaching) others	1	2	3	2	1
Yes	No	Traveling (any means, locally, globally)	1	2	3	2	1
Yes	No	Storytelling	1	2	3	2	1

Indices

Assessment Index

Author Index

Subject Index

Financial Disclosures

Dr. Jennifer Allison has no financial or proprietary interest in the materials presented herein.

Sue Baptiste has no financial or proprietary interest in the materials presented herein.

Dr. Carolyn M. Baum has no financial or proprietary interest in the materials presented herein.

Marie-Louise F. Blount is coeditor of the journal *Occupational Therapy in Mental Health*.

Dr. Brent Braveman has no financial or proprietary interest in the materials presented herein.

Dr. Catana Brown receives royalties for the Adolescent Adult Sensory Profile from the Psychological Corporation and for the Test of Grocery Shopping Skills from the American Occupational Therapy Association.

Dr. Ann Chapleau has no financial or proprietary interest in the materials presented herein.

Dr. Lisa Tabor Connor has no financial or proprietary interest in the materials presented herein.

Brock Cook has no financial or proprietary interest in the materials presented herein.

Dr. Mary V. Donohue is the author of *Social Profile: Assessment of Social Participation in Children, Adolescents, and Adults*, published by AOTA Press.

Catherine A. Earhart, as primary developer of the Allen Diagnostic Module (2nd Edition), receives royalties on sales of these products from S&S Worldwide, as well as for other Allen cognitive assessments (ACLS-5) sold through S&S Worldwide. She receives royalties on electronic downloaded assessments (ADM-2) sold through the Allen Cognitive Group website.

Dr. Glen Gillen has no financial or proprietary interest in the materials presented herein.

Dr. Kristine Haertl has no financial or proprietary interest in the materials presented herein.

Ashley Hartman has no financial or proprietary interest in the materials presented herein.

Dr. Barbara J. Hemphill has no financial or proprietary interest in the materials presented herein.

Dr. Margo B. Holm has no financial or proprietary interest in the materials presented herein.

Dr. Michael K. Iwama has no financial or proprietary interest in the materials presented herein.

Dr. Celeste Januszewski has no financial or proprietary interest in the materials presented herein.

Dr. Noomi Katz has no financial or proprietary interest in the materials presented herein.

Dr. Lisa Mahaffey has no financial or proprietary interest in the materials presented herein.

Dr. Kathleen Matuska has no financial or proprietary interest in the materials presented herein.

Deane B McCraith has no financial or proprietary interest in the materials presented herein.

Dr. Christine Raber has no financial or proprietary interest in the materials presented herein.

Dr. Emily Raphael-Greenfield has no financial or proprietary interest in the materials presented herein.

Dr. Nadine Revheim has no financial or proprietary interest in the materials presented herein.

Dr. Joan C. Rogers has no financial or proprietary interest in the materials presented herein.

Jane Ryan has no financial or proprietary interest in the materials presented herein.

Dr. Victoria Schindler has no financial or proprietary interest in the materials presented herein.

Dr. Emily Schulz has no financial or proprietary interest in the materials presented herein.

Dr. Mary P. Shotwell has no financial or proprietary interest in the materials presented herein.

Dr. Franklin Stein has no financial or proprietary interest in the materials presented herein.

Linda Kohlman Thomson has no financial or proprietary interest in the materials presented herein.

Dr. Joan Toglia is the author of the Weekly Calendar Planning Activity and receives royalties from the publisher, AOTA Press.

Dr. Carolyn A. Unsworth has no financial or proprietary interest in the materials presented herein.

Dr. Christine K. Urish has no financial or proprietary interest in the materials presented herein.

Dr. Janet Watts has no financial or proprietary interest in the materials presented herein.

Suzanne White has no financial or proprietary interest in the materials presented herein.

Dr. Timothy J. Wolf has no financial or proprietary interest in the materials presented herein.

Printed in the United States
by Baker & Taylor Publisher Services

Appendix I

Alternative Force Expressions

Summary

It is very useful to formulate expressions for forces alternative to the usual force
theorem of Section 3.3. The basic idea is that since the wavefunction is required to be
at a variational minimum, the energy is invariant to *any* change in the wavefunction
to linear order. The usual force theorem assumes that the wavefunction remains
unchanged when a parameter is changed, but there are an infinite number of other
possibilities. An important example involves core electrons; it is much more physical
and leads to simpler expressions if the core states are assumed to be rigidly attached
to nuclei when a nucleus moves or the crystal is strained. This leads to very useful
expressions for forces, stress (pressure), and generalized forces that are energy
differences taken to first order for various changes.

The "force theorem" or "Hellmann–Feynman theorem," Eqs. (3.19) or (7.39),

$$\mathbf{F}_I = -\frac{\partial E}{\partial \mathbf{R}_I} = -\int d^3 r \, n(\mathbf{r}) \frac{\partial V_{\text{ext}}(\mathbf{r})}{\partial \mathbf{R}_I} - \frac{\partial E_{II}}{\partial \mathbf{R}_I}, \tag{I.1}$$

or the generalized form, Eq. (3.25),

$$\frac{\partial E}{\partial \lambda} = \left\langle \Psi_\lambda \left| \frac{\partial \hat{H}}{\partial \lambda} \right| \Psi_\lambda \right\rangle, \tag{I.2}$$

applies to any variation and to nonlocal potentials as in Eq. (13.3) for pseudopotentials.
The same fundamental ideas lead to the "stress theorem," Eq. (3.23), and the practical
expression in Appendix G. These expressions follow from first-order variation of the
energy, assuming all the electronic degrees of freedom are at the variational minimum.
The expressions correspond to evaluating the force as the derivative of the energy with
respect to the parameter λ, keeping the electrons fixed. This is illustrated on the left-hand
side of Fig. I.1.

The subject of this appendix is alternative formulas that take advantage of the fact that
the electronic degrees of freedom are at a variational minimum. Because the derivative of
the energy with respect to any of these variables vanishes, any linear change can be added

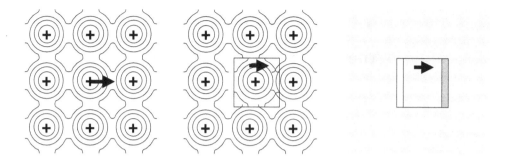

Figure I.1. Illustration of two ways of calculating forces. Left: the usual force theorem, Eq. (I.1), follows if the electron density is held constant to first order as the nucleus moves. Center: a region of charge is moved rigidly with the nucleus. Right: definition of the region B that is "cut out" and moved rigidly leading to the changed density in region C.

with no change in the force. The resulting degrees of freedom can be used to transform the expressions into different forms that can be more useful in specific cases. An extreme form – that is useful in practice – is shown in the center of Fig. I.1 and explained in Section I.1.

There are two general approaches for choosing alternative expressions:

- *Use of the variational principle, involving the effective potential and density* to reexpress Eq. (I.1) in forms that involve changes in the density $n(\mathbf{r})$ and/or changes in the total internal potential $V_{\text{eff}}(\mathbf{r})$. The advantage is that the resulting expressions may be easier to evaluate.
- *Geometric relations* that relate the force acting on the nucleus to the force *transferred across a boundary that surrounds the nucleus.* This can be formulated in terms of a stress field, which is a force per unit area, establishing relations with the stress density field. Actual expressions can often be shown to be equivalent to specific choices of variations of $n(\mathbf{r})$ and $V_{\text{eff}}(\mathbf{r})$.

I.1 Variational Freedom and Forces

The usual form of the "force theorem" follows immediately since the first-order change in energy can be considered to arise solely from the term $\int d\mathbf{r}\ V_{\text{ext}}(\mathbf{r})n(\mathbf{r})$ in Eq. (7.16) with all other changes summing to zero. Alternative formulations for force in density functional theory can be understood using the functionals derived in Section 7.3. Different expression can be derived using the most general functional, Eq. (7.26), which is *variational with respect to both the effective potential and the density* for a given external potential [361, 363, 367, 368, 1049].

The essential point for our purpose is that one can add *any change in* $V_{\text{eff}}(\mathbf{r})$ *or* $n(\mathbf{r})$ *with no change in the force.* The disadvantage of this approach is that one must calculate the first-order change in the individual terms in Eq. (7.26); the advantage is that difficult problems can be greatly reduced or eliminated. For example, consider the force acting on a nucleus. The usual expression is derived by displacing the nucleus while holding the density constant, *even the density of core electrons of that nucleus* as illustrated on the left-hand side of Fig. I.1.

An alternative approach is to displace the electron density in a region around the nucleus rigidly with the nucleus; then there are no changes in the large core–nucleus interaction and one arrives at the physically appealing picture that the force is due to the nucleus and core moving together relative to the other atoms. It is important to note that *this is not an approximation*; it is merely a rearrangement of terms. How can this be done? One way that at first appears extremely artificial is to "cut out a region of space" and displace it. This leaves a slice of vacuum on one side and double density on the other, as shown on the right-hand side of Fig. I.1. The effect in the case of moving a nucleus is shown in the center of the figure.

Despite the totally unphysical nature of this change of density, the final consequences are physical and there are advantages in the way the equations can be formulated as first shown by Mackintosh and Andersen [498] and described by Heine [499]. A very simple derivation has been presented by Jacobsen, Norskov, and Puska ([367] appendix A) using the properties of the functional, Eq. (7.26), where we can choose any variation of the density and effective potential. Since the densities are frozen, it is straightforward to evaluate all the terms involving the electron density to linear order:

$$\delta E^{CC} = \delta E^{CC}_{A \leftrightarrow B} + \int_C n(\mathbf{r}) V^{CC}_{A+B}(\mathbf{r}),$$

$$\delta E_{xc} = \int_C n(\mathbf{r}) \epsilon_{xc}[n(\mathbf{r})], \tag{I.3}$$

$$\delta T = \delta \left[\sum_i \varepsilon_i \right] - \int_C n(\mathbf{r}) V_{eff}(\mathbf{r}),$$

where $\delta E^{CC}_{A \leftrightarrow B}$ denotes classical Coulomb interactions *between* regions A and B (interactions inside A and B do not change); V^{CC}_{A+B} is the potential due to regions A and B (that due to region C is higher order); δE_{xc} is only considered in the local density approximation; and δT is the change in kinetic energy. Then the total change is (Exercise I.1)

$$\delta E_{total} = \delta \left[\sum_i \varepsilon_i \right] + \delta E^{CC}_{A \leftrightarrow B} + \int_C n(\mathbf{r}) \left\{ V^{CC}_{A+B}(\mathbf{r}) \epsilon_{xc}[n(\mathbf{r})] - V_{eff}(\mathbf{r}) \right\}. \tag{I.4}$$

Finally, one has freedom to choose $V_{eff}(\mathbf{r})$ in region C and a clever choice is to make [367] the last term vanish. This means simply to *define* $V_{eff}(\mathbf{r})$ to have an added term $\epsilon_{xc}(n(\mathbf{r}) - V_{xc}(n(\mathbf{r}))$ only in region C. With this definition of the derivative, $\partial V_{eff}(\mathbf{r})/\partial \mathbf{R}_I$ is a delta function on the boundary on region B, and for this change in V_{eff}, the force is given strictly in terms of the eigenvalues plus the force from electrostatic interactions *that cross the A–B boundary*:

$$-\frac{\partial E_{total}}{\partial \mathbf{R}_I} = -\frac{\partial \sum_i \varepsilon_i}{\partial \mathbf{R}_I} - \frac{\partial E^{CC}_{A \leftrightarrow B}}{\partial \mathbf{R}_I}. \tag{I.5}$$

I.2 Energy Differences

The expressions for "force" in terms of the eigenvalue sums are actually most useful for calculation of small, but finite, energy differences between cases that involve small changes in the potential. Thus a convenient way of calculating the energy difference due to a small change (adding an external field, change of volume or shape, displacement of an atom, etc.) using standard programs is to calculate the finite energy difference

$$\Delta E_{\text{total}} = \Delta \sum_i \varepsilon_i + \Delta E_{A \leftrightarrow B}^{\text{CC}} \tag{I.6}$$

for potentials as defined above. Perhaps the simplest example in solid state physics – which is also very useful – is the difference in energy between fcc, hcp, and bcc structure metals. In each case the potential is well approximated as neutral and spherical – i.e., the ASA of Section 16.6. Then the Coulomb terms vanish and the energy difference is just

$$\Delta E_{\text{total}} \rightarrow \Delta \sum_i \varepsilon_i, \tag{I.7}$$

where *it is essential not to use the self-consistent potential for each structure: instead the eigenvalues ε_i for each structure are calculated using the same potential!* To linear order of accuracy, the difference, Eq. (I.7), can be evaluated using the potential from any one of the structures. Since the differences are small, this procedure is very useful, taking advantage of the variational freedom to make the calculation more accurate and at the same time easier!

I.3 Pressure

The same ideas apply for any derivative – e.g., stress and pressure – as described in general in Section H.2. Figure H.1 illustrates the choice of "pulling apart" rigid units in a crystal, leaving space in between. From appropriate derivatives of the total energy one can calculate the stress on the boundaries. Furthermore, the stress on a boundary that cuts all space into two parts (e.g., a boundary drawn through the spaces in Fig. H.1) can be used to define the *macroscopic stress*: because all forces between the two half-spaces must cross the boundary, the average stress on the boundary is rigorously the macroscopic stress with no nonunique gauge terms [162].

An extremely useful application of the alternative form of the force theorem is the calculation of pressure in an isotropic situation. In a crystal, this means the ASA (Section 16.5, especially Fig. 16.9). Also the idea is useful for liquids and matter at high pressure and temperature where the average environment is spherical [496–499]. This is the fortunate situation in which the electrostatic terms vanish because there are no Coulomb fields outside a neutral sphere. The pressure is given simply by the change in sum of eigenvalues for the change in effective potential defined following Eq. (I.4). The resulting expression can be written in terms of the wavefunctions as [496, 499] (see Exercise I.2)

$$3P\Omega = \int d\mathbf{S} \cdot \left\{ \sum_i \left[\nabla \psi_i^* (\mathbf{r} \cdot \nabla \psi_i) - \psi_i^* \nabla (\mathbf{r} \cdot \nabla \psi_i) + \text{c.c.} \right] + \frac{1}{3} n \epsilon_{\text{xc}} \mathbf{r} \right\}. \tag{I.8}$$

Using the fact that ψ_i is a solution of the Kohn–Sham equations in spherical geometry, it was shown by Pettifor [499, 1046] that the expression can be rewritten as

$$4\pi S^2 P = \sum_l \int dE n_l(E)\psi_l^2(S,E)$$

$$\left\{ [E - V_{xc}(S)]S^2 + (D_l - l)(D_l + l + 1) + \frac{1}{3}\epsilon_{xc}(S)S^2 \right\}. \qquad (I.9)$$

These expressions are particularly convenient for calculation of the equation of state of materials in the ASA approximation because they give the experimentally measurable pressure P directly instead of the total energy (which is very large since it includes all the core electrons). The equilibrium volume Ω is for $P(\Omega) = 0$; the bulk modulus is the slope $B = -dP/d\Omega$; the cohesive energy as a function of volume can be found as the integral $\Delta E_{total} = \int P d\Omega$; and, finally, the absolute total energy is the cohesive energy plus the total energy of the atom that can be found separately.

Expressions for the pressure in the ASA can also be derived from the stress density (Section H.2) as was shown by Nielsen and Martin [162] and as can be seen in Eq. (H.21). There is no ambiguity of the stress field in this case because it is a one-dimensional (radial) problem, and the pressure is the radial stress – i.e., the force per unit area. Also, Eq. (H.21) simplifies because there are no Coulomb terms at the sphere boundary so that the final expressions involve only kinetic and exchange–correlation terms, finally leading to expressions equivalent to those above [162].

I.4 Force and Stress

An alternative expression [162, 1050] for the total force *on a volume* is given by the well-known relation that a force field is a divergence of a stress field [806]

$$f_\alpha(\mathbf{r}) = \sum_\beta \nabla_\beta \sigma_{\alpha,\beta}(\mathbf{r}). \qquad (I.10)$$

By integrating over a volume containing a nucleus – e.g., region B in Fig. I.1 – and using Gauss's theorem, the total force on the region is given in terms of a surface integral of the stress field

$$F_\alpha^{total} = \sum_\beta \int_S dS \hat{S}_\beta \sigma_{\alpha,\beta}(\mathbf{r}), \qquad (I.11)$$

where S is the surface of the volume and $\hat{S}$ is the outward normal unit vector. Although there are nonunique terms in the stress field (Section H.2), the force is well defined and gauge invariant because such terms vanish in the divergence or in the integral (see also Section H.3).

Grafenstein and Ziesche [1050] have shown that Eq. (I.11) leads to the form of the generalized force expression given in Eq. (I.5) for the particular case of the local density approximation. This provides an additional way of understanding the meaning of the terms, since it does not depend on the seemingly arbitrary tricks used in the derivation of Eq. (I.5).

In addition, the relation to the stress field provides a simple interpretation valid for both independent-particle and many-body problems. First, since the system is assumed to be in equilibrium, the force on the region is the force of constraint – i.e., the external force that is needed to hold the nucleus fixed. This is the same as in the application of the usual force theorem, but here it is essential to add that there are no other constraints on the system in the volume considered. The expression for the stress (e.g., see Appendix H) is a sum of potential and kinetic terms. The kinetic term is due to particles *crossing the surface* and is present in classical systems at finite temperature and quantum systems at all temperatures. The potential terms are due to interactions *crossing the surface*; interactions within the region – e.g., a nucleus with its own core electrons – are not counted. For electrostatic interactions, this is simply the force on the multipoles inside the region due to fields from outside, which can be conveniently written as volume integrals over the sphere. Finally, the exchange–correlation contribution is the effect of the exchange–correlation hole extending across the surface; for the LDA this is a delta function.

I.5 Force in APW-Type Methods

An approach to calculation of forces in APW and LAPW methods has been developed by Soler and Williams [706] and by Yu, Singh, and Krakauer [707]. The general idea is quite close to the spirit of the alternative force approaches described above, but the implementation is very different. These authors work directly with the APW or LAPW expressions for the total energy and calculate a force from the derivative of the total energy with respect to the displacement of an atom *relative to the rest of the lattice*, or equivalently *the displacement of the rest of the lattice relative to the given atom*. There are many choices for the change in the wavefunction with displacement of the nucleus, and the latter interpretation suggests a most convenient one. The sphere and all it contents (nucleus, core electrons, etc.) are held fixed, and the energy changes only because of the change in boundary conditions on the sphere and Coulomb potentials that propagate into the sphere. The change in energy to first order can be found straightforwardly [706] by differentiating each of the terms in the expression for the APW or LAPW total energy with respect to the position of the sphere, evaluated for the unchanged wavefunction. This avoids any need to evaluate the derivative of the large Coulomb energy of interaction of the nucleus with the change density in its sphere; the effect is replaced by forces on the sphere due to its displacement relative to surrounding spheres.

SELECT FURTHER READING

An intuitive discussion of the meaning of the terms in alternative expressions:

Heine, V., in *Solid State Physics*, vol. 35, edited by H. Ehenreich, H., F. Seitz, F., and D. Turnbull (Academic Press, New York, 1980), p. 1.
A simple, compact derivation of the basic ideas using the variational properties of functions:
Jacobsen, K. W., Norskov, J. K., and Puska, M. J., "Interatomic interactions in the effective-medium theory," *Phys. Rev. B* 35:7423–7442, 1987, app. A.

Exercises

I.1 Show that the expression, (I.4), for an energy difference to first order follows from the form of the energy functional given in Eq. (7.26). Use this result with the special choice for the change in potential to derive the final result, Eq. (I.5).

I.2 Using the fact that ψ_i is a solution of the Kohn–Sham equations in a spherical geometry, show that the potential can be eliminated and the expression for pressure can be written in terms of the wavefunction and its derivatives as in Eq. (I.8). Also show that there is an added term for exchange and correlation that can be written in the form in Eq. (I.8) in the local approximation. Hint: the first part can be done by partial integration and the second is the correction due to the fact that the potential is not fixed as the spherical system is scaled.

Appendix J

Scattering and Phase Shifts

Summary

Scattering and phase shifts play a central role in many fields of physics and are especially relevant for electronic structure in the properties of pseudopotentials (Chapter 11) and the formulation of augmented and multiple-scattering KKR methods (Chapters 16 and 17). The purpose of this appendix is to collect the formulas together and to make added connections to scattering cross sections and electrical resistivity.

J.1 Scattering and Phase Shifts for Spherical Potentials

Scattering plays an essential role in interesting physical properties of electronic systems and in basic electronic structure theory. Scattering due to defects leads to such basic phenomena as resistivity in metals and is the basis for pseudopotential theory (Chapter 11) and all the methods that involve augmentation (Chapter 16). The basic element is the scattering from a single center, which we will consider here only in the spherical approximation, although the formulation can be extended to general symmetries (see [684]). A schematic figure of the scattering of plane waves is shown in Fig. J.1.

Consider the problem of scattering from a potential that is localized. This applies to a neutral atom (and charged ions with appropriate changes) and to the problem of a single muffin-tin potential, where the potential is explicitly set to a constant outside the muffin-tin sphere of radius S. Since the problem is inherently spherical, scattering of plane waves is described by first transforming to spherical functions using the well-known identity [10, 480, 996]

$$e^{i\mathbf{q}\cdot\mathbf{r}} = 4\pi \sum_{L} i^l \, j_l(qr) \, Y_L^*(\hat{\mathbf{q}}) \, Y_L(\hat{\mathbf{r}}), \tag{J.1}$$

where $j_l(qr)$ are spherical Bessel functions (Section K.1) and $Y_L(\hat{r}) \equiv Y_{l,m}(\theta,\phi)$ denotes a spherical harmonic with $\{l,m\} \equiv L$ (Section K.2). Since there is no dependence on the angle around the axis defined by $\hat{r}$, this can also be written as a function of r and θ,

$$e^{i\mathbf{q}\cdot\mathbf{r}} = e^{iqr\cos(\theta)} = \sum_{l}(2l+1) \, i^l \, j_l(qr) \, P_l[\cos(\theta)], \tag{J.2}$$

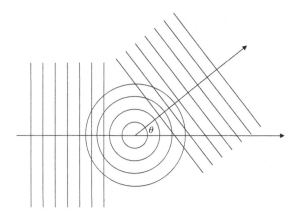

Figure J.1. Schematic illustration of scattering of a plane wave by a spherical potential.

where $P_l(x)$ are the Legendre polynomials (Section K.2). Using spherical symmetry, the scattering can be classified in terms of wavefunctions of angular momentum $L \equiv \{l,m\}$, which can be written as

$$\psi_L(\mathbf{r}) = i^l \psi_l(r) Y_L(\theta,\phi) = i^l r^{-1} \phi_l(r) Y_L(\theta,\phi), \tag{J.3}$$

as in Eq. (10.1). Inside the region, where the potential is nonzero, radial function $\psi_l(r)$ or $\phi_l(r)$ can be found by numerical integration of the radial Schrödinger equation, (10.12). Outside the region at large r the solution must be a linear combination of regular and irregular solutions – i.e., spherical Bessel and Neumann functions $j_l(\kappa r)$ and $n_l(\kappa r)$,

$$\psi_l^>(\varepsilon,r) = C_l \left[j_l(\kappa r) - \tan\eta_l(\varepsilon) \, n_l(\kappa r) \right], \tag{J.4}$$

where $\kappa^2 = \varepsilon$. The energy-dependent phase shifts $\eta_l(\varepsilon)$ are determined by the condition that $\psi_l^>(\varepsilon, S)$ must match the inner solution $\psi_l(\varepsilon, S)$ in value and slope at the chosen radius S. In terms of the dimensionless logarithmic derivative of the inner solution (see Eq. (11.20))

$$D_l(\varepsilon,r) \equiv r\psi_l'(r)/\psi_l(r) = r\frac{d}{dr}\ln\psi_l(r); \tag{J.5}$$

this leads to the result

$$\tan\eta_l(\varepsilon) = \frac{S\dfrac{d}{dr}j_l(\kappa r)|_S - D_l(\varepsilon)\,j_l(\kappa S)}{S\dfrac{d}{dr}n_l(\kappa r)|_S - D_l(\varepsilon)\,n_l(\kappa S)}. \tag{J.6}$$

The scattering cross-section for a single site at positive energies can be expressed in terms of the phase shift. Using asymptotic forms of the Bessel and Neumann functions at positive energies $\varepsilon = \frac{1}{2}k^2$, the wave function, Eq. (J.4), at large radius approaches [306, 787, 996]

$$\psi_l^>(\varepsilon,r) \rightarrow \frac{C_l}{kr}\sin\left[kr + \eta_l(\varepsilon) - \frac{l\pi}{2}\right], \tag{J.7}$$

which shows that each η_l is a phase shift for a partial wave. The full scattered function can be written

$$\psi_l^>(\varepsilon,r) \rightarrow e^{i\mathbf{q}\cdot\mathbf{r}} + i\frac{e^{iqr}}{qr} \sum_l (2l+1)e^{i\eta_l} \sin(\eta_l) P_l[\cos(\theta)], \qquad \text{(J.8)}$$

and the scattering cross-section is then given by the scattered flux per unit solid angle (see, e.g., [306, 787, 996])

$$\frac{d\sigma}{d\Omega} = \frac{1}{q^2} \left| \sum_l (2l+1)e^{i\eta_l} \sin(\eta_l) P_l[\cos(\theta)] \right|^2, \qquad \text{(J.9)}$$

and the total cross-section by

$$\sigma_{\text{total}} = 2\pi \int \sin(\theta)d\theta \frac{d\sigma}{d\Omega} = \frac{4\pi}{q^2} \sum_l (2l+1)\sin^2(\eta_l). \qquad \text{(J.10)}$$

For negative energy, κ is imaginary and the Neumann function should be replaced by the Hankel function (Section K.1) $h_l^{(1)} = j_l + in_l$, which has the asymptotic form $i^{-l}e^{-|\kappa|r}/|\kappa|r$. The condition for a bound state is that $tan(\eta_l(\varepsilon)) \rightarrow \infty$, so that the coefficient of the Bessel function vanishes in Eq. (J.4) and the Hankel solution is the solution in all space outside the sphere. The bound-state wavefunctions are thus real if one adopts a convention of inclusion of a factor i^l in the wavefunction as in Eq. (16.36), for example.

SELECT FURTHER READING

Basic formulas for phase shifts and scattering:

Shankar, R., *Principles of Quantum Mechanics* (Plenum Publishing, New York, 1980).

Thijssen, J. M., *Computational Physics* (Cambridge University Press, Cambridge, 2000).

References on augmented and multiple scattering methods:

Kübler, J., *Theory of Itinerant Electron Magnetism* (Oxford University Press, Oxford, 2001).

Kübler, J. and Eyert, V., in *Electronic and Magnetic Properties of Metals and Ceramics*, edited by K. H. J. Buschow (VCH-Verlag, Weinheim, Germany, 1992), p. 1.

Lloyd, P. and Smith, P. V., "Multiple scattering theory in condensed materials," *Adv. Phys.* 21:29, 1972.

Appendix K

Useful Relations and Formulas

Summary

Here are given some of the functions and relationships used in this book.

K.1 Bessel, Neumann, and Hankel Functions

Spherical Bessel, Neumann, and Hankel functions are radial solutions of the Helmholtz equation in three dimensions. Spherical Bessel and Neumann functions are related to the half-order functions and can be represented as

$$j_m(x) = \sqrt{\frac{\pi}{2x}} J_{m+\frac{1}{2}}(x) = (-1)^m x^m \left(\frac{d}{x dx}\right)^m \frac{\sin(x)}{x}, \tag{K.1}$$

and

$$n_m(x) = \sqrt{\frac{\pi}{2x}} N_{m+\frac{1}{2}}(x) = -(-1)^m x^m \left(\frac{d}{x dx}\right)^m \frac{\cos(x)}{x}. \tag{K.2}$$

Examples are

$$j_0(x) = \frac{\sin(x)}{x}, x) = -\frac{\cos(x)}{x},$$

$$j_1(x) = \frac{\sin(x)}{x^2} - \frac{\cos(x)}{x}, x) = -\frac{\cos(x)}{x^2} - \frac{\sin(x)}{x},$$

$$j_2(x) = \left(\frac{3}{x^3} - \frac{1}{x}\right)\sin(x) - \frac{3}{x^2}\cos(x), n_2(x) = \left(-\frac{3}{x^3} + \frac{1}{x}\right)\cos(x) - \frac{3}{x^2}\sin(x). \tag{K.3}$$

Hankel functions are defined by $h_l^{(1)} = j_l + i n_l$ and $h_l^{(2)} = j_l - i n_l$, which are convenient combinations for many problems. In particular, for positive imaginary arguments, $h_l^{(1)}$ has the asymptotic form $i^{-l} e^{-|\kappa|r}/|\kappa|r$ corresponding to a bound-state solution.

K.2 Spherical Harmonics and Legendre Polynomials

Spherical harmonics are the angular part of the solutions of the Laplace equation in spherical coordinates. They are given by[1]

$$Y_{l,m}(\theta,\phi) = \sqrt{\frac{2l+1}{4\pi}\frac{(l-m)!}{(l+m)!}}P_l^m[\cos(\theta)]e^{im\phi}, \tag{K.4}$$

which define an orthonormal representation on a sphere

$$\int_0^\pi d\theta \sin(\theta)\int_0^{2\pi} d\phi Y_{l,m}^*(\theta,\phi)Y_{l',m'}(\theta,\phi) = \delta_{ll'}\delta_{mm'}. \tag{K.5}$$

The functions $P_l^m(\cos(\theta))$ are associated Legendre polynomials, which are related to the ordinary Legendre polynomials $P_l(x)$ by

$$P_l^m(x) = (-1)^m(1-x^2)^{m/2}\frac{d^m P_l(x)}{dx^m}, m = 0,\ldots,l. \tag{K.6}$$

The Legendre polynomials $P_l(x)$ are defined to be orthogonal on the interval $[-1,1]$; a compact expression valid for any order is (Rodrigues formula)

$$P_l(x) = \frac{1}{2^l l!}\frac{d^l(x^2-1)^l}{dx^l}. \tag{K.7}$$

Using the Rodrigues formula for $P_l(x)$, a definition for $P_l^m(x)$ can be derived valid for both negative and positive m (see previous footnote regarding the factor $(-1)^m$).

$$P_l^m(x) = \frac{(-1)^m}{2^l l!}(1-x^2)^{m/2}\frac{d^{l+m}(x^2-1)^l}{dx^{l+m}}. \tag{K.8}$$

It can be shown that

$$P_l^{-m}(x) = (-1)^m\frac{(l-m)!}{(l+m)!}P_l^m(x). \tag{K.9}$$

It is helpful to give explicit examples for low orders in terms of angles with $P_l^m \equiv P_l^m(\cos(\theta))$:

$$P_0^0 = 1, P_1^0 = \cos(\theta), \quad P_2^0 = \tfrac{1}{2}[3\cos^2(\theta)-1], P_3^0 = \tfrac{1}{2}\cos(\theta)[5\cos^2(\theta)-3],$$

$$P_1^1 = -\sin(\theta), P_2^1 = -3\sin(\theta)\cos(\theta), P_3^1 = -\tfrac{3}{2}\sin(\theta)[5\cos^2(\theta)-1],$$

$$P_2^2 = 3\sin^2(\theta), \qquad\qquad P_3^2 = 15\cos(\theta)\sin^2(\theta),$$

$$P_3^3 = -15\sin^3(\theta). \tag{K.10}$$

[1] The definitions here are the same as given by Condon and Shortley [1051], Jackson [480], and in *Numerical Recipes* [776]. However, some authors define $Y_{l,m}$ with a factor $(-1)^m$ and omit the factor $(-1)^m$ in the associated Legendre polynomials, Eq. (K.6). Of course, the final form for $Y_{l,m}$ is the same, but one must be careful to use consistent definitions.

K.3 Real Spherical Harmonics

It is often convenient to work with real functions instead of $Y_{l,m}(\theta,\phi)$ that are eigenfunctions of angular momentum. The general definition is simply the normalized real and imaginary parts of $Y_{l,m}(\theta,\phi)$, which can be denoted $S_{l,m}(\theta,\phi)$ given by

$$S_{l,m}^{+}(\theta,\phi) = \frac{1}{\sqrt{2}}[Y_{l,m}(\theta,\phi) + Y_{l,m}^{*}(\theta,\phi)],$$

$$S_{l,m}^{-}(\theta,\phi) = \frac{1}{\sqrt{2}i}[Y_{l,m}(\theta,\phi) - Y_{l,m}^{*}(\theta,\phi)]. \tag{K.11}$$

These functions are used, e.g., in Chapter 14.

K.4 Clebsch–Gordon and Gaunt Coefficients

The Clebsch–Gordan coefficients are extensively used in the quantum theory of angular momentum and play an important role in the decomposition of reducible representations of a rotation group into irreducible representations. Clebsch–Gordan coefficients are given in terms of Wigner $3jm$ symbols by the expression

$$C_{j_1 m_1, j_2 m_2}^{j_3 m_3} = (-1)^{j_1 - j_2 + m_3}\sqrt{2j_3 + 1}\begin{pmatrix} j_1 & j_2 & j_3 \\ m_1 & m_2 & -m_3 \end{pmatrix}, \tag{K.12}$$

where the Wigner $3jm$ symbol is defined by

$$\begin{pmatrix} j_1 & j_2 & j_3 \\ m_1 & m_2 & m_3 \end{pmatrix} = \delta_{m_1 + m_2 + m_3, 0}(-1)^{j_1 - j_2 - m_3}$$

$$\times \left[\frac{(j_3 + j_1 - j_2)!\,(j_3 - j_1 + j_2)!\,(j_1 + j_2 - j_3)!\,(j_3 - m_3)!\,(j_3 + m_3)!}{(j_1 + j_2 + j_3 + 1)!\,(j_1 - m_1)!\,(j_1 + m_1)!\,(j_2 - m_2)!\,(j_2 + m_2)!}\right]^{1/2}$$

$$\times \sum_k \frac{(-1)^{k + j_2 + m_2}(j_2 + j_3 - m_1 - k)!\,(j_1 - m_1 + k)!}{k!\,(j_3 - j_1 + j_2 - k)!\,(j_3 - m_3 - k)!\,(k + j_1 - j_2 + m_3)!}. \tag{K.13}$$

The summation over k is over all integers for which the factorials are nonnegative.

The Gaunt coefficients [1052] (also given by Condon and Shortley [1051], pp. 178–179) are defined as

$$c^{l''}(l\,m, l'\,m') = \sqrt{\frac{2}{2l'' + 1}}\int_0^\pi d\theta\,\sin(\theta)\Theta(l'', m - m')\,\Theta(l, m)\,\Theta(l', m'), \tag{K.14}$$

where $\Theta(l, m)$ are given by

$$\Theta(l, m) = \sqrt{\frac{2l + 1}{2}\frac{(l - m)!}{(l + m)!}}P_l^m[\cos(\theta)]. \tag{K.15}$$

Like the Clebsch–Gordan coefficients, the Gaunt coefficients can be expressed in terms of the Wigner $3jm$ symbols

$$c^{l''}(l\,m,l'\,m') = (-1)^m \left[\frac{(2l+1)(2l'+1)}{2l''+1}\right]^{1/2}$$

$$\times \begin{pmatrix} l & l' & l'' \\ 0 & 0 & 0 \end{pmatrix} \begin{pmatrix} l & l' & l'' \\ m & -m' & -m+m' \end{pmatrix}. \tag{K.16}$$

The product of two Wigner $3jm$ symbols is associated with the coupling of two angular momentum vectors. In order to make the connection between the two coefficients more transparent we express the Gaunt coefficients in terms of the Clebsch–Gordan

$$c^{l''}(l\,m,l'\,m') = (-1)^{m'} \frac{\left[(2l+1)(2l'+1)\right]^{1/2}}{2l''+1}\, C^{l''0}_{l0,l'0} C^{l''m-m'}_{lm,l'-m'}. \tag{K.17}$$

K.5 Chebyshev Polynomials

A Taylor series is a direct expansion in powers of the variable

$$f(x) \to c_0 + c_1 x + c_2 x^2 + \cdots + c_M x^M. \tag{K.18}$$

In operator expansions, such as needed in Eq. (18.20), this has the advantage that each successive term is simply obtained recursively using $x^{n+1} = x x^n$; however, for high powers there can be problems with instabilities and the expansion becomes worse as x increases. On the other hand, Chebyshev polynomials of type I, $T_n(x)$, are defined to be orthogonal on the interval $[-1, +1]$, so that any function on this interval can be expanded as a unique linear combination of $T_n(x)$. Furthermore, the expansion has the property that it fits the function $f(x)$ over the entire interval in a least-squares sense, and the polynomials can be computed recursively. The polynomials can be expressed by defining the first two and all others by the recursion relation [776]

$$T_0(x) = 1; \quad T_1(x) = x; \quad T_{n+1}(x) = 2x T_n(x) - T_{n-1}(x). \tag{K.19}$$

The resulting expansion is

$$f(x) \to \frac{c_0}{2} + \sum_{n=1}^{M_p} c_n T_n(x). \tag{K.20}$$

It is a simple exercise to derive the first few polynomials and to demonstrate the orthogonality.

Appendix L
Numerical Methods

Summary

The methods described here are widely used in numerical analysis, selected because of their importance in electronic structure calculations. These methods are used primarily in iterative improvements of the wavefunctions (iterative diagonalization), updates of the charge density in the Kohn–Sham self-consistency loop, and displacements of atoms in structure relaxation. Because the size and nature of the problems are so varied, different methods are more appropriate for different cases.

L.1 Numerical Integration and the Numerov Method

Equations (10.8) and (10.12) are examples of second-derivative equations that play a prominent role in physics, e.g., the Poisson equation, which we also need to solve in finding the self-consistent solution of the full Kohn–Sham or Hartree–Fock equations. These equations can be written in the general form

$$\frac{d^2}{dr^2}u_l(r) + k_l^2(r)u_l(r) = S_l(r), \tag{L.1}$$

where $S = 0$ for Schrödinger-like equations. For the Poisson equation, $u_l(r)$ is the electrostatic potential and $S_l(r) = 4\pi\rho_l(r)$ is the l angular momentum component of the charge density. The equations may be discretized on a grid and integrated using a numerical approximation for the second derivative. (A good description can be found in [485].) An efficient approach is to use the Numerov algorithm [1053] to integrate the equations outward from the origin, and inward from infinity to a matching point. The solution is given by requiring that the wavefunction and its derivative match at a chosen radius R_c. Since the amplitude of the wavefunction can be required to match (only the overall amplitude is set by normalization), actually it is required only to match the ratio $x(r) \equiv (d\phi_l(r)/dr)/\phi_l(r)$, which is the logarithmic derivative of $d\phi_l(r)$.

We want to discretize the differential equation (L.1) on a grid with spacing h. The second-derivative operator can be expressed as (here we drop the subscript l and denote discrete points by $r_j \to j$)

$$\frac{d^2}{dr^2}u(j) = \frac{u(j+1) - 2u(j) + u(j-1)}{h^2} + \frac{h^2}{12}\frac{d^4}{dr^4}u(r) + O(h^4). \tag{L.2}$$

Here we have explicitly written out the leading error, which is $O(h^2)$ (see Exercise L.1). Direct application of this discretized derivative allows one to calculate all values of $u(j)$ recursively given two initial values, say $u(1)$ and $u(2)$. The error in calculating the new $u(j)$ at each step is of order h^4. However, with a little extra work we can obtain a method that is of order h^6, a substantial improvement known as the Numerov method.

The leading error in the second-derivative formula Eq. (L.2) is from the fourth derivative of the function. But this can be found by differentiating the differential equation, (Eq. (L.1)), twice, which leads to the relation $\frac{d^4}{dr^4}u(r) = \frac{d^2}{dr^2}(S(r) - k^2(r)u(r))$. That is, knowledge about the curvature of the source and potential terms leads to a more accurate integration scheme. Substituting this expression into Eq. (L.2), defining $F(r) = S(r) - k^2(r)u(r)$, and using Eq. (L.2) to lowest order for $\frac{d^2}{dr^2}F(r)$, we find the improved formula (Exercise L.2)

$$\frac{d^2}{dr^2}u(j) = \frac{u(j+1) - 2u(j) + u(j-1)}{h^2} + \frac{F(j+1) - 2F(j) + F(j-1)}{12} + O(h^4). \tag{L.3}$$

Substituting this into the original equation leads to the final formula (here $a \equiv h^2/12$)

$$[1 + ak^2(j+1)]u(j+1) - 2[1 - 5ak^2(j)]u(j) + [1 + ak^2(j-1)]u(j-1)$$

$$= a[S(j+1) - 2S(j) + S(j-1)] + O(h^6), \tag{L.4}$$

which can be solved recursively (forward or backward) starting with u at two grid points.

The idea behind the Numerov method can be extended to any dimension, where the pattern of points is given the name "Mehrstellen" (see [576], which cites [577], p. 164). The key point is the use of the differential equation itself to find an expression for both kinetic and potential terms valid to higher order than the original finite difference expression.

L.2 Steepest Descent

Minimization of a function $F(\{x_i\})$ in space of variables x_i, $i = 1, N$ is a widely studied problem in numerical anlysis [776, 1054, 1055].[1] In the absence of any other information the best choice for a direction of displacement from a point x_i^0 to reach the minimum is the steepest descent (SD) direction

$$g_i^0 = -\frac{\partial F}{\partial x_i}\Big|_{x_i = x_i^0}, \tag{L.5}$$

which is shown by the initial direction from point 0 in Fig. L.1. The lowest energy along this direction can be found by "line minimization" in one-dimensional space, i.e., the minimum

---

[1] For simplicity we assume that there is only one minimum, which is valid in large classes of problems in electronic structure. For special cases, such as level crossing at transition states, one may need to adopt special measures.

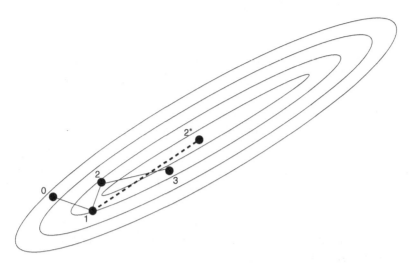

Figure L.1. Schematic illustration of minimization of a function in two dimensions. The steps $1, 2, 3, \ldots$, denote the steepest descent steps, and the point 2^* denotes the conjugate gradient path that reaches the exact solution after two steps if the functional is quadratic.

of F as a function of α^1, where $x_i^1 = x_i^0 + \alpha^1 g_i^0$. Of course, a series of such steps must be taken to approach the absolute minimum, generating the sets of points $x_i^0, x_i^1, x_i^2, \ldots$. This process is illustrated in Fig. L.1 for a very simple function of two variables $F(x_1, x_2) = A(x_1)^2 + B(x_2)^2$, with $B \gg A$. We see that even though the function F decreases at each step, the steps do not move directly to the minimum. Furthermore, the method suffers from a real version of the "Zeno paradox" and one never reaches the minimum exactly. The SD method is particularly bad if the function F has very different dependence on the different variables so that the region around the minimum forms a long narrow valley.

L.3 Conjugate Gradient

Although it may seem surprising, there is a faster way to reach the minimum than to always follow the "downhill" steepest descent direction. After the first step, one not only has the gradient F at the present point, but also the value and gradient at previous points. The additional information can be used to choose a more optimal direction along which the line minimization will lead to a lower energy. In fact, for a quadratic functional in N dimensions, the conjugate gradient (CG) method is guaranteed to reach the minimum in N steps [776, 787, 1054, 1055]. We will consider this case explicitly to illustrate the power of method. In addition, CG can be applied to more complicated functionals (such as the Kohn–Sham functional) and we expect many advantages still to accrue since the functional is quadratic near the minimum.

Consider the quadratic functional

$$F(\{x_i\}) \equiv F(\mathbf{x}) = \frac{1}{2}\mathbf{x} \cdot \mathbf{H} \cdot \mathbf{x}, \qquad \text{(L.6)}$$

with gradients

$$\mathbf{g} = -\frac{\partial F}{\partial \mathbf{x}} = -\mathbf{H} \cdot \mathbf{x}. \tag{L.7}$$

The first step is the same as steepest descent, i.e., minimization of F along a line $\mathbf{x}^1 = \mathbf{x}^0 + \alpha^1 \mathbf{d}^0$, where $\mathbf{d}^0 = \mathbf{g}^0$. For this and for all steps, the minimum occurs for

$$\mathbf{d}^n \cdot \mathbf{g}(\mathbf{x}^{n+1}) = 0. \tag{L.8}$$

For the $n + 1$ step the best choice is to move in a direction where the gradient along the previous direction $\mathbf{d}^n$ remains zero. Since the change in gradient as we move in the new direction $\mathbf{d}^{n+1}$ is $\Delta \mathbf{g} = \alpha^{n+1} \mathbf{H} \cdot \mathbf{d}^{n+1}$, it follows that the desired condition is satisfied if

$$\mathbf{d}^n \cdot \mathbf{H} \cdot \mathbf{d}^{n+1} = 0. \tag{L.9}$$

This equation defines the "conjugate direction" in the sense of orthogonality in the space with metric $\mathbf{H} = H_{ij}$. If this condition is satisfied at each step, then it can be shown (Exercise L.3) that the conjugate condition is maintained for *all steps*

$$\mathbf{d}^{n'} \cdot \mathbf{H} \cdot \mathbf{d}^{n+1} = 0, \text{ for all } n' \leq n. \tag{L.10}$$

The key point is that (unlike SD) each line minimization *preserves* the minimization done in all previous steps and only adds independent (i.e., conjugate) variations. This is manifested in the fact that (unlike the SD method that never reaches the minimum) for a quadratic functional the conjugate gradient method reaches the minimum *exactly* in N steps, where N is the dimension of the space x_i, $i = 1, N$. This is illustrated in Fig. L.1 where the exact solution is reached in two steps for a problem with two variables.

For actual calculations it is useful to specify the new conjugate gradient direction $\mathbf{d}^{n+1}$ in terms of the quantities at hand, the current gradient and the previous direction,

$$\mathbf{d}^{n+1} = \mathbf{g}^{n+1} + \gamma^{n+1} \mathbf{d}^n. \tag{L.11}$$

Also available is the quantity $\mathbf{y}^n = \mathbf{d}^n \cdot \mathbf{H}$, which is needed for the evaluation of F in the line minimization for direction $\mathbf{d}^n$. Using Eqs. (L.8), (L.11) can be written

$$\gamma^{n+1} = -\frac{\langle \mathbf{y}^n | \mathbf{g}^{n+1} \rangle}{\langle \mathbf{y}^n | \mathbf{d}^n \rangle}. \tag{L.12}$$

It is straightforward to show (Exercise L.4) that the directions are also given by

$$\gamma^{n+1} = \frac{\mathbf{g}^{n+1} \cdot \mathbf{g}^{n+1}}{\mathbf{g}^n \cdot \mathbf{g}^n}, \tag{L.13}$$

with the definition $\gamma^1 = 0$. These forms[2] are equivalent for the quadratic case; however, they are different in the applications needed for electronic structure, where there are constraints or nonlinearities (Appendix M).

---

[2] Equation (L.12) is often called the Hestens–Steifel form; Eq. (L.13) is the Fletcher–Reeves expression; and an alternative Pollak–Ribiere form is particularly useful for nonquadratic functionals [776].

How does one apply the CG method to problems that are not quadratic? The basic idea is to define conjugate directions as above, but to carry out the line minimization for the given nonlinear functional. This is essential for the CG algorithm since one must reach the line minimum in order for the new gradient to be perpendicular to the present direction, so that the functional is fully minimized along each direction in turn.

L.4 Quasi-Newton–Raphson Methods

Consider the problem of solving the equation

$$\mathbf{F}(\mathbf{x}) = \mathbf{x}, \tag{L.14}$$

where $\mathbf{x}$ denotes a vector in many dimensions. For example, this could be the problem in Section 7.4 of finding the solution of the Kohn–Sham equations where the output density $n^{out}(\mathbf{r})$ (which is a function of the input density $n^{in}(\mathbf{r})$) is equal to the input density $n^{in}(\mathbf{r})$. This problem has exactly the form of Eq. (L.14) if the density is expanded in a set of M functions $n^{in}(\mathbf{r}) = \sum_k^M x^k h^k(\mathbf{r})$, with $\mathbf{x} = \{x^k\}$. This becomes a minimization problem for the norm of the residual $|\mathbf{R}[\mathbf{x}]|$, where

$$\mathbf{R}[\mathbf{x}] \equiv \mathbf{F}(\mathbf{x}) - \mathbf{x}. \tag{L.15}$$

In Eqs. (7.34) and (13.7) it was shown how to solve this problem if one is in a region where $\mathbf{R}$ is a linear function of $\mathbf{x}$ and the Jacobian,

$$\mathbf{J} \equiv \frac{\delta \mathbf{R}}{\delta \mathbf{x}}, \tag{L.16}$$

is known. Then one can follow the Quasi-Newton–Raphson approach to minimize the residual. In terms of $\mathbf{x}_i$ at step i, the value that would give $\mathbf{r}_{i+1} = 0$ at the next iteration is

$$\mathbf{x}_{i+1} = \mathbf{x}_i - \mathbf{J}^{-1}\mathbf{R}_i. \tag{L.17}$$

The problem is that, in general, the Jacobian is not known (or it is hard to invert) and one needs to resort to other methods that iterate to the solution in a space of functions, i.e., a Krylov subspace.

L.5 Pulay DIIS Full-Subspace Method

The idea behind the discrete inversion in the iterative subspace method[3] [1057, 1058] is to minimize the residual at any step i by using the best possible combination of all previously generated vectors, i.e., making use of the full Krylov subspace.

$$\mathbf{x}_{i+1} = \sum_{j=0}^{i} a_j \mathbf{x}_j = c_0 \mathbf{x}_0 + \sum_{j=1}^{i} c_j \delta \mathbf{x}_j. \tag{L.18}$$

---

[3] Also called the Pulay method; the present discussion follows [1056].

If we assume linearity of the residual near the solution, then

$$\mathbf{R}[\mathbf{x}_{i+1}] = \mathbf{R}\left[\sum_{j=0}^{i} a_j \mathbf{x}_j\right] = \sum_{j=0}^{i} a_j \mathbf{R}[\mathbf{x}_j]. \tag{L.19}$$

The condition is that $\mathbf{x}_{i+1}$ be chosen to minimize the square norm of the residual

$$\langle \mathbf{R}[\mathbf{x}_{i+1}] | \mathbf{R}[\mathbf{x}_{i+1}] \rangle = \sum_{j,k} a_j a_k A_{j,k}; \ A_{j,k} = \langle \mathbf{R}[\mathbf{x}_j] | \mathbf{R}[\mathbf{x}_k] \rangle, \tag{L.20}$$

subject to any auxiliary conditions. In electronic structure problems, the two most relevant conditions are

- electronic bands, where one requires orthonormalization of eigenvectors;
- density mixing, where $\sum_{j=0}^{i} a_j = 1$ for charge conservation.

In the latter case the solution is [1056]

$$a_i = \sum_j A_{j,i}^{-1} \Big/ \sum_{j,k} a_j a_k A_{j,k}^{-1}. \tag{L.21}$$

Through Eq. (L.18), this provides the optimal new vector at each step i in terms of the results of all previous steps. For extremely large problems, such as many eigenvectors for the Schrödinger equation, it is not feasible to store many sets of vectors. However, for density mixing, especially for only a few troublesome components of the density, one can store several previous densities.

Kresse and Furthmüller [1056] have shown that the Pulay DIIS method described above is equivalent to updating a Jacobian that is closely related to the modified Broyden schemes [380, 381]. In addition, van Lenthe and Pulay have shown that it is possible to carry out the Davidson and DIIS algorithms with only three vectors at each step [1059].

L.6 Broyden Jacobian Update Methods

The Broyden method [374] is a way to generate the inverse Jacobian successively in the course of an iterative process.[4] The modified Broyden method [380, 381] given at the end is similar to the result of the DIIS method, except that it explicitly involves only the two states at a time. This method is widely used and it is illuminating to derive the form in steps that show the relevant points.

The method starts with a reasonable guess $\mathbf{J}_0^{-1}$ (e.g., that for linear mixing $\mathbf{J}_0^{-1} = \alpha \mathbf{1}$ [376]). The approximate form may be used for several steps after which the inverse $\mathbf{J}^{-1}$ is improved at subsequent steps. Since the Jacobian is not exact at any step, Eq. (L.17) and the actual calculation at step i provide two quantities: (1) the prediction from Eq. (L.17) for step i, $\delta \mathbf{x}_i = \mathbf{x}_i - \mathbf{x}_{i-1} = -\mathbf{J}_{i-1}^{-1} \mathbf{R}_{i-1}$; and (2) the actual result from step i, the change in

---

[4] The description here follows that of Pickett in [372].

the residual $\delta \mathbf{R}_i = \mathbf{R}_i - \mathbf{R}_{i-1}$. The new, improved $\mathbf{J}_i^{-1}$ is chosen by requiring that at each step i the $\mathbf{J}_i^{-1}$ be able to reproduce the result of the iteration just completed, i.e.,

$$0 = \delta \mathbf{x}_i - \mathbf{J}_i^{-1} \delta \mathbf{R}_i. \tag{L.22}$$

This provides M equations for the M^2 components of $\mathbf{J}_i^{-1}$. The other conditions are fixed by requiring the norm of the change in the Jacobian matrix

$$Q = ||\mathbf{J}_i^{-1} - \mathbf{J}_{i-1}^{-1}|| \tag{L.23}$$

be minimized. The last may be accomplished by the method of Lagrange multipliers and is equivalent to the condition that $\mathbf{J}_i^{-1}$ produces the same result as $\mathbf{J}_{i-1}^{-1}$ acting on *all* vectors orthogonal to the current change $\delta \mathbf{R}_i$. The result is [372, 376] (see Exercise L.8)

$$\mathbf{J}_i^{-1} = \mathbf{J}_{i-1}^{-1} \frac{(\delta \mathbf{x}_i - \mathbf{J}_i^{-1} \delta \mathbf{R}_i) \delta \mathbf{R}_i}{\langle \delta \mathbf{R}_i | \delta \mathbf{R}_i \rangle}. \tag{L.24}$$

As it stands, Eq. (L.24) can be used if the Jacobian matrix is small, e.g., in plane wave methods where only a few troublesome components of the density need to be treated in this way. However, it is not useful in cases where storage of a full Jacobian matrix is not feasible, e.g., in the update of the charge density on a large grid needed in many calculations. Srivastava [376] introduced a way to avoid storage of the matrices completely by using Eq. (L.24) to write the predicted change $\delta \mathbf{x}_{i+1}$ in terms of a sum over all the previous steps involving only the initial $\mathbf{J}_0^{-1}$ (see also [377]).

A modified Broyden method has been proposed by Vanderbilt and Louie [380] and adapted by Johnson [381] to include the advantages of Srivistava's method [376], which requires less storage. The idea is that the requirement that the immediate step be reproduced exactly is too restrictive, and an improved algorithm can take into account information from previous iterations. Then one finds $\mathbf{J}_i^{-1}$ by minimizing a weighted norm

$$Q^{\text{modified}} = \sum_{j=1}^{i} w_j |\delta \mathbf{x}_j - \mathbf{J}_i^{-1} \delta \mathbf{R}_j|^2 + w_0 ||\mathbf{J}_i^{-1} - \mathbf{J}_0^{-1}||. \tag{L.25}$$

This has the advantage that the weights w_j can be chosen to emphasize the most relevant prior steps and the term w_0 adds stability. Vanderbilt and Louie [380] showed a simple example in which the modified method approached the exact Jacobian rapidly, compared to a slower approach using the original Broyden scheme. Clearly, there are strong resemblances to the Pulay DIIS algorithm of the previous section.

L.7 Moments, Maximum Entropy, Kernel Polynomial Method, and Random Vectors

The direct determination of the spectral properties of a Hermitian matrix via conventional Householder tridiagonalization has computational cost scaling as N^3. However, if one is interested only in the density of states of such a matrix (whatever its origin – dynamical matrix, Hamiltonian matrix, etc.), then there are more efficient schemes based on the relative ease of extracting *power moments* of the spectral densities. The utility of moments in physical calculations was recognized before the era of quantum mechanics, when Thirring used moments of the dynamical matrix to estimate thermodynamic quantities [1060]. Montroll employed moments to compute vibrational state densities as referenced in Born and Huang [91], p. 74.

The moments of the eigenvalue spectrum about an energy E_0 are defined as

$$\langle [H - E_0]^n \rangle = \sum_i [\varepsilon_i - E_0]^n = \int d\varepsilon [\varepsilon - E_0]^n n(\varepsilon), \tag{L.26}$$

where $n(\varepsilon)$ is the density of states (see Section 4.7)

$$n(\varepsilon) = \sum_i \delta(\varepsilon - \varepsilon_i). \tag{L.27}$$

The zeroth moment is the total number of states; the first moment, the average eigenvalue; the second, a measure of the spectral width; the third moment, a measure of the spectral asymmetry about E_0; etc. From many moments, one can approximately reconstruct the density of states. Similarly, local information is derived using the local projected density of states, such as the angular momentum projected density around an atomic site in Eq. (16.32) or the basis function projection in Eq. (18.17). Thus the fundamental quantities in electronic structure can be determined from the moments if there are useful ways to compute the moments and there are stable algorithms to reconstruct the spectrum.

The first aspect, finding the moments given the hamiltonian matrix, is beautifully solved by the recursion method [753]. The expressions given in Eq. (18.17) relate the moments to the coefficients generated in the Lanczos algorithm, which have the interpretation of creating a "chain" of hops whereby the hamiltonian connects one state to the next. If the hamiltonian matrix is localized in space (short-range hops) this means that information about the local density of states at a site can be efficiently generated in a small number of applications of the hamiltonian because only hops within some local range are needed, as explained in Chapter 18.

If the global (rather than projected) DOS is needed, one can compute approximate moments of the global DOS by repeated matrix-on-vector operations where the vectors needed have random components (a suitable choice is to sample each component independently from the unit normal distribution). For the global DOS for large matrices, very few vectors are needed to provide moments leading to accurate spectra (there is a "self-averaging," which requires *fewer* vectors for larger system sizes [757]). Very accurate determination of partial integrals of the DOS is another matter and requires more careful convergence of the moment data with respect to random vectors. Much of this was grasped earlier with characteristic prescience by Lanczos [1061].

The second aspect, reconstructing the spectrum, is a long-standing problem in applied mathematics in the nineteenth and twentieth centuries called the "classical moment problem" [1062]:

> Given a finite number of moments over some interval of a nonnegative function, find the function from which the moments arose.

Two classes of practical solutions have emerged. Most naturally, one may adopt a polynomial solution using polynomials suitably orthogonal on the interval. With a sufficient number of moments, it is possible to obtain very accurate reconstructions, e.g., with plausible jagged spikes approximating δ functions. The method is numerically robust [762] and has been extended to nonorthogonal bases [1063]. It is routine in these computations to work with several hundred or more moments.

Alternately, one can seek to find a "best" solution given incomplete information (a finite moment sequence). A modern method that has been applied to this problem is the method of maximum entropy, which utilizes a variational principle to maximize the "entropy" $-\int n(\varepsilon)\ln(n(\varepsilon))$ subject to the constraints that the moment conditions are satisfied [1064]. The utility of maximum entropy for moments was shown with examples by Mead and Papanicolaou [1065]; Skilling [1064] used maximum entropy with random vectors to extract state densities of large matrices; Drabold and Sankey [757] applied the method to electronic structure problems and introduced "importance sampling" in selecting vectors to improve the convergence of integrated quantities (like the band energy for determining Fermi level); and Stephan, Drabold, and Martin [778] demonstrated that this scheme was useful in density functional schemes for determining the Fermi level order-N in several thousand atom models. An example of calculation of the phonon density of states from a sparse dynamical matrix is given in Fig. 18.4. Maximum entropy converges much faster than the orthogonal polynomial solution, but is more delicate numerically and it is difficult to use more than a few hundred moments in current maximum entropy schemes.

SELECT FURTHER READING

Computational physics books:

Koonin, S. E. and Meredith, D. C., *Computational Physics* (Addison Wesley, Menlo Park, CA, 1990).

Press, W. H. and Teukolsky, S. A., *Numerical Recipes* (Cambridge University Press, Cambridge, 1992).

Thijssen, J. M., *Computational Physics* (Cambridge University Press, Cambridge, 2000).

Numerical analysis:

Booten, A. and van der Vorst, H., "Cracking large scale eigenvalue problems, part I: Algorithms," *Comp. in Phys.* 10:239–242 (1996).

Booten, A. and van der Vorst, H., "Cracking large scale eigenvalue problems, part II: Implementations," *Comp. in Phys.* 10:331–334 (1996). [941]

Golub, G. H. and Van Loan, C. F., *Matrix Computations* (Johns Hopkins University Press, Baltimore, MD, 1980).

Heath, M. T., *Scientific Computing: An Introductory Survey* (McGraw-Hill, New York, 1997).

Parlett, B. N., *The Symmetric Eigenvalue Problem* (Prentice Hall, Engelwood Cliffs, NJ, 1980).

Exercises

L.1 Derive the leading error in the finite difference approximation to the second derivative that is $O(h^2)$ and is given explicitly in Eq. (L.2).

L.2 Derive the Numerov expressions (L.3) and (L.4) and show the leading error in the solutions are, respectively, $O(h^4)$ and $O(h^6)$.

L.3 Show that the conjugate gradient minimization equations, Eqs. (L.8) and (L.9), follow from differentiating the functional and assuming it is quadratic. Then derive the key equation, (L.10), that if each direction is made conjugate to the previous one, then it is also conjugate to all previous directions. This can be shown by induction given that each direction is defined to be conjugate to the previous direction and it is a linear combination only of the new steepest descent gradient and the previous direction, as in Eq. (L.11).

L.4 For the quadratic functional Eq. (L.6), show that the conjugate directions Eq. (L.12) are also given by Eq. (L.13).

L.5 Consider a two-dimensional case $F(x, y) = Ax^2 + By^2$, with $B = 10A$. Show that the CG method reaches the exact minimum in two steps, starting from any point (x, y), whereas SD does not. What is the value of F in the SD method after two steps starting from $x = 1$; $y = 1$.

L.6 As the simplest three-dimensional example, consider $F(x, y, z) = Ax^2 + By^2 + Cz^2$, and show that the third direction $\mathbf{d}^3$ is conjugate to the first direction $\mathbf{d}^1 = \mathbf{g}^1$.

L.7 Make a short computer program to do the CG minimization of a function $F = \mathbf{G} \cdot \mathbf{x} + \mathbf{x} \cdot \mathbf{G} \cdot \mathbf{x}$ in any dimension for any $\mathbf{G}$ and $\mathbf{H}$.

L.8 The Broyden method generates a new approximation to the inverse Jacobian $\mathbf{J}_i^{-1}$ at each step i based on the conditions outlined before Eq. (L.24). Verify that $\mathbf{J}_i^{-1}$, defined by Eq. (L.24), satisfies Eq. (L.22) and that $\mathbf{J}_i^{-1} - \mathbf{J}_{i-11}^{-1}$ gives a null result when acting on any residual orthogonal to $\delta \mathbf{R}_i$.

Appendix M

Iterative Methods in Electronic Structure

Summary

This appendix describes technical aspects of advances that have brought entire new classes of problems and properties under the umbrella of *ab initio* electronic structure. The methods belong to general classes of iterative algorithms that have a long history in eigenvalue problems, even though their widespread use in electronic structure in condensed matter followed the work of Car and Parrinello. This chapter is devoted to features particularly relevant to electronic structure, and aspects that are inherent to general numerical algorithms are the topic of Appendix L. The methods may be classified in many ways: as minimization of the energy versus minimization of a residual, single vector update versus full iterative subspace methods, etc. Nevertheless, they can all be brought into a common framework, in which the key features are to

- replace matrix diagonalization by iterative equations for the wavefunctions ψ_i in an iterative (Krylov) subspace;
- find new ψ_i^{n+1} using ψ_i^n (and possibly previous $\psi_i^{n'}$, $n' < n$) and the gradient $dE/d\psi_i^{n*} = H_{KS}\psi_i^n$ (the algorithms for this step is where methods differ); and
- for plane waves, replace dense matrix multiplications with fast Fourier transforms (FFTs).

M.1 Why Use Iterative Methods?

Electronic structure methods can be grouped into two camps differentiated by the types of basis functions. Methods such as LCAO and LMTO are predicated upon the goal of constructing a *minimal basis* of size N_b; the work goes into constructing the basis, which may be highly optimized for a given class of problems. Except for very large systems (see Chapter 18), the hamiltonian is expressed as a small, dense matrix of size $N_b \times N_b$, for which it is appropriate to employ traditional dense matrix diagonalization techniques, for which the computational effort scales as N_b^3 or as $N_e N_b^2$, where N_e is the number of desired eigenvectors.

On the other hand, methods that use general bases such as plane waves[1] and grids often involve a much larger number of basis functions than the number of desired eigenstates ($N_b \gg N_e$); the hamiltonian is very simple to construct and it can be made sparse, i.e., mainly zero elements so that only the nonzero elements need to be calculated and/or stored. Except for small problems, it is much more efficient to use iterative methods, in which the $N_b \times N_b$ hamiltonian is never explicitly constructed and the computational effort scales as $N_e^2 N_b$ or as $N_e^2 N_b \ln(N_b)$. These approaches have been applied most successfully to plane waves (where they are built upon the pioneering work of Car and Parrinello [85] using fast Fourier transforms and regular grids as described in Section M.11), and real-space methods [568]: finite difference [569–572], finite element [585, 586]; multigrid [576, 582, 584]; and wavelets [1066, 1067]. See [572] for a review of methods.

The iterative methods described in this appendix have much in common with the problem of finding the self-consistent Kohn–Sham potential, which is in general an iterative process as described in Chapter 7, and "order-N" approaches of Chapter 18, which are useful for very large systems with iterative methods employed that take advantage of the sparseness of the hamiltonian. Since many of the methods employed are useful in many contexts, the general forms for the methods are discussed in Appendix L and their application to calculations of eigenvalues and eigenvectors emphasized in this appendix.

We first consider the problem of solving the Schrödinger equation for a fixed hamiltonian

$$(H - \varepsilon)|\psi\rangle = 0. \tag{M.1}$$

This is the problem in many-body simulations where the hamiltonian never changes, and it is the inner loop in a Kohn–Sham problem where the effective independent-particle hamiltonian may be taken as fixed during the iterations (the solution inside of the loop in Fig. 7.2) to find the eigenvalues and eigenvectors of that effective hamiltonian. Iterative methods also have the advantage that the hamiltonian can be updated simultaneously with improvements to the wavefunctions (e.g., in the Car–Parrinello unified method, Chapter 19) to achieve self-consistency as well as to solve the Schrödinger equations. However, logically it is simpler to first consider the case of a fixed hamiltonian after which the extension is not difficult.

M.2 Simple Relaxation Algorithms

The algorithm [1068] proposed by Jacobi in 1848 is in many ways the grandfather of iterative eigenvalue methods. The basic idea is to iterate a from of the equation

$$(H - \varepsilon^n)|\psi^n\rangle = |R[\psi^n]\rangle, \tag{M.2}$$

where n is the iteration step, $|\psi^n\rangle$ and ε^n are approximate eigenvectors and eigenvalues, and $|R[\psi^n]\rangle$ is a "residual" vector. The iterations continue with a particular choice of the

---

[1] The APW, LAPW, and PAW methods are in some ways intermediate and it may be possible to take advantage of both types of approaches.

improved eigenvector $|\psi^{n+1}\rangle$ and eigenvalue ε^{n+1} until the eigenvalue is converged or the norm of the residual vanishes to within some tolerance [1069].

If the matrix is diagonally dominant (as is the case for the hamiltonian expressed in the bases most commonly chosen in electronic structure calculations) then we can rewrite the eigenvalue problem, Eq. (M.1), as

$$|\psi\rangle = D^{-1}(H - \varepsilon)|\psi\rangle + |\psi\rangle, \tag{M.3}$$

where D is a non-singular matrix. This form suggests many variations and the choice of D can be viewed as a "preconditioning" of the hamiltonian operator, as discussed below. If we define the iteration sequence [1069]

$$\varepsilon^n = \frac{\langle\psi^n|H|\psi^n\rangle}{\langle\psi^n|\psi^n\rangle},$$

$$\delta\psi^{n+1} = D^{-1}(H - \varepsilon^n)\psi^n,$$

$$\psi^{n+1} = \psi^n + \delta\psi^{n+1}, \tag{M.4}$$

then the middle equation of Eq. (M.4) is just the linear set of equations

$$D\delta\psi^{n+1} = R^n \text{ or } \delta\psi^{n+1} = D^{-1}R^n \equiv KR^n, \tag{M.5}$$

where R^n is the residual at step n and $K \equiv D^{-1}$.

The sequence Eqs. (M.4) with (M.5) corresponds to updates of ψ using the residual R multiplied by a "preconditioning" matrix K (see Section M.3). For the methods to be efficient, the matrix D must be easier to invert than the original matrix $(H - \varepsilon)$, and yet be chosen so that the change $\delta\psi^{n+1}$ is as close as possible to the improvement needed to bring ψ^n to the correct eigenvector. From perturbation theory we know that if the hamiltonian is diagonally dominant a good choice is D equal to the diagonal part of H (the choice made by Jacobi). If D is the lower (or upper) triangular part of H, then this becomes the Gauss–Seidel relaxation method [776, 1070], which is useful in "sweep methods" where the points on one side have already been updated. At each iteration the new vector is updated with only information from the previous step.

M.3 Preconditioning

The basic idea behind "preconditioning" is to modify the functional dependence on the variables to be more "isotropic," i.e., to make the curvature more similar for the different variables, which is exactly the idea behind the improved convergence in Eq. (M.5). For the problems encountered in electronic structure, it often happens that the original formulation is very badly conditioned; but on physical grounds it is simple to see how to improve the conditioning. In general, the choice of formula depends on the problem and we will be content to list two characteristic examples.

The simplest example is the energy expressed in a plane wave basis, where the functions are expressed as $\psi_{i,\mathbf{k}}(\mathbf{r}) = \exp(i\mathbf{k} \cdot \mathbf{r})u_{i,\mathbf{k}}(\mathbf{r})$, with u the Bloch function given in Eq. (12.12), where $c_{i,m}^n(\mathbf{k})$ are the $m = 1, N_{PW}$ variables describing the $i = 1, N_e$ eigenvectors at step n. Because high Fourier components $|\mathbf{k} + \mathbf{G}_m|$ have high kinetic energy, the total energy varies much more rapidly as a function of coefficients $c_{i,m}^n(\mathbf{k})$ with large $|\mathbf{G}_m|$ than for coefficients with small $|\mathbf{G}_m|$. Preconditioning can be used to modify the gradients and cancel this effect; a simple form suggested in [1071] is

$$K(x) = \frac{27 + 18x + 12x^2 + 8x^3}{27 + 18x + 12x^2 + 8x^3 + 16x^4}, \tag{M.6}$$

where

$$x_i^n(\mathbf{G}_m) = \frac{1}{2}\frac{|\mathbf{k} + \mathbf{G}_m|^2}{T_i^n}, \tag{M.7}$$

which multiplies each steepest descent vector $g_i^n(\mathbf{G}_m)$. Here $x_i^n(\mathbf{G}_m)$ is the ratio of the kinetic energy of the $|\mathbf{k} + \mathbf{G}_m|$ Fourier component to the kinetic energy T_i^n of the state i at step n. Since $K \propto 1/|\mathbf{G}_m|^2$ for large $|\mathbf{G}_m|$, this cancels the increase in $g_i^n(\mathbf{G}_m)$, which grows as $|\mathbf{G}_m|^2$.

Seitsonen [1072] proposed to precondition the steepest descent vector in real-space methods by extending the form of Eq. (M.6) to represent a local kinetic energy at point $\mathbf{r}$. The variable x in Eq. (M.6) is defined to be

$$x_i^n(\mathbf{r}) = A\frac{|\varepsilon_i^m - V(\mathbf{r})|}{T_i^n}, \tag{M.8}$$

which is the ratio of the local kinetic energy $|\varepsilon_i^n - V(r)|$ to the total kinetic energy for state i, $T_i^n = \langle \psi_i^n|\nabla^2|\psi_i^n\rangle$, and A is an adjustable parameter. At each step n the factor $K(x_i^n(\mathbf{r}))$ multiplies the residual for state i at each point $\mathbf{r}$ of the real-space grid as in Eq. (M.5).

M.4 Iterative (Krylov) Subspaces

Iterative methods are based on repeated application of some operator A to generate new vectors. Starting from a trial vector ψ^0, a set of vectors $A^n\psi^0$ is generated by recursive application of A. Linear combinations of the vectors can be chosen to construct the set $\{\psi^0, \psi^1, \psi^2, \ldots\}$, which forms a Krylov subspace [1073]. In many cases, an accurate solution for desired states can be found in terms of a number of states in this new basis that is much smaller than the number of states in the original basis. The distinction between the various methods is the choice of operator A and the way that new vectors ψ^{n+1} are created at each step using $A\psi^n$ and the previously generated $\psi^i, i = 0, n$.

There are three choices for A that are most directly applicable to problems related to electronic structure: the (shifted) hamiltonian, $A = [H - \varepsilon]$; the shifted inverse hamiltonian operator, $A = [H - \varepsilon]^{-1}$; and the imaginary time propagator, $A = \exp(-\delta\tau(H - \varepsilon))$. Each of these choices has important advantages. The first is closely related to the variational Schrödinger and Kohn–Sham equations, Eqs. (3.13) and (7.11), which leads to helpful physical interpretations and suggests solution in terms of well-established minimization techniques and subspace matrix diagonalization techniques [1054, 1073, 1074]. The second choice, employing inverse powers, is especially appropriate for finding eigenvectors close to a trial eigenvalue ε. The inverse is useful for proofs of principle, but in practice one uses approximations with easily invertible operators; these are closely related to perturbation expansions for the wavefunctions and eigenvalues. Imaginary time projection has the advantage that it is closely related to real-time methods for time-dependent phenomena (see Chapter 21) and to statistical mechanics involving thermal expectation values, where $\beta = 1/k_B T \to \delta\tau$.

Methods differ in the extent of the Krylov subspace explicitly treated at each iteration. Simple relaxation methods such as the Jacobi algorithm find the new approximate eigenvector ψ^{n+1} in terms of the previous ψ^n only. This is analogous to steepest descent minimization. Others, such as the Lanczos, Davidson, and the RMM–DIIS (Section M.7) methods consider the entire subspace generated up to the given iteration. In general, a great price must be paid to keep the entire Krylov subspace for very large problems; however, the widely used Lanczos and conjugate gradient (CG) minimization methods are full subspace methods, able to generate a new vector orthogonal (or conjugate) to *all* previous vectors even though ψ^{n+1} is found only in terms of the previous two vectors ψ^n and ψ^{n-1}. Thus these methods can be much more powerful than simple relaxation methods, with only a moderate increase in requirements at each step of the iteration. The original Davidson method [1075] requires keeping the entire subspace, but it can also be cast in a form requiring only three vectors using a CG approach [1059].

M.5 The Lanczos Algorithm and Recursion

The Lanczos method [1076] was one of the first iterative methods used by modern computers to solve eigenvalue problems. It is remarkably simple and amazingly powerful as a tool to bring out physical interpretations and analogies. The algorithm automatically generates an orthogonal basis (a Krylov or iterative subspace) in which the given operator A is tridiagonal. (In electronic structure problems $A = H$, where H is often the hamiltonian.) It is especially powerful for generating a number of the lowest (or highest) eigenvectors of large matrices. The simplest version suffers from the "Lanczos disease" of spurious solutions due to numerical rounding errors as the number of desired eigenvectors increases; however, this can be easily controlled by orthogonalizing after a number of iterative steps. In addition, it can be formulated as a continued fraction, which leads to powerful methods for finding moments of the spectral distribution.

The Lanczos algorithm proceeds as follows (good descriptions can be found in [485] and [1077]): starting with a normalized trial vector ψ_1, form a second vector $\psi_2 = C_2 [A\psi_1 - A_{11}\psi_1]$, where $A_{11} = \langle\psi_1|A|\psi_1\rangle$ and C_2 is chosen so that ψ_2 is normalized. It is easy to see that ψ_2 is orthogonal to ψ_1. Subsequent vectors are constructed recursively by

$$\psi_{n+1} = C_{n+1}\left[A\psi_n - A_{nn}\psi_n - A_{nn-1}\psi_{n-1}\right]. \tag{M.9}$$

The matrix $A_{nn'}$ is explicitly tridiagonal since Eq. (M.9) shows that A operating on ψ_n yields only terms proportional to ψ_n, ψ_{n-1}, and ψ_{n+1}. Furthermore, each vector ψ_n is orthogonal to *all* the other vectors, as may be shown by induction (see Exercise M.1). Going to step M yields a tridiagonal matrix

$$
A = \begin{bmatrix}
\alpha_1 & \beta_2 & & & & \\
\beta_2 & \alpha_2 & \beta_3 & & & \\
& \beta_3 & \alpha_3 & \cdot & & \\
& & & \cdot & \cdot & \cdot \\
& & & & \cdot & \cdot & \beta_M \\
& & & & & \beta_M & \alpha_M
\end{bmatrix}, \tag{M.10}
$$

where α and β are given by Eq. (M.9). Standard routines exist to find eigenvalues of an order-M tridiagonal matrix in time order-M. (The ideas are straightforward and can be cast in the form of the roots of a function defined by a recursive set of polynomials [485]. See Exercise M.2.) Eigenvectors can easily be found by inverse iteration if the eigenvalues are known. If the original basis contains N vectors, then N steps are required to generate the full hamiltonian in this tridiagonal form.

The importance of the method is that eigenvectors and eigenvalues near the bottom and top of the spectrum can be determined with great accuracy *without generating the entire matrix*. One can understand why the highest and lowest vectors are generated first by noting that if one starts with a trial vector ψ_1 that is a linear combination of eigenvectors, each step of Eq. (M.9) is an operation by H that increases the weight of those eigenvectors that are farthest away in energy from the average energy of the trial state. Since the average energy must be somewhere in the middle of the spectrum the states at the edges are projected out with greatest efficiency. In typical cases involving millions of states, a few steps of the algorithm are sufficient to find the ground state with great precision [1077].

There are many variations in the way the Lanczos algorithm can be used. For example, the recursive relation Eq. (M.9) can be used to generate a matrix of size $M \times M$, which is diagonalized to find the desired state, e.g., the lowest eigenstate. The state thus found can be used as the starting vector for the next iteration, etc., until the desired accuracy is achieved. This is particularly stable [1077] and useful in a block form for finding several states. This approach may even be used for M as small as $M = 2$, which makes a particularly efficient algorithm for the ground state that does not require storing many vectors.

The Lanczos algorithm is widely used for a few extreme eigenvalues in extremely large problems such as many-body problems where it is synonymous with "exact diagonalization." The most complete application in large-scale electronic structure calculations has been presented by Wang and Zunger [1078], who have incorporated procedures for avoiding spurious states.

The Arnoldi method [776] is a variation of Lanczos that explicitly orthogonalizes each vector ψ_n to all the previous vectors by a Gram–Schmidt procedure. This eliminates the instability and allows calculation of as many eigenvectors as desired. This approach can be applied to nonhermitian matrices.

An elegant consequence of the Lanczos tridiagonal form is a "continued fraction" representation of the spectrum for any dynamical correlation function, expressed as a function of complex frequency z. This leads to the recursion method [732, 753], for which pertinent aspects are summarized in Section 18.4.

M.6 Davidson Algorithms

Davidson [1059, 1075, 1079–1081] has devised methods that are now widely applied to electronic structure problems. There are a number of variations that cannot be covered here. A primary point is that the Davidson approach is closely related to the Lanczos algorithm, but adapted to be more efficient for problems in which the operator is diagonally dominant. This is often the case in electronic structure problems, e.g., plane wave algorithms.

The flavor of the Davidson methods can be illustrated by defining the diagonal part of the hamiltonian matrix as $D_{mm'} = H_{mm}\delta_{mm'}$ and rewriting the eigenvalue problem $H\psi = \varepsilon\psi$ as

$$(H - D)\psi = (\varepsilon I - D)\psi, \tag{M.11}$$

or

$$\psi = (\varepsilon I - D)^{-1}(H - D)\psi. \tag{M.12}$$

Here I is the unit matrix, inversion of $I - D$ is trivial, and $H - D$ involves only off-diagonal elements. The latter equation is very similar to perturbation theory and suggests iterative procedures that converge rapidly if the diagonal part of the hamiltonian is dominant. An algorithm has been suggested by Lenthe and Pulay [1059] that involves three vectors at each step of the iteration.

M.7 Residual Minimization in the Subspace – RMM–DIIS

The approaches described up to now (and the minimization methods described below) converge to the lowest state with no problems because the ground state is an absolute minimum. In order to find higher states, they must ensure orthogonality, either implicitly as in the Lanczos methods or by explicit orthogonalization. The residual minimization method (RMM) proposed by Pulay [1057, 1058] avoids this requirement and converges to the state in the spectrum with eigenvalue closest to the trial eigenvalue ε because it minimizes the norm of a "residual vector" instead of the energy. Since the approach of Pulay minimizes the residual in the full Krylov iterative space generated by previous iterations, the method is known as RMM–DIIS for "residual minimization method by direct inversion in the iterative subspace." The general idea is to replace the last equation in Eq. (M.5) with

$$\psi^{n+1} = c_0\psi^0 + \sum_{j=1}^{n+1} c_j\delta\psi^j, \tag{M.13}$$

where the entire set of c_j is chosen to minimize the norm of the residual R^{n+1}. (Preconditioning can also be applied at each step [1056] to speed the convergence.) The c_j coefficients can be obtained by diagonalizing the hamiltonian in the iterative subspace $\{\psi^0, \psi^1, \psi^2, \ldots, \psi^n\}$, which is a miniscule operation since the number of vectors is at most 10 or so. The time-consuming step is the operation $H\psi$, which is a matrix operation requiring, in general, $O(N_b^2)$ operations for each eigenvector ψ, where N_b is the size of the basis. However, for sparse operations this reduces to $O(N_b)$ for large bases, and to $O(N_b \ln(N_b))$ if FFTs are used as described in Section M.11. In practice, for large problems, it is prohibitive to store many vectors and only small matrices are actually diagonalized corresponding to only a few steps n before restarting the process.

The application of this approach in electronic structure was initiated by Wood and Zunger [1082] and used subsequently by many authors in various modifications [1056, 1069, 1083]. The DIIS method involves construction of a full matrix of the size of the subspace, which can be efficient so long as the matrix is small and all the vectors spanning the space can be stored. This can be achieved in solving the Kohn–Sham equations in two regimes. If the number of eigenstates needed is small, then all states can be generated at once using the RMM–DIIS approach. If the number of eigenstates needed is large, then the problem can be broken up into energy ranges, and a few states with eigenvalues nearest the chosen energy can be generated by solving a small matrix equation. In this case, care must be taken not to miss or to overcount eigenstates [1056]. A great advantage of this method compared to the conjugate gradient methods of Section M.8 is that any eigenvector can be found even in the middle of the spectrum with no explicit need to require orthogonality to the other vectors.

M.8 Solution by Minimization of the Energy Functional

The energy minimization approach has the virtue that it parallels exactly the physical picture of minimizing the total energy and the analytic variational equations Eqs. (3.10)–(3.12) and (7.8), which is also given below in Eq. (M.15). To accomplish the minimization one can utilize the steepest descent (SD) and conjugate gradient (CG) algorithms, which are general minimization methods widely used in numerical analysis [776, 1054] and in electronic structure calculations [369, 385, 1071, 1084, 1085]. As in all iterative methods, one starts from trial functions ψ_i^0, for the $i = 1, N$ orbitals, and generates improved functions ψ_i^n by n successive iterations. The basic SD and CG algorithms are described in Appendix L; however, applications in electronic structure require special choices and modifications due to the *constraint of orthonormality* of the functions ψ_i^n. The explicit equations and the sequence of operations in electronic structure calculations are given in Fig. M.1 which is described in this section.

Minimization Algorithm with Constraints

The analytic variational equations, Eqs. (3.10)–(3.12) and (7.8), including the constraint of orthonormality follow from the Lagrange multiplier formulation[2] with

$$\mathcal{L} = E[\psi_i] - \sum_{ij} \Lambda_{ij} \left(\int d\mathbf{r} \psi_i^*(\mathbf{r}) \psi_j(\mathbf{r}) - \delta_{ij} \right), \qquad (M.14)$$

---

[2] Note the similarity to the lagrangian in the Car–Parrinello method, Chapter 19, where there the "fictitious electronic mass" is also added.

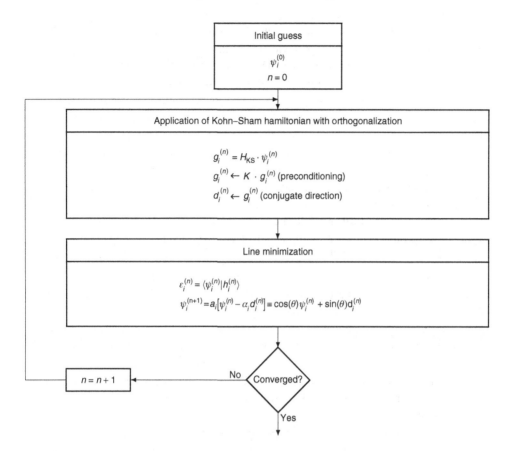

Figure M.1. Iterative loop for solving the non-self-consistent Schrödinger equation in the "band-by-band" conjugate gradient method [385, 1071] (or steepest descent where $d_i = g_i$), using the notation of Appendix L. For unconstrained functionals of nonorthonormal orbitals (Eq. (M.16) or Eq. (18.26)), this is the usual SD or CG method and no other steps are needed. If the constraint of orthonormality is explicitly imposed, then in addition to the steps shown there are orthonormalization operations $g_i^{(n)} \leftarrow g_i^{(n)} \perp (\psi_1, \psi_2, \ldots, \psi_{i-1}; \psi_i^{(n)})$; $d_i^{(n)} \leftarrow d_i^{(n)} \perp (\psi_1, \psi_2, \ldots, \psi_{i-1}; \psi_i^{(n)})$.

where $E[\psi_i]$ is the usual Kohn–Sham expression for energy, Eq. (7.5). The derivative of the lagrangian gives the steepest descent direction including the constraint

$$\frac{\delta \mathcal{L}}{\delta \psi_i^*} = H_{KS}\psi_i - \sum_j \Lambda_{ij}\psi_j. \qquad (M.15)$$

This is completely sufficient for infinitesimal variations; however, for finite steps in a numerical procedure additional steps must be taken to conserve orthonormality.

In Car–Parrinello MD simulations (Chapter 19), constraints are enforced using a Lagrange multiplier in a way that conserves energy [788]. Minimization methods have the opposite philosophy: the goal is *energy minimization*, by loosing energy as efficiently as possible to reach the ground state (which of course must obey the constraints). In SD and CG minimization, the constraint is violated at each step, so that orthonormalization is needed after each of the intermediate steps. The most common method is the Gram–Schmidt procedure, which produces one of the possible sets of orthonormal vectors.

There are two basic approaches for SD or CG minimization in electronic structure: "band-by-band" [1071] and "all-bands" [1085]. The former approach diagonalizes the hamiltonian, i.e., all the desired eigenvalues and vectors are found. The latter finds vectors that span the desired subspace, which is sufficient for many purposes; subspace diagonalization can be added if needed. We will describe the steps in the "band-by-band" method; the only change needed for "all bands" is that all desired eigenvectors $i = 1, N_e$ are treated together as a "supervector" in each line minimization. The basic strategy is outlined in Fig. M.1 and further details are given in [385, 1071]. The algorithm for finding the direction in Hilbert space for minimization of ψ_i^n, the ith vector at step n, is as follows: calculate the SD gradient $g_i^{(n)} = H_{KS}\psi_i^n$ as in Fig. M.1; orthogonalize $g_i^{(n)}$ to all the previously calculated eigenvectors ψ_j, $j < i$, and to the present vector ψ_i^n; precondition and orthonormalize; find the conjugate direction $d_i^{(n)}$ in the case of CG minimization followed by another orthonormalization.

The next step is line minimization, i.e., $\psi_i^n \to \psi_i^{n+1} = a\psi + b\Delta\psi$ to find the minimum eigenvalue ε_i as a function of a and b. A simple procedure to maintain normalization is to construct the new vector as $\cos(\theta)\psi + \sin(\theta)\Delta\psi$, *and* minimize as a function of θ. Since both ψ and $\Delta\psi$ are orthogonal to the previous vectors by construction, this maintains orthonormalization along the line. Repeating for $i = 1, N_e$, produces the desired set of eigenvectors ψ_i, $i = 1, N_e$.

The CG method is well known to speed convergence greatly in some problems, as discussed in Appendix L. However, the basic ideas of CG are violated by the constraints or for nonlinear functionals (as is the case for the unconstrained quadratic functionals in Section M.8); there is no proof that the new direction is conjugate to all previous directions. Furthermore, the two formulas for the CG direction, Eqs. (L.12) and (L.13), are no longer equivalent and tests must be made to find the most efficient approach in any given problem.[3]

Finally, there is another important choice: when to update the density $n(\mathbf{r})$ and the potential $V_{\text{eff}}(\mathbf{r})$ in the Kohn–Sham or any other self-consistent method. The "band-by-band" method has the advantage that one can update during or after the line minimization for each band. If there are many bands, each update of the density is a small perturbation, which can improve convergence (see Section 7.4). If the update is done after all bands are completed, then various extrapolation techniques can be used to choose a new $V_{\text{eff}}^{n+1}(\mathbf{r})$ given the potential and/or density at previous steps $n, n - 1, \ldots$. In addition, there are

---

[3] The widely used form in Eq. (L.13) does not converge for the simplest case of a fixed hamiltonian; however, it may still be useful if one only needs inaccurate solutions for a given hamiltonian in a self-consistency cycle.

choices of the way to update the density most effectively during iterations toward self-consistency or when the atoms move [1086].

Functionals of Nonorthogonal Orbitals

One can also construct functionals that do not require orthonormal orbitals so that the SD and CG methods can be used directly. One approach is the CG method of [1084], where the density and energy are defined using well-known expressions in terms of the inverse overlap matrix S_{ij}^{-1}, where $S_{ij}^{n} = \langle \psi_i^n | \psi_j^n \rangle$ at step n (see also Section 18.6). Using the expressions in Section 7.3, such as Eq. (7.20) the energy can be written as

$$E_{KS} = \sum_{ij} \langle \psi_i | H_{KS} | \psi_j \rangle S_{ij}^{-1} + G[n]. \tag{M.16}$$

Another approach is described in Chapter 18: to define a modified functional, Eq. (18.26), that can be minimized with no constraint and which equals the Kohn–Sham energy at the minimum. The new functional is closely related to Eq. (M.16), except that the inverse matrix is replaced by $S^{-1} = [1 + (S - 1)]^{-1} \rightarrow [1 - (S - 1)] = 2 - S$. This can be viewed as the first term [768] in the expansion of S^{-1} or as an interpretation [769] of the Lagrange equations, (M.15).

Nonextremal Eigenstates

How can one use minimization methods to find states in the middle of a spectrum? The first and simplest approach follows by noting that the eigenfunctions of the "folded" operator $(H - \varepsilon)^2$ are the same as those of H, and the eigenvalues are always positive with absolute minimum for the state with eigenvalue closest to ε. Any minimization method or power method (such as Lanczos) that rapidly converges to extreme states can be used to find the states closest to ε. However, there is a problem with this approach due to poor convergence that is inherent in the use of the "folded" operator $(H - \varepsilon)^2$. The eigenvalue spectrum of the squared operator is compressed $\propto (\varepsilon_i - \varepsilon)^2$ close to the chosen energy ε, making the problem poorly conditioned and leading to difficulties in separating the states in the desired energy range near ε. Nevertheless, there is an important case where the method is effective: the states closest to the gap (the HOMO and LUMO) in a semiconductor or insulator [1087] can be found choosing ε in the gap. Since there are no states with very small values of $\varepsilon_i - \varepsilon$, the spectrum has a positive lower bound and there is no essential difficulty. More than one state can be found if orthonormalization is explicitly required or if a "block" method of several states is used.

A much more robust method is the "shift and invert" approach often attributed to Ericsson and Ruhe [1088], which is a transformation of the Lanczos method. There is a price to pay for the inversion, but the full inverse is not required – only the operation of the inverse on vectors. The advantage is that the spectrum is spread out near the desired energy ε making it easier to obtain the eigenstates near ε. In fact, if the eigenvalues are separated by $\approx \Delta E$, the separation of the eigenvalues of the shift-invert operator is $\propto \Delta E / (\varepsilon_i - \varepsilon)^2$.

M.9 Comparison/Combination of Methods: Minimization of Residual or Energy

A comparison of the CG and RMM–DIIS methods has been presented by Kresse and Furthmüller [1056]. The methods require very similar operations except that CG minimization requires explicit orthonormalization of each vector at each step. They report that for large systems, orthonormalization becomes the dominant factor because one vector must be orthonormalized to a large number of other vectors at every single band update. This requires access to memory, which then dominates over the cost of the floating point operations. The RMM–DIIS method operates on each vector separately and needs no such orthonormalization, except at intervals during the iterations because the vectors may become nonorthogonal due to numerical error. However, for small systems, the cost can be comparable. The main disadvantage of RMM–DIIS is that it always finds the vector closest to the trial vector, so that care must be taken to find all the vectors.

Various algorithms are used in the VASP code [1056] and many examples of convergence are given in [1056] and in the documentation at the VASP website.

M.10 Exponential Projection in Imaginary Time

The Schrödinger equation in imaginary time $\tau = it$ is

$$-\frac{\mathrm{d}\psi}{\mathrm{d}\tau} = H\psi, \tag{M.17}$$

which has the formal solution

$$\psi(\tau) = \mathrm{e}^{-H\tau}\psi(0). \tag{M.18}$$

It is straightforward to see that the operation in Eq. (M.18) projects out of the ground state as $\tau \to \infty$.

This is a widely used approach in many problems (e.g., many-body quantum Monte Carlo simulations) and it has the conceptual advantage that it is closely related to time-dependent phenomena and to statistical mechanics. It has not been widely applied in solving the Kohn–Sham equations for condensed matter, but has been adapted to calculations on electrons confined to "quantum dot" structures [764].

M.11 Algorithmic Complexity: Transforms and Sparse Hamiltonians

All iterative methods replace diagonalization of the hamiltonian matrix by the application of an operator $\hat{A}$, such as the hamiltonian $\hat{H}$ or a function of $\hat{H}$,

$$H_{\mathrm{KS}}\psi_i = \frac{\delta E_{\mathrm{KS}}}{\delta \psi_i^*} \equiv -F_i^e, \tag{M.19}$$

to approximate wavefunctions, where we have omitted spin and space labels. The interpretation as a gradient of the total energy follows from the Kohn–Sham equations, Eqs. (7.8) and (7.12), which can be considered as a the negative of a generalized "force" on the electrons $-F_i^e$. The solution at the minimum is that the force be zero, and iterative procedures arrive at this condition in various ways.

In this appendix we will consider plane waves as the primary example for iterative methods. (It is straightforward to translate the arguments and algorithms for other bases, e.g., real-space grids treated in Section 12.8.) The explicit form of Eq. (M.19) needed for plane waves is given by (using Eq. (12.9))

$$-F_i(\mathbf{G}_m) = \sum_{m'} H_{m,m'}(\mathbf{k}) c_{i,m'}(\mathbf{k}), \tag{M.20}$$

where the variables in the wavefunctions are the $c_{n,m}(\mathbf{k})$ coefficients in the Bloch functions (see Eq. (12.12)),

$$u_{i\mathbf{k}}(\mathbf{r}) = \frac{1}{\sqrt{\Omega_{\text{cell}}}} \sum_m c_{i,m}(\mathbf{k}) \exp(i\mathbf{G}_m \cdot \mathbf{r}). \tag{M.21}$$

Here $i = 1, N_e$, where N_e is the number of desired eigenvectors (often the number of filled bands) and $m = 1, N_{\text{PW}}$, where $N_{\text{PW}} = N_b$ is the number of plane waves included in the basis. Applied straightforwardly, however, this does *not* lead to an efficient algorithm for plane waves. The reason is that the matrix operator form for $H_{m,m'}(\mathbf{k})$ in plane waves $\mathbf{G}_m$, $\mathbf{G}_{m'}$ given in Eq. (12.10) is a dense matrix due to the fact that the potential part $V_{\text{eff}}(\mathbf{G}_m - \mathbf{G}_{m'})$ is, in general, nonzero for all $\mathbf{G}_m$, $\mathbf{G}_{m'}$. Multiplication by a full square matrix on each of the N_e eigenvectors requires $N_e N_{\text{PW}}^2$ operations. In addition, there are other operations such as construction of the charge density in real space that require convolutions in Fourier space that involve $O(N_e N_{\text{PW}}^2)$ operations if done by the direct sums over $\mathbf{G}$ vectors as Eq. (12.29).

How can an efficient *sparse* algorithm be created for plane waves? The idea has already been used in Section 12.7 to calculate the density from the wavefunctions using fast Fourier transforms (FFTs) and the fact that the density is easily expressed in real space as $n(\mathbf{r}_j) = \sum_{i,\mathbf{k}} |u_{i,\mathbf{k}}(\mathbf{r}_j)|^2$. If each wavefunction is expanded in N_{PW} plane waves, the density requires a larger number of Fourier components $\bar{N}_{\text{PW}}$ (see explanation below). In order to calculate the density each wavefunction is represented by $c_{i,m}(\mathbf{k})$ with $m = 1, N_{\text{PW}}$ nonzero components and the other $\bar{N}_{\text{PW}} - N_{\text{PW}}$ components set equal to zero. This expanded $c_{i,m}(\mathbf{k})$ is then transformed using an FFT to a grid in real space, leading to the Bloch function Eq. (M.21) on a grid of $\bar{N}_{\text{grid}} = \bar{N}_{\text{PW}}$ regularly spaced points $\mathbf{r}_j$. The density is then simply the sum of squares of the wavefunctions at each point, as shown in Fig. 12.4.

Now consider the operation $H\psi_i$ needed in Eq. (M.20) (and the corresponding equations (19.14), (M.2), or (M.15)). Multiplication of the kinetic energy term is very simple since the kinetic energy part of $H_{m,m'}(\mathbf{k})$ given by Eq. (12.10) is a diagonal matrix in Fourier space. On the other hand, multiplication by V is simple in real space, where V is diagonal. The operations are done by FFTs as shown in the sequence of steps in Fig. M.2 very much like the operations for the charge density. The FFTs are done on an expanded grid with $\bar{N}_{\text{PW}}$ points and the new wavefunction is truncated to the original size N_{PW} when

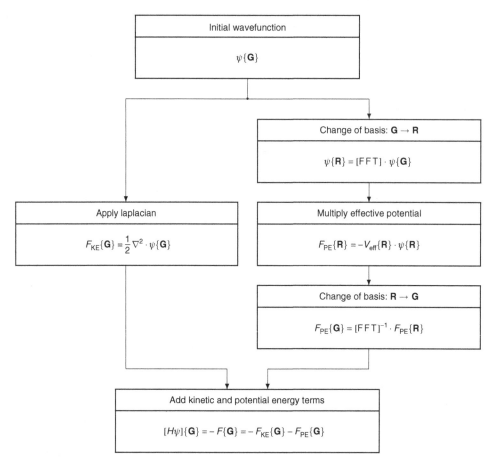

Figure M.2. Schematic representation describing the application of the hamiltonian using Fourier transforms (FFTs). The "force" in Eq. (M.19) is denoted by F_i. The operations are diagonal in each space respectively as long as the potential is local; nonlocal pseudopotentials require generalization to a nonlocal expression on the grid points in real space.

the results are collected in Fourier space. This procedure can be used in any of the iterative plane wave methods described here as well as in the Car–Parrinello method of Chapter 19.

Clearly, this approach can be applied to any operator A involving the hamiltonian. In general, additional applications of the FFT will be needed; however, this need not be a major increase in complexity. In particular, powers of H may be treated by repeated application of the FFT.

Aliasing and the FFT Transforms

When is the FFT operation exact? Clearly, the Fourier analysis is a mathematical identity if done with an infinite number of plane waves. But the question is: What is required for the FFT operations to give the exact answers for a given finite basis of plane waves? One of the great advantages of the plane wave method is that it truly is a basis, i.e., it is variational and the energy always decreases as more plane waves are added. We do not want to add some uncontrolled approximation that would destroy this property. See Exercise M.3 for further discussion.

For the density, it is easy to see the required conditions. If the wavefunction is limited to Fourier components with $|\mathbf{G}| < |\mathbf{G}_{max}|$, then the density can have components up to $|2\mathbf{G}_{max}|$. If the box for the FFT is defined to be *greater than twice as large as* $|\mathbf{G}_{max}|$ *in all directions*, then every Fourier component will be calculated exactly. Note that in three dimensions, this means a box of size *at least* as large as $2^3 = 8$ times larger than the smallest box that contains the sphere of $\mathbf{G}$ vectors, i.e., N_{PW}^* is larger than N_{PW} by at least a factor of $8\pi/3 = 8.4$, *roughly an order of magnitude*. Despite this fact, it is still much more efficient to carry out the operations using the FFT for all but the smallest problems.

Note that the estimate for the size of the FFT box depends on the assumption that the problem is roughly isotropic so that the $\mathbf{G}$ vectors are defined in a cube. If one chooses nonorthorhombic primitive vectors of the reciprocal lattice, then the number of $\mathbf{G}$ vectors will be larger than the above estimate in order to circumscribe a sphere of radius $|2\mathbf{G}_{max}|$. Fortunately, for large systems, where the methods are most useful, the cell can usually be chosen so that the FFT operations are efficient.

The condition for multiplication of the potential times the wavefunction does not appear so obvious at first sight. There is no reason to suppose that $V(\mathbf{G})$ has a limited number of Fourier components; the ionic potential has a $1/G^2$ form, which is reduced by screening but not to zero. The Hartree potential has exactly the same range as the density due to the Poisson equation; however, there is no such limitation on the exchange–correlation potential (more on this below). Thus $V\psi$ extends to all $\mathbf{G}$ vectors even if ψ is limited. *Nevertheless, the range up to* $|2\mathbf{G}_{max}|$ *is sufficient for an exact calculation.* The reason is that only the Fourier components of $V\psi$ with $|\mathbf{G}| < |\mathbf{G}_{max}|$ are relevant for the Schrödinger equation. This is easily seen from the definition of the matrix elements of the potential, Eq. (12.8), which involves only components of V up to $|2\mathbf{G}_{max}|$ if the wavefunctions extend up to $|\mathbf{G}_{max}|$. In an iterative approach, the potential enters by explicit multiplication of V times a trial vector; even though multiplication would give Fourier components with $|\mathbf{G}| > |\mathbf{G}_{max}|$, *only those with* $|\mathbf{G}| < |\mathbf{G}_{max}|$ *are relevant.* Even if the higher Fourier components are calculated, the contribution to the wavefunction is explicitly omitted. *In fact, it is essential that such components be omitted; otherwise one violates the original statement of the problem: the solution of the Schrödinger equation with wavefunctions expanded in a fixed finite basis set.*

The algorithm shown in Fig. M.2 denotes the operations on a wavefunction $\psi(\mathbf{G})$ defined on a set of N_{PW} Fourier components. The algorithm, in fact, generates the product $V\psi$ on a large grid of size N_{PW}^* and the product is explicitly truncated to produce the "force" $F(\mathbf{G})$ defined on the small set of N_{PW} Fourier components. This force is then used to update the wavefunction in any of the iterative methods described in this chapter.

A few words are in order regarding the exchange–correlation energy and potential. There is no simple relation of the reciprocal space and real-space formulations since $\epsilon_{xc}(n)$ is a nonlinear function of n. For example, the fact that exchange involves $n^{1/3}$ means that a single Fourier component of $n(\mathbf{G})$ gives rise to an infinite set of components of $\epsilon_{xc}(\mathbf{G})$ and $V_{xc}(\mathbf{G})$. Thus the problem is in $\mathbf{G}$ space formulation: direct sums in $\mathbf{G}$ space can never give exact $\epsilon_{xc}(\mathbf{G})$ and $V_{xc}(\mathbf{G})$ in terms of $n(\mathbf{G})$. However, FFT formulation allows the exchange–correlation terms to be treated in real space with no problem. So long as one includes all components up to $|2\mathbf{G}_{max}|$, the resulting $\epsilon_{xc}(\mathbf{G})$ and $V_{xc}(\mathbf{G})$ can be used to *define* those terms in a way that is sufficiently accurate for the solution of Kohn–Sham equations (Exercise M.3).

SELECT FURTHER READING

See references for numerical methods at the end of Appendix L.

Reviews focused on methods:

Beck, T. L., "Real-space mesh techniques in density-functional theory," *Rev. Mod. Phys.* 72:1041–1080, 2000.

Payne, M. C., Teter, M. P., Allan, D. C., Arias, T. A., and Joannopoulos, J. D., "Iterative minimization techniques for *ab initio* total-energy calculations: Molecular dynamics and conjugate gradients," *Rev. Mod. Phys.* 64:1045–1097, 1992.

Saad, Y., Chelikowsky, J., and Shontz, S., "Numerical methods for electronic structure calculations of materials," *SIAM Review*, 52:3–54, 2010.

Exercises

M.1 Show by induction that each vector ψ_n generated by the Lanczos algorithm is orthogonal to *all* the other vectors, and that the hamiltonian has tridiagonal form, Eq. (M.10). Regarding the problem that orthogonality is guaranteed only for infinite numerical precision, show how errors in each step can accumulate in the deviations from orthogonality.

M.2 The solution for the eigenvalues of the tridiagonal matrix H in Eq. (M.10) is given by $|H_{ij} - \lambda\delta_{ij}| = 0$, which is polynomial $P_M(\lambda)$ of degree M. This may be solved in a recursive manner starting with the subdeterminant with $M = 1$. The first two polynomials are $P_1(\lambda) = \alpha_1 - \lambda$ and $P_2(\lambda) = (\alpha_2 - \lambda)P_1(\lambda) - \beta_2^2$. Show that the general relation for higher polynomials is

$$P_n(\lambda) = (\alpha_n - \lambda)P_{n-1}(\lambda) - \beta_n^2[P_{n-2}(\lambda)], \qquad (M.22)$$

and thus that the solution can be found by root tracing (varying λ successively to reach condition $P_M(\lambda) = 0$ in computer time proportional to M for each eigenvalue).

M.3 Consider a plane wave calculation with the wavefunction limited to Fourier components with $|\mathbf{G}| < |\mathbf{G}_{max}|$. Show that all Fourier components of the external potential and the Hartree potential are given exactly (with no "aliasing") by the FFT algorithm, so long as the FFT extends to $|2\mathbf{G}_{max}|$. For the nonlinear exchange–correlation potential, show that there is no exact expression but the use in the Kohn-Sham equation is exact as stated in the text.

Appendix N

Two-Center Matrix Elements: Expressions for Arbitrary Angular Momentum l

Summary

The expressions given here are not used in the theory or codes for tight binding used in this book, but they can be useful for higher angular momentum states.

Two-center matrix elements for any particular angular momenta can be worked out [1089], with increasing effort for increasing L. Is it possible to make an algorithm that works for any angular momenta? By using rotation operator algebra, the rotations (analogous to those shown explicitly for p states in Fig. 14.2) can be generated to define the quantization axis for the orbitals along the line between the atoms.[1] The general formulation is most easily cast in terms of the complex orbitals that are eigenfunctions of L_z, where the z-axis is the same for all orbitals. (It is straightforward at the end to convert back to real orbitals.) Thus the two orbitals involved in any matrix element are l, m and l', m'. These orbitals must be written in a representation quantized along the z'-axis, which is parallel to the direction $\hat{\mathbf{R}}$. The transformation is applied to the set of orbitals $-l \leq m \leq l$ for a given l, since the transformation preserves the angular momentum l but the different m components are mixed. Let the set of $2l + 1$ states for a given l be denoted by $|l\{m\}\rangle$. The rotation is a unitary transformation given by [1090]

$$|l\{m'\}\rangle = e^{-i\theta \hat{L}_y} e^{-i\phi \hat{L}_z} |l\{m\}\rangle, \tag{N.1}$$

where the rotation angles θ and ϕ are defined by

$$\hat{\mathbf{R}} = \sin\theta(\hat{\mathbf{x}}\cos\phi + \hat{\mathbf{y}}\sin\phi) + \hat{\mathbf{z}}\cos\theta. \tag{N.2}$$

The two exponential operators in Eq. (N.1) rotate the quantization axis first about the z-axis, and then about the new y'-axis to define the quantization axis along z'. Then the matrix elements for the $(2l + 1) \times (2l' + 1)$ block of the K matrix corresponding to l and l' can be written

$$K_{l\{m\},l'\{m'\}} = \langle l\{m\}|e^{i\phi \hat{L}_z} e^{i\theta \hat{L}_y} \hat{K} e^{-i\theta \hat{L}_y} e^{-i\phi \hat{L}_z}|l'\{m'\}\rangle, \tag{N.3}$$

---

[1] This formulation is due to N. Romero and T. Arias.

where the right-hand side is expressed in terms of the operator $\hat{K}$ (e.g., the overlap), which is diagonal in the azimuthal quantum number m defined about the z'-axis.

The operations involving $\hat{L}_z$ are straightforward; the states are eigenfunctions of $\hat{L}_z$ so that $e^{-i\phi\hat{L}_z}|l,m\rangle = e^{-im\phi}|l,m\rangle$, which is diagonal in the set $\{m\}$. However, $\hat{L}_y$ is more difficult. The matrix elements of $\hat{L}_y$ are well known [1090]

$$
\langle l,m|\hat{L}_y|l',m'\rangle = \frac{1}{2i}\delta_{ll'}
$$
$$
\times \left[\sqrt{l(l+1) - m'(m'+1)}\,\delta_{m,m'+1} - \sqrt{l(l+1) - m'(m'-1)}\,\delta_{m,m'-1}\right],
$$

$$(N.4)$$

but there is still a difficulty since this nondiagonal operator appears in an exponential. This can be solved by diagonalizing the matrix, Eq. (N.4), for the $\hat{L}_y$ operator in the basis of eigenfunctions $|l,m\rangle$ of $\hat{L}_z$ for each l. Standard numerical routines can be used to find the eigenvalues and eigenvectors so that the $\hat{L}_y$ operator can be written as

$$
\hat{L}_y = M_y L_z M_y^\dagger,
$$

$$(N.5)$$

where M_y is a matrix whose columns are the eigenstates of the $\hat{L}_y$ operator written in $\hat{L}_z$ basis. Using the identity $e^{VAV^\dagger} = Ve^A V^\dagger$, where V is unitary, the resulting expression for the matrix elements takes the form

$$
K_{l\{m\},l'\{m'\}} = \langle l\{m\}|e^{i\phi\hat{L}_z}M_y e^{i\theta\hat{L}_z}M_y^\dagger \hat{K} M_y e^{-i\theta\hat{L}_y}M_y^\dagger e^{-i\phi\hat{L}_z}|l\{m'\}\rangle.
$$

$$(N.6)$$

Finally, it is a small step to transform $K_{l\{m\},l'\{m'\}}$ to a representation with real orbitals $S_{l,m}^\pm$ that are combinations of $\pm m$ and $\pm m'$ give in Eq. (K.11).

Appendix O

Dirac Equation and Spin–Orbit Interaction

almost by sheer cerebration [mental reasoning]

John Ziman

Summary

The Dirac equation is a stroke of genius that has profound effects in all of physics. One is the spin–orbit interaction and in Section O.2 we discuss the profound consequences for electronic structure, where it leads to effects that are qualitatively different from anything that can be produced by a potential. Fortunately, it is usually sufficient in solids to describe the spin–orbit interaction by the usual Schrödinger equation with an added term $\hat{H}_{SO}$ in Eq. (O.10). In Section O.3 is the derivation starting from the full four-component Dirac equation. The spin–orbit interaction has come to the fore in the theory of condensed matter with the discovery of topological insulators in Chapters 25–28.

In much of this book, the focus is on the nonrelativistic Schrödinger equation in which the goal is to take into account the large spin-independent effects of the nuclear potentials and the electron–electron Coulomb interactions, which is essential in any realistic calculation. The theory is developed assuming spin is quantized ↑ and ↓ along a chosen axis; spin can be taken into account with spin-independent Schrödinger equation and a factor of two whenever it is needed to account for the spin degeneracy, or two equations for ↑ and ↓ for magnetic systems. For many purposes this is sufficient; however, it cannot be complete. The Schrödinger equation is first order in the derivative with respect to time $i\hbar \partial/\partial t$, but second order in momenta $p_x = i\hbar \nabla$, and a correct theory must involve space and time in the same way in order to be Lorentz invariant. This leads to spin–orbit interactions and other effects that play a special role in the band structure of bulk crystals and surface states, with the largest consequences in solids containing heavy atoms where velocities can be a significant fraction of the speed of light. The effects can be very large; for example, Fig. 17.7 shows the large shift in the conduction band s state due to the scalar relativistic effects. Although it has long been recognized that it must be taken into account in molecules and the band structures of crystals, the advent of topological insulators has brought spin–orbit interaction to the forefront of condensed matter theory and new classifications of electronic structure of crystals in terms of topology, as described in Chapters 25–28.

0.1 The Dirac Equation

The papers by Dirac in 1928 [26, 27] are a magnificent example of creativity that brought together the principles of quantum mechanics and special relativity.[1] The Dirac equation is linear in time and momenta in order for it to be Lorentz invariant. Dirac found that the coefficients had to obey commutation rules that can be satisfied only by matrices and a wavefunction with four components (spinors). From this reasoning emerged a very simple equation with the remarkable prediction that such a particle is a fermion with spin 1/2 and an antiparticle discovered only later by experiments.

The Dirac equation for a free particle can be written

$$i\hbar \frac{\partial \psi}{\partial t} = (c\boldsymbol{\gamma} \cdot \mathbf{p} + \gamma_0 mc^2)\psi, \tag{O.1}$$

where $\mathbf{p} = i\frac{\partial}{\partial \mathbf{r}}$ for the three spatial coordinates. The γ's are 4×4 matrices, which can be chosen in different ways.[2] A choice that describes fermions is given by

$$\gamma_i = \begin{bmatrix} 0 & \sigma_i \\ -\sigma_i & 0 \end{bmatrix}, \quad i = 1, 2, 3, \quad \text{and} \quad \gamma_0 = \begin{bmatrix} 1 & 0 \\ 0 & -1 \end{bmatrix}, \tag{O.2}$$

where the σ_i are the three Pauli matrices and $\mathbf{1}$ is the 2×2 unit matrix,

$$\sigma_1 = \sigma_x = \begin{bmatrix} 0 & 1 \\ 1 & 0 \end{bmatrix}, \quad \sigma_2 = \sigma_y = \begin{bmatrix} 0 & -i \\ i & 0 \end{bmatrix}, \quad \sigma_3 = \sigma_z = \begin{bmatrix} 1 & 0 \\ 0 & -1 \end{bmatrix}, \quad \text{and} \quad \mathbf{1} = \begin{bmatrix} 1 & 0 \\ 0 & 1 \end{bmatrix}. \tag{O.3}$$

It is convenient to write the solution in the form

$$\psi(x^\mu) = e^{-iEt/\hbar} \begin{pmatrix} \psi(\mathbf{r}) \\ \chi(\mathbf{r}) \end{pmatrix}, \tag{O.4}$$

where $x^\mu = (\mathbf{r}, t)$, and $\psi(\mathbf{r})$ and $\chi(\mathbf{r})$ are time-independent two-component spinors describing the spatial and spin degrees of freedom. Thus the Dirac equation (O.1) becomes coupled equations for ψ and χ,

$$c(\sigma \cdot \mathbf{p})\chi = (E - mc^2)\psi,$$
$$c(\sigma \cdot \mathbf{p})\psi = (E + mc^2)\chi. \tag{O.5}$$

The equations for the interaction of an electron with electric and magnetic fields can be derived by the replacements $\mathbf{p} \to \boldsymbol{\pi} = \mathbf{p} - (e/c)\mathbf{A}$ and $mc^2 \to mc^2 + eV$ where $\mathbf{A}$ and V are the vector and scalar potentials, which in general are functions of space and time.

---

[1] See *The Principles of Quantum Mechanics* by Dirac published in 1930 [1091]. In his pithy, informative book [1092], Ziman says that Dirac formulated his theory "almost by sheer cerebration," i.e., by sheer mental reasoning.

[2] A different choice is matrices that are purely real, which can describe a Majorana fermion that is its own antiparticle.

0.2 The Spin–Orbit Interaction in the Schrödinger Equation

For electrons (positive energy solutions) with energy $\varepsilon = E - mc^2 > 0$ much less than the rest mass energy,[3] ψ is the large component and χ is smaller by a factor $\propto \varepsilon/mc^2$, and the equation for ψ can be written as a 2×2 equation with the effect of χ included as a perturbation. The result (See Section O.3 for a derivation.) is a Schrödinger-like equation that is the same as the nonrelativistic form except that is for a two-component wavefunction ψ that can be expressed in terms of two spin states along a chosen axis,

$$\psi = \begin{bmatrix} \psi_\uparrow(\mathbf{r}) \\ \psi_\downarrow(\mathbf{r}) \end{bmatrix}. \tag{O.6}$$

and there are two added terms in the hamiltonian:[4]

$$i\hbar \frac{\partial \psi}{\partial t} = H\psi = \left[\frac{\pi^2}{2m} + V + H_Z + H_{SO} \right] \psi, \tag{O.7}$$

where $\boldsymbol{\pi} = \mathbf{p} - (e/c)\mathbf{A}$ acts on the spatial part of the wavefunction in the presence of a magnetic field (the same as in the usual Schrödinger equation), $H_Z = \mu_B \boldsymbol{\sigma} \cdot \mathbf{B}$ is the Zeeman term, and H_{SO} is the spin–orbit interaction

$$H_{SO} = \frac{e\hbar}{4m^2c^2} (\mathbf{p} \times \nabla V) \cdot \boldsymbol{\sigma}. \tag{O.8}$$

It is instructive to note that the magnetic moment $\mu_B = e\hbar/2mc$ and spin–orbit interactions have a common origin: the spin–orbit interaction can be viewed as the result of an electron with momentum $\mathbf{p}$ and spin σ moving in an electric field (the gradient of the potential ∇V), which is equivalent to a magnetic field in the rest frame of the electron.

Equation (O.7) is the generalization of the basic equation (3.36) for noninteracting electrons to include the magnetic field and H_{SO}. The only term that couples the two spins is H_{SO} so that the hamiltonian can always be written as terms that are diagonal in the spin $\uparrow$ and $\downarrow$ plus H_{SO} that can be written as

$$H_{SO} = \begin{bmatrix} H_{SO}(\uparrow\uparrow) & H_{SO}(\downarrow\uparrow) \\ H_{SO}(\uparrow\downarrow) & H_{SO}(\downarrow\downarrow) \end{bmatrix}, \tag{O.9}$$

Spherical Geometry

For a general problem with no symmetry, one must calculate the matrix elements of the operator $(\mathbf{p} \times \nabla V)$. However, in solids made of atoms the largest effects of spin–orbit interaction occur deep in the core near the nucleus where ∇V is large, and the derivation can be done in an atom-like spherical geometry. In that case the gradient is purely radial $\nabla V = \hat{\mathbf{r}} dV/dr$, and Equation (O.8) can be written as

---

[3] The solution for the full four-component wavefunctions is given in Section O.3 for a spherical potential.

[4] In addition, there are the mass-velocity and Darwin terms (see Section O.3), which are spin-independent scalar fields that are not written explicitly here.

$$\hat{H}_{SO} = \frac{\hbar^2}{4M^2c^2} \frac{1}{r} \frac{dV}{dr} \mathbf{L} \cdot \sigma,$$ (O.10)

where $\mathbf{L} = \mathbf{r} \times \mathbf{p}$ is the angular momentum operator. The sense in which the linear momentum is perpendicular to the electric field is depicted in the lower left part of Fig. O.1, and the diagram at the lower right indicates the spin–orbit splitting for the states with total angular momentum $J = L \pm 1/2$, which is described by a single parameter for each L. The expression in terms of the angular momentum operator carries over to the solid where matrix elements of Equation (O.10) can be calculated by projecting out the different angular momentum states in the wavefunction for the solid. This is straightforward to do in methods that work directly with a basis of atom-centered states with well-defined angular momenta. In a pseudopotential calculation the spin–orbit interaction can be taken into account by the construction of the pseudopotential in the atom including the spin–orbit interaction and the resulting angular momentum projectors (see Section 11.8). In an empirical tight-binding calculation one only needs to specify the parameter for each L, for example, the expressions for the hamiltonian for p states ($L = 1$) in Eq. (14.12) and the calculations in Sections 27.5 and 27.6.

Planar Geometry

The top part of Fig. O.1 illustrates a planar geometry that is a model for a surface or interface. This provides a vivid example of the fact that the velocity-dependent spin–orbit interaction leads to effects that are qualitatively different from anything that can be produced by a potential. The linear dispersion occurs because of the low symmetry of the surface, and it can be expected in many problems where there is not a center of inversion. This is an

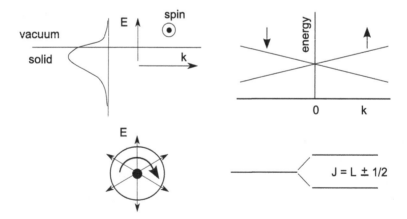

Figure O.1. Consequences of the spin–orbit interaction. Top: dispersion of a surface state is linear in momentum **k** along the surface with opposite sign for spin ↑ and ↓ in the direction perpendicular to **k** due to the electric field (gradient of the potential) normal, which is nonzero by symmetry at a surface. Bottom: a depiction of the redial electroic field around a nucleus and the resulting splitting of the total angular momentum components for $\mathbf{J} = \mathbf{L} + \mathbf{S}$.

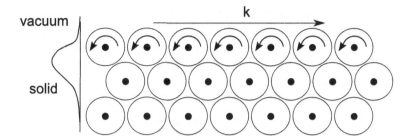

Figure O.2. Illustration of a surface state with momentum **k** where the linear momentum **k** results in angular momentum around surface atoms because the wavefunction is not symmetric around the nucleus. The schematic curve at the left indicates a function that is smaller in the vacuum than inside the material. This leads to a coupling to the spin through the spin–orbit interaction and the dispersion of the surface bands, e.g., in gold as shown in Fig. 22.3.

example of the Rashba effect [870, 871] and it occurs for any surface state whether or not it is related to topology. The linear dispersion is a critical aspect of topological insulators, and examples are shown in Figs. 27.3, 27.7 and 27.9,[5] and in the calculations for topological surface states for gold in Fig. 22.3 and Bi_2Se_3 in Figs. 2.27 and 28.5.

The consequence of the effect can be much larger at an actual surface that is made of atoms with large spin–orbit interaction. It can be understood as shown in Fig. O.2, which shows the layers of atoms and a schematic picture of a surface state that is not symmetric around the surface atoms. The asymmetry leads to a coupling of linear and angular momenta as indicated: for momentum **k** in one direction the spin out of the page is favored and for **k** in the opposite direction the opposite spin is favored.

0.3 Relativistic Equations and Calculation of the Spin–Orbit Interaction in an Atom

In this section we give the equations for solution of the Dirac equation (O.1) for the full four-component wavefunction spherical potential $V(r)$, and the demonstration that for energy small compared to the rest mass it reduces to the expressions for $\hat{H}_{SO}$ in Eq. (O.10). In the case of a spherical potential $V(r)$, one can make use of conservation of parity and total angular momentum denoted by the quantum numbers jm. Then the wavefunction for each principle quantum number n can be written in terms of radial and angular-spin functions (see [1093], section 4.4),

$$\psi_{njm}^l = \begin{pmatrix} g_{nj}(r)\varphi_{jm}^l \\ if_{nj}(r)\frac{\sigma \cdot \mathbf{r}}{r}\varphi_{jm}^l \end{pmatrix}, \tag{O.11}$$

---

[5] It might seem surprising that such effects would occur in a tight-binding model where there is no electric field in the model. However, the essential point is that there is no inversion symmetry around a surface atom, and there is the implicit effect of the nuclear electric field that is manifested in the value and sign of the spin–orbit interaction parameter.

which defines two functions with the same jm but opposite parity for the two possible values $l = j \pm \frac{1}{2}$. The two-component functions φ^l_{jm} can be written explicitly as

for $j = l + \dfrac{1}{2}$,

$$\varphi^l_{jm} = \sqrt{\frac{l + \frac{1}{2} + m}{2l + 1}} Y^{m - \frac{1}{2}}_l (\uparrow) + \sqrt{\frac{l + \frac{1}{2} - m}{2l + 1}} Y^{m + \frac{1}{2}}_l (\downarrow),$$

for $j = l - \dfrac{1}{2}$,   (O.12)

$$\varphi^l_{jm} = \sqrt{\frac{l + \frac{1}{2} - m}{2l + 1}} Y^{m - \frac{1}{2}}_l (\uparrow) - \sqrt{\frac{l + \frac{1}{2} + m}{2l + 1}} Y^{m + \frac{1}{2}}_l (\downarrow).$$

The resulting equations for the radial functions are simplified if we define a radially varying mass,

$$M(r) = m + \frac{\varepsilon - V(r)}{2c^2},$$ (O.13)

and the quantum number κ,

$$\kappa = \pm \left(j + \frac{1}{2} \right) \qquad \begin{cases} +, \text{ if } l = j + \frac{1}{2} \Rightarrow \kappa = l, \\ -, \text{ if } l = j - \frac{1}{2} \Rightarrow \kappa = -(l + 1). \end{cases}$$ (O.14)

Note that $\kappa(\kappa + 1) = l(l + 1)$ in either case. Then the coupled equations can be written in the form of the radial equations [157, 673, 1094, 1095]

$$-\frac{\hbar^2}{2M} \frac{1}{r^2} \frac{d}{dr} \left(r^2 \frac{dg_{n\kappa}}{dr} \right) + \left[V + \frac{\hbar^2}{2M} \frac{l(l + 1)}{r^2} \right] g_{n\kappa},$$

$$-\frac{\hbar^2}{4M^2c^2} \frac{dV}{dr} \frac{dg_{n\kappa}}{dr} - \frac{\hbar^2}{4M^2c^2} \frac{dV}{dr} \frac{(1 + \kappa)}{r} g_{n\kappa} = \varepsilon g_{n\kappa},$$ (O.15)

and

$$\frac{df_{n\kappa}}{dr} = \frac{1}{\hbar c}(V - \varepsilon)g_{n\kappa} + \frac{(\kappa - 1)}{r} f_{n\kappa}.$$ (O.16)

These are the general equations for a spherical potential; no approximations have been made thus far. Equation (O.15) is the same as an ordinary Schrödinger equation except that the mass M is a function of radius and there are two added terms on the left-hand side, which are, respectively, the Darwin term and the spin–orbit coupling. The latter can be written out explicitly in terms of the spin using the relation

$$\mathbf{L} \cdot \sigma \varphi_{\kappa m} = -\hbar(1 + \kappa)\varphi_{\kappa m},$$ (O.17)

where $\varphi_{\kappa m}$ is the appropriate φ^l_{jm} determined by κ.

Scalar Relativistic Equation and Spin–Orbit Coupling

If we make the approximation that the spin–orbit term is small, then we can omit it in the radial equations for g and f and treat it by perturbation theory. Then Eqs. (O.15) and (O.16) depend only on the principle quantum number n and orbital angular momentum l and can be written in terms of the approximate functions, $\tilde{g}_{nl}$ and $\tilde{f}_{nl}$. The result is an equation exactly like the usual Schrödinger equation for an atom in Eq. (10.4) with the addition of the spin–orbit interaction (the last term on the left side),

$$-\frac{\hbar^2}{2M}\frac{1}{r^2}\frac{d}{dr}\left(r^2\frac{d\tilde{g}_{nl}}{dr}\right) + \left[V + \frac{\hbar^2}{2M}\frac{l(l+1)}{r^2}\right]\tilde{g}_{nl} - \frac{\hbar^2}{4M^2c^2}\frac{dV}{dr}\frac{d\tilde{g}_{nl}}{dr} = \varepsilon\tilde{g}_{nl} \quad (O.18)$$

and

$$\tilde{f}_{nl} = \frac{\hbar}{2Mc}\frac{d\tilde{g}_{nl}}{dr}, \quad (O.19)$$

with the normalization condition

$$\int (\tilde{g}_{nl}^2 + \tilde{f}_{nl}^2)r^2 dr = 1. \quad (O.20)$$

Equation (O.18) is the scalar relativistic radial equation, which can be solved by the same techniques as the usual nonrelativistic equation, and the other equations can then be treated easily on the radial grid following the approach of MacDonald et al. [1095]. In actual calculations in materials it is usually sufficient to set $M = m$, the electron rest mass, and ignore the small component so that Eq. (O.20) is just the standard normalization condition for $\tilde{g}$. Then $\tilde{g}$ can be identified as the radial wavefunction ψ and, together with Eq. (O.17), Eq. (O.18) becomes the usual nonrelativistic Schrödinger equation with the addition of the spin–orbit interaction $\hat{H}_{SO}$ in Eq. (O.10).

Appendix P

Berry Phase, Curvature, and Chern Numbers

Summary

In this appendix the Berry phase and topological invariant Chern number are derived from the principle of superposition in quantum mechanics. Expressions are given in both discrete and continuous forms; the former is most convenient for numerical calculations and the latter provides the elegant expressions in terms of the gauge invariant Berry curvature. The explicit expressions most useful for applications to crystals are given in Chapter 25.

P.1 Overview

A Berry phase[1] is the phase difference acquired by a wavefunction that depends on parameters that are varied a closed loop, for example, the ground state of a hamiltonian determined by parameters that vary continuously so that it is the same at the start and finish. In general the phase of a wavefuntion is arbitrary; however, the relative phase of the function carried around a loop and compared to the phase of the starting wavefunction is well defined. The change in phase may be larger than 2π but the Berry phase is defined to be in the range 0 to 2π, i.e., the actual phase accumulated along the path is the Berry phase modulo 2π. The Berry phase is gauge invariant, i.e., it is not changed by a gauge transformation in which the phase of the wavefunction along the path is varied, even though the total phase may change by multiples of 2π.

A familiar example that illustrates the physical consequence of the relative phase is the double slit experiment in which a particle can follow two paths to the same point;

---

[1] It can also be referred to as a "geometric phase" or a "Pancharatnam phase," after early work by Pancharatnam in 1956, and there are various precedents such as the Aharonov–Bohm effect [1096], which is discussed in Section P.6. The concepts were codified in the 1980s, in seminal papers by Berry in 1984 [177] and other work, for example by Simon in 1983 [1097]. (Simon learned about Berry's work and refers to "the Berry phase" even though his paper was published before Berry's.) See the volume edited by Wilczek and Shapere [1098] for subsequent papers by Berry and others. A description of Berry phases in a way that is particularly appropriate for readers of this book can be found in the book by Vanderbilt [918].

the interference is determined by the relative phase in the range 0 to 2π. Another is the Aharonov–Bohm effect in Section P.6, which is determined by the relative phase of the wavefunction of a particle that encircles a magnetic flux. This illustrates the Berry phase due to the vector potential in the hamiltonian and provides an instructive example of the way that Berry phases can be viewed as analogous to electromagnetism, but with additional possibilities since the behavior of the phase of a quantum wavefunctions is not constrained to obey Maxwell's equations.

A Berry phase is not the expectation value of an operator, and yet it can have physical consequences. Because it is a change of phase along a path that is directed, a Berry phase changes sign if the path is traversed in the opposite direction. Thus we can already realize that time plays a key role in understanding the consequences and we can expect that the Berry phase may be closely related to time-reversal symmetry. This might lead us to expect that the Berry phase can be nonzero only in systems that do not have time-reversal symmetry, for example, a system in a magnetic field or a topological insulator where spin–orbit interaction plays an essential role, as shown in Chapters 27 and 28. However, Berry phases can be also nonzero for physical properties that are actual changes, i.e., the difference between two states of a system where the change can be considered as a function of time or some other parameter that governs the hamiltonian between the two states, even if the hamiltonian has time-reversal symmetry at all times. Indeed, this is the proper way to determine the physically measurable electric polarization in condensed matter, as discussed in Chapter 24. Thus Berry phases provide a unified theory of such diverse phenomena as the quantum Hall effect, topological insulators, and electric polarization; it even unifies condensed matter and particle physics, although that is not the topic of this volume.[2]

The use of Berry phases in condensed matter is most directly applicable to insulators. This is because the energy of the ground state is separated by an energy gap from all other eigenstates of the hamiltonian, and we can readily identify the transitions between insulating states with different topologies as the points where the gap vanishes. In general the ground state is a many-body wavefunction that is characterized by a single phase. In the independent particle approximation the ground state is a determinant, and an important part of practical methods is to determine the phase in terms of the phases of the individual single-particle functions.

P.2 Berry Phase and Berry Connection

Berry Phase for a Discrete Path

Consider a set of normalized wavefunctions u_j that can be considered as functions of a parameter that varies to return to the starting point.[3] This can be represented by a loop like

---

[2] See, for example, the article "Particle physics and condensed matter: The saga continues" by Frank Wilczek [952].

[3] The notation u is adopted because the main applications considered later are to solids where u_k is the periodic part of the Bloch function, but at this point the theory is completely general.

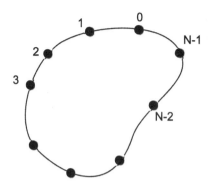

Figure P.1. Schematic illustration of a discrete set of steps along a path.

that illustrated in Fig. P.1, which depicts a discrete set of steps $j = 0$ to $j = N$ that define a path in the order shown. It is important that the function at the last step, the one after step $N - 1$, is the same as the initial function labeled 0. The relative phases of the wavefunctions at any two adjacent points can be expressed as

$$\Delta\phi_{j, j+1} = \text{Im} \ln[\langle u_j | u_{j+1} \rangle], \tag{P.1}$$

using the relation that $\text{Im} \ln z$ is the phase α of $z = |z| e^{i\alpha}$, restricted to be in the range 0 to 2π. With this definition the Berry phase for the path can be written as[4]

$$\phi = -\text{Im} \ln[\langle u_0 | u_1 \rangle \langle u_1 | u_2 \rangle \langle u_2 | \ldots | u_{N-2} \rangle \langle\langle u_{N-2} | u_{N-1} \rangle \langle u_{N-1} | u_0 \rangle]. \tag{P.2}$$

This is a convenient form for taking the continuum limit and for showing the gauge invariance, which is essential if it is to have a physical meaning. The phase of the wavefunction at each point along the loop is arbitrary and yet gauge invariance means that the resulting Berry phase for the loop must be invariant even if the phase of the wavefunction at any step is varied. This can be seen in Eq. (P.2) since every function appears in both a a ket $|u_j\rangle$ and a bra $\langle u_j|$. At this point it might seem that the Berry phase must always be zero! But we shall see that this is not the case and it contains physically meaningful information depending on the way the phases vary for a physical problem.

Continuum Limit and the Berry Connection

The choice of the definition in Eq. (P.2) allows us to have a well-defined continuum limit as a function of a variable x if we require that u_x be a smooth, differentiable function of x.[5] Then each step becomes

$$\ln\langle u_x | u_{x+dx} \rangle = \ln[1 + dx \langle u_x | \partial_x u_x \rangle + \cdots \to dx \langle u_x | \partial_x u_x \rangle. \tag{P.3}$$

---

[4] The minus sign is the convention in the Vanderbilt book [918], but it is omitted by some authors.

[5] In the literature the continuous variable is often denoted λ (for example in [918]). Here we use x to avoid confusion with the use of λ in the text.

Now $dx\langle u_x|\partial_x u_x\rangle$ is purely imaginary (see Exercise P.1) so that

$$\phi = -\text{Im} \oint dx\langle u_x|\partial_x u_x\rangle = \oint dx\langle u_x|i\partial_x u_x\rangle, \tag{P.4}$$

where $\oint$ denotes a line integral along a closed path. The last expression is the famous expression for the Berry phase in a continuous form [177, 1098]. Notice that unlike the definition in Eq. (P.2), the phase ϕ is not restricted to 0 to 2π and it should regarded as the Berry phase modulo 2π.

The Berry connection is the integrand in Eq. (P.4),

$$\mathcal{A}(x) = \langle u_x|i\partial_x u_x\rangle, \tag{P.5}$$

so that

$$\phi = \oint dx\mathcal{A}(x). \tag{P.6}$$

The notation $\mathcal{A}$ is used because it is analogous to the vector potential $\mathbf{A}$ in electrodynamics, as brought out in the example of the Aharonov–Bohm effect in Section P.6. The Berry connection $\mathcal{A}$ is also called the "Berry potential" and, like the vector potential $\mathbf{A}$, it is not gauge invariant.

It is useful to see effect of a gauge transformation (see also Eq. (23.2))

$$|\tilde{u}_x\rangle = e^{i\alpha(x)}|u_x\rangle, \tag{P.7}$$

where $\alpha(x)$ is a continuous real function of x, so that

$$\tilde{\mathcal{A}}(x) = \mathcal{A}(x) + \frac{d\alpha(x)}{dx}. \tag{P.8}$$

The condition on $\alpha(x)$ is that the phase difference around the loop is the same for $\tilde{u}_x$ and u_x, so that the only possibility for the integral in Eqs. (P.4) or (P.6) is that

$$\oint dx\alpha(x) = 2n\pi; \tag{P.9}$$

the total phase ϕ may be changed by multiples of 2π, leaving the Berry phase unchanged. We will refer to ϕ as the Berry phase with the understanding that it is gauge-invariant Berry phase modulo 2π. This is exactly what we anticipate and this provides one way of understanding how the added factors of 2π can occur.

P.3 Berry Flux and Curvature

Up to this point we have considered only a line integral. A geometrical theory and topological classification can be formulated for cases where the parameters span a two-dimensional space, which can be defined by $\mathbf{x} = (x_1, x_2)$, as illustrated in Fig. P.2. The notation is meant to be general, for example, momentum in one dimension and a parameter (k, λ) or two components of the momentum (k_x, k_y) in a two-dimensional space, as shown in

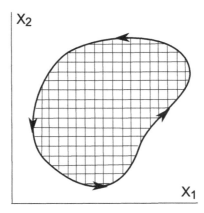

Figure P.2. Schematic illustration of the area bounded by a loop in two dimensions. See Fig. 25.1 for the corresponding figure used for calculation of polarization and topology in crystals.

Fig. 25.1.[6] Similarly, we define the two-component vector Berry connection $\mathcal{A} = (\mathcal{A}_1, \mathcal{A}_2)$ where

$$\mathcal{A}_i(\mathbf{x}) = -\text{Im}\langle u_{\mathbf{x}}|\partial_i u_{\mathbf{x}}\rangle, \quad i = 1, 2, \tag{P.10}$$

where $\partial_i = \partial_{x_i}$, and the Berry phase becomes the line integral around a loop in the x_1, x_2 plane

$$\phi = \oint \mathcal{A}(\mathbf{x}) \cdot d\mathbf{x}, \tag{P.11}$$

as depicted in Fig. P.2.

Although the Berry phase is gauge independent, the expressions so far have given it only as a sum or integral of quantities that are gauge dependent. Much is gained by expressing the Berry phase in terms of an integral over a function that is gauge invariant. Consider the Berry phase integrated around one of the small squares of the grid in Fig. P.2, which called the Berry flux through the square. If the variation of the phase is continuous, then for small enough squares the change of phase around the loop is small and it is gauge invariant with no uncertainly of factors of 2π. The Berry curvature $\Omega(\mathbf{x})$ is defined to be the Berry flux per unit area in the continuum limit, and it is straightforward to show that in two dimensions[7]

$$\Omega(\mathbf{x}) = \partial_1 \mathcal{A}_2 - \partial_2 \mathcal{A}_1 = -2\text{Im}\langle \partial_1 u(\mathbf{x})|\partial_2 u(\mathbf{x})\rangle, \tag{P.12}$$

where the last form can be derived using the condition that the wavefunction is normalized as shown in Exercise P.2.

---

[6] We consider two-dimensional spaces that are sufficient for the applications in Chapters 24–27, and provide the basis for the extension to three dimensions in Chapter 28.

[7] Note that Ω without subscripts is defined to be Ω_{12} and $\Omega_{21} = -\Omega_{12}$. The concept of curvature generalizes to any dimension with Ω an antisymmetric tensor with elements $\Omega_{\alpha\beta}(\mathbf{x}) = \partial_\alpha \mathcal{A}_\beta - \partial_\beta \mathcal{A}_\alpha = -2\text{Im}\langle \partial_\alpha u(\mathbf{x})|\partial_\beta u(\mathbf{x})\rangle$.

The total Berry flux is the Berry curvature integrated over the area bounded by the loop. If we identify the expression (P.12) for the curvature as a curl of $\mathcal{A}$ and $\boldsymbol{\Omega}$ as a pseudovector in three dimensions in the direction perpendicular to x and y, i.e., normal to the surface, then if the curvature is sufficiently smooth over the entire surface (see below for counterexamples), Stokes theorem leads to the expression the flux through the surface as the integral over the surface

$$\Phi = \int_S \boldsymbol{\Omega}(\mathbf{x}) \cdot d\mathbf{S}$$

$$= \oint \mathcal{A} \cdot d\mathbf{x} \mod(2\pi) \tag{P.13}$$

where $\mathbf{S}$ is the area vector directed along the normal to the surface. The first line of Eq. (P.13) defines the flux by the surface integral of gauge invariant quantities, but the second line is the gauge invariant Berry flux plus multiples of 2π. The full information can only be determined by the integral over the area. Nevertheless, the relationship in Eq. (P.13) establishes facts about the line integral that are invaluable for all the theoretical development to follow. The problem can be divided into two parts:

- The gauge invariant Berry phase can be established by the line integral around the boundary. The Berry phase is essential to determine quantities like polarization in Chapter 24.
- The integer multiples of 2π can be determined from the surface integral. For a closed surface, the integers are topological invariants that are the basis for the analysis in Chapters 25–28.

P.4 Chern Number and Topology

A Chern number is defined for a closed surface as an integer C that is the total Berry flux Φ divided by 2π. If there is a smooth gauge defined everywhere, then C must be zero because the integral of the curvature is equal to the line integral, which vanishes for a closed surface where there is no boundary. However, there are cases where it is not possible to find a gauge that is smooth everywhere, in which case C is nonzero.[8] All possible surfaces are classified by C, which is a topological invariant. Note that this is *not* the topology of the surface illustrated in Fig. P.2; it is the topology of the curvature Ω defined on the surface.

The topological classification is determined by the Chern number C and a key point is that a smooth gauge can be found over the entire surface only if $C = 0$. This is called a "trivial topology" analogous to a sphere. However, $C \neq 0$ is analogous to a surfaces with holes, which occurs if there is no gauge in which the wavefunction can be defined as a smooth function everywhere on the surface. An example is the wavefunction for a spin on

---

[8] The relation to topology is embodied by the Gauss–Bonnet theorem, which states that the total gaussian curvature of a closed surface is equal to 2π times the Euler characteristic of the surface, which equals $2 - g$ where g is the genus of the surface. Any such surface without boundary is topologically equivalent to a sphere with "handles" attached, where each handle adds one hole in the surface, and g counts the number of handles.

the surface of a sphere that encloses a source term analogous to a magnetic monopole. As discussed in Section P.7, this illustrates a case where one cannot find a gauge in which the wavefunction can be defined to be a smooth function everywhere on the sphere.

P.5 Adiabatic Evolution

The previous sections have developed the theory of Berry phases in a general framework that applies to many problems. Even the specialization to crystals in Section 25.4 only defines the notation and uses properties of the Brillouin zone. If we consider the case of a wavefunction where $u(\mathbf{k})$ is the ground state of the hamiltonian, the Berry phase can be expressed in terms of the eigenstates of hamiltonian, which leads to another consideration: the physical requirements that the system remain in the instantaneous ground state of the hamiltonian at each point of the variation.[9] This is called the adiabatic condition, and the physical requirement is that the evolution is sufficiently slow that frequency is much less than the excitation energies. There are many cases where the physical problem is a variation that is slow compared to electronic excitation energies but not zero, e.g., for phonons, where this is called the adiabatic approximation (see Appendix C). For uses considered here this is not an approximation because we can consider the limit as the speed of the variation goes to zero.

An example of the formulation is the current that flows as a function of "time" in Section 24.3. Equations (24.6) is the expression for the current in terms of excited states, which is transformed to a Berry curvature in Eq. (24.9) in terms of only the ground state.

P.6 Aharonov–Bohm Effect

The Berry phase and connection can be illustrated by the famous Aharonov–Bohm effect, which predated the work of Berry and which is often used as the textbook example of a surprising quantum effect that has no classical analogue. The effect is the phase acquired by a charge particle as it encircles a magnetic flux even though the particle is never in a region where there is a magnetic field. This is indicated in Fig. P.3 where the magnetic field $\mathbf{B}$ is nonzero only inside the tube and there is no field anywhere along the path of the particle. However, the vector potential $\mathbf{A}$ is related to the magnetic field by $\nabla \times \mathbf{A} = \mathbf{B}$, which is nonzero outside the tube and by the Stokes theorem the line integral of $\mathbf{A}$ is the total flux Φ, so that

$$\Phi = \int_S \mathbf{B} \cdot d\mathbf{S} = \oint \mathbf{A}(\mathbf{r}) \cdot d\mathbf{r}, \tag{P.14}$$

where $\mathbf{S}$ is the surface enclosed by the path. Note that both the path and the surface are directed, e.g., in this example the path is the counterclockwise sense and the surface normal is directed upward.

---

[9] As pointed out before, the Chern number is nonzero only if time reversal is broken; however, that does not preclude application to adiabatic evolution. Even if the variation is infinitely slow, it still has a direction and the Berry phase changes sign if the direction is reversed.

In the thought-experiment problem a particle is moved around the circle by confining it to a small box at position $\mathbf{r}$ so the $\mathbf{r}$ is the parameter that is varied in a loop and it enters the hamiltonian as the parameter in $\mathbf{A}(\mathbf{r})$, which can be written (giving the constants $\hbar$, e, and m explicitly for clarity)

$$H = \frac{1}{2m}\left(\mathbf{p} - \frac{e}{c}\mathbf{A}(\mathbf{r})\right)^2 = \frac{\hbar^2}{2m}\left(-i\nabla - \frac{e}{\hbar c}\mathbf{A}(\mathbf{r})\right)^2 = -\frac{\hbar^2}{2m}\left(\nabla - i\frac{e}{\hbar c}\mathbf{A}(\mathbf{r})\right)^2 \quad \text{(P.15)}$$

and the wavefunction for the particle has an additional phase acquired as the particle moves around the flux

$$\frac{e}{\hbar c}\oint \mathbf{A}(\mathbf{r})\cdot d\mathbf{r} = \frac{e}{\hbar c}\Phi \quad\quad\quad \text{(P.16)}$$

due to the vector potential, which is analogous to the factor of $e^{i\mathbf{k}\cdot\mathbf{r}}$ in the Bloch function for a crystal.

The same result is found using the definition of the Berry phase and Berry connection in Eqs. (P.10) and (P.11); in this case the parameter is $\mathbf{r}$ with $\mathcal{A}$ given by the vector potential $\mathbf{A}$ multiplied by $e/\hbar c$. The fact that the Berry phase is determined only up to factors of 2π has an important consequence that is illustrated in this case. It follows from Eq. (P.16) that Φ is determined only up to a fundamental unit of magnetic flux $\Phi_0 = 2\pi\hbar c/e = hc/e$.

The relation to the vector potential $\mathbf{A}$ and Berry connection $\mathcal{A}$ is the reason that $\mathcal{A}$ is also called the "Berry potential." The parallel between Eqs. (P.13) and (P.14) is striking and it brings out the relation of the curvature $\mathbf{\Omega}$ and the magnetic field $\mathbf{B}$, both of which are gauge invariant even though the potentials are not. We can also see from this example and the illustration in Fig. P.3 that we may expect that the Berry phase may lead to important, physical effects for cases where the path encloses a singularity like the singularity in the vector potential $\mathbf{A} = \nabla \times \mathbf{B}$ if the region of the magnetic field is reduced to a point in the surface S enclosed by the path.

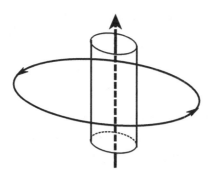

Figure P.3. Illustration of the Aharonov–Bohm effect for a charged particle following a path around a magnetic field that is confined to the region inside the tube, such as can be generated by a solenoid. Even though the magnetic field is zero at the position of the particle, the vector potential $\mathbf{A}$ is nonzero and the line integral of $\mathbf{A}$ on the circle is equal to the flux as indicated in Eq. (P.14).

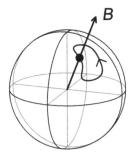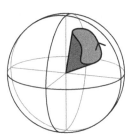

Figure P.4. Magnetic field pointed radially with direction that forms a closed loop. A spin in the ground state is oriented along the field direction, with wavefunction described in the text. The Berry phase is 1/2 the solid angle enclosed by the loop indicated at the right. Provided by D. H. Vanderbilt.

P.7 Dirac Magnetic Monopoles and Chern Number

In 1931 Dirac [1099] posed the question: Suppose there are magnetic monopoles in nature; what would be the consequences? Although monopoles of magnetic charge have not been discovered, the beautiful mathematical description has inspired many theoretical ideas and now we know that monopoles exactly like this have been lurking in Brillouin zones of crystals just waiting to be discovered. The relation of Berry curvature and connection $\mathcal{A}$ to the magnetic field and vector potential **A** provides many insights, but the Berry fields are not required to obey by Maxwell's equations where there are no magnetic monopoles. For a wavefunction defined in Brillouin zone there can be monopoles with quantized values given by the Chern number.

Consider the lowest-energy eigenstate of a spin 1/2 in a magnetic field for a monopole that radiates in all directions as indicated in Fig. P.4. (The same ideas apply to any two-level system, such as the ground state for one occupied and one empty band in a crystal, as a function of the momentum and/or other parameters in the hamiltonian.) The key result is that so long as the field varies continuously the integral of the Berry curvature is 1/2 the solid angle enclosed by the loop. By Stoke's theorem this is the Berry phase around the loop (modulo 2π). If the hamiltonian vector is defined relative to the z axis by the azimuthal and polar angles ϕ and θ, one choice for the eigenvectors is[10]

$$\psi^- = \begin{bmatrix} cos(\theta/2)e^{-i\phi/2} \\ sin(\theta/2)e^{i\phi/2} \end{bmatrix}, \text{ and } \psi^+ = \begin{bmatrix} -sin(\theta/2)e^{-i\phi/2} \\ cos(\theta/2)e^{i\phi/2} \end{bmatrix}. \tag{P.17}$$

This choice has singularities at both the south and north poles and is continuous at the equator. The Berry phase for an equatorial circle is the phase difference π, i.e., a change of sign of the wavefunction for a full rotation of 2π.

---

[10] The derivation is given in many texts on quantum mechanics, e.g., Shankar, pp. 390–391, gives the eigenvectors in this form.

Another choice given in the book by Vanderbilt [918] is

$$\psi^- = \begin{bmatrix} cos(\theta/2) \\ sin(\theta/2)e^{i\phi} \end{bmatrix}, \text{ and } \psi^+ = \begin{bmatrix} -sin(\theta/2) \\ cos(\theta/2)e^{i\phi} \end{bmatrix}, \tag{P.18}$$

which is smooth everywhere except at the south pole. The radial magnetic field at one end of a long thin solenoid acts like a monopole, and Eq. (P.18) could describe such a physical system with a solenoid that enters the sphere at the south pole. On the other hand the solenoid could enter at the north pole and a choice like Eq. (P.18), except with the ϕ dependence in the first component, is continuous at the south pole but not the north pole. What happens if one takes the two choices that are each smooth in one hemisphere and "glues them together" at the equator? For a real magnetic field this is just a way to move the singularity to the equator and there is no allowed smooth gauge. It might appear that same conclusions apply for the Berry phase for a two-band system; however, there is a difference because the Berry phase is defined as modulo 2π. This is an allowed gauge so long as the phase difference at the equator is a multiple of 2π. The symmetric choice is for the Berry phase at the equator to be $\pm\pi$ for the two hemispheres: an integral around the sphere just below (above) the equator would be π ($-\pi$) or vice versa, which is equivalent to the result for the choice in Eq. (P.17). In each case the total flux is 1/2 the solid angle, i.e., 1/2 of 4π.

Berry Phase around the Equator and Winding Numbers in One Dimension

The winding number for a one-dimensional problem is illustrated in Fig. 26.5, where the left side is a case that does not wind and the right one that winds once around the origin. The fact that this corresponds to a Berry phase of 0 or $\pm\pi$ follows from the present analysis of the Berry flux through the upper or lower parts of the sphere. The Berry phase for the ground-state wavefunction in Section 26.4 is an integral around the Brillouin zone, which is equivalent to the integral around the equator in Fig. P.4 where the result is 0 for the case of winding number zero (that does not enclose a zero-gap point) and $\pm\pi$ for the case of winding number one.

Explicit Example of Calculation of the Flux

Consider a path on the sphere in Fig. P.4 that traces out an octant: from $\hat{z}$ to $\hat{x}$ to $\hat{y}$ and back to $\hat{z}$. A triangle of the three points is a starting approximation to the continuous path, and it turns out to be exact [918]. Then the Berry phase is given by (see Exercise P.3)

$$\phi = -Im \ln[\langle\uparrow z| \uparrow x\rangle\langle\uparrow x| \uparrow y\rangle\langle\uparrow y| \uparrow z\rangle], \tag{P.19}$$

where $| \uparrow x\rangle$ denotes a state with spin up in the $\mathbf{x}$ direction, etc. If we chose the low-energy state with spin pointing along the magnetic field normal to the sphere, ϕ^- as represented in Eq. (P.18), the states are

$$| \uparrow x\rangle = \frac{1}{\sqrt{2}} \begin{pmatrix} 1 \\ 1 \end{pmatrix}, \; | \uparrow y\rangle = \frac{1}{\sqrt{2}} \begin{pmatrix} 1 \\ i \end{pmatrix}, \text{ and } | \uparrow z\rangle = \begin{pmatrix} 1 \\ 0 \end{pmatrix}. \tag{P.20}$$

Inserting these functions into Eq. (P.19) we find $\phi = -Im \ln[(1)(1+i)(1)] = \pi/4$, which is 1/2 the solid angle enclosed, the exact value. In Exercise P.4 you are asked to work out the corresponding result for a path that also visits the south pole $| \uparrow -z\rangle$.

SELECT FURTHER READING

See the list at the end of Chapter 25 of books with pedagogical overview of Berry phases.

Exercises

P.1 Show that $\langle u_x | \partial_x u_x \rangle$ needed in Eq. (P.3) is purely imaginary.

P.2 Derive the first equality in expression for $\Omega(\mathbf{k})$ in Eq. (P.12) from the expressions for the Berry phases in the previous equations. Discuss when there might be added factors of 2π. Show that the second equality follows from the normalization condition for the wavefunctions.

P.3 Work out the expressions for the eigenvectors Eq. (P.20) and verify the result $\phi = \pi/4$.

P.4 Calculate the Berry phase for the loop with four states from $\hat{\mathbf{z}}$ to $\hat{\mathbf{x}}$ to $-\hat{\mathbf{z}}$ to $\hat{\mathbf{y}}$ and back to $\hat{\mathbf{z}}$.

Appendix Q
Quantum Hall Effect and Edge Conductivity

Summary

The quantum Hall effect (QHE) illustrates the bulk-boundary correspondence, where quantization of the edge current is a necessary consequence of the topology of the electronic system in the bulk. The QHE serves as both a model for topological arguments and a direct demonstration of edge currents, which is a model for related currents in topological insulators.

Q.1 Quantum Hall Effect and Topology

The quantum Hall effect[1] occurs in two-dimensional systems with a large perpendicular magnetic field so that only one spin is occupied. The eigenstates are Landau levels (see texts such as Kittel [285] and Ashcroft and Mermin [280]), which are circular orbits as depicted in Fig. Q.1. The understanding of the QHE was a major theoretical development that was one of the first uses of topological characterization of bands in condensed matter.

The QHE is of great practical consequence and it is now the international standard of resistance. The Hall coefficient has units of resistance and the fact that current follows with zero resistance only at very precise quantized values of the Hall coefficient defines the value of resistance in units of fundamental quantities that is the standard.

In the QHE the bulk is an insulator if a set of Landau levels is filled and there is a gap to the next level. There is no net current in the interior of the material since the currents from different Landau states cancel as depicted in Fig. Q.1. However, the energy of the states at the edge are increased to lie in the gap of the bulk insulator [1101]; if the Fermi energy is in the gap there are partially filled states that are confined to the edge and move only in one direction. The current flows with no resistance since an electron cannot scatter to lose momentum because it only moves in one direction. If there is a defect the current simply goes around it as depicted in Fig. 25.3. This makes an intuitive picture of edge currents, but it does not show the remarkable feature that the current is very precisely quantized.

---

[1] See, e.g., the book by Prange and Giorvin [1100].

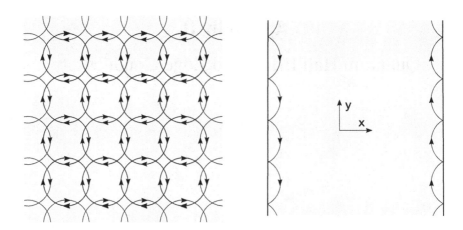

Figure Q.1. Schematic illustration of the QHE where there are circulating currents in the states in a filled Landau level in a homogeneous two-dimensional system in a magnetic field. The currents cancel in the interior but form the circulating current at the edges. See the corresponding Fig. 27.2 for a Chern insulator, which is termed a quantum anomalous Hall effect.

The proof was provided in a two-page paper by Laughlin [1102], who showed that the conductance must be an integral multiple of the fundamental unit of conductance e^2/h due to gauge invariance.

Topological classification Z and Chern numbers

Thouless, Kohmoto, Nightingale, and den Nijs (TKNN) [89] considered the problem of the QHE in a crystal with a periodic potential and they showed that the precise quantization is a topological property of the bands of the crystal, and the number of edge bands is equal to the Chern number, which is an example of bulk-boundary correspondence. This established the relation of the topology of the bands and the quantization of the edge state conductance, so that the edge currents are "topologically protected" and must occur even for materials that have defects and disorder. The classification is denoted Z, the set of integers, since the number of modes can be any integer. (This was one of the original works for which the 2016 Nobel prize was awarded to Haldane, Kosterlitz, and Thouless.)

Q.2 Nature of the Surface States in the QHE

It is instructive to see how the effect comes about in terms of the properties of the surface bands along with the effect of "pumping" of electrons that changes the number of electrons is the surface band. First, it is interesting to see how unique it is to have a Hall effect in an insulator! The Hall effect was discovered in metals in 1879 when graduate student Edwin H. Hall observed that a small transverse voltage appeared across a current-carrying thin metal strip in an applied magnetic field [1103]. It is explained in textbooks by the fact that for a magnetic field applied perpendicular to the plane of the strip, the current carrying particles are pushed to one side of the strip by the force $q\mathbf{v} \times \mathbf{B}$. This must be balanced by a force $q\mathbf{E}$ that can be detected as a voltage across the strip. It is a transport effect and the explanations involve the carier density and in general the mean free path that depends on extrinsic effects, etc. The Hall effect is characterized by the conductivity σ_{xy} for electric field in the y direction and current in the x direction along the strip. The final result that the Hall resistance (voltage divided by current) is $R_{Hall} = 1/(nqc)$ if there is only one type of carrier with charge q and density n.

How could a Hall effect occur in an insulator? The answer is that it can happen in a system that is insulating in the bulk only if it *must* have a conducting band or bands along the surface. Furthermore, it can happen in such a system only if it has quantized values. In the quantum Hall effect this happens when the Fermi energy is in a gap between Landau levels in the bulk but band bending leads to fractional occupied surface band(s). The effect can be visualized as in Fig. Q.1 where there is current flowing in opposite directions on the two edges. The following analysis applies also to a two-dimensional Chern insulator since the edge bands have the same form (see Section 27.2).

From this point on it is easy to see the affect – easier than in a metal! It is an intrinsic effect determined solely by the existence of the one-way edge bands independent of all details. Consider a long strip of width W with a voltage applied across the strip. (Since it is an insulator, there can be an electric field $\mathbf{E}$ in the bulk and a voltage difference $V = |\mathbf{E}|W$.) An applied field shifts the Fermi energy $\pm V/2$ on the two edges so that the number of electrons is increased on one side and decreased on the other; since the electrons flow in opposite directions on the two edges, the change of the current is the same magnitude and direction on the two edges. The penultimate step is the remarkable fact that the edge current is determined solely by the Fermi energy independent of the details of the edge band. Consider the current in the band due to particles in range k to $k + \Delta k$ as shown in Fig. Q.2,

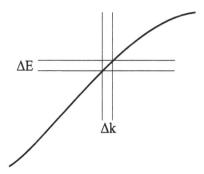

Figure Q.2. Illustration of the dispersion of a surface state in the quantum Hall effect, where electrons can move in only one direction along an edge. The slope $d\varepsilon/dk$ is the integrand in Eq. (Q.1), which provides a heuristic justification of the quantization of the conductance in Eq. (Q.2). The same logic applies to the edge states in one edge of a Chern insulator for each spin in a topological insulator in Chapter 27.

$$\Delta I = \frac{e}{2\pi} \int_k^{k+\Delta k} dk v_g = \frac{e}{2\pi h} \int_k^{k+\Delta k} dk \frac{d\varepsilon}{dk} = \frac{e}{h} \Delta E_F, \qquad (Q.1)$$

where q and ε are the charge and energy of the particles, v_g is the group velocity, and the maximum energy of the occupied states is the Fermi energy. Finally, in equilibrium ΔE_F is eV, and the result can be summarized as a universal value of the conductance for one edge, the current divided by the transverse voltage,

$$G = \frac{I}{V} = \frac{e^2}{h}, \qquad (Q.2)$$

which is determined solely by fundamental constants. The QHE is normally expressed in terms of the Hall resistance, but here it is most useful to recognize Eq. (Q.2) to be the quantum of conductance for a single channel.[2]

Even though this makes a intuitive picture with the correct final result, we should keep in mind that it is the topological character that guarantees the precise quantization.

---

[2] Often the quantum of conductance is defined to be $2e^2/h$ where the factor of 2 includes the spin degeneracy of electrons that is appropriate for phenomena that involve the sum of currents of the two spins, but here it is a single spin that is involved. For a topological insulator with time-reversal symmetry the two spins cancel and there is no net charge current, but they add leading to a net spin current (in the approximation that spin is conserved – see discussion of the quantum spin Hall effect).

Appendix R

Codes for Electronic Structure Calculations for Solids

Below is a list of codes that were used in work presented, or referred to, in this book. At the date this book was written, each was available. Almost all are free and open-source. Much more complete lists of software for electronic structure calculations can be found at sites such as https://psi-k.net/software/ and https://dft.sandia.gov/Quest/.

Tutorial codes:
- TBPW is a modular code intended for pedagogical purposes. It consists of modules for TB (tight-binding), PW (empirical pseudopotential plane waves) and features common for all methods (structure, Brillouin zone, etc.).
  Available at http://www.mcc.uiuc.edu/software/.
- Codes at nanoHUB.org that can treat empirical pseudopotential and tight-binding at many levels from simple models to semiconductor device simulation. Also many other codes.
- PythTB (Python Tight Binding) is a software package providing a Python implementation of tight-binding for arbitrary dimension (crystals, slabs, ribbons, clusters, etc.), with features for computing Berry phases and related properties. Not actually used in this book, but there are extensive examples in the book by Vanderbilt [918].
  Available at http://www.physics.rutgers.edu/pythtb/.

Plane wave codes:
- ABINIT [1104] is a package of open-source codes for density functional calculations using pseudopotentials (or PAW) and a plane wave basis, including phonons and molecular dynamics. It includes methods for many-body perturbation theory and dynamical mean field theory.
- CASTEP [1105] is a plane wave code for calculations of energetics, structure, vibrational, and other properties, including infrared and Raman spectroscopies, NMR, and core level spectra.
- Qbox is a plane wave, pseudopotential code designed especially for first-principles molecular dynamics for operation on large parallel computers.
- quantum-ESPRESSO [1106] is an integrated suite of open-source computer codes for density functional theory using plane waves and pseudopotentials. It includes phonons, molecular dynamics, and other codes.

- VASP [1056] package for plane wave calculations using either pseudopotentials or the projector augmented wave method.

(L)APW codes:
- ELK is an open-source all-electron full-potential linearized augmented plane wave (LAPW) code for density functional calculations designed to be as simple as possible so that new developments can be added quickly and reliably.
- WIEN2k is a package of codes for all-electron calculations based on the full-potential (linearized) augmented plane wave ((L)APW) + local orbitals (lo) method.

Local orbital codes:
- CRYSTAL [1107] Hartree–Fock calculations for periodic compounds using gaussian basis functions.
- DMol [655] uses numerical radial function basis set for periodic and molecular systems.
- FHI-aims [113] is all-electron, full-potential code with numeric atom-centered orbitals defined in Section 15.4, for periodic and nonperiodic systems.
- FPLO [654] is an all-electron, full-potential, local-orbital electronic structure code using a fixed atomic-like basis set with periodic or open boundary conditions.
- SIESTA [646] is a code for density functional calculations with numerical atomic orbitals defined in Section 15.4 (see also $O(N)$ codes).

Real-space codes:
- DFT-FE [586] – a real-space DFT code based on adaptive finite-element discretization for all-electron and pseudopotential calculations, periodic and nonperiodic.
- PARSEC [571] – finite difference pseudopotential codes for computing the electronic properties of periodic and nonperiodic materials.
- RMGDFT [584] is an open-source Real Space Multigrid code for density functional theory using real space basis and pseudopotentials. It is designed for scalability; it has been run on hundreds of thousands of CPU cores.
- SPARC [573] (Simulation Package for Ab-initio Real-space Calculations), a finite-difference formulation for extended systems.

Time-dependent DFT:
- Most of the plane wave, real space, and local orbitals codes listed above, and many other codes, also can perform TDFT calculations.
- OCTOPUS [1108] is a software package for performing density functional (DFT) and time-dependent density functional (TDDFT) calculations using pseudopotentials and real-space numerical grids.
- turboTDDFT [844] – a code for the simulation of molecular spectra using the Liouville–Lanczos approach to time-dependent density functional perturbation theory.

Linear scaling $O(N)$ codes:
These are codes written especially for linear scaling. These codes can also be used for usual nonlinear scaling calculations, and other codes may also be used in a linear scaling way.

- BigDFT [592] is a code for DFT using a wavelet basis set, designed to be massively parallel.
- CONQUEST [1109] can treat tight binding up to full DFT with plane wave accuracy using Blip functions (b-splines).
- ONETEP [1110, 1111] – linear-scaling density functional theory with plane waves,
- SIESTA [646] is a linear scaling code for DFT calculations with numerical atomic orbitals.

Wannier functions:
- WANNIER90 [1112] – a tool for obtaining maximally localized Wannier functions.

Structure searching:
- AIRSS (Ab initio Random Structure Searching) [130] is a simple, yet powerful and highly parallel, approach to structure prediction.
- CALYPSO (Crystal structure AnaLYsis by Particle Swarm Optimization) [1113] is a structure prediction method using particle swarm optimization.
- USPEX (Universal Structure Predictor: Evolutionary Xtallography) – code for crystal structure prediction using evolutionary techniques.

References

[1] R. M. Martin, L. Reining, and D. M. Ceperley, *Interacting Electrons: Theory and Computational Approaches*, Cambridge University Press, Cambridge, UK, 2016.

[2] H. A. Lorentz, *Theory of Electrons*, reprint of volume of lectures given at Columbia University in 1906, Dover, New York, 1952.

[3] P. Zeeman, "The effect of magnetisation on the nature of light emitted by a substance," translated by Arthur Stanton from the Proceedings of the Physical Society of Berlin, *Nature* 55:347, 1897.

[4] J. J. Thomson, "Cathode rays," *Phil. Mag., Series 5* 44:310–312, 1897.

[5] J. J. Thomson, "Cathode rays," *The Electrician: A Weekly Illustrated Journal of Electrical Engineering, Industry and Science* 39, 1897.

[6] E. Rutherford, "The scattering of α and β particles by matter and the structure of the atom," *Phil. Mag., Series 6* 21:669–688, 1911.

[7] N. Bohr, "On the constitution of atoms and molecules," *Phil. Mag., Series 6* 26:1–25, 1913.

[8] M. Jammer, *The Conceptual Development of Quantum Mechanics*, McGraw-Hill, New York, 1966.

[9] *Sources of Quantum Mechanics*, edited by B. L. van de Waerden, North Holland, Amsterdam, 1967.

[10] A. Messiah, *Quantum Mechanics*, vol. I, Wiley, New York, 1964.

[11] L. Hoddeson and G. Baym, "The development of the quantum-mechanical electron theory of metals: 1900–1928," *Proc. Roy. Soc. A* 371:8, 1987.

[12] L. Hoddeson and G. Baym, "The development of the quantum-mechanical electron theory of metals: 1928–1933," *Rev. Mod. Phys.* 59:287, 1987.

[13] L. Hoddeson, E. Braun, J. Teichmann, and S. Weart, *Out of the Crystal Maze*, chapters for the history of solid state physics, Oxford University Press, New York, Oxford, 1992.

[14] O. Stern, "Ein Weg zur experimentellen Prüfung der Richtungsquantelung im Magnetfeld" [Experiment to test the applicability of the quantum theory to the magnetic field], *Z. Physik* 7:249–253, 1921.

[15] W. Gerlach and O. Stern, "Der experimentelle Nachweis der Richtungsquantelung im Magnetfeld (Experimental test of the applicability of the quantum theory to the magnetic field)," *Z. Physik* 9:349–352, 1922.

[16] A. H. Compton, "Possible magnetic polarity of free electrons: Estimate of the field strength of the electron," *Z. Phys.* 35:618–625, 1926.

[17] S. A. Goudschmidt and G. H. Uhlenbeck, "Die Kopplungsmöglichkeiten der Quantenvektoren im Atom," *Z. Phys.* 35:618–625, 1926.

[18] W. Pauli, "Uber den Zusammenhang des Abschlusses der Elektronengruppen im Atom mit der Komplex Struktur der Spektren," *Z. Phys.* 31:765, 1925.

[19] E. C. Stoner, "The distribution of electrons among atomic levels," *Phil. Mag.* 48:719, 1924.

[20] E. Fermi, "Zur Quantelung des Idealen Einatomigen Gases," *Z. Phys.* 36:902, 1926.

[21] S. N. Bose, "Plancks Gesetz und Lichtquanten-hypothese," *Z. Phys.* 26:178, 1924.

[22] A. Einstein, "Quantheorie des Idealen Einatomigen Gases," *Sber. preuss Akad. Wiss.* p. 261, 1924.

[23] W. Heisenberg, "Mehrkorperproblem und Resonanz in der Quantenmechanik," *Z. Phys.* 38:411, 1926.

[24] P. A. M. Dirac, "On the theory of quantum mechanics," *Proc. R. Soc. A* 112:661, 1926.

[25] J. C. Slater, "The theory of complex spectra," *Phys. Rev.* 34:1293, 1929.

[26] P. A. M. Dirac, "The quantum theory of the electron," *Proc. R. Soc. A* 117:610–624, 1928.

[27] P. A. M. Dirac, "The quantum theory of the electron. Part II," *Proc. R. Soc. A* 118:351–361, 1928.

[28] G. N. Lewis, "The atom and the molecule," *J. Am. Chem. Soc.* 38:762–786, 1916.

[29] W. Heitler and F. London, "Wechselwirkung neutraler Atome und homopolare Bindung nach der Quantenmechanik," *Z. Phys.* 44:455, 1927.

[30] W. Pauli, "Uber Gasentartung und Paramagnetismus," *Z. Phys.* 41:91, 1927.

[31] A. Sommerfeld, "Zur Elektronen Theorie der Metalle auf Grund der Fermischen Statistik," *Z. Phys.* 47:43, 1928.

[32] P. Drude, "Bestimmung optischer Konstanten der Metalle," *Wied. Ann.* 39:481–554, 1897.

[33] P. Drude, *Lehrbuch der Optik (Textbook on Optics)*, S. Hirzel, Leipzig, 1906.

[34] H. Bethe, "Theorie der Beugung von Elektronen in Kristallen," *Ann. Phys. (Leipzig)* 87:55, 1928.

[35] F. Bloch, "Uber die Quantenmechanik der Elektronen in Kristallgittern," *Z. Phys.* 52:555, 1928.

[36] R. E. Peierls, "Zur Theorie der galvanomagnetischen Effekte," *Z. Phys.* 53:255, 1929.

[37] R. E. Peierls, "Zur Theorie der electrischen und thermischen Leitfähigkeit von Metallen," *Ann. Phys. (Leipzig)* 4:121, 1930.

[38] A. H. Wilson, "The theory of electronic semiconductors," *Proc. R. Soc. A* 133:458, 1931.

[39] A. H. Wilson, "The theory of electronic semiconductors – II," *Proc. R. Soc. A* 134:277, 1931.

[40] F. Seitz, *The Modern Theory of Solids*, McGraw-Hill Book Company, New York, 1940, reprinted in paperback by Dover Press, New York, 1987.

[41] G. E. Kimball, "The electronic structure of diamond," *J. Chem. Phys.* 3:560, 1935.

[42] W. Shockley, "On the surface states associated with a periodic potential," *Phys. Rev.* 56: 317–323, 1939.

[43] W. Shockley, "Energy band structure of sodium cloride," *Phys. Rev.* 50:754–759, 1937.

[44] D. Pines, *The Many Body Problem*, Advanced Book Classics, originally published in 1961, Addison-Wesley, Reading, MA, 1997.

[45] A. A. Abrikosov, L. P. Gorkov, and I. E. Dzyaloshinski, *Methods of Quantum Field Theory in Statistical Physics*, Prentice-Hall, Englewood Cliffs, NJ, 1963.

[46] J. M. Luttinger and J. C. Ward, "Ground-state energy of a many-fermion system. II," *Phys. Rev.* 118:1417–1427, 1960.

[47] J. M. Luttinger, "Fermi surface and some simple equilibrium properties of a system of interacting fermions," *Phys. Rev.* 119:1153–1163, 1960.

[48] J. C. Slater, *Solid-State and Molecular Theory: A Scientific Biography*, John Wiley & Sons, New York, 1975.

[49] D. R. Hartree, *The Calculation of Atomic Structures*, John Wiley & Sons, New York, 1957.

[50] D. R. Hartree, "The wave mechanics of an atom with non-Coulombic central field: Parts I, II, III," *Proc. Cambridge Phil. Soc.* 24:89,111,426, 1928.

[51] E. Hylleraas, "Neue Berectnumg der Energie des Heeliums im Grundzustande, sowie tiefsten Terms von Ortho-Helium," *Z. Phys.* 54:347, 1929.

[52] E. A. Hylleraas, "Uber den Grundterm der Zweielektronenprobleme von H^-, He, Li^+, Be^+ usw.," *Z. Phys.* 65:209, 1930.

[53] V. Fock, "Naherungsmethode zur Losung des quanten-mechanischen Mehrkorperprobleme," *Z. Phys.* 61:126, 1930.

[54] E. P. Wigner and F. Seitz, "On the constitution of metallic sodium," *Phys. Rev.* 43:804, 1933.

[55] A. Sommerfeld and H. Bethe, "Elektronentheorie der Metalle," *Handbuch der Physik* 24/2:333, 1933.

[56] J. C. Slater, "The electronic structure of metals," *Rev. Mod. Phys.* 6:209–280, 1934.

[57] E. P. Wigner and F. Seitz, "On the constitution of metallic sodium II," *Phys. Rev.* 46:509, 1934.

[58] J. C. Slater, "Electronic energy bands in metals," *Phys. Rev.* 45:794–801, 1934.

[59] F. Herman and J. Callaway, "Electronic structure of the germanium crystal," *Phys. Rev.* 89:518–519, 1953.

[60] H. M. Krutter, "Energy bands in copper," *Phys. Rev.* 48:664, 1935.

[61] J. C. Slater, "Wave function in a periodic potential," *Phys. Rev.* 51:846–851, 1937.

[62] J. C. Slater, "An augmented plane wave method for the periodic potential problem," *Phys. Rev.* 92:603–608, 1953.

[63] M. M. Saffren and J. C. Slater, "An augmented plane wave method for the periodic potential problem II," *Phys. Rev.* 92:1126, 1953.

[64] W. C. Herring, "A new method for calculating wave functions in crystals," *Phys. Rev.* 57:1169, 1940.

[65] E. Fermi, "Displacement by pressure of the high lines of the spectral series," *Nuovo Cimento* 11:157, 1934.

[66] H. Hellmann, "A new approximation method in the problem of many electrons," *J. Chem. Phys.* 3:61, 1935.

[67] H. Hellmann, "Metallic binding according to the combined approximation procedure," *J. Chem. Phys.* 4:324, 1936.

[68] F. Herman, "Theoretical investigation of the electronic energy band structure of solids," *Rev. Mod. Phys.* 30:102, 1958.

[69] F. Herman, "Elephants and mahouts – Early days in semiconductor physics," *Phys. Today* June, 1984:56, 1984.

[70] W. Heisenberg, "The theory of ferromagnetism," *Z. Phys.* 49:619–636, 1928.

[71] P. A. M. Dirac, "Quantum mechanics of many-electron systems," *Proc. R. Soc. A* 123: 714–733, 1929.

[72] N. Bohr, Studier over Metallernes Elektrontheori (thesis), 1911.

[73] H. J. van Leeuwen, Vraagstukken uit de Electrontheorie van het Magnetisme (thesis), 1911.

[74] H. J. van Leeuwen, "Problemes de la Theorie Electronique du Magnetisme," *J. Phys. Radium* 6:361, 1921.

[75] L. Pauling, *The Nature of the Chemical Bond,* 3rd ed., Cornell University Press, Ithaca, NY, 1960.

[76] E. P. Wigner, "On the interaction of electrons in metals," *Phys. Rev.* 46:1002–1011, 1934.

[77] N. F. Mott and R. Peierls, "Discussion of the paper by De Boer and Verwey," *Proc. Phys. Soc. A* 49:72, 1937.

[78] N. F. Mott, "The basis of the theory of electron metals, with special reference to the transition metals," *Proc. Phys. Soc. A* 62:416, 1949.

[79] N. F. Mott, *Metal–Insulator Transitions*, Taylor & Francis, London/Philadelphia, 1990.

[80] J. H. de Boer and E. J. W Verwey, "Semi-conductors with partially and with completely filled 3d-lattice bands," *Proc. Phys. Soc.* 49:59–71, 1937.

[81] P. W. Anderson, "More is different: Broken symmetry and the nature of the heirachical styrurcture of science," *Science* 177:393–396, 1972.

[82] *More Is Different: Fifty Years of Condensed Matter Physics*, edited by N.-P. Ong and R. Bhatt, Princeton University Press, Princeton, NJ, 2001.

[83] P. Hohenberg and W. Kohn, "Inhomogeneous electron gas," *Phys. Rev.* 136:B864–871, 1964.

[84] W. Kohn and L. J. Sham, "Self-consistent equations including exchange and correlation effects," *Phys. Rev.* 140:A1133–A1138, 1965.

[85] R. Car and M. Parrinello, "Unified approach for molecular dynamics and density functional theory," *Phys. Rev. Lett.* 55:2471–2474, 1985.

[86] C. L. Kane and E. J. Mele, "Z_2 topological order and the quantum spin Hall effect," *Physical Review Letters* 95:146802, 2005.

[87] C. L. Kane and E. J. Mele, "Quantum spin Hall effect in graphene," *Physical Review Letters* 95:226801, 2005.

[88] B. Andrei Bernevig and S.-C. Zhang, "Quantum spin Hall effect," *Phys. Rev. Lett.* 96:106802, 2006.

[89] D. J. Thouless, M. Kohmoto, M. P. Nightingale, and M. den Nijs, "Quantized Hall conductance in a two-dimensional periodic potential," *Phys. Rev. Lett.* 49:405–408, 1982.

[90] M. Born and J. R. Oppenheimer, "Zur Quantentheorie der Molekeln," *Ann. Physik* 84:457, 1927.

[91] M. Born and K. Huang, *Dynamical Theory of Crystal Lattices*, Oxford University Press, Oxford, 1954.

[92] J. S. Rowlinson, "Legacy of van der Waals," *Nature* 244:414–417, 1973.

[93] J. D. van der Waals, *Nobel Lectures in Physics*, Elsevier, Amsterdam, 1964, pp. 254–265.

[94] S. C. Wang, "The problem of the normal hydrogen molecule in the new quantum mechanics," *Phys. Rev.* 31:579–586, 1928.

[95] J. C. Slater and J. G. Kirkwood, "The van der Waals forces in gases," *Phys. Rev.* 37:682–697, 1931.

[96] R. Eisenschitz and F. London, "Uber das Verhaltnis der van der Waalsschen Krafte zu den homopolaren Bindungskraften," *Z. Phys.* 60:491–527, 1930.

[97] F. London, "Zur Theorie und Systematik der Molekularkrafte," *Z. Phys. A* 63:245–279, 1930.

[98] P. M. Chaikin and T. C. Lubensky, *Principles of Condensed Matter Physics*, Cambridge University Press, Cambridge, UK, 1995.

[99] J. M. Zuo, P. Blaha, and K. Schwarz, "The theoretical charge density of silicon: Experimental testing of exchange and correlation potentials," *J. Phys. Condens. Matter.* 9:7541–7561, 1997.

[100] Z. W. Lu, A. Zunger, and M. Deutsch, "Electronic charge distribution in crystalline diamond, silicon, and germanium," *Phys. Rev. B* 47:9385–9410, 1993.

[101] M. T. Yin and M. L. Cohen, "Theory of static structural properties, crystal stability, and phase transformations: Application to Si and Ge," *Phys. Rev. B* 26:5668–5687, 1982.

[102] O. H. Nielsen and R. M. Martin, "Stresses in semiconductors: *Ab initio* calculations on Si, Ge, and GaAs," *Phys. Rev. B* 32(6):3792–3805, 1985.

[103] V. L. Moruzzi, A. R. Williams, and J. F. Janak, "Local density theory of metallic cohesion," *Phys. Rev. B* 15:2854–2857, 1977.

[104] V. L. Moruzzi, J. F. Janak, and A. R. Williams, *Calculated Electronic Properties of Metals*, Pergamon Press, New York, 1978.

[105] F. D. Murnaghan, "The compressibility of media under extreme pressures," *Proc. Nat. Acad. Sci. USA* 50:244–247, 1944.

[106] L. P. Howland, "Band structure and cohesive energy of potassium chloride," *Phys. Rev.* 109:1927, 1958.

[107] P. D. DeCicco, "Self-consistent energy bands and cohesive energy of potassium chloride," *Phys. Rev.* 153:931, 1967.

[108] W. E. Rudge, "Variation of lattice constant in augmented-plane-wave energy-band calculation for lithium," *Phys. Rev.* 181:1033, 1969.

[109] M. Ross and K. W. Johnson, "Augmented-plane-wave calculation of the total energy, bulk modulus, and band structure of compressed aluminum," *Phys. Rev. B* 2:4709, 1970.

[110] E. C. Snow, "Total energy as a function of lattice parameter for copper via the self-consistent augmented-plane-wave method," *Phys. Rev. B* 8:5391, 1973.

[111] J. F. Janak, V. L. Moruzzi, and A. R. Williams, "Ground-state thermomechanical proerties of some cubic elements in the local-density formalism," *Phys. Rev. B* 12:1257–1261, 1975.

[112] G.-X. Zhang, A. M. Reilly, A. Tkatchenko, and M. Scheffler, "Performance of various density-functional approximations for cohesive properties of 64 bulk solids," *New J. Phys.* 20:063020, 2018.

[113] V. Blum, R. Gehrke, F. Hanke, P. Havu, V. Havu, X. Ren, K. Reuter, and M. Scheffler, "*Ab initio* molecular simulations with numeric atom-centered orbitals," *Comput. Phys. Commun.* 180:2175–2196, 2009.

[114] E. B. Isaacs and C. Wolverton, "Performance of the strongly constrained and appropriately normed density functional for solid-state materials," *Phys. Rev. Materials* 2:063801, 2018.

[115] M Marsman, J Paier, A Stroppa, and G Kresse, "Hybrid functionals applied to extended systems," *J. Phys. Condens. Matter* 20:064201, 2008.

[116] Y. Fu and D. J. Singh, "Applicability of the strongly constrained and appropriately normed density functional to transition-metal magnetism," *Phys. Rev. Lett.* 121:207201, 2018.

[117] H.-K. Mao, X.-J. Chen, Y. Ding, B. Li, and L. Wang, "Solids, liquids, and gases under high pressure," *Rev. Mod. Phys.* 90:015007, 2018.

[118] R. Biswas, R. M. Martin, R. J. Needs, and O. H. Nielsen, "Complex tetrahedral structures of silicon and carbon under pressure," *Phys. Rev. B* 30(6):3210–3213, 1984.

[119] M. T. Yin, "Si-III (BC-8) crystal phase of Si and C: Structural properties, phase stabilities, and phase transitions," *Phys. Rev. B* 30:1773–1776, 1984.

[120] G. J. Ackland, "High-pressure phases of group IV and III–V semiconductores," *Rep. Prog. Phys.* 64:483–516, 2001.

[121] A. Mujica, A. Rubio, A. Munoz, and R. J. Needs, "High-pressure phases of group IVa, IIIa–Va and IIb–VIa compounds," *Rev. Mod. Phys.* 75:863–912, 2003.

[122] J. S. Kasper and Jr. R. H. Wentorf, "The crystal structures of new forms of silicon and germanium," *Acta Cryst.* 17:752, 1964.

[123] R. J. Needs and A. Mujica, "Theoretical description of high-pressure phases of semiconductors," *High Press. Res.* 22:421, 2002.

[124] H. Olijnyk, S. K. Sikka, and W. B. Holzapfel, "Structural phase transitions in Si and Ge under pressures up to 50 GPa," *Phys. Lett.* 103A:137, 1984.

[125] J. Z. Hu and I. L. Spain, "Phases of silicon at high pressure," *Solid State Commun.* 51:263, 1984.

[126] A. K. McMahan, "Interstitial-sphere linear muffin-tin orbital structural calculations for C and Si," *Phys. Rev. B* 30:5835–5841, 1984.

[127] B. Xiao, J. Sun, A. Ruzsinszky, J. Feng, R. Haunschild, G. E. Scuseria, and J. P. Perdew, "Testing density functionals for structural phase transitions of solids under pressure: Si, SiO_2, and Zr," *Phys. Rev. B* 88:184103, 2013.

[128] C. Shahi, J. Sun, and J. P. Perdew, "Accurate critical pressures for structural phase transitions of group IV, III–V, and II–VI compounds from the SCAN density functional," *Phys. Rev. B* 97:094111, 2018.

[129] N. Sengupta, J. E. Bates, and A. Ruzsinszky, "From semilocal density functionals to random phase approximation renormalized perturbation theory: A methodological assessment of structural phase transitions," *Phys. Rev. B* 97:235136, 2018.

[130] C. J. Pickard and R. J. Needs, "*Ab initio* random structure searching," *J. Phys. Condens. Matter* 23:053201, 2011.

[131] R. J. Needs and C. J. Pickard, "Perspective: Role of structure prediction in materials discovery and design," *APL Materials* 4:053210, 2016.

[132] D. H. Wolpert and W. G. Macready, "No free lunch theorems for optimization," *IEEE Trans. Evol. Comput.* 1:67–82, 1997.

[133] S. Kirkpatrick, C. D. Gelatt, and M. P. Vecchi, "Optimization by simulated annealing," *Science* 220:671–680, 1983.

[134] X.-S. Yang, in *Nature-Inspired Optimization Algorithms*, edited by X.-S. Yang, Elsevier, Oxford, 2014, pp. 99–110.

[135] J. Kennedy and R. C. Eberhart, in *Proceedings of the IEEE International Conference on Neural Networks, Piscataway, NJ, 1995*, edited by X.-S. Yang, Available at IEEE Xplore Digital Library, ieeexplore.ieee.org.

[136] T. Back, *Evolutionary Algorithms in Theory and Practice: Evolution Strategies, Evolutionary Programming, Genetic Algorithm*, Oxford University Press, Oxford, U.K., 1990.

[137] A. O. Lyakhov, A. R. Oganov, H. T. Stokes, and Q. Zhu, "New developments in evolutionary structure prediction algorithm USPEX," *Comput. Phys. Commun.* 184:1172–1182, 2013.

[138] A. R. Oganov and C. W. Glass, "Crystal structure prediction using *ab initio* evolutionary techniques: Principles and applications," *J. Chem. Phys.* 124:244704, 2006.

[139] C. Mailhiot, L. H. Yang, and A. K. McMahan, "Polymeric nitrogen," *Phys. Rev. B* 46:14419–14435, 1992.

[140] M. I. Eremets, A. G. Gavriliuk, I. A. Trojan, D. A. Dzivenko, and R. Boehler, "Single-bonded cubic form of nitrogen," *Nat. Mater.* 3:558–563, 2004.

[141] M. I. Eremets, A. G. Gavriliuk, N. R. Serebryanaya, I. A. Trojan, D. A. Dzivenko, R. Boehler, H. K. Mao, and R. J. Hemley, "Structural transformation of molecular nitrogen to a single-bonded atomic state at high pressures," *J. Chem. Phys.* 121:11296–11300, 2004.

[142] E. M. Benchafia, Z. Yao, G. Yuan, Tsengmin Chou, H. Piao, X. Wang, and Z. Iqbal, "Cubic gauche polymeric nitrogen under ambient conditions," *Nat. Commun.* 8:930, 2017.

[143] C. J. Pickard and R. J. Needs, "High-pressure phases of nitrogen," *Phys. Rev. Lett.* 102:125702, 2009.

[144] J. M. McMahon, M. A. Morales, C. Pierleoni, and D. M. Ceperley, "The properties of hydrogen and helium under extreme conditions," *Rev. Mod. Phys.* 84:1607–1653, 2012.

[145] N. W. Ashcroft, "Hydrogen dominant metallic alloys: High temperature superconductors?," *Phys. Rev. Lett.* 92:187002, 2004.

[146] D. Duan, Y. Liu, F. Tian, D. Li, X. Huang, Z. Zhao, H. Yu, B. Liu, W. Tian, and T. Cui, "Pressure-induced metallization of dense $(H_2S)_2H_2$ with high-Tc superconductivity," *Sci. Rep.* 4:6968, 2014.

[147] Y. Li, J. Hao, H. Liu, Y. Li, and Y. Ma, "The metallization and superconductivity of dense hydrogen sulfide," *J. Chem. Phys.* 140:174712, 2014.

[148] A. P. Drozdov, M. I. Eremets, I. A. Troyan, V. Ksenofontov, and S. I. Shylin, "Conventional superconductivity at 203 Kelvin at high pressures in the sulfur hydride system," *Nature* 525:73, 2015.

[149] M. Einaga, M. Sakata, T. Ishikawa, K. Shimizu, M. I. Eremets, A. P. Drozdov, I. A. Troyan, N. Hirao, and Y. Ohishi, "Crystal structure of the superconducting phase of sulfur hydride," *Nat. Phys.* 12:835, 2016.

[150] N. Bernstein, C. Stephen Hellberg, M. D. Johannes, I. I. Mazin, and M. J. Mehl, "What superconducts in sulfur hydrides under pressure and why," *Phys. Rev. B* 91:060511, 2015.

[151] D. A. Papaconstantopoulos, B. M. Klein, M. J. Mehl, and W. E. Pickett, "Cubic H_3S around 200 GPa: An atomic hydrogen superconductor stabilized by sulfur," *Phys. Rev. B* 91:184511, 2015.

[152] D. Duan, X. Huang, F. Tian, D. Li, H. Yu, Y. Liu, Y. Ma, B. Liu, and T. Cui, "Pressure-induced decomposition of solid hydrogen sulfide," *Phys. Rev. B* 91:180502, 2015.

[153] M. Benoit, A. H. Romero, and D. Marx, "Reassigning hydrogen-bond centering in dense ice," *Phys. Rev. Lett.* 89:145501, 2002.

[154] H. Liu, I. I. Naumov, R. Hoffmann, N. W. Ashcroft, and R. J. Hemley, "Potential high-Tc superconducting lanthanum and yttrium hydrides at high pressure," *Proc. Natl. Acad. Sci. U.S.A.* 114:6990–6995, 2017.

[155] F. Peng, Y. Sun, C. J. Pickard, R. J. Needs, Q. Wu, and Y. Ma, "Hydrogen clathrate structures in rare earth hydrides at high pressures: Possible route to room-temperature superconductivity," *Phys. Rev. Lett.* 119:107001, 2017.

[156] M. Somayazulu, M. Ahart, A. K. Mishra, Z. M. Geballe, M. Baldini, Y. Meng, V. V. Struzhkin, and R. J. Hemley, "Evidence for superconductivity above 260 K in lanthanum superhydride at megabar pressures," *Phys. Rev. Lett.* 122:027001, 2019.

[157] J. Kübler and V. Eyert, in *Electronic and Magnetic Properties of Metals and Ceramics*, edited by K. H. J. Buschow, VCH-Verlag, Weinheim, Germany, 1992, p. 1.

[158] E. C. Stoner, "Collective electron ferromagnetism. II. Energy and specific heat," *Proc. Roy. Soc. A* 169:339–371, 1939.

[159] C. Herring, in *Magnetism IV: Exchange Interactions among Itinerant Electrons*, edited by G. Rado and H. Suhl, Academic Press, New York, 1966.

[160] Q. Niu and L. Kleinman, "Spin-wave dynamics in real crystals," *Phys. Rev. Lett.* 80:2205–2208, 1998.

[161] R. Gebauer and S. Baroni, "Magnons in real materials from density-functional theory," *Phys. Rev. B* 61:R6459–R6462, 2000.

[162] O. H. Nielsen and R. M. Martin, "Quantum-mechanical theory of stress and force," *Phys. Rev. B* 32(6):3780–3791, 1985.

[163] O. H. Nielsen and R. M. Martin, "First-principles calculation of stress," *Phys. Rev. Lett.* 50(9):697–700, 1983.

[164] O. H. Nielsen, "Optical phonons and elasticity of diamond at megabar stresses," *Phys. Rev. B* 34:5808–5819, 1986.

[165] *Lattice Dynamics*, edited by R. F. Wallis, Pergamon Press, London, 1965.

[166] *Dynamical Properties of Solids,* vol. 3, edited by G. K. Horton and A. A. Maradudin, North-Holland, Amsterdam, 1979.

[167] K. Kunc and R. M. Martin, "Density-functional calculation of static and dynamic properties of GaAs," *Phys. Rev. B* 24(4):2311–2314, 1981.

[168] P. Ordejon, E. Artacho, R. Cachau, J. Gale, A. Garcia, J. Junquera, J. Kohanoff, M. Machado, D. Sanchez-Portal, J. M. Soler, and R. Weht, "Linear scaling DFT calculations with numerical atomic orbitals," *Mat. Res. Soc. Symp. Proc.* 677, 2001.

[169] R. E. Cohen and H. Krakauer, "Electronic-structure studies of the differences in ferroelectric behavior of $BaTi_xO_3$ and $PbTi_xO_3$," *Ferroelectrics* 136:65, 1992.

[170] K.-M. Ho, C.-L. Fu, and B. N. Harmon, "Vibrational frequencies via total-energy calculations: Applications to transition metals," *Phys. Rev. B* 29:1575–1587, 1984.

[171] D. J. Chadi and R. M. Martin, "Calculation of lattice dynamical properties from electronic energies: Application to C, Si and Ge," *Solid State Commun.* 19(7):643–646, 1976.

[172] H. Wendel and R. M. Martin, "Theory of structural properties of covalent semiconductors," *Phys. Rev. B* 19(10):5251–5264, 1979.

[173] U. V. Waghmare and K. M. Rabe, "*Ab initio* statistical mechanics of the ferroelectric phase transition in $PbTiO_3$," *Phys. Rev. B* 55:6161–6173, 1997.

[174] P. García-Fernández, J. C. Wojdeł, J. Íñiguez, and J. Junquera, "Second-principles method for materials simulations including electron and lattice degrees of freedom," *Phys. Rev. B* 93:195137, 2016.

[175] R. D. King-Smith and D. H. Vanderbilt, "Theory of polarization of crystalline solids," *Phys. Rev. B* 47:1651–1654, 1993.

[176] R. Resta, "Macroscopic polarization in crystalline dielectrics: the geometric phase approach," *Rev. Mod. Phys.* 66:899–915, 1994.

[177] M. V. Berry, "Quantal phase factors accompanying adiabatic changes," *Proc. R. Soc. A* 392:45–47, 1984.

[178] P. D. De Cicco and F. A. Johnson, "The quantum theory of lattice dynamics. IV," *Proc. R. Soc. A* 310:111–119, 1969.

[179] L. J. Sham, "Electronic contribution to lattice dynamics in insulating crystals," *Phys. Rev.* 188:1431–1439, 1969.

[180] R. Pick, M. H. Cohen, and R. M. Martin, "Microscopic theory of force constants in the adiabatic approximation," *Phys. Rev. B* 1:910–920, 1970.

[181] S. Baroni, S. de Gironcoli, and A. Dal Corso, "Phonons and related properties of extended systems from density-functional perturbation theory," *Rev. Mod. Phys.* 73:515–562, 2001.

[182] P. Giannozzi, S. de Gironcoli, P. Pavoni, and S. Baroni, "*Ab initio* calculation of phonon dispersion in semiconductors," *Phys. Rev. B* 43:7231, 1991.

[183] T. Tsuchiya, J. Tsuchiya, K. Umemoto, and R. M. Wentzcovitch, "Phase transition in $MgSiO_3$ perovskite in the earth's lower mantle," *Earth Planet. Sc. Lett.* 224:241–248, 2004.

[184] M. J. Gillan, D. Alfe, J. Brodholt, L. Vocadlo, and G. D. Price, "First-principles modelling of earth and planetary materials at high pressures and temperatures," *Rep. Prog. Phys.* 69:2365–2441, 2006.

[185] R. Wentzcovitch and L. Stixrude, "Theoretical and computational methods in mineral physics: Geophysical applications," *Rev. Mineral Geochem.* 71:iii–vi, 2010.

[186] D. Alfè, G. Kresse, and M. J. Gillan, "Structure and dynamics of liquid iron under Earth's core conditions," *Phys. Rev. B* 61:132–142, 2000.

[187] H. K. Mao, Y. Wu, L. C. Chen, J. F. Shu, and A. P. Jephcoat, "Static compression of iron to 300 GPa and $Fe_{0.8}Ni_{0.2}$ alloy to 260 GPa: Implications for composition of the core," *J. Geophys. Res. B* 95:21737–21742, 1990.

[188] D. Alfe, "Iron at Earth core conditions from first principles calculations," *Rev. Mineral Geochem.* 71:337–354, 2010.

[189] E. Schwegler, G. Galli, F. Gygi, and R. Q. Hood, "Dissociation of water under pressure," *Phys. Rev. Lett.* 87:265501, 2001.

[190] L. Pauling, "The structure and entropy of ice and of other crystals with some randomness of atomic arrangement," *J. Am. Chem. Soc.* 157:2680, 1935.

[191] A. Jeffery, *An Introduction to Hydrogen Bonding*, Oxford University Press, Oxford, UK, 1997.

[192] A. Luzar and D. Chandler, "Hydrogen-bond kinetics in liquid water," *Nature* 379:55–57, 1996.

[193] T. A. Pham, T. Ogitsu, E. Y. Lau, and E. Schwegler, "Structure and dynamics of aqueous solutions from PBE-based first-principles molecular dynamics simulations," *J. Chem. Phys.* 145:154501, 2016.

[194] A. P. Gaiduk, J. Gustafson, F. Gygi, and G. Galli, "First-principles simulations of liquid water using a dielectric-dependent hybrid functional," *J. Phys. Chem. Lett.* 9:3068–3073, 2018.

[195] M. Chen, H.-Y. Ko, R. C. Remsing, Marcos F. Calegari A., B. Santra, Z. Sun, A. Selloni, R. Car, M. L. Klein, J. P. Perdew, and X. Wu, "*Ab initio* theory and modeling of water," *Proc. Natl. Acad. Sci. U.S.A.* 114:10846–10851, 2017.

[196] L. B. Skinner, C. Huang, D. Schlesinger, L. G. M. Pettersson, A. Nilsson, and C. J. Benmore, "Benchmark oxygen-oxygen pair-distribution function of ambient water from X-ray diffraction measurements with a wide q-range," *J. Chem. Phys.* 138:074506, 2013.

[197] M. J. Gillan, D. Alfe, and A. Michaelides, "Perspective: How good is DFT for water?," *J. Chem. Phys.* 144:130901, 2016.

[198] R. A. DiStasio, B. Santra, Z. Li, X. Wu, and R. Car, "The individual and collective effects of exact exchange and dispersion interactions on the *ab initio* structure of liquid water," *J. Chem. Phys.* 141:084502, 2014.

[199] A. F. Goncharov, V. V. Struzhkin, H.-K. Mao, and R. J. Hemley, "Raman spectroscopy of dense H_2O and the transition to symmetric hydrogen bonds," *Phys. Rev. Lett.* 83:1998–2001, 1999.

[200] C. Lee, D. Vanderbilt, Kari Laasonen, R. Car, and M. Parrinello, "*Ab initio* studies on high pressure phases of ice," *Phys. Rev. Lett.* 69:462–465, 1992.

[201] M. Boero, M. Parrinello, and K. Terakura, "First principles molecular dynamics study of Ziegler–Natta heterogeneous catalysis," *J. Am. Chem. Soc.* 120:746–2752, 1998.

[202] M. Boero, M. Parrinello, S. Huffer, and H. Weiss, "First principles study of propene polymerization in Ziegler–Natta heterogeneous catalysis," *J. Am. Chem. Soc.* 122:501–509, 2000.

[203] E. Penev, P. Kratzer, and M. Scheffler, "Effect of the cluster size in modeling the H_2 desorption and dissociative adsorption on Si(001)," *J. Chem. Phys.* 110:3986–3994, 1999.

[204] W. A. Harrison, "Theory of polar semiconductor surfaces," *J. Vac. Sci. Technol.* 16:1492–1496, 1979.

[205] R. M. Martin, "Atomic reconstruction at polar interfaces of semiconductors," *J. Vac. Sci. Technol.* 17(5):978–981, 1980.

[206] A. A. Wilson, *Thermodynamics and Statistical Mechanics*, Cambridge University Press, Cambridge, U.K., 1957.

[207] A. A. Wilson, *Fundamentals of Statistical and Thermal Physics*, McGraw-Hill, New York, 1965.

[208] G. X. Qian, R. M. Martin, and D. J. Chadi, "First-principles calculations of atomic and electronic structure of the GaAs (110) surface," *Phys. Rev. B* 37:1303, 1988.

[209] A. Garcia and J. E. Northrup, "First-principles study of Zn- and Se-stabilized ZnSe(100) surface reconstructions," *J. Vac. Sci. Technol. B* 12:2678–2683, 1994.

[210] J. E. Northrup and S. Froyen, "Structure of GaAs(001) surfaces: The role of electrostatic interactions," *Phys. Rev. B* 50:2015, 1994.

[211] A. Franciosi and C. G. Van de Walle, "Heterojunction band offset engineering," *Surf. Sci. Rep.* 25:1, 1996.

[212] C. G. Van de Walle and R. M. Martin, "Theoretical study of band offsets at semiconductor interfaces," *Phys. Rev. B* 35:8154–8165, 1987.

[213] C. G. Van de Walle and R. M. Martin, "'Absolute' deformation potentials: Formulation and *ab initio* calculations for semiconductors," *Phys. Rev. Lett.* 62:2028–2031, 1989.

[214] A. Ohtomo and H. Y. Hwang, "A high-mobility electron gas at the $LaAlO_3/SrTiO_3$ heterointerface," *Nature* 427:423, 2004.

[215] S. Vaziri, et al., "Ultrahigh thermal isolation across heterogeneously layered two-dimensional materials," *Sci. Adv.* 5, 2019.

[216] T. Li and G. Galli, "Electronic properties of MoS_2 nanoparticles," *J. Phys. Chem. C* 111:16192–16196, 2007.

[217] K. F. Mak, C. Lee, J. Hone, J. Shan, and T. F. Heinz, "Atomically thin MoS_2: A new direct-gap semiconductor," *Phys. Rev. Lett.* 105:136805, 2010.

[218] Jason K. Ellis, Melissa J. Lucero, and G. E. Scuseria, "The indirect to direct band gap transition in multilayered MoS2 as predicted by screened hybrid density functional theory," *Appl. Phys. Lett.* 99:261908, 2011.

[219] A. K. Geim and I. V. Grigorieva, "Perspective: Van der Waals heterostructures," *Nature* 499:419, 2013.

[220] f K. S. Novoselov, A. Mishchenko, A. Carvalho, and A. H. Castro Neto, "2D materials and van der Waals heterostructures," *Science* 353, 2016.

[221] W. D. Knight, K. Clemenger, W. A. de Heer, W. A. Saunders, M. Y. Chou, and M. L. Cohen, "Electronic shell structure and abundances of sodium clusters," *Phys. Rev. Lett.* 52:2141, 1984.

[222] M. Brack, "The physics of simple metal clusters: Self-consistent jellium model and semiclassical approaches," *Rev. Mod. Phys.* 65:677–732, 1993.

[223] U. Rothlisberger, W. Andreoni, and P. Giannozzi, "Thirteen-atom clusters: Equilibrium geometries, structural transformations, and trends in Na, Mg, Al, and Si," *J. Chem. Phys.* 92:1248, 1992.

[224] J. C. Phillips, "Electron-correlation energies and the structure of Si_{13}," *Phys. Rev. B* 47:14132, 1993.

[225] J. C. Grossman and L. Mitas, "Quantum Monte Carlo determination of elecronic and structural properties of Si_n clusters ($n \leq 20$)," *Phys. Rev. Lett.* 74:1323–1325, 1995.

[226] J. C. Grossman and L. Mitas, "Family of low-energy elongated Si_n ($n \leq 50$) clusters," *Phys. Rev. B* 52:16735–16738, 1995.

[227] H. W.Kroto, J. R. Heath, S. C. O'Brien, R. F. Curl, and R. E. Smalley, "C_{60}: Buckminsterfullerene," *Nature* 318:162, 1985.

[228] S. Iijima, "Helical microtubules of graphitic carbon," *Nature* 354:56, 1991.

[229] K. S. Novoselov, A. K. Geim, S. V. Morozov, D. Jiang, Y. Zhang, S. V. Dubonos, I. V. Grigorieva, and A. A. Firsov, "Electric field effect in atomically thin carbon films," *Science* 306:666–669, 2004.

[230] W. Kratschmer, L.D. Lamb, K. Fostiropoulos, and D.R. Huffman, "Solid C_{60}: A new form of carbon," *Nature* 347:354, 1990.

[231] R. C. Haddon, et al., "Conducting films of C_{60} and C_{70} by alkali-metal doping," *Nature* 350:320, 1991.

[232] N. Hamada, S. Sawada, and A. Oshiyama, "New one-dimensional conductors: Graphitic microtubules," *Phys. Rev. Lett* 68:1579–1581, 1992.

[233] R. Saito, M. Fujita, G. Dresselhaus, and M. S. Dresselhaus, "Electronic structure of graphene tubules based on C_{60}," *Phys. Rev. B* 46:1804–1811, 1992.

[234] R. Saito, G. Dresselhaus, and M. S. Dresselhaus, *Physical Properties of Carbon Nanotubes*, Imperial College Press, London, 1998.

[235] D. J. Rizzo, G. Veber, T. Cao, C. Bronner, T. Chen, F. Zhao, H. Rodriguez, S. G. Louie, M. F. Crommie, and Felix R. Fischer, "Topological band engineering of graphene nanoribbons," *Nature* 560:204–208, 2018.

[236] T. Cao, F. Zhao, and S. G. Louie, "Topological phases in graphene nanoribbons: Junction states, spin centers, and quantum spin chains," *Phys. Rev. Lett.* 119:076401, 2017.

[237] A. Damascelli, Z.-X. Shen, and Z. Hussain, "Angle-resolved photoemission studies of the cuprate superconductors," *Rev. Mod. Phys.* 75:473, 2003.

[238] H. Ibach and H. Luth, *Solid State Physics: An Introduction to Theory and Experiment*, Springer-Verlag, Berlin, 1991.

[239] S. Huffner, *Photoelectron Spectroscopy*, 2nd ed., Springer-Verlag, Berlin, 1995.

[240] M. Imada, A. Fujimori, and Y. Tokura, "Metal-insulator transitions," *Rev. Mod. Phys.* 70:1039–1263, 1998.

[241] L. Hedin and S. Lundquist, in *Solid State Physics*, vol. 23, edited by H. Ehenreich, F. Seitz, and D. Turnbull, Academic Press, New York, 1969, p. 1.

[242] A. J. Garza and G. E. Scuseria, "Predicting band gaps with hybrid density functionals," *J. Phys. Chem. Lett.* 7:4165–4170, 2016.

[243] Z.-H. Yang, H. Peng, J. Sun, and J. P. Perdew, "More realistic band gaps from meta-generalized gradient approximations: Only in a generalized Kohn–Sham scheme," *Phys. Rev. B* 93:205205, 2016.

[244] J. H. Skone, M. Govoni, and G. Galli, "Self-consistent hybrid functional for condensed systems," *Phys. Rev. B* 89:195112, 2014.

[245] A. Zangwill and P. Soven, "Density-functional approach to local-field effects in finite systems: Photoabsorption in the rare gases," *Phys. Rev. A* 21:1561, 1980.

[246] E. Runge and E. K. U. Gross, "Density-functional theory for time-dependent systems," *Phys. Rev. Lett.* 52:997–1000, 1984.

[247] K. Burke, J. Werschnik, and E. K. U. Gross, "Time-dependent density functional theory: Past, present, and future," *J. Chem. Phys.* 123:062206, 2005.

[248] *Time-Dependent Density Functional Theory, Lecture Notes in Physics,* vol. 706, edited by M. A. L. Marques, C. A. Ullrich, F. Nogueira, A. Rubio, K. Burke, and E. K. U. Gross, Springer, Berlin, 2006.

[249] C. Ullrich, *Time-Dependent Density-Functional Theory: Concepts and Applications*, Oxford University Press, Oxford, UK, 2012.

[250] *Density-Functional Methods for Excited States* (Topics in Current Chemistry), edited by N. Ferre, M. Filatov, and M. Huix-Rotllant, Springer International, Switzerland, 2016.

[251] M. Staedele, M. Moukara, J. A. Majewski, P. Vogl, and A. Gorling, "Exact exchange Kohn–Sham formalism applied to semiconductors," *Phys. Rev. B* 59:10031–10043, 1999.

[252] J. Paier, M. Marsman, and G. Kresse, "Dielectric properties and excitons for extended systems from hybrid functionals," *Phys. Rev. B* 78:121201, 2008.

[253] S. Refaely-Abramson, M. Jain, S. Sharifzadeh, J. B. Neaton, and L. Kronik, "Solid-state optical absorption from optimally tuned time-dependent range-separated hybrid density functional theory," *Phys. Rev. B* 92:081204, 2015.

[254] J. Bardeen, "Theory of the work function. II. The surface double layer," *Phys. Rev.* 49:653, 1936.

[255] Y. L. Chen, J.-H. Chu, J. G. Analytis, Z. K. Liu, K. Igarashi, H.-H. Kuo, X. L. Qi, S. K. Mo, R. G. Moore, D. H. Lu, M. Hashimoto, T. Sasagawa, S. C. Zhang, I. R. Fisher, Z. Hussain, and Z. X. Shen, "Massive Dirac fermion on the surface of a magnetically doped topological insulator," *Science* 329:659–662, 2010.

[256] D. J. Thouless, "Quantization of particle transport," *Phys. Rev. B* 27:6083–6087, 1983.

[257] H. Zhang, C.-X. Liu, X.-L. Qi, X. Dai, Z. Fang, and S.-C. Zhang, "Topological insulators in $Bi_2Se_3, Bi_2Te_3, Sb_2Te_3$ with a single Dirac cone on the surface," *Nat. Phys.* 5:438–442, 2009.

[258] W. Ritz, "Uber eine neue Methode zur Losung Gewisser Variationsprobleme der mathema-tischen Physik," *Reine Angew. Math.* 135:1, 1908.

[259] J. W. Strutt (Lord Rayleigh), *Theory of Sound*, Dover Publications, New York, 1945. First published in 1877.

[260] W. Jones and N. H. March, *Theoretical Solid State Physics,* vol. 1, John Wiley & Sons, New York, 1976.

[261] J. Matthews and R. L. Walker, *Mathematical Methods of Physics*, W. A. Benjamin, Inc., New York, 1964.

[262] G. B. Arfken, H. J. Weber, and F. E. Harris, *Mathematical Methods of Physics*, 7th ed., Academic Press, Waltham, MA, 2012.

[263] P. Ehrenfest, "Bemurkung über die angenäherte Gültigkeit der klassischen Mechanik inner-halb der Quantenmechanik," *Z. Phys.* 45:455, 1927.

[264] M. Born and V. Fock, "Beweis des Adiabatensatzes," *Z. Phys.* 51:165, 1928.

[265] P. Güttiger, "Das Verhalten von Atomen im magnetischen Drefeld," *Z. Phys.* 73:169, 1931.

[266] W. Pauli, *Handbuch der Physik*, Springer, Berlin, 1933. Pages 83–272 relate to force and stress.

[267] H. Hellmann, *Einfuhrung in die Quantumchemie*, Franz Duetsche, Leipzig, 1937.

[268] R. P. Feynman, "Forces in molecules," *Phys. Rev.* 56:340, 1939.

[269] P. Pulay, "*Ab initio* calculation of force constants and equilibrium geometries in polyatomic molecules. I. Theory," *Mol. Phys.* 17:197–204, 1969.

[270] V. Fock, "Naherungsmethode zur Losung des quanten-mechanischen Mehrkorperprobleme," *Z. Phys.* 63:855, 1930.

[271] J. Harris, "Adiabatic-connection approach to Kohn–Sham theory," *Phys. Rev. A* 29:1648, 1984.

[272] O. Gunnarsson and B. I. Lundqvist, "Exchange and correlation in atoms, molecules, and solids by the spin-density-functional formalism," *Phys. Rev. B* 13:4274–4298, 1976.

[273] R. G. Parr and W. Yang, *Density-Functional Theory of Atoms and Molecules*, Oxford University Press, New York, 1989.

[274] A. Szabo and N. S. Ostlund, *Modern Quantum Chemistry: Introduction to Advanced Elec-tronic Structure Theory*, Dover, Mineola, New York, 1996. Unabridged reprinting of 1989 version.

[275] R. D. McWeeny and B. T. Sutcliffe, *Methods of Molecular Quantum Mechanics,* 2nd ed., Academic Press, New York, 1976.

[276] C. A. White, B. G. Johnson, P. M.W. Gill, and M. Head-Gordon, "Linear scaling density functional calculations via the continuous fast multipole method," *Chem. Phys. Letters* 253:268–278, 1996.

[277] T. Koopmans, "Uber die Zuordnung von Wellenfunktionen und Eigenwerten zu den Einzel-nen Elektronen Eines Atoms," *Physica* 1:104–113, 1934.

[278] E. M. Landau and L. P. Pitaevskii, *Statistical Physics: Part 1*, Pergamon Press, Oxford, U.K., 1980.

[279] J. K. L. MacDonald, "Successive approximations by the Rayleigh–Ritz variation method," *Phys. Rev.* 43:830, 1933.

[280] N. W. Ashcroft and N. D. Mermin, *Solid State Physics*, W. B. Saunders Company, Philadel-phia, PA, 1976.

[281] V. Heine, *Group Theory*, Pergamon Press, New York, 1960.

[282] M. Tinkham, *Group Theory and Quantum Mechanics*, McGraw-Hill, New York, 1964.

[283] M. J. Lax, *Symmetry Principles in Solid State and Molecular Physics*, Wiley, New York, 1974.

[284] J. C. Slater, *Symmetry and Energy Bands in Crystals*, Dover, New York, 1972. Corrected and reprinted version of 1965 *Quantum Theory of Molecules and Solids*, vol. 2.

[285] C. Kittel, *Introduction to Solid State Physics*, John Wiley & Sons, New York, 1996.

[286] J. Moreno and J. M. Soler, "Optimal meshes for integrals in real- and reciprocal-space unit cells," *Phys. Rev. B* 45:13891–13898, 1992.

[287] H. J. Monkhorst and J. D. Pack, "Special points for Brillouin-zone integrations," *Phys. Rev. B* 13:5188–5192, 1976.

[288] A. H. MacDonald, "Comment on special points for Brillouin-zone integrations," *Phys. Rev. B* 18:5897–5899, 1978.

[289] A. Baldereschi, "Mean-value point in the Brillouin zone," *Phys. Rev. B* 7:5212–5215, 1973.

[290] D. J. Chadi and M. L. Cohen, "Electronic structure of $Hg_{1-x}Cd_x Te$ alloys and charge-density calculations using representative k points," *Phys. Rev. B* 8:692–699, 1973.

[291] J. F. Janak, in *Computational Methods in Band Theory*, edited by P. M. Marcus, J. F. Janak, and A. R. Williams, Plenum, New York, 1971, pp. 323–339.

[292] P. E. Blöchl, O. Jepsen, and O. K. Andersen, "Improved tetrahedron method for Brillouin-zone integrations," *Phys. Rev. B* 49:16223–16233, 1994.

[293] G. Gilat, "Analysis of methods for calculating spectral properties in solids," *J. Comput. Phys.* 10:432–65, 1972.

[294] G. Gilat, "Methods of Brillouin zone integration," *Methods Comput. Phys.* 15:317–70, 1976.

[295] A. H. MacDonald, S. H. Vosko, and P. T. Coleridge, "Extensions of the tetrahedron method for evaluating spectral properties of solids," *J. Phys. C: Solid State Phys.* 12:2991–3002, 1979.

[296] L. Van Hove, "The occurrence of singularities in the elastic frequency distribution of a crystal," *Phys. Rev.* 89:1189–1193, 1953.

[297] D. Pines, *Elementary Excitations in Solids*, Wiley, New York, 1964.

[298] D. Pines and P. Nozières, *The Theory of Quantum Liquids*, vol. 1 (Advanced Book Classics), Addison-Wesley Inc., Redwood City, CA, 1989. Originally published in 1966.

[299] N. Moll, M. Bockstedte, M. Fuchs, E. Pehlke, and M. Scheffler, "Application of generalized gradient approximations: The diamond-beta-tin phase transition in Si and Ge," *Phys. Rev. B* 52:2550–2556, 1995.

[300] M. Marder, *Condensed Matter Physics*, John Wiley & Sons, New York, 2000.

[301] R. M. Martin, "Fermi-surface sum rule and its consequences for periodic Kondo and mixed-valence systems," *Phys. Rev. Lett.* 48:362–365, 1982.

[302] S. Goedecker, "Decay properties of the finite-temperature density matrix in metals," *Phys. Rev. B* 58:3501–3502, 1998.

[303] J. W. Gibbs, "Fourier series," *Nature* (letter to the editor) 59:200, 1898.

[304] S. Ismail-Beigi and T. A. Arias, "Locality of the density matrix in metals, semiconductors and insulators," *Phys. Rev. Lett.* 82:2127–2130, 1999.

[305] U. von Barth and L. Hedin, "A local exchange–correlation potential for the spin polarized case: I," *J. Phys. C* 5:1629, 1972.

[306] G. D. Mahan, *Many-Particle Physics,* 3rd ed., Kluwer Academic/Plenum Publishers, New York, 2000.

[307] E. P. Wigner, "Effects of the electron interaction on the energy levels of electrons in metals," *Trans. Faraday Soc.* 34:678, 1938.

[308] M. Gell-Mann and K. A. Brueckner, "Correlation energy of an electron gas at high-density," *Phys. Rev.* 106:364, 1957.

[309] W. J. Carr and A.A. Maradudin, "Ground state energy of a high-density electron gas," *Phys. Rev.* 133:371, 1964.

[310] W. J. Carr, "Energy, specific heat, and magnetic properties of the low-density electron gas," *Phys. Rev.* 122:1437, 1961.

[311] D. M. Ceperley and B. J. Alder, "Ground state of the electron gas by a stochastic method," *Phys. Rev. Lett.* 45:566–569, 1980.

[312] S. Vosko, L. Wilk, and M. Nusair, "Accurate spin-dependent electron liquid correlation energies for local spin density calculations: A critical analysis," *Can. J. Phys.* 58:1200, 1983.

[313] J. P. Perdew and A. Zunger, "Self-interaction correction to density-functional approximations for many-electron systems," *Phys Rev. B* 23:5048, 1981.

[314] B. Holm, "Total energies from GW calculations," *Phys. Rev. Lett.* 83:788–791, 1999.

[315] G. Ortiz and P. Ballone, "Correlation energy, structure factor, radial distribution function and momentum distribution of the spin-polarized uniform electron gas," *Phys. Rev. B* 50:1391–1405, 1994.

[316] Y. Kwon, D. M. Ceperley, and R. M. Martin, "Effects of backflow correlation in the three-dimensional electron gas: Quantum Monte Carlo study," *Phys. Rev. B* 58:6800–6806, 1998.

[317] E. Maggio and G. Kresse, "Correlation energy for the homogeneous electron gas: Exact bethe-salpeter solution and an approximate evaluation," *Phys. Rev. B* 93:235113, 2016.

[318] P. Gori-Giorgi, F. Sacchetti, and G. B. Bachelet, "Analytic structure factors and pair correlation functions for the unpolarized electron gas," *Phys. Rev. B* 61:7353–7363, 2000.

[319] G. Ortiz, M. Harris, and P. Ballone, "Correlation energy, structure factor, radial density distribution function, and momentum distribution of the spin-polarized electron gas," *Phys. Rev. Lett.* 82:5317–5320, 1999.

[320] J. C. Slater, "Cohesion in monovalent metals," *Phys. Rev.* 35:509, 1930.

[321] W. G. Aulbur, L. Jonsson, and J. W. Wilkins, "Quasiparticle calculations in solids," *Solid State Physics* 54:1–218, 2000.

[322] I.-W. Lyo and E. W. Plummer, "Quasiparticle band structure of Na and simple metals," *Phys. Rev. Lett.* 60:1558–1561, 1988.

[323] E. Jensen and E. W. Plummer, "Experimental band structure of Na," *Phys. Rev. Lett.* 55:1912, 1985.

[324] J. Lindhard, "On the properties of a gas of charged particles," *Kgl. Danske Videnskab. Selskab, Mat.-fys. Medd.* 28:1–57, 1954.

[325] D. Pines and P. Nozières, *The Theory of Quantum Liquids,* vol. 1 (Advanced Book Classics), Westview Press, Boulder, CO, 1999. Originally published W. A. Benjamin, New York, 1966.

[326] N. David Mermin, "Thermal properties of the inhomogeneous electron gas," *Phys. Rev.* 137:A1441–1443, 1965.

[327] L. H. Thomas, "The calculation of atomic fields," *Proc. Cambridge Phil. Roy. Soc.* 23:542–548, 1927.

[328] E. Fermi, "Un metodo statistico per la determinazione di alcune priorieta dell'atome," *Rend. Accad. Naz. Lincei* 6:602–607, 1927.

[329] P. A. M. Dirac, "Note on exchange phenomena in the Thomas–Fermi atom," *Proc. Cambridge Phil. Roy. Soc.* 26:376–385, 1930.

[330] C. F. von Weizsacker, "Zur Theorie der Kernmassen," *Z. Phys.* 96:431, 1935.

[331] E. Teller, "On the stability of molecules in the Thomas–Fermi theory," *Rev. Mod. Phys.* 34:627–631, 1962.

[332] W. Kohn, in *Highlights in Condensed Matter Theory*, edited by F. Bassani, F. Fumi, and M. P. Tosi, North Holland, Amsterdam, 1985, p. 1.

[333] M. Levy, "Universal variational functionals of electron densities, first-order density matrices, and natural spin-orbitals and solution of the n-representability problem," *Proc. Natl. Acad. Sci. U.S.A.* 76:6062, 1979.

[334] M. Levy, "Electron densities in search of hamiltonians," *Phys. Rev. A* 26:1200, 1982.

[335] M. Levy and J. P. Perdew, in *Density Functional Methods in Physics*, edited by R. M. Dreizler and J. da Providencia, Plenum, New York, 1985, p. 11.

[336] E. Lieb, in *Physics as Natural Philosophy*, edited by A. Shimony and H. Feshbach, MIT Press, Cambridge, 1982, p. 111.

[337] E. Lieb, "Density functionals for Coulomb systems," *Int. J. Quant. Chem.* 24:243, 1983.

[338] E. Lieb, in *Density Functional Methods in Physics*, edited by R. M. Dreizler and J. da Providencia, Plenum, New York, 1985, p. 31.

[339] T. L. Gilbert, "Hohenberg-Kohn theorem for nonlocal external potentials," *Phys. Rev. B* 12:2111, 1975.

[340] O. Gunnarsson, B. I. Lundqvist, and J. W. Wilkins, "Contribution to the cohesive energy of simple metals: Spin-dependent effect," *Phys. Rev. B* 10:1319–1327, 1974.

[341] R. O. Jones and O. Gunnarsson, "The density functional formalism, its applications and prospects," *Rev. Mod. Phys.* 61:689–746, 1989.

[342] G. Vignale and M. Rasolt, "Current- and spin-density-functional theory for inhomogeneous electronic systems in strong magnetic fields," *Phys. Rev. B* 37:10685–10696, 1988.

[343] G. Vignale and W. Kohn, "Current-dependent exchange–correlation potential for dynamical linear response theory," *Phys. Rev. Lett.* 77:2037–2040, 1996.

[344] K. Capelle and E. K. U. Gross, "Spin-density functionals from current-density functional theory and vice versa: A road towards new approximations," *Phys. Rev. Lett.* 78:1872–1875, 1997.

[345] R. van Leeuwen, "Causality and symmetry in time-dependent density-functional theory," *Phys. Rev. Lett.* 80:1280–1283, 1998.

[346] J. P. Perdew, R. G. Parr, M. Levy, and Jr. J. L. Balduz, "Density-functional theory for fractional particle number: Derivative discontinuities of the energy," *Phys. Rev. Lett.* 49:1691–1694, 1982.

[347] N. T. Maitra, I. Souza, and K. Burke, "Current-density functional theory of the response of solids," *Phys. Rev. B* 68:045109, 2003.

[348] G. Wannier, "Dynamics of band electrons in electric and magnetic fields," *Rev. Mod. Phys.* 34:645, 1962.

[349] G. Nenciu, "Dynamics of band electrons in electric and magnetic fields: Rigorous justification of the effective hamiltonians," *Rev. Mod. Phys.* 63:91, 1991.

[350] X. Gonze, Ph. Ghosez, and R. W. Godby, "Density-polarization functional theory of the response of a periodic insulating solid to an electric field," *Phys. Rev. Lett.* 74:4035–4038, 1995.

[351] R. M. Martin and G. Ortiz, "Functional theory of extended coulomb systems," *Phys. Rev. B* 56:1124–1140, 1997.

[352] R. M. Martin and G. Ortiz, "Recent developments in the theory of polarization in solids," *Solid State Commun.* 102:121–126, 1997.

[353] J. E. Harriman, "Orthonormal orbitals for the representation of an arbitrary density," *Phys. Rev. A* 24:680–682, 1981.

[354] W. A. Harrison, *Electronic Structure and the Properties of Solids*, Dover, New York, 1989.

[355] V. P. Antropov, M. I. Katsnelson, M. van Schilfgaarde, and B. N. Harmon, "Exchange-coupled spin-fluctuation theory: Application to Fe, Co, and Ni," *Phys. Rev. Lett.* 75:729–732, 1995.

[356] M. Uhl and J. Kübler, "*Ab initio* spin dynamics in magnets," *Phys. Rev. Lett.* 77:334–337, 1996.

[357] T. Oda, A. Pasquarello, and R. Car, "Fully unconstrained approach to noncollinear magnetism: Application to small fe clusters," *Phys. Rev. Lett.* 80:3622–3625, 1998.

[358] D. M. Bylander, Q. Niu, and L. Kleinman, "Fe magnon dispersion curve calculated with the frozen spin-wave method," *Phys. Rev. B* 61:R11875–R11878, 2000.

[359] J. Harris, "Simplified method for calculating the energy of weakly interacting fragments," *Phys. Rev. B* 31:1770–1779, 1985.

[360] M. Weinert, R. E. Watson, and J. W. Davenport, "Total-energy differences and eigenvalue sums," *Phys. Rev. B* 32:2115–2119, 1985.

[361] W. M. C. Foulkes and R. Haydock, "Tight-binding models and density-functional theory," *Phys. Rev. B* 39:12520–12536, 1989.

[362] O. F. Sankey and D. J. Niklewski, "*Ab initio* multicenter tight-binding model for molecular dynamics simulations and other applications in covalent systems," *Phys. Rev. B* 40:3979–3995, 1989.

[363] M. Methfessel, "Independent variation of the density and potential in density functional methods," *Phys. Rev. B* 52:8074, 1995.

[364] A. J. Read and R. J. Needs, "Tests of the Harris energy functional," *J. Phys. Condens. Matter* 1:7565, 1989.

[365] E. Zaremba, "Extremal properties of the Harris energy functional," *J. Phys. Condens. Matter* 2:2479, 1990.

[366] I. J. Robertson and B. Farid, "Does the Harris energy functional possess a local maximum at the ground-state density?," *Phys. Rev. Lett.* 66:3265–3268, 1991.

[367] K. W. Jacobsen, J. K. Norskov, and M. J. Puska, "Interatomic interactions in the effective-medium theory," *Phys. Rev. B* 35:7423–7442, 1987.

[368] D. M. C. Nicholson, G. M. Stocks, Y. Wang, W. A. Shelton, Z. Szotek, and W. M. Temmerman, "Stationary nature of the density-functional free energy: Application to accelerated multiple-scattering calculations," *Phys. Rev. B* 50:14686–14689, 1994.

[369] M. J. Gillan, "Calculation of the vacancy formation energy in aluminum," *J. Phys. Condens. Matter* 1:689, 1989.

[370] N. Marzari, D. Vanderbilt, and M. C. Payne, "Ensemble density-functional theory for *ab initio* molecular dynamics of metals and finite-temperature insulators," *Phys. Rev. Lett.* 79:1337–1340, 1997.

[371] P. H. Dederichs and R. Zeller, "Self-consistency iterations in electronic-structure calculations," *Phys. Rev. B* 28:5462, 1983.

[372] W. E. Pickett, "Pseudopotential methods in condensed matter applications," *Comput. Phys. Commun.* 9:115, 1989.

[373] K.-M. Ho, J. Ihm, and J. D. Joannopoulos, "Dielectric matrix scheme for fast convergence in self-consistent electronic-structure calculations," *Phys. Rev. B* 25:4260–4262, 1982.

[374] C. G. Broyden, "A class of methods for solving nonlinear simulataneous equations," *Math. Comput.* 19:577–593, 1965.

[375] P. Bendt and A. Zunger, "New approach for solving the density-functional self-consistent-field problem," *Phys. Rev. B* 26:3114–3137, 1982.

[376] G. P. Srivastava, "Broyden's method for self-consistent field convergence acceleration," *J. Phys. A* 17:L317, 1984.

[377] D. Singh, H. Krakauer, and C. S. Wang, "Accelerating the convergence of self-consistent linearized augmented-plane-wave calculations," *Phys. Rev. B* 34:8391–8393, 1986.

[378] A. J. Garza and G. E. Scuseria, "Comparison of self-consistent field convergence acceleration techniques," *J. Chem. Phys.* 137:054110, 2012.

[379] Masahiko Nakano, Junji Seino, and Hiromi Nakai, "Assessment of self-consistent field convergence in spin-dependent relativistic calculations," *Chem. Phys. Letters* 657:65–71, 2016.

[380] D. Vanderbilt and S. G. Louie, "Total energies of diamond (111) surface reconstructions by a linear combination of atomic orbitals method," *Phys. Rev. B* 30:6118, 1984.

[381] D. D. Johnson, "Modified Broyden's method for accelerating convergence in self-consistent calculations," *Phys. Rev. B* 38:12807–12813, 1988.

[382] M. Allen and D. Tildesley, *Computer Simulation of Liquids*, Oxford University Press, New York, Oxford, 1989.

[383] M. Parrinello and A. Rahman, "Crystal structure and pair potentials: A molecular-dynamics study," *Phys. Rev. Lett.* 45:1196–1199, 1980.

[384] I. Souza and J. L. Martins, "Metric tensor as the dynamical variable for variable-cell-shape molecular dynamics," *Phys. Rev. B* 55:8733–8742, 1997.

[385] M. C. Payne, M. P. Teter, D. C. Allan, T. A. Arias, and J. D. Joannopoulos, "Iterative minimization techniques for *ab initio* total-energy calculations: molecular dynamics and conjugate gradients," *Rev. Mod. Phys.* 64:1045–1097, 1992.

[386] O. Gritsenko, R. van Leeuwen, and E. J. Baerends, "Analysis of electron interaction and atomic shell structure in terms of local potentials," *J. Chem. Phys.* 101:8455, 1994.

[387] J. P. Perdew and M. Levy, "Physical content of the exact Kohn–Sham orbital energies: Band gaps and derivative discontinuities," *Phys. Rev. Lett.* 51:1884–1887, 1983.

[388] L. J. Sham and M. Schlüter, "Density-functional theory of the energy gap," *Phys. Rev. Lett.* 51:1888–1891, 1983.

[389] C. Almbladh and U. von Barth, "Exact results for the charge and spin densities, exchange–correlation potentials, and density-functional eigenvalues," *Phys. Rev. B* 31:3231, 1985.

[390] M. Levy, J. P. Perdew, and V. Sahni, "Exact differential equation for the density and ionization energy of a many-particle system," *Phys. Rev. A* 12:2745–2748, 1984.

[391] A. Gorling, "Density-functional theory for excited states," *Phys. Rev. A* 54:3912–3915, 1996.

[392] J. F. Janak, "Proof that $\partial e/\partial n_i = \epsilon_i$ in density-functional theory," *Phys. Rev. B* 18:7165, 1978.

[393] D. Mearns, "Inequivalence of physical and Kohn–Sham Fermi surfaces," *Phys. Rev. B* 38:5906, 1988.

[394] C. A. Ullrich, "Time-dependent density-functional theory beyond the adiabatic approximation: Insights from a two-electron model system," *J. Chem. Phys.* 125:234108, 2006.

[395] N. T. Maitra, "Perspective: Fundamental aspects of time-dependent density functional theory," *J. Chem. Phys.* 144:220901, 2016.

[396] H. J. F. Jansen, "Many-body properties calculated from the Kohn–Sham equations in density-functional theory," *Phys Rev. B* 43:12025, 1991.

[397] L. N. Oliveira, E. K. U. Gross, and W. Kohn, "Density-functional theory for superconductors," *Phys. Rev. Lett.* 60:2430–2433, 1988.

[398] M. Lüders, M. A. L. Marques, N. N. Lathiotakis, A. Floris, G. Profeta, L. Fast, A. Continenza, S. Massidda, and E. K. U. Gross, "*Ab initio* theory of superconductivity. I. Density functional formalism and approximate functionals," *Phys. Rev. B* 72:024545, 2005.

[399] M. A. L. Marques, M. Lüders, N. N. Lathiotakis, G. Profeta, A. Floris, L. Fast, A. Continenza, E. K. U. Gross, and S. Massidda, "*Ab initio* theory of superconductivity. II. Application to elemental metals," *Phys. Rev. B* 72:024546, 2005.

[400] A. Seidl, A. Görling, P. Vogl, J. A. Majewski, and M. Levy, "Generalized Kohn–Sham schemes and the band-gap problem," *Phys. Rev. B* 53:3764–3774, 1996.

[401] M. Levy and J. P. Perdew, "Hellmann-Feynman, virial, and scaling requisites for the exact universal density functionals: Shape of the correlation potential and diamagnetic susceptibility for atoms," *Phys. Rev. A* 32:2010–2021, 1985.

[402] O. Gunnarsson, M. Jonson, and B. I. Lundqvist, "Descriptions of exchange and correlation effects in inhomogeneous electron systems," *Phys. Rev. B* 20:3136, 1979.

[403] W. Kolos and L. Wolniewicz, "Potential-energy curves for the X $^1\sigma_g^+$, b $^3\sigma_u^+$, and C $^1\pi_u$ states of the hydrogen molecule," *J. Chem. Phys.* 43:2429, 1965.

[404] C. O. Almbladh and A. C. Pedroza, "Density-functional exchange–correlation potentials and orbital eigenvalues for light atoms," *Phys. Rev. A* 29:2322–2330, 1984.

[405] R. Q. Hood, M. Y. Chou, A. J. Williamson, G. Rajagopal, R. J. Needs, and W. M. C. Foulkes, "Exchange and correlation in silicon," *Phys. Rev. B* 57:8972–8982, 1998.

[406] K. Lejaeghere, et al., "Reproducibility in density functional theory calculations of solids," *Science* 351, 2016.

[407] F. Herman, J. P. Van Dyke, and I. P. Ortenburger, "Improved statistical exchange approximation for inhomogeneous many-electron systems," *Phys. Rev. Lett.* 22:807, 1969.

[408] P. S. Svendsen and U. von Barth, "Gradient expansion of the exchange energy from second-order density response theory," *Phys. Rev. B* 54:17402–17413, 1996.

[409] J. P. Perdew and K. Burke, "Comparison shopping for a gradient-corrected density functional," *Int. J. Quant. Chem.* 57:309–319, 1996.

[410] A. D. Becke, "Density-functional exchange-energy approximation with correct asymptotic behavior," *Phys. Rev. A* 38:3098–3100, 1988.

[411] J. P. Perdew and Y. Wang, "Accurate and simple analytic representation of the electron-gas correlation energy," *Phys. Rev. B* 45:13244–13249, 1992.

[412] J. P. Perdew, K. Burke, and M. Ernzerhof, "Generalized gradient approximation made simple," *Phys. Rev. Lett.* 77:3865–3868, 1996.

[413] W. Koch and M. C. Holthausen, *A Chemists' Guide to Density Funcitonal Thoery*, Wiley-VCH, Weinheim, 2001.

[414] S.-K. Ma and K. A. Brueckner, "Improved statistical exchange approximation for inhomogeneous many-electron systems," *Phys. Rev.* 165:18–31, 1968.

[415] N. Mardirossian and M. Head-Gordon, "Thirty years of density functional theory in computational chemistry: An overview and extensive assessment of 200 density functionals," *Mol. Phys.* 115:2315–2372, 2017.

[416] C. Lee, W. Yang, and R. G. Parr, "Development of the Colle–Salvetti correlation-energy formula into a functional of the electron density," *Phys. Rev. B* 37:785–789, 1988.

[417] R. Colle and O. Salvetti, "Approximate calculation of the correlation energy for the closed and open shells," *Theo. Chim. Acta* 53:59–63, 1979.

[418] J. B. Krieger, Y. Chen, G. J. Iafrate, and A. Savin, "Construction of an accurate SIC-corrected correlation energy functional based on an electron gas with a gap," preprint, 2000.

[419] J. Rey and A. Savin, "Virtual space level shifting and correlation energies," *Int. J. Quant. Chem.* 69:581–587, 1998.

[420] M. D. Towler, A. Zupan, and M. Causa, "Density functional theory in periodic systems using local gaussian basis sets," *Comput. Phys. Commun.* 98:181–205, 1996.

[421] D. R. Hamann, "Generalized gradient theory for silica phase transitions," *Phys. Rev. Lett.* 76:660–663, 1996.

[422] J. A. White and D. M. Bird, "Implementation of gradient-corrected exchange-correlation potentials in Car-Parrinello total-energy calculations," *Phys. Rev. B* 50:4954–4957, 1994.

[423] Y.-H. Kim, I.-H. Lee S. Nagaraja, J. P. Leburton, R. Q. Hood, and R. M. Martin, "Two-dimensional limit of exchange–correlation energy functional approximations," *Phys. Rev. B* 61:5202–5211, 2000.

[424] Y. Zhao and D. G. Truhlar, "The M06 suite of density functionals for main group thermochemistry, thermochemical kinetics, noncovalent interactions, excited states, and transition elements: two new functionals and systematic testing of four M06-class functionals and 12 other functionals," *Theor. Chem. Acc.* 120:215–241, 2008.

[425] J. C. Snyder, M. Rupp, K. Hansen, K.-R. Müller, and K. Burke, "Finding density functionals with machine learning," *Phys. Rev. Lett.* 108:253002, 2012.

[426] Axel D. Becke, "Perspective: Fifty years of density-functional theory in chemical physics," *J. Chem. Phys.* 140:301, 2014.

[427] S. Kummel and L. Kronik, "Orbital-dependent density functionals: Theory and applications," *Rev. Mod. Phys.* 80:3–60, 2008.

[428] J. P. Perdew and K. Schmidt, "Jacob's ladder of density functional approximations for the exchange–correlation energy," *AIP Conf. Proc.* 577:1–20, 2001.

[429] L. J. Sham and M. Schlüter, "Density functional theory of the band gap," *Phys. Rev. B* 32:3883, 1985.

[430] J. P. Perdew, W. Yang, K. Burke, Z. Yang, Eberhard K. U. Gross, M. Scheffler, G. E. Scuseria, T. M. Henderson, I. Y. Zhang, A. Ruzsinszky, H. Peng, J. Sun, E. Trushin, and A. Görling, "Understanding band gaps of solids in generalized Kohn–Sham theory," *Proc. Natl. Acad. Sci. U.S.A.* 114:2801–2806, 2017.

[431] R. Baer and L. Kronik, "Time-dependent generalized Kohn–Sham theory," *Eur. Phys. J. B* 91:170, 2018.

[432] A. D. Becke, "A new mixing of Hartree–Fock and local density-functional theories," *J. Chem. Phys.* 98:1372–1377, 1993.

[433] J. P. Perdew, M. Ernzerhof, and K. Burke, "Rationale for mixing exact exchange with density functional approximations," *J. Chem. Phys.* 105:9982–9985, 1996.

[434] M. A. L. Marques, J. Vidal, M. J. T. Oliveira, L. Reining, and S. Botti, "Density-based mixing parameter for hybrid functionals," *Phys. Rev. B* 83:035119, 2011.

[435] J. Heyd, G. E. Scuseria, and M. Ernzerhof, "Hybrid functionals based on a screened coulomb potential," *J. Chem. Phys.* 118:8207–8215, 2003.

[436] J. Heyd, G. E. Scuseria, and M. Ernzerhof, "Erratum: Hybrid functionals based on a screened Coulomb potential [*J. Chem. Phys.* 118, 8207 (2003)]," *J. Chem. Phys.* 124:219906, 2006.

[437] A. V. Krukau, O. A. Vydrov, A. F. Izmaylov, and G. E. Scuseria, "Influence of the exchange screening parameter on the performance of screened hybrid functionals," *J. Chem. Phys.* 125:224106, 2006.

[438] W. Chen, G. Miceli, G.-M. Rignanese, and A. Pasquarello, "Nonempirical dielectric-dependent hybrid functional with range separation for semiconductors and insulators," *Phys. Rev. Materials* 2:073803, 2018.

[439] A. Tkatchenko and M. Scheffler, "Accurate molecular van der Waals interactions from ground-state electron density and free-atom reference data," *Phys. Rev. Lett.* 102:073005, 2009.

[440] R. Baer, E. Livshits, and U. Salzner, "Tuned range-separated hybrids in density functional theory," *Annu. Rev. Phys. Chem.* 61:85–109, 2010.

[441] J. P. Perdew, J. Sun, R. M. Martin, and B. Delley, "Semilocal density functionals and constraint satisfaction," *Int. J. Quant. Chem.* 116:847–851, 2016.

[442] A. D. Becke and M. R. Roussel, "Exchange holes in inhomogeneous systems: A coordinate-space model," *Phys. Rev. A* 39:3761–3767, 1989.

[443] J. Tao, J. P. Perdew, V. N. Staroverov, and G. E. Scuseria, "Climbing the density functional ladder: Nonempirical meta–generalized gradient approximation designed for molecules and solids," *Phys. Rev. Lett.* 91:146401, 2003.

[444] J. Sun, A. Ruzsinszky, and J. P. Perdew, "Strongly constrained and appropriately normed semilocal density functional," *Phys. Rev. Lett.* 115:036402, 2015.

[445] J. G. Brandenburg, J. E. Bates, J. Sun, and J. P. Perdew, "Benchmark tests of a strongly constrained semilocal functional with a long-range dispersion correction," *Phys. Rev. B* 94:115144, 2016.

[446] R. T. Sharp and G. K. Horton, "A variational approach to the unipotential many-electron problem," *Phys. Rev.* 90:317, 1953.

[447] M. E. Casida, in *Recent Developments and Applications of Density Functional Theory*, edited by J. M. Seminario, Elsevier, Amsterdam, 1996, p. 391.

[448] D. M. Bylander and L. Kleinman, "The optimized effective potential for atoms and semiconductors," *Int. J. Mod. Phys.* 10:399–425, 1996.

[449] T. Grabo, T. Kreibich, S. Kurth, and E. K. U. Gross, in *Strong Coulomb Correlations in Electronic Structure: Beyond the Local Density Approximation*, edited by V. I. Anisimov, Gordon & Breach, Tokyo, 1998.

[450] J. B. Krieger, Y. Li, and G. J. Iafrate, "Exact relations in the optimized effective potential method employing an arbitrary $E_{xc}[\{\psi_{i\sigma}\}]$," *Phys. Lett. A* 148:470–473, 1990.

[451] J. B. Krieger, Y. Li, and G. J. Iafrate, "Construction and application of an accurate local spin-polarized Kohn–Sham potential with integer discontinuity: Exchange-only theory," *Phys. Rev. A* 45:101, 1992.

[452] J. B. Krieger, Y. Li, and G. J. Iafrate, in *Density Functional Theory*, edited by E. K. U. Gross and R. M. Dreizler, Plenum Press, New York, 1995, p. 191.

[453] J. C. Slater, "A simplification of the Hartree–Fock method," *Phys. Rev.* 81:385–390, 1951.

[454] A. Svane and O. Gunnarsson, "Localization in the self-interaction-corrected density-functional formalism," *Phys Rev. B* 37:9919, 1988.

[455] A. Svane and O. Gunnarsson, "Transition-metal oxides in the self-interaction-corrected density functional formalism," *Phys Rev. Lett.* 65:1148–1151, 1990.

[456] W. M. Temmerman, Z. Szotek, and H. Winter, "Self-interaction corrected electronic structure of La_2CuO_4," *Phys Rev. B* 47, 1993.

[457] A. Svane, Z. Szotek, W. M. Temmerman, J. Lægsgaard, and H. Winter, "Electronic structure of cerium pnictides under pressure," *J. Phys. Condens. Matter* 10:5309–5325, 1998.

[458] V. I. Anisimov, J. Zaanen, and O. K. Andersen, "Band theory and Mott insulators: Hubbard U instead of Stoner I," *Phys. Rev. B* 44:943, 1991.

[459] V. I. Anisimov, F. Aryasetiawan, and A. I. Lichtenstein, "First principles calculations of the electronic structure and spectra of strongly correlated systems: The LDA + U method," *J. Phys. Condens. Matter* 9:767–808, 1997.

[460] J. Hubbard, "Electron correlations in narrow energy bands. IV. The atomic representation," *Proc. R. Soc. Lond. A* 285:542–560, 1965.

[461] D. Baeriswyl, D. K. Campbell, J. M. P. Carmelo, and F. Guinea, *The Hubbard Model*, Plenum Press, New York, 1995.

[462] I. Dabo, A. Ferretti, N. Poilvert, Y. Li, N. Marzari, and M. Cococcioni, "Koopmans' condition for density-functional theory," *Phys. Rev. B* 82:115121, 2010.

[463] N. L. Nguyen, N. Colonna, A. Ferretti, and N. Marzari, "Koopmans-compliant spectral functionals for extended systems," *Phys. Rev. X* 8:021051, 2018.

[464] D. C. Langreth and J. P. Perdew, "Exchange–correlation energy of a metallic surface: Wave-vector analysis," *Phys. Rev. B* 15:2884–2901, 1977.

[465] X. Ren, P. Rinke, C. Joas, and M. Scheffler, "Random-phase approximation and its applications in computational chemistry and materials science," *J. Mater. Sci.* 47:7447–7471, 2012.

[466] R. A DiStasio Jr., V. V. Gobre, and A. Tkatchenko, "Many-body van der Waals interactions in molecules and condensed matter," *J. Phys. Condens. Matter* 26:213202, 2014.

[467] J. Harl, L. Schimka, and G. Kresse, "Assessing the quality of the random phase approximation for lattice constants and atomization energies of solids," *Phys. Rev. B* 81:115126, 2010.

[468] M. Dion, H. Rydberg, E. Schröder, D. C. Langreth, and B. I. Lundqvist, "Van der Waals density functional for general geometries," *Phys. Rev. Lett.* 92:246401, 2004.

[469] H. B. G. Casimir and D. Polder, "The influence of retardation on the London–van der Waals forces," *Phys. Rev.* 73:360–372, 1948.

[470] S. Grimme, J. Antony, S. Ehrlich, and H. Krieg, "A consistent and accurate *ab initio* parametrization of density functional dispersion correction (DFT-D) for the 94 elements H-Pu," *J. Chem. Phys.* 132:154104, 2010.

[471] T. Brinck, J. S. Murray, and P. Politzer, "Polarizability and volume," *J. Chem. Phys.* 98:4305–4306, 1993.

[472] F. L. Hirshfeld, "Bonded-atom fragments for describing molecular charge densities," *Theoret. Chim. Acta* 44:129–138, 1977.

[473] Guillermo Román-Pérez and José M. Soler, "Efficient implementation of a van der Waals density functional: Application to double-wall carbon nanotubes," *Phys. Rev. Lett.* 103:096102, 2009.

[474] O. A. Vydrov and T. Van Voorhis, "Improving the accuracy of the nonlocal van der Waals density functional with minimal empiricism," *J. Chem. Phys.* 130:104105, 2009.

[475] O. A. Vydrov and T. Van Voorhis, "Nonlocal van der Waals density functional: The simpler the better," *J. Chem. Phys.* 133:244103, 2010.

[476] A. D. Becke and E. R. Johnson, "A simple effective potential for exchange," *J. Chem. Phys.* 124:221101, 2006.

[477] F. Tran and P. Blaha, "Accurate band gaps of semiconductors and insulators with a semilocal exchange–correlation potential," *Phys. Rev. Lett.* 102:226401, 2009.

[478] D. Waroquiers, et al., "Band widths and gaps from the Tran–Blaha functional: Comparison with many-body perturbation theory," *Phys. Rev. B* 87:075121, 2013.

[479] S. Kurth, J.P. Perdew, and P. Blaha, "Molecular and solid-state tests of density functional approximations: LSD, GGAs, and meta-GGAs," *Int. J. Quantum Chem.* 75:889, 1999.

[480] J. D. Jackson, *Classical Electrodynamics*, Wiley, New York, 1962.

[481] F. Herman and S. Skillman, *Atomic Structure Calculations*, Prentice-Hall, Engelwood Cliffs, NJ, 1963.

[482] C. F. Fischer, *The Hartree–Fock Method for Atoms: A Numerical Approach*, John Wiley & Sons, New York, 1977.

[483] J. C. Slater, *Quantum Theory of Atomic Structure,* vol. 1, McGraw-Hill, New York, 1960.

[484] J. C. Slater, *Quantum Theory of Atomic Structure,* vol. 2, McGraw-Hill, New York, 1960.

[485] S. E. Koonin and D. C. Meredith, *Computational Physics*, Addison Wesley, Menlo Park, CA, 1990.

[486] M. S. Hybertsen and S. G. Louie, "Spin–orbit splitting in semiconductors and insulators from the *ab initio* pseudopotential," *Phys. Rev. B* 34:2920, 1986.

[487] G. Theurich and N. A. Hill, "Self-consistent treatment of spin–orbit coupling in solids using relativistic fully separable *ab initio* pseudopotentials," *Phys. Rev. B* 64:073106, 1986.

[488] F. R. Vukajlovic, E. L. Shirley, and R. M. Martin, "Single-body methods in 3d transition-metal atoms," *Phys. Rev. B* 43:3994, 1991.

[489] J. C. Slater, *The Self-Consistent Field Theory for Molecules and Solids: Quantum Theory of Molecules and Solids,* vol. 4, McGraw-Hill, New York, 1974.

[490] A. K. McMahan, R. M. Martin, and S. Satpathy, "Calculated effective hamiltonian for La2Cu04 and solution in the Anderson impurity approximation," *Phys. Rev. B* 38:6650, 1988.

[491] J. F. Herbst, D. N. Lowy, and R. E. Watson, "Single-electron energies, many-electron effects, and the renormalized-atom scheme as applied to rare-earth metals," *Phys. Rev. B* 6:1913–1924, 1972.

[492] J. F. Herbst, R. E. Watson, and J. W. Wilkins, "Relativistic calculations of 4f excitation energies in the rare-earth metals: Further results," *Phys. Rev. B* 17:3089–3098, 1978.

[493] O. K. Andersen and O. Jepsen, "Explicit, first-principles tight-binding theory," *Physica* 91B:317, 1977.

[494] G. K. Straub and Walter A. Harrison, "Analytic methods for the calculation of the electronic structure of solids," *Phys. Rev. B* 31:7668–7679, 1985.

[495] O. K. Andersen, "Simple approach to the band structure problem," *Solid State Commun.* 13:133–136, 1973.

[496] D. A. Liberman, "Virial theorem in self-consistent-field calculations," *Phys. Rev. B* 3:2081–2082, 1971.

[497] J. F. Janak, "Simplification of total-energy and pressure calculations in solids," *Phys. Rev. B* 20:3985–3988, 1974.

[498] A. R. Mackintosh and O. K. Andersen, in *Electrons at the Fermi Surface*, edited by M. Springford, Cambridge Press, Cambridge, 1975, p. 149.

[499] V. Heine, in *Solid State Physics*, edited by H. Ehenreich, F. Seitz, and D. Turnbull, Academic Press, New York, 1980, Vol. 35, p. 1.

[500] E. Amaldi, O. D'Agostino, E. Fermi, B. Pontecorvo, F. Rasetti, and E. Segre, "Artificial radioactivity induced by neutron bombardment – II," *Proc. R. Soc. Lond. A* 149:522–558, 1935.

[501] J. Callaway, "Electron energy bands in sodium," *Phys. Rev.* 112:322, 1958.

[502] E. Antoncik, "A new formulation of the method of nearly free electrons," *Czech. J. Phys.* 4:439, 1954.

[503] E. Antoncik, "Approximate formulation of the orthogonalized plane-wave method," *J. Phys. Chem. Solids* 10:314, 1959.

[504] J. C. Phillips and L. Kleinman, "New method for calculating wave functions in crystals and molecules," *Phys. Rev.* 116:287, 1959.

[505] W. C. Herring and A. G. Hill, "The theoretical constitution of metallic beryllium," *Phys. Rev.* 58:132, 1940.

[506] V. Heine, in *Solid State Physics*, edited by H. Ehrenreich, F. Seitz, and D. Turnbull, Academic, New York, 1970, p. 1.

[507] M. L. Cohen and V. Heine, in *Solid State Physics*, edited by H. Ehrenreich, F. Seitz, and D. Turnbull, Academic, New York, 1970, p. 37.

[508] W. A. Harrison, *Pseudopotentials in the Theory of Metals*, Benjamin, New York, 1966.

[509] P. E. Blöchl, "Generalized separable potentials for electronic-structure calculations," *Phys. Rev. B* 41:5414–5416, 1990.

[510] D. Vanderbilt, "Soft self-consistent pseudopotentials in a generalized eigenvalue formalism," *Phys. Rev. B* 41:7892, 1990.

[511] F. Herman, "Calculation of the energy band structures of the diamond and germanium crystals by the method of orthogonalized plane waves," *Phys. Rev.* 93:1214, 1954.

[512] T. O. Woodruff, "Solution of the Hartree–Fock–Slater equations for silicon crystal by the method of orthogonalized plane waves," *Phys. Rev.* 98:1741, 1955.

[513] F. Herman, "Speculations on the energy band structure of Ge–Si alloys," *Phys. Rev.* 95:847, 1954.

[514] F. Bassani, "Energy band structure in silicon crystals by the orthogonalized plane-wave method," *Phys. Rev.* 263:1741, 1957.

[515] B. Lax, "Experimental investigations of the electronic band structure of solids," *Rev. Mod. Phys.* 30:122, 1958.

[516] M. H. Cohen and V. Heine, "Cancellation of kinetic and potential energy in atoms, molecules, and solids," *Phys. Rev.* 122:1821, 1961.

[517] N. W. Ashcroft, "Electron–ion pseudopotentials in metals," *Phys. Lett.* 23:48–53, 1966.

[518] I. V. Abarenkov and V. Heine, "The model potential for positive ions," *Phil. Mag.* 12:529, 1965.

[519] A. O. E. Animalu, "Non-local dielectric screening in metals," *Phil. Mag.* 11:379, 1965.

[520] A. O. E. Animalu and V. Heine, "The screened model potential for 25 elements," *Phil. Mag.* 12:1249, 1965.

[521] P. A. Christiansen, Y. S. Lee, and K. S. Pitzer, "Improved *ab initio* effective core potentials for molecular calculations," *J. Chem. Phys.* 71:4445–4450, 1979.

[522] M. Krauss and W. J. Stevens, "Effective potentials in molecular quantum chemistry," *Ann. Rev. Phys. Chem* 35:357, 1984.

[523] D. R. Hamann, M. Schlüter, and C. Chiang, "Norm-conserving pseudopotentials," *Phys. Rev. Lett.* 43:1494–1497, 1979.

[524] W. C. Topp and J. J. Hopfield, "Chemically motivated pseudopotential for sodium," *Phys. Rev.* 7:1295–1303, 1973.

[525] E. Engel, A., R. N. Schmid, R. M.Dreizler, and N. Chetty, "Role of the core-valence interaction for pseudopotential calculations with exact exchange," *Phys. Rev. B* 64:125111–125122, 2001.

[526] E. L. Shirley, D. C. Allan, R. M. Martin, and J. D. Joannopoulos, "Extended norm-conserving pseudopotentials," *Phys. Rev. B* 40:3652, 1989.

[527] G. Lüders, "Zum zusammenhang zwischen S-Matrix und Normierungsintegrassen in der Quantenmechanik," *Z. Naturforsch.* 10a:581, 1955.

[528] G. B. Bachelet, D. R. Hamann, and M. Schlüter, "Pseudopotentials that work: From H to Pu," *Phys. Rev. B* 26:4199, 1982.

[529] D. Vanderbilt, "Optimally smooth norm-conserving pseudopotentials," *Phys. Rev. B* 32:8412, 1985.

[530] G. P. Kerker, "Non-singular atomic pseudopotentials for solid state applications," *J. Phys. C* 13:L189, 1980.

[531] N. Troullier and J. L. Martins, "Efficient pseudopotentials for plane-wave calculations," *Phys. Rev. B* 43:1993–2006, 1991.

[532] A. M. Rappe, K. M. Rabe, E. Kaxiras, and J. D. Joannopoulos, "Optimized pseudopotentials," *Phys. Rev. B* 41:1227, 1990.

[533] G. Kresse, J. Hafner, and R. J. Needs, "Optimized norm-conserving pseudopotentials," *J. Phys. Condens. Matter* 4:7451, 1992.

[534] S. G. Louie, S. Froyen, and M. L. Cohen, "Nonlinear ionic pseudopotentials in spin-density-functional calculations," *Phys. Rev. B* 26:1738–1742, 1982.

[535] D. R. Hamann, "Optimized norm-conserving Vanderbilt pseudopotentials," *Phys. Rev. B* 88:085117, 2013.

[536] S. Goedecker and K. Maschke, "Transferability of pseudopotentials," *Phys. Rev. A* 45:88–93, 1992.

[537] M. Teter, "Additional condition for transferability in pseudopotentials," *Phys. Rev. B* 48:5031–5041, 1993.

[538] A. Filippetti, D. Vanderbilt, W. Zhong, Y. Cai, and G. B. Bachelet, "Chemical hardness, linear response, and pseudopotential transferability," *Phys. Rev. B* 52:11793–11804, 1995.

[539] L. Kleinman and D. M. Bylander, "Efficacious form for model pseudopotentials," *Phys. Rev. Lett.* 48:1425–1428, 1982.

[540] X. Gonze, R. Stumpf, and M. Scheffler, "Analysis of separable potentials," *Phys. Rev. B* 44:8503, 1991.

[541] M.J. van Setten, M. Giantomassi, E. Bousquet, M. J. Verstraete, D. R. Hamann, X. Gonze, and G.-M. Rignanese, "The pseudodojo: Training and grading a 85 element optimized norm-conserving pseudopotential table," *Comput. Phys. Commun.* 226:39–54, 2018.

[542] P. E. Blöchl, "Projector augmented-wave method," *Phys. Rev. B* 50:17953–17979, 1994.

[543] N. A. W. Holzwarth, G. E. Matthews, A. R. Tackett, and R. B. Dunning, "Comparison of the projector augmented-wave, pseudopotential, and linearized augmented-plane-wave formalisms for density-functional calculations of solids," *Phys. Rev. B* 55:2005–2017, 1997.

[544] G. Kresse and D. Joubert, "From ultrasoft pseudopotentials to the projector augmented-wave method," *Phys. Rev. B* 59:1758–1775, 1999.

[545] M. Marsman and G. Kresse, "Relaxed core projector-augmented-wave method," *J. Chem. Phys.* 125:104101, 2006.

[546] P. E. Blöchl, "The projector augmented wave method: Algortithm and results," Conference of the Asian Consortium for Computational Materials Science, Bangalore, India, 2001.

[547] S. Baroni and R. Resta, "*Ab initio* calculation of the macroscopic dielectric constant in silicon," *Phys. Rev. B* 33:7017, 1986.

[548] M. S. Hybertsen and S. G. Louie, "*Ab initio* static dielectric matrices from the density-functional approach. I. Formulation and application to semiconductors and insulators," *Phys. Rev. B* 35:5585, 1987.

[549] C. P. Slichter, *Principles of Magnetic Resonance,* 3rd ed., Springer Verlag, Berlin, 1996.

[550] F. Mauri, B. G. Pfrommer, and S. G. Louie, "*Ab initio* theory of NMR chemical shifts in solids and liquids," *Phys. Rev. Lett.* 77:5300–5303, 1996.

[551] T. Gregor, F. Mauri, and R. Car, "A comparison of methods for the calculation of NMR chemical shifts," *J. Chem. Phys.* 111:1815–1822, 1999.

[552] G. B. Bachelet, D. M. Ceperley, and M. G. B. Chiocchetti, "Novel pseudo-hamiltonian for quantum Monte Carlo simulations," *Phys. Rev. Lett.* 62:2088–2091, 1989.

[553] M. W. C. Foulkes and M. Schlüter, "Pseudopotentials with position-dependent electron masses," *Phys. Rev. B* 42:11505–11529, 1990.

[554] A. Bosin, V. Fiorentini, A. Lastri, and G. B. Bachelet, "Local norm-conserving pseudo-hamiltonians," *Phys. Rev. A* 52:236, 1995.

[555] E. L. Shirley and R. M. Martin, "GW quasiparticle calculations in atoms," *Phys. Rev. B* 47:15404–15412, 1993.

[556] E. L. Shirley and R. M. Martin, "Many-body core-valence partitioning," *Phys. Rev. B* 47:15413–15427, 1993.

[557] M. Dolg, U. Wedig, H. Stoll, and H. Preuss, "Energy-adjusted *ab initio* pseudopotentials for the first row transition elements," *J. Chem. Phys.* 86:866–872, 1987.

[558] B. Segall, "Energy bands of aluminum," *Phys. Rev.* 124:1797–1806, 1961.

[559] V. Heine, "The band structure of aluminum III. A self-consistent calculation," *Proc. Roy. Soc. (London)* A240:361, 1957.

[560] V. Heine and D. Weaire, in *Solid State Physics*, edited by H. Ehrenreich, F. Seitz, and D. Turnbull, Academic, New York, 1970, p. 249.

[561] M. L. Cohen and J. R. Chelikowsky, *Electronic Structure and Optical Properties of Semiconductors*, 2nd ed., Springer-Verlag, Berlin, 1988.

[562] J. Ihm, A. Zunger, and M. L. Cohen, "Momentum-space formalism for the total energy of solids," *J. Phys. C* 12:4409, 1979.

[563] T. C. Chiang, J. A. Knapp, M. Aono, and D. E. Eastman, "Angle-resolved photoemission, valence-band dispersions e(k), and electron and hole lifetimes for GaAs," *Phys. Rev. B* 21:3513–3522, 1980.

[564] K. C. Pandey and J. C. Phillips, "Nonlocal pseudopotentials for Ge and GaAs," *Phys. Rev. B* 9:1552–1559, 1974.

[565] P. Y. Yu and M. Cardona, *Fundamentals of Semiconductors: Physics and Materials Properties*, Springer-Verlag, Berlin, 1996.

[566] L. W. Wang and A. Zunger, "Solving Schrödinger's equation around a desired energy: Application to silicon quantum dots," *J. Chem. Phys.* 48:2394–2397, 1994.

[567] L. W. Wang, J. Kim, and A. Zunger, "Electronic structures of [110]-faceted self-assembled pyramidal InAs/GaAs quantum dots," *Phys. Rev. B* 59:5678–5687, 1999.

[568] T. L. Beck, "Real-space mesh techniques in density-functional theory," *Rev. Mod. Phys.* 72:1041–1080, 2000.

[569] J. R. Chelikowsky, N. Troullier, Y. Saad, and K. Wu, "Finite-difference-pseudopotential method: Electronic structure calculations without a basis," *Phys. Rev. Lett.* 72:1240–1243, 1994.

[570] J. R. Chelikowsky, N. Troullier, and Y. Saad, "Higher-order finite-difference pseudopotential method: An application to diatomic molecules," *Phys. Rev. B* 50:11355–11364, 1994.

[571] L. Kronik, et al., "PARSEC the pseudopotential algorithm for real-space electronic structure calculations: Recent advances and novel applications to nano-structures," *Phys. Stat. Sol. B* 243:1063–1079, 2006.

[572] Y. Saad, J. Chelikowsky, and S. Shontz, "Numerical methods for electronic structure calculations of materials," *SIAM Review* 52:3–54, 2010.

[573] S. Ghosh and P. Suryanarayana, "SPARC: Accurate and efficient finite-difference formulation and parallel implementation of density functional theory: Extended systems," *Comput. Phys. Commun.* 216:109–125, 2017.

[574] B. Fornberg and D. Sloan, in *Acta Numerica 94*, edited by A. Iserles, Cambridge Press, Cambridge, 1994, pp. 203–267.

[575] J. R. Chelikowsky I. Vasiliev and R. M. Martin, "Surface oxidation effects on the optical properties of silicon nanocrystals," *Phys. Rev. B* 65:121302, 2002.

[576] E. L. Briggs, D. J. Sullivan, and J. Bernholc, "Real-space multigrid-based approach to large-scale electronic structure calculations," *Phys. Rev. B* 54:14362–14375, 1996.

[577] L. Collatz, *The Numerical Treatment of Differential Equations*, 3rd ed., Springer-Verlag, Berlin, 1960.

[578] G. Schofield, J. R. Chelikowsky, and Y. Saad, "A spectrum slicing method for the Kohn Sham problem," *Comput. Phys. Commun.* 183:497–505, 2012.

[579] L. Lin, J. Lu, L. Ying, and E. W. Weinan, "Adaptive local basis set for Kohn Sham density functional theory in a discontinuous Galerkin framework I: Total energy calculation," *Journal of Computational Physics* 231:2140–2154, 2012.

[580] Q. Xu, P. Suryanarayana, and J. E. Pask, "Discrete discontinuous basis projection method for large-scale electronic structure calculations," *J. Chem. Phys.* 149:094104, 2018.

[581] A. Brandt, "Multi-level adaptive solutions to boundary-value problems," *Mat. Comp.* 31:333–390, 1977.

[582] E. L. Briggs, D. J. Sullivan, and J. Bernholc, "Large-scale electronic-structure calculations with multigrid acceleration," *Phys. Rev. B* 52:R5471–R5474, 1995.

[583] M. Heiskanen, T. Torsti, M. J. Puska, and R. M. Nieminen, "Multigrid method for electronic structure calculations," *Phys. Rev. B* 63:245106, 2001.

[584] J. Bernholc, M. Hodak, and W. Lu, "Recent developments and applications of the real-space multigrid method," *J. Phys. Condens. Matter* 20:294205, 2008.

[585] J. E. Pask and P. A. Sterne, "Finite element methods in *ab initio* electronic structure calculations," *Model. Simul. Mater. Sci. Eng.* 13:R71–R96, 2005.

[586] P. Motamarri, S. Das, S. Rudraraju, K. Ghosh, D. Davydov, and V. Gavini, "DFT-FE: A massively parallel adaptive finite-element code for large-scale density functional theory calculations," *Comput. Phys. Commun.*, 246:106853, 2020.

[587] K. Ghosh, H. Ma, V. Gavini, and G. Galli, "All-electron density functional calculations for electron and nuclear spin interactions in molecules and solids," *Phys. Rev. Mater.* 3:043801, 2019.

[588] S. Mohr, L. E. Ratcliff, R. Boulanger, L. Genovese, D. Caliste, T. Deutsch, and S. Goedecker, "Daubechies wavelets for linear scaling density functional theory," *J. Chem. Phys.* 140:204110, 2014.

[589] I. Daubechies, *Ten Lectures on Wavelets*, SIAM, Philadelphia, PA, 1992.

[590] S. Wei and M. Y. Chou, "Wavelets in self-consistent electronic structure calculations," *Phys. Rev. Lett.* 76:2650–2653, 1996.

[591] K. Cho, A. Arias, J. D. Joannopoulos, and P. K. Lam, "Wavelets in electronic structure calculations," *Phys. Rev. Lett.* 71:1808–1811, 1994.

[592] S. Mohr, L. E. Ratcliff, L. Genovese, D. Caliste, R. Boulanger, S. Goedecker, and T. Deutsch, "Accurate and efficient linear scaling dft calculations with universal applicability," *Phys. Chem. Chem. Phys.* 17:31360–31370, 2015.

[593] F. Gygi, "Electronic-structure calculations in adaptive coordinates," *Phys. Rev. B* 48:11692–11700, 1993.

[594] D. R. Hamann, "Application of adaptive curvilinear coordinates to the electronic structure of solids," *Phys. Rev. B* 51:7337–7340, 1995.

[595] F. Gygi and G. Galli, "Real-space adaptive-coordinate electronic-structure calculations," *Phys. Rev. B* 52:R2229–R2232, 1995.

[596] N. A. Modine, G. Zumbach, and E. Kaxiras, "Adaptive-coordinate real-space electronic-structure calculations for atoms, molecules, and solids," *Phys. Rev. B* 55:10289–10301, 1997.

[597] D. R. Hamann, "Comparison of global and local adaptive coordinates for density-functional calculations," *Phys. Rev. B* 63:075107, 2001.

[598] L. Mihaly and M. C. Martin, *Solid State Physics: Problems and Solutions,* 2nd ed., Wiley-VCH, Berlin, Germany, 2009.

[599] M. T. Yin and M. L. Cohen, "Theory of *ab initio* pseudopotential calculations," *Phys. Rev. B* 25:7403–7412, 1982.

[600] W. C. Herring and M. H. Nichols, "Thermionic emission," *Rev. Mod. Phys.* 21:185–270, 1949.

[601] K. Kunc and R. M. Martin, "Atomic structure and properties of polar Ge-GaAs(100) interfaces," *Phys. Rev. B* 24(6):3445–3455, 1981.

[602] E. Wimmer, H. Krakauer, M. Weinert, and A. J. Freeman, "Full-potential self-consistent linearized-augmented-plane-wave method for calculating the electronic structure of molecules and surfaces: O_2 molecule," *Phys. Rev. B* 24:864–875, 1981.

[603] K. Laasonen, R. Car, C. Lee, and D. Vanderbilt, "Implementation of ultrasoft pseudopotentials in *ab initio* molecular dynamics," *Phys. Rev. B* 43:6796, 1991.

[604] F. Gygi and A. Baldereschi, "Self-consistent Hartree–Fock and screened-exchange calculations in solids: Application to silicon," *Phys. Rev. B* 34:4405–4408, 1986.

[605] S. Chawla and G. A. Voth, "Exact exchange in *ab initio* molecular dynamics: An efficient plane-wave based algorithm," *J. Chem. Phys.* 108:4697–4700, 1998.

[606] A. Sorouri, W. M. C. Foulkes, and N. D. M. Hine, "Accurate and efficient method for the treatment of exchange in a plane-wave basis," *J. Chem. Phys.* 124:064105, 2006.

[607] X. Wu, A. Selloni, and R. Car, "Order-N implementation of exact exchange in extended insulating systems," *Phys. Rev. B* 79:085102, 2009.

[608] K. Kunc and R. M. Martin, "*Ab initio* force constants in GaAs: A new approach to calculation of phonons and dielectric properties," *Phys. Rev. Lett.* 48(6):406–409, 1982.

[609] M. T. Yin and M. L. Cohen, "*Ab initio* calculation of the phonon dispersion relation: Application to Si," *Phys. Rev. B* 25:4317–4320, 1982.

[610] S. Wei and M. Y. Chou, "*Ab initio* calculation of force constants and full phonon dispersions," *Phys. Rev. Lett.* 69:2799–2802, 1992.

[611] N. Marzari and D. J. Singh, "Dielectric response of oxides in the wieghted density approximation," *Phys. Rev. B* 62:12724–12729, 2000.

[612] V. Meunier, C. Roland, J. Bernholc, and M. Buongiorno Nardelli, "Electronic and field emission properties of boron nitride/carbon nanotube superlattices," *Appl. Phys. Lett.* 81:46, 2002.

[613] J. C. Slater and G. F. Koster, "Simplified LCAO method for the periodic potential problem," *Phys. Rev.* 94:1498–1524, 1954.

[614] H. Jones, N. Mott, and Skinner, "A theory of the form of the X-ray emission bands of metals," *Phys. Rev.* 45:379, 1934.

[615] W. A. Harrison, *Elementary Electronic Structure*, World Publishing, Singapore, 1999.

[616] D. A. Papaconstantopoulos, *Handbook of Electronic Structure of Elemental Solids*, Plenum, New York, 1986.

[617] M. D. Stiles, "Generalized Slater-Koster method for fitting band structures," *Phys. Rev. B* 55:4168–4173, 1997.

[618] S. G. Louie, in *Carbon Nanotubes,* edited by M. S. Dresselhaus, G. Dresselhaus, and Ph. Avouris, Springer-Verlag, Berlin, 2001, pp. 113–145.

[619] C. H. Xu, C. Z. Wang, C. T. Chan, and K. M. Ho, "A transferable tight-binding potential for carbon," *J. Phys. Condens. Matter* 4:6047, 1992.

[620] X. Blase, L. X. Benedict, E. L. Shirley, and S. G. Louie, "Are fullerene tubules metallic?," *Phys. Rev. Lett* 72:1878–1881, 1994.

[621] M. Machon, S. Reich, C. Thomsen, D. Sanchez-Portal, and P. Ordejon, "*Ab initio* calculations of the optical properties of 4-a-diameter single-walled nanotubes," *Phys. Rev. B* 66:155410, 2002.

[622] D. A. Papaconstantopoulos, M. J. Mehl, J. C. Erwin, and M. R. Pederson, in *Tight-Binding Approach to Computational Materials Science*, edited by P. E. A. Turchi, A. Gonis, and L. Columbo, Materials Research Society, Warrendale, PA, 1998.

[623] A. Rubio, J. L. Corkill, and M. L. Cohen, "Theory of graphitic boron nitride nanotubes," *Phys. Rev. B* 49:5081–5084, 1994.

[624] N. G. Chopra, R. J. Luyken, K. Cherrey, V. H. Crespi, M. L. Cohen, S. G. Louie, and A. Zettl, "Boron nitride nanotubes," *Science* 269:966, 1995.

[625] E. J. Mele and P. Kral, "Electric polarization of heteropolar nanotubes as a geometric phase," *Phys. Rev. Lett.* 88:056803, 2002.

[626] M. S. Hybertsen, M. Schlüter, and N. E. Christensen, "Calculation of Coulomb interaction parameters for La_2CuO_4 using a constrained-density-functional approach," *Phys. Rev. B* 39:9028, 1989.

[627] P. Vogl, H. P. Hjalmarson, and J. D. Dow, "A semi-empirical tight-binding theory of the electronic structure of semiconductors," *Europhys. Lett.* 44:365, 1983.

[628] D. A. Papaconstantopoulos, *Handbook of the Band Structure of Elemental Solids: From Z = 1 to Z = 112*, 2nd ed. Springer, New York, 2015.

[629] L. Shi and D. A. Papaconstantopoulos, "Modifications and extensions to Harrison's tight-binding theory," *Phys. Rev. B* 70:205101, 2004.

[630] O. F. Sankey and D. J. Niklewski, "*Ab initio* multicenter tight-binding model for molecular-dynamics simulations and other applications in covalent systems," *Phys. Rev. B* 40:3979, 1989.

[631] R. E. Cohen, M. J. Mehl, and D. A. Papaconstantopoulos, "Tight-binding total-energy method for transition and noble metals," *Phys. Rev. B* 50:14694–14697, 1994.

[632] D. Porezag, Th. Frauenheim, Th. Köhler, G. Seifert, and R. Kaschner, "Construction of tight-binding-like potentials on the basis of density-functional theory: Application to carbon," *Phys. Rev. B* 51:12947–12957, 1995.

[633] L. Goodwin, A. J. Skinner, and D. G. Pettifor, "Generating transferable tight-binding parameters – Application to silicon," *Europhys. Lett.* 9:701, 1989.

[634] I. Kwon, R. Biswas, C. Z. Wang, K. M. Ho, and C. M. Soukoulis, "Transferable tight-binding models for silicon," *Phys. Rev. B* 49:7242, 1994.

[635] T. J. Lenosky, J. D. Kress, I. Kwon, A. F. Voter, B. Edwards, D. F. Richards, S. Yang, and J. B. Adams, "Highly optimized tight-binding model of silicon," *Phys. Rev. B* 55:1528–1544, 1997.

[636] C. Z. Wang, B C Pan, and K. M. Ho, "An environment-dependent tight-binding potential for Si," *J. Phys. Condens. Matter* 11:2043–2049, 1999.

[637] J. Kim, J. W. Wilkins, F. S. Khan, and A. Canning, "Extended Si [311] defects," *Phys. Rev. B* 55:16186, 1997.

[638] J. Kim, F. Kirchhoff, J. W. Wilkins, and F. S. Khan, "Stability of Si-interstitial defects: From point to extended defects," *Phys. Rev. Lett.* 84:503, 2000.

[639] N. Bernstein, M. J. Mehl, D. A. Papaconstantopoulos, N. I. Papanicolaou, M. Z. Bazant, and E. Kaxiras, "Energetic, vibrational, and electronic properties of silicon using a nonorthogonal tight-binding model," *Phys. Rev. B* 62:4477–4487, 2000.

[640] N. C. Bacalis, D. A. Papaconstantopoulos, M. J. Mehl, and M. Lach-hab, "Transferable tight-binding parameters for ferromagnetic and paramagnetic iron," *Physica B* 296:125–129, 2001.

[641] F. Jensen, *An Introduction to Computational Chemistry*, John Wiley & Sons, New York, 1998.

[642] C. J. Cramer, *Essentials of Computational Chemistry: Theories and Models*, Wiley, New York, 2002.

[643] H. Eschrig, *Optimized LCAO Methods*, Springer, Berlin, 1987.

[644] R. Orlando, R. Dovesi, C. Roetti, and V. R. Saunders, "*Ab initio* Hartree–Fock calculations for periodic compounds: application to semiconductors," *J. Phys. Condens. Matter* 2:7769, 1990.

[645] V. R. Saunders, R. Dovesi, C. Roetti, M. Causa, N. M. Harrison, R. Orlando, and C. M. Zicovich-Wilson, *CRYSTAL User's Manual* (University of Torino, Torino). See http://www.theochem.unito.it/, 2003.

[646] J. M. Soler, E. Artacho, J. Gale, A. Garcia, J. Junquera, P. Ordejon, and D. Sanchez-Portal, "The SIESTA method for *ab intio* order-N materials simulations," *J. Phys. Condens. Matter* 14:2745–2779, 2002.

[647] S. F. Boys, "Electron wave functions I. A general method for calculation for the stationary states of any molecular system," *Proc. R. Soc. Lond. A* 200:542, 1950.

[648] Y. H. Shao, C. A. White, and M. Head-Gordon, "Efficient evaluation of the Coulomb force in density-functional theory calculations," *J. Chem. Phys.* 114:6572–6577, 2001.

[649] J. K. Perry, J. Tahir-Kheli, and W. A. Goddard, "Antiferromagnetic band structure of La_2CuO_4: Becke-3-Lee-Yang-Parr calculations," *Phys. Rev. B* 63:144510, 2001.

[650] K. N. Kudin, G. E. Scuseria, and R. L. Martin, "Hybrid density-functional theory and the insulating gap of UO_2," *Phys. Rev. Lett.* 89:266402, 2002.

[651] M. Rohlfing, P. Krüger, and J. Pollmann, "Quasiparticle band structures of clean, hydrogen- and sulfur-terminated Ge(001) surfaces," *Phys. Rev. B* 54:13759–13766, 1996.

[652] G. E. Scuseria, "Linear scaling density functional calculations with gaussian orbitals," *J. Phys. Chem. A* 103:4782–4790, 1999.

[653] B. Delley, "An all-electron numerical method for solving the local density functional for polyatomic molecules," *J. Chem. Phys.* 92:508–517, 1990.

[654] K. Koepernik and H. Eschrig, "Full-potential nonorthogonal local-orbital minimum-basis band-structure scheme," *Phys. Rev. B* 59:1743–1757, 2000.

[655] B. Delley, "From molecules to solids with the DMol3 approach," *J. Chem. Phys.* 113:7756–7764, 2000.

[656] J. Junquera, O. Paz, D. Sanchez-Portal, and E. Artacho, "Numerical atomic orbitals for linear-scaling calculations," *Phys. Rev. B* 64:235111, 2001.

[657] M. R. Pederson and K. A. Jackson, "Variational mesh for quantum-mechanical simulations," *Phys. Rev. B* 41:7453–7461, 1990.

[658] A. D. Becke, "A multicenter numerical integration scheme for polyatomic molecules," *J. Chem. Phys.* 88:2547–2553, 1988.

[659] P. Ordejón, E. Artacho, and J. M. Soler, "Selfconsistent order-N density-functional calculations for very large systems," *Phys. Rev. B* 53:R10441–R10444, 1996.

[660] G. A. Baraff and M. Schluter, "Self-consistent Green's-function calculation of the ideal Si vacancy," *Phys. Rev. Lett.* 41:892, 1978.

[661] J. Bernholc, N. O. Lipari, and S. T. Pantelides, "Self-consistent method for point defects in semiconductors: Application to the vacancy in silicon," *Phys. Rev. Lett.* 41:895, 1978.

[662] P. J. Feibelman, "First-principles total-energy calculation for a single adatom on a crystal," *Phys. Rev. Lett.* 54:2627–2630, 1985.

[663] P. J. Feibelman, "Force and total-energy calculations for a spatially compact adsorbate on an extended, metallic crystal surface," *Phys. Rev. B* 35:2626–2646, 1987.

[664] S. G. Louie, K.-M. Ho, and M. L. Cohen, "Self-consistent mixed-basis approach to the electronic structure of solids," *Phys. Rev. B* 19:1774–1782, 1979.

[665] G. Li and Y. Chang, "Planar-basis pseudopotential calculations of the Si(001)2 x 1 surface with and without hydrogen passivation," *Phys. Rev. B* 48:12032–12036, 1993.

[666] T. Loucks, *The Augmented Plane Wave Method*, Benjamin, New York, 1967.

[667] J. O. Dimmock, in *Solid State Physics*, vol. 26, edited by H. Ehenreich, F. Seitz, and D. Turnbull, Academic Press, New York, 1971, pp. 104–274.

[668] M. I. Chodorow, "Energy band structure of copper," *Phys. Rev.* 55:675, 1939.

[669] G. A. Burdick, "Energy band structure of copper," *Phys. Rev.* 129:138–150, 1963.

[670] P. Thiry, D. Chandesris, J. Lecante, C. Guillot, R. Pinchaux, and Y. Petroff, "E vs k and inverse lifetime of Cu(110)," *Phys. Rev. Lett.* 43:82–85, 1979.

[671] L. F. Mattheiss, "Energy bands for the iron transition series," *Phys. Rev.* 134:A970–A973, 1964.

[672] J. C. Slater, "Magnetic effects and the Hartree–Fock equation," *Phys. Rev.* 82:538–541, 1951.

[673] J. Kübler, *Theory of Itinerant Electron Magnetism*, Oxford University Press, Oxford, 2001.

[674] V. Heine, "s–d interaction in transition metals," *Phys. Rev.* 153:673–682, 1967.

[675] J. W. D. Connolly, "Energy bands in ferromagnetic nickel," *Phys. Rev.* 159:415, 1967.

[676] J. Ziman, in *Solid State Physics*, vol. 26, edited by H. Ehenreich, F. Seitz, and D. Turnbull, Academic Press, New York, 1971, pp. 1–101.

[677] J. Korringa, "On the calculation of the energy of a Bloch wave in a metal," *Physica* 13:392, 1947.

[678] W. Kohn and N. Rostocker, "Solution of the Schrodinger equation in periodic lattices with an application to metallic lithium," *Phys. Rev.* 94:1111, 1954.

[679] J. W. Strutt [Lord Rayleigh], "On the influence of obstacles arranged in rectangular order upon the properties of a medium," *Phil. Mag. Series 5* 34:481–502, 1892.

[680] R. Zeller, P. H. Dederichs, B. Ujfalussy, L. Szunyog, and P. Weinberger, "Theory and convergence properties of the screened Korringa–Kohn–Rostoker method," *Phys. Rev. B* 52:8807–8812, 1995.

[681] T. Huhne, C. Zecha, H. Ebert, P. H. Dederichs, and R. Zeller, "Full-potential spin-polarized relativistic Korringa–Kohn–Rostoker method implemented and applied to bcc Fe, fcc Co, and fcc Ni," *Phys. Rev. B* 58:10236, 1998.

[682] W. H. Butler, P. H. Dederichs, A. Gonis, and R. L. Weaver, *Applications of Multiple Scattering Theory to Material Science*, Materials Research Society, Pittsburg, Penn., 1992.

[683] E.N. Economou, *Green's Functions in Quantum Physics*, 2nd ed., Springer-Verlag, Berlin, 1992.

[684] P. Lloyd and P. V. Smith, "Multiple scattering theory in condensed materials," *Adv. Phys.* 21:29, 1972.

[685] B. L. Gyorffy, in *Applications of Multiple Scattering Theory to Material Science*, edited by W. H. Butler, P. H. Dederichs, A. Gonis, and R. L. Weaver, Materials Research Society, Pittsburgh, PA, 1992, pp. 5–25.

[686] P. Lloyd, "Wave propagation through an assembly of spheres II: The density of single particle eigenstates," *Proc. Phys. Soc, London* 90:207–216, 1967.

[687] S. Müller and A. Zunger, "Structure of ordered and disordered alpha-brass," *Phys. Rev. B* 63:094204, 2001.

[688] P. Soven, "Coherent-potential model of substitutional disordered alloys," *Phys. Rev.* 156:809–813, 1967.

[689] B. Velicky, S. Kirkpatrick, and H. Ehrenreich, "Single-site approximations in the electronic theory of simple binary alloys," *Phys. Rev.* 175:747–766, 1968.

[690] M. Lax, "Multiple scattering of waves," *Rev. Mod. Phys.* 23:287–310, 1951.

[691] J. L. Beeby, "Electronic structure of alloys," *Phys. Rev.* 135:A130, 1964.

[692] G. M. Stocks, W. M. Temmerman, and B. L. Gyorffy, "Complete solution of the Korringa–Kohn–Rostocker coherent-potential-approximation equations: Cu–Ni alloys," *Phys. Rev. Lett.* 41:339–343, 1978.

[693] J. S. Faulkner and G. M. Stocks, "Calculating properties with the coherent-potential approximation," *Phys. Rev. B* 21:3222–3244, 1980.

[694] W. H. Butler, "Theory of electronic transport in random alloys: Korringa–Kohn–Rostoker coherent-potential approximation," *Phys. Rev. B* 31:3260, 1985.

[695] D. D. Johnson, D. M. Nicholson, F. J. Pinski, B. L. Gyorffy, and G. M. Stocks, "Total-energy and pressure calculations for random substitutional alloys," *Phys. Rev. B* 41:9701–9716, 1990.

[696] A. F. Tatarchenko, V. S. Stepanyuk, W. Hergert, P. Rennert, R. Zeller, and P. H. Dederichs, "Total energy and magnetic moments in disordered Fe_xCu_{1-x} alloys," *Phys. Rev. B* 57:5213–5219, 1998.

[697] J. B. Staunton, J. Poulter, B. Ginatempo, E. Bruno, and D. D. Johnson, "Incommensurate and commensurate antiferromagnetic spin fluctuations in Cr and Cr alloys from *ab initio* dynamical spin susceptibility calculations," *Phys. Rev. Lett.* 82:3340–3343, 1999.

[698] O. K. Andersen, in *Computational Methods in Band Theory*, edited by P. M. Marcus, J. F. Janak, and A. R. Williams, Plenum, New York, 1971, p. 178.

[699] H. Skriver, *The LMTO Method*, Springer, New York, 1984.

[700] O. K. Andersen, "Linear methods in band theory," *Phys. Rev. B* 12:3060–3083, 1975.

[701] O. K. Andersen and O. Jepsen, "Explicit, first-principles tight-binding theory," *Phys. Rev. Lett.* 53:2571–2574, 1984.

[702] J. Keller, "Modified muffin tin potentials for the band structure of semiconductors," *J. Phys. C: Solid State Phys.* 13:L85–L87, 1980.

[703] D. Glötzel, B. Segall, and O. K. Andersen, "Self-consistent electronic structure of Si, Ge and diamond LMTO-ASA method," *Solid State Commun.* 36:403, 1980.

[704] Y. Wang, G. M. Stocks, W. A. Shelton, D. M. C. Nicholson, Z. Szotec, and W. M. Temmerman, "Order-N multiple scattering approach to electronic structure calculations," *Phys. Rev. Lett.* 75:2867–2870, 1995.

[705] O. K. Andersen, Z. Pawlowska, and O. Jepsen, "Illustration of the LMTO tight-binding representation: Compact orbitals and charge density in Si," *Phys. Rev. B* 34:5253–5269, 1986.

[706] J. M. Soler and A. R. Williams, "Augmented-plane-wave forces," *Phys. Rev. B* 42:9728–9731, 1990.

[707] R. Yu, D. Singh, and H. Krakauer, "All-electron and pseudopotential force calculations using the linearized-augmented-plane-wave method," *Phys. Rev. B* 93:6411–6422, 1991.

[708] S. Mishra and S. Satpathy, "Kronig-penny model with the tail-cancellation method," *Am. J. Phys.* 69:512–513, 2001.

[709] D. J. Singh, *Planewaves, Pseudopotentials, and the APW Method*, Kluwer Academic Publishers, Boston, 1994, and references therein.

[710] A. R. Williams, J. Kübler, and Jr. C. D. Gelatt, "Cohesive properties of metallic compounds: Augmented-spherical-wave calculations," *Phys. Rev. B* 19:6094–6118, 1979.

[711] D. D. Koelling and G. O. Arbman, "Use of energy derivative of the radial solution in an augmented plane wave method: application to copper," *J. Phys. F: Met. Phys.* 5:2041–2054, 1975.

[712] H. Krakauer, M. Posternak, and A. J. Freeman, "Linearized augmented plane-wave method for the electronic band structure of thin films," *Phys. Rev. B* 19:1706–1719, 1979.

[713] M. Weinert, E. Wimmer, and A. J. Freeman, "Total-energy all-electron density functional method for bulk solids and surfaces," *Phys. Rev. B* 26:4571–4578, 1982.

[714] L. F. Mattheiss and D. R. Hamann, "Linear augmented-plane-wave calculation of the structural properties of bulk Cr, Mo, and W," *Phys. Rev. B* 33:823–840, 1986.

[715] P. Blaha, K. Schwarz, P. Sorantin, and S.B. Trickey, "Full-potential, linearized augmented plane wave programs for crystalline systems," *Comput. Phys. Commun.* 59(2):399, 1990.

[716] W. E. Pickett, "Electronic structure of the high-temperature oxide superconductors," *Rev. Mod. Phys.* 61:433, 1989.

[717] H. J. F. Jansen and A. J. Freeman, "Total-energy full-potential linearized augmented-plane-wave method for bulk solids: Electronic and structural properties of tungsten," *Phys. Rev. B* 30:561–569, 1984.

[718] R. E. Cohen, W. E. Pickett, and H. Krakauer, "Theoretical determination of strong electron–phonon coupling in $YBa_2Cu_3O_7$," *Phys. Rev. Lett.* 64:2575–2578, 1990.

[719] H. Krakauer, W. E. Pickett, and R. Cohen, "Analysis of electronic structure and charge density of the high-temperature superconductor $YBa_2Cu_3O_7$," *J. Superconductivity* 1:111, 1988.

[720] M. Methfessel, "Elastic constants and phonon frequencies of Si calculated by a fast full-potential linear-muffin-tin-orbital method," *Phys. Rev. B* 38:1537, 1988.

[721] M. Methfessel, C. O. Rodriguez, and O. K. Andersen, "Fast full-potential calculations with a converged basis of atom-centered linear muffin-tin orbitals: Structural and dynamic properties of silicon," *Phys. Rev. B* 40:2009, 1989.

[722] M. Methfessel and M. van Schilfgaarde, in *Electronic Strcuture and Physical Properties of Solids: The Uses of the LMTO Method*, edited by H. Dreysse, Springer, Heidelberg, 1999, pp. 114–147.

[723] O. Jepsen, O. K. Andersen, and A. R. Mackintosh, "Electronic structure of hcp transition metals," *Phys. Rev. B* 12:3084–3103, 1977.

[724] T. Fujiwara, "Electronic structure calculations for amorphous alloys," *J. Non-crystalline Solids* 61-62:1039–48, 1984.

[725] H. J. Nowak, O. K. Andersen, T. Fujiwara, O. Jepsen, and P. Vargas, "Electronic-structure calculations for amorphous solids using the recursion method and linear muffin-tin orbitals: Application to $Fe_{80}B_{20}$," *Phys. Rev. B* 44:3577–3598, 1991.

[726] S. K. Bose, O. Jepsen, and O. K. Andersen, "Real-space calculation of the electrical resistivity of liquid 3d transition metals using tight-binding linear muffin-tin orbitals," *Phys. Rev. B* 48:4265–4275, 1993.

[727] G. B. Bachelet and N. E. Christensen, "Relativistic and core-relaxation effects on the energy bands of gallium arsenide and germanium," *Phys. Rev. B* 31:879–887, 1985.

[728] S. Satpathy and Z. Pawlowska, "Construction of bond-centered Wannier functions for silicon bands," *Phys. Stat. Sol. (b)* 145:555–565, 1988.

[729] N. E. Christensen, "Dipole effects and band offsets at semiconductor interfaces," *Phys. Rev. B* 37:4528, 1988.

[730] W. R. L. Lambrecht, B. Segall, and O. K. Andersen, "Self-consistent dipole theory of heterojunction band offsets," *Phys. Rev. B* 41:2813, 1990.

[731] J. C. Duthi and D. G. Pettifor, "Correlation between d-band occupancy and crystal structure in the rare earths," *Phys. Rev. Lett.* 38:564–567, 1977.

[732] R. Haydock, in *Recursion Method and Its Applications*, edited by D. G. Pettifor and D. L. Weaire, Springer-Verlag, Berlin, 1985.

[733] J. Friedel, "Electronic structure of primary solid solutions in metals," *Adv. Phys.* 3:446, 1954.

[734] O. K. Andersen, T. Saha-Dasgupta, R. Tank, C. Arcangeli, O. Jepsen, and G. Krier, in *Electronic Structure and Physical Properties of Solids*, edited by H. Dreysse, Springer, Berlin, 1998, pp. 3–84.

[735] O. K. Andersen and T. Saha-Dasgupta, "Muffin-tin orbitals of arbitrary order," *Phys. Rev. B* 62:R16219–R16222, 2000.

[736] K. H. Weyrich, "Full-potential linear muffin-tin-orbital method," *Phys. Rev. B* 37:10269–10282, 1988.

[737] L. Greengard, "Fast algorithms for classical physics," *Science* 265:909–914, 1994.

[738] P. Fulde, *Electron Correlation in Molecules and Solids*, 2nd ed., Springer-Verlag, Berlin, 1993.

[739] D. R. Bowler and T. Miyazaki, "O(N) methods in electronic structure calculations," *Rep. Prog. Phy.* 75:036503, 2012.

[740] Mark S. Gordon, Dmitri G. Fedorov, Spencer R. Pruitt, and Lyudmila V. Slipchenko, "Fragmentation methods: A route to accurate calculations on large systems," *Chem. Rev.* 112:632–672, 2012.

[741] D. J. Cole and Nicholas D. M. Hine, "Applications of large-scale density functional theory in biology," *J. Phys. Condens. Matter* 28:393001, 2016.

[742] W. Kohn, "Density functional and density matrix method scaling linearly with the number of atoms," *Phys. Rev. Lett.* 76:3168–3171, 1996.

[743] J. Aarons, M. Sarwar, D. Thompsett, and C.-K. Skylaris, "Perspective: Methods for large-scale density functional calculations on metallic systems," *J. Chem. Phys.* 145:220901, 2016.

[744] R. Baer and M. Head-Gordon, "Sparsity of the density matrix in Kohn–Sham density functional theory and an assessment of linear system-size scaling methods," *Phys. Rev. Lett.* 79:3962–3965, 1997.

[745] W. Hierse and E. Stechel, "Order-N methods in self-consistent density-functional calculations," *Phys. Rev. B* 50:17811–17819, 1994.

[746] W. T. Yang, "Absolute-energy-minimum principles for linear-scaling electronic-structure calculations," *Phys. Rev. B* 56:9294–9297, 1997.

[747] A. L. Ankudinov, C. E. Bouldin, J. J. Rehr, J. Sims, and H. Hung, "Parallel calculation of electron multiple scattering using Lanczos algorithms," *Phys. Rev. B* 65:104107, 2002.

[748] G. Galli and M. Parrinello, in *Computer Simulations in Material Science*, edited by M. Meyer and V. Pontikis, Kluwer, Dordrecht, 1991, pp. 283–304.

[749] C. M. Goringe, D. R. Bowler, and E. Hernandez, "Tight-binding modelling of materials," *Rep. Prog. Phys.* 60:1447–1512, 1997.

[750] D. G. Pettifor, "New many-body potential for the bond order," *Phys. Rev. Lett.* 63:2480–2483, 1989.

[751] M. Aoki, "Rapidly convergent bond order expansion for atomistic simulations," *Phys. Rev. Lett.* 71:3842, 1993.

[752] A. P. Horsfield, "A comparison of linear scaling tight-binding methods," *Mater. Sci. Eng.* 5:199, 1996.

[753] R. Haydock, in *Solid State Physics*, vol. 35, edited by H. Ehenreich, F. Seitz, and D. Turnbull, Academic Press, New York, 1980, p. 1.

[754] R. Haydock, V. Heine, and M. J. Kelly, "Electronic structure based on the local atomic environment for tight-binding bands: II," *J. Phys. C* 8:2591–2605, 1975.

[755] D. A. Drabold, P. Ordejon, J. J. Dong, and R. M. Martin, "Spectral properties of large fullerenes: from cluster to crystal," *Solid State Commun.* 96:833, 1995.

[756] C. H. Xu and G. Scuseria, "An O(N) tight-binding study of carbon clusters up to C_{8640}: The geometrical shape of the giant icosahedral fullerenes," *Chem. Phys. Lett.* 262:219, 1996.

[757] D. A. Drabold anf O. F. Sankey, "Maximum entropy approach for linear scaling in the electronic structure problem," *Phys. Rev. Lett.* 70:3631–3634, 1993.

[758] P. Ordejón, D. A. Drabold, R. M. Martin, and S. Itoh, "Linear scaling method for phonon calculations from electronic structure," *Phys. Rev. Lett.* 75:1324–1327, 1995.

[759] W. T. Yang, "Direct calculation of electron density in density functional theory," *Phys. Rev. Lett.* 66:1438–1441, 1991.

[760] S. Goedecker and L. Colombo, "Efficient linear scaling algorithm for tight-binding molecular dynamics," *Phys. Rev. Lett.* 73:122–125, 1994.

[761] A. F. Voter, J. D. Kress, and R. N. Silver, "Linear-scaling tight binding from a truncated-moment approach," *Phys. Rev. B* 53:12733–12741, 1996.

[762] R. N. Silver and H. Roder, "Calculation of densities of states and spectral functions by Chebyshev recursion and maximum entropy," *Phys. Rev. E* 56:4822–4829, 1997.

[763] S. Goedecker, "Low complexity algorithms for electronic structure calculations," *J. Comp. Phys.* 118, 1995.

[764] D. Jovanovic and J. P. Leburton, "Self-consistent analysis of single-electron charging effects in quantum-dot nanostructures," *Phys. Rev. B* 49:7474, 1994.

[765] A. Alavi, Parrinello, and D. Frenkel, "*Ab initio* calculation of the sound velocity of dense hydrogen: Implications for models of Jupiter," *Science* 269:1252–4, 1995.

[766] J. L. Corkill and K. M. Ho, "Electronic occupation functions for density-matrix tight-binding methods," *Phys. Rev. B* 54:5340–5345, 1996.

[767] X.-P. Li, R. W. Nunes, and D. Vanderbilt, "Density-matrix electronic-structure method with linear system-size scaling," *Phys. Rev. B* 47:10891–10894, 1993.

[768] F. Mauri, G. Galli, and R. Car, "Orbital formulation for electronic structure calculation with linear system-size scaling," *Phys. Rev. B* 47:9973–9976, 1993.

[769] P. Ordejón, D. A. Drabold, M. P. Grumbach, and R. M. Martin, "Unconstrained minimization approach for electronic computations that scales linearly with system size," *Phys. Rev. B* 48:14646–14649, 1993.

[770] J. Kim, F. Mauri, and G. Galli, "Total-energy global optimizations using nonorthogonal localized orbitals," *Phys. Rev. B* 52:1640–1648, 1995.

[771] R. W. Nunes and D. Vanderbilt, "Generalization of the density-matrix method to a nonorthogonal basis," *Phys. Rev. B* 50:17611–17614, 1994.

[772] S. Itoh, P. Ordejón, D. Drabold, and R. M. Martin, "Structure and energetics of giant fullerenes: An order-N molecular dynamics study," *Phys. Rev. B* 53:2132–2140, 1996.

[773] S. Y. Qiu, C. Z. Wang, K. M. Ho, and C. T. Chan, "Tight-binding molecular dynamics with linear system-size scaling," *J. Phys. Condens. Matter* 6:9153, 1994.

[774] S. Liu, J. M. Perez-Jorda, and W. Yang, "Nonorthogonal localized molecular orbitals in electronic structure theory," *J. Chem. Phys.* 112:1634, 2000.

[775] E. B. Stechel, A. R. Williams, and P. J. Feibelman, "N-scaling algorithm for density-functional calculations of metals and insulators," *Phys. Rev. B* 49:10088–10101, 1994.

[776] W. H. Press and S. A. Teukolsky, *Numerical Recipes*, Cambridge University Press, Cambridge, 1992.

[777] U. Stephan and D. A. Drabold, "Order-N projection method for first-principles computations of electronic quantities and Wannier functions," *Phys. Rev. B* 57:6391–6407, 1998.

[778] U. Stephan, D. A. Drabold, and R. M. Martin, "Improved accuracy and acceleration of variational order-N electronic-structure computations by projection techniques," *Phys. Rev. B* 58:13472–13481, 1998.

[779] U. Stephan, R. M. Martin, and D. A. Drabold, "Extended-range computation of Wannier-like functions in amorphous semiconductors," *Phys. Rev. B* 62:6885–6888, 2000.

[780] P. J. de Pablo, F. Moreno-Herrero, J. Colchero, J. G. Herrero, P. Herrero, A. M. Baro, P. Ordejon, J. M. Soler, and E. Artacho, "Absence of DC-conductivity in lambda-DNA," *Phys. Rev. Lett.* 85:4992–4995, 2000.

[781] E. Hernandez and M. J. Gillan, "Self-consistent first-principles technique with linear scaling," *Phys. Rev. B* 51:10157–10160, 1995.

[782] J.-L. Fattebert and J. Bernholc, "Towards grid-based O(N) density-functional theory methods: Optimized nonorthogonal orbitals and multigrid acceleration," *Phys. Rev. B* 62:1713–1722, 2000.

[783] P. D. Haynes and M. C. Payne, "Localized spherical-wave basis set for O(N) total energy pseudopotential calculations," *Comput. Phys. Commun.* 102:17–27, 1997.

[784] D. Marx and J. Hutter, *Ab Initio Molecular Dynamics: Basic Theory and Advanced Methods*, Cambridge University Press, Cambridge, UK, 2009.

[785] M. C. Payne, J. D. Joannopoulos, D. C. Allan, M. P. Teter, and D. M. Vanderbilt, "Molecular dynamics and *ab initio* total energy calculations," *Phys. Rev. Lett.* 56:2656, 1986.

[786] O. F. Sankey and R. E. Allen, "Atomic forces from electronic energies via the Hellmann-Feynman theorem, with application to semiconductor (110) surface relaxation," *Phys. Rev. B* 33:7164–7171, 1986.

[787] J. M. Thijssen, *Computational Physics*, Cambridge University Press, Cambridge, U.K., 2000.

[788] J. P. Ryckaert, G. Ciccotti, and H. J. C. Berendsen, "Numerical integration of the cartesian equations of motion of a system with constraints: Molecular dynamics of n-alkanes," *J. Comput. Phys.* 23:327, 1977.

[789] R. Car and M. Parrinello, in *Simple Molecular Systems at Very High Density*, edited by A. Polian, P. Loubeyre, and N. Boccara, Plenum, New York, 1989, p. 455.

[790] D. K. Remler and P. A. Madden, "Molecular dynamics without effective potentials via the Car-Parrinello approach," *Mol. Phys.* 70:921, 1990.

[791] G. Pastore, E. Smargiassi, and F. Buda, "Theory of *ab initio* molecular-dynamics calculations," *Phys. Rev. A* 44:6334, 1991.

[792] M. C. Payne, "Error cancellation in the molecular dynamics method for total energy calculations," *J. Phys. Condens. Matter* 1:2199–2210, 1989.

[793] R. Car, M. Parrinello, and M. Payne, "Comment on 'error cancellation in the molecular dynamics method for total energy calculations,'" *J. Phys. Condens. Matter* 3:9539–9543, 1991.

[794] M. P. Grumbach and R. M. Martin, "Phase diagram of carbon at high pressures and temperatures," *Phys. Rev. B* 54:15730–15741, 1996.

[795] M. E. Tuckerman and M. Parrinello, "Integrating the Car-Parrinello equations. I. Basic integration techniques," *J. Chem. Phys.* 101:1302, 1994.

[796] M. E. Tuckerman and M. Parrinello, "Integrating the Car-Parrinello equations. II. Multiple time scale techniques," *J. Chem. Phys.* 101:1316, 1994.

[797] G. Galli, R. M. Martin, R. Car, and M. Parrinello, "*Ab initio* calculation of properties of carbon in the amorphous and liquid states," *Phys. Rev. B* 42:7470, 1990.

[798] M. Elstner, D. Porezag, G. Jungnickel, J. Elsner, M. Haugk, Th. Frauenheim, S. Suhai, and G. Seifert, "Self-consistent-charge density-functional tight-binding method for simulations of complex materials properties," *Phys. Rev. B* 58:7260–7268, 1998.

[799] A. A. Correa, S. A. Bonev, and G. Galli, "Carbon under extreme conditions: Phase boundaries and electronic properties from first-principles theory," *Proc. Natl. Acad. Sci. U.S.A.* 103:1204–1208, 2006.

[800] X. Wang, S. Scandolo, and R. Car, "Carbon phase diagram from *ab initio* molecular dynamics," *Phys. Rev. Lett.* 95:185701, 2005.

[801] J. H. Eggert, et al., "Melting temperature of diamond at ultrahigh pressure," *Nat. Phys.* 6:40–43, 2010.

[802] F. P. Bundy, W. A. Bassettand, M. S. Weathers, R. J. Hemley, H. K. Mao, and A. F. Goncharov, "The pressure-temperature phase and transformation diagram for carbon; updated through 1994," *Carbon* 34:141–153, 1996.

[803] G. Galli, R. M. Martin, R. Car, and M. Parrinello, "Melting of diamond at high pressure," *Science* 250:1547, 1990.

[804] A. C. Mitchell, J. W. Shaner, and R. N. Keller, "The use of electrical-conductivity experiments to study the phase diagram of carbon," *Physica* 139:386, 1986.

[805] O. Sugino and R. Car, "*Ab initio* molecular dynamics study of first-order phase transitions: Melting of silicon," *Phys. Rev. Lett.* 74:1823–1826, 1995.

[806] L. D. Landau and E. M. Lifshitz, *Theory of Elasticity*, Pergamon Press, Oxford, U.K., 1958.

[807] J. F. Nye, *Physical Properties of Crystals*, Oxford University Press, Oxford, U.K., 1957.

[808] H. Wendel and R. M. Martin, "Charge density and structural properties of covalent semiconductors," *Phys. Rev. Lett.* 40(14):950–953, 1978.

[809] K.-M. Ho, C.-L. Fu, B. N. Harmon, W. Weber, and D. R. Hamann, "Vibrational frequencies and structural properties of transition metals via total-energy calculations," *Phys. Rev. Lett.* 49:673–676, 1982.

[810] V. Heine and J. H. Samson, "Magnetic, chemical and structural ordering in transition metals," *J. Phys. F* 13:2155, 1983.

[811] S. Baroni, P. Giannozzi, and A. Testa, "Green's function approach to linear response in solids," *Phys. Rev. Lett.* 58:1861–1864, 1987.

[812] A. A. Quong and B. M. Klein, "Self-consistent-screening calculation of interatomic force constants and phonon dispersion curves from first principles," *Phys. Rev. B* 46:10734–10737, 1992.

[813] X. Gonze and J. P. Vigneron, "Density functional approach to non-linear response coefficients in solids," *Phys. Rev. B* 39:13120, 1989.

[814] S. Y. Savrasov and D. Y. Savrasov, "Linear-response theory and lattice dynamics: A muffin-tin-orbital approach," *Phys. Rev. B* 54:16470–16486, 1996.

[815] R. M. Sternheimer, "Electronic polarizabilities of ions from the Hartree–Fock wave functions," *Phys. Rev.* 96:951, 1954.

[816] X. Gonze, "Perturbation expansion of variational principles at arbitrary order," *Phys. Rev. A* 52:1086–1095, 1995.

[817] X. Gonze, "Adiabatic density-functional perturbation theory," *Phys. Rev. A* 52:1096–1114, 1995.

[818] S. de Gironcoli, "Lattice dynamics of metals from density-functional perturbation theory," *Phys. Rev. B* 51:6773, 1995.

[819] R. Resta and K. Kunc, "Self-consistent theory of electronic states and dielectric response in semiconductors," *Phys. Rev. B* 34:7146–7157, 1986.

[820] P. B. Littlewood, "On the calculation of the macroscopic polarisation induced by an optic phonon," *J. Phys. C* 13:4893, 1980.

[821] R. Resta, M. Posternak, and A. Baldereschi, "Towards a quantum theory of polarization in ferroelectrics: The case of $KNbO_3$," *Phys. Rev. Lett.* 70:1010–1013, 1993.

[822] Ph. Ghosez, X. Gonze, Ph. Lambin, and J.-P. Michenaud, "Born effective charges of barium titanate: Band-by-band decomposition and sensitivity to structural features," *Phys. Rev. B* 51:6765–6768, 1995.

[823] W. Zhong, R. D. King-Smith, and D. Vanderbilt, "Giant LO–TO splittings in perovskite ferroelectrics," *Phys. Rev. Lett.* 72:3618–3621, 1994.

[824] P. B. Allen and B. Mikovic, in *Solid State Physics*, vol. 37, edited by H. Ehrenreich, F. Seitz, and D. Turnbull, Academic, New York, 1982, p. 1.

[825] D. Rainer, *Progress in Low Temperature Physics*, vol. 10, North-Holland, Amsterdam, 1986, pp. 371–424.

[826] O. E. Gunnarsson, "Superconductivity in fullerides," *Rev. Mod. Rev.* 69:575–606, 1997.

[827] G. M. Eliashberg, "Interactions between electrons and lattice vibrations in a superconductor [translation: *Sov. Phys. JETP* 11, 696 (1960)]," *Zh. Eksp. Teor. Fiz.* 38:966, 1960.

[828] G. D. Gaspari and B. L. Gyorffy, "Electron–phonon interactions, d resonances, and superconductivity in transition metals," *Phys. Rev. Lett.* 28:801–805, 1972.

[829] J. J. Hopfield, "Angular momentum and transition-metal superconductivity," *Phys. Rev.* 186:443–451, 1969.

[830] S. Y. Savrasov and D. Y. Savrasov, "Electron–phonon interactions and related physical properties of metals from linear-response theory," *Phys. Rev. B* 54:16487–16501, 1996.

[831] M. M. Dacorogna, M. L. Cohen, and P. K. Lam, "Self-consistent calculation of the q dependence of the electron–phonon coupling in aluminum," *Phys. Rev. Lett.* 55:837–840, 1985.

[832] J. F. Cooke, "Neutron scattering from itinerant-electron ferromagnets," *Phys. Rev. B* 7:1108–1116, 1973.

[833] S. Y. Savrasov, "Linear response calculations of spin fluctuations," *Phys. Rev. Lett.* 81:2570–2573, 1998.

[834] L. J. P. Ament, M. van Veenendaal, T. P. Devereaux, J. P. Hill, and J. van den Brink, "Resonant inelastic X-ray scattering studies of elementary excitations," *Rev. Mod. Phys.* 83:705–767, 2011.

[835] D. J. Thouless and J. G. Valatin, "Time-dependent Hartree–Fock equations and rotational states of nuclei," *Nucl. Phys.* 31:211, 1962.

[836] T. Ando, A. Fowler, and F. Stern, "Density-functional calculation of sub-band structure in accumulation and inversion layers," *Phys. Rev. B* 13:3468–3477, 1976.

[837] C. A. Ullrich, U. J. Gossmann, and E. K. U. Gross, "Density-functional approach to atoms in strong laser-pulses," *Ber. Bunsenges. Phys. Chem* 99:488–497, 1995.

[838] *Fundamentals of Time-Dependent Density Functional Theory,* Vol. 837 of Lecture Notes in Physics, edited by M. A. Marques, N. T. Maitra, F. M. Nogueira, E. Gross, and A. Rubio, Springer, Berlin, Heidelberg, 2012.

[839] R. van Leeuwen, "Causality and symmetry in time-dependent density-functional theory," *Phys. Rev. Lett.* 80:1280–1283, 1998.

[840] M. Caro, A. A. Correa, E. Artacho, and A. Caro, "Stopping power beyond the adiabatic approximation," *Sci. Rep.* 7:2618, 2017.

[841] G. Onida, L. Reining, and A. Rubio, "Electronic excitations: Density-functional versus many-body Green's-function approaches," *Rev. Mod. Phys.* 74:601, 2002.

[842] B. Walker, A. M. Saitta, R. Gebauer, and S. Baroni, "Efficient approach to time-dependent density-functional perturbation theory for optical spectroscopy," *Phys. Rev. Lett.* 96:113001, 2006.

[843] D. Rocca, R. Gebauer, Y. Saad, and S. Baroni, "Turbo charging time-dependent density-functional theory with Lanczos chains," *J. Chem. Phys.* 128:154105, 2008.

[844] O. B. Malcolu, R. Gebauer, D. Rocca, and S. Baroni, "turboTDDFT: A code for the simulation of molecular spectra using the Liouville–Lanczos approach to time-dependent density-functional perturbation theory," *Comput. Phys. Commun.* 182:1744–1754, 2011.

[845] H. Flocard, S. Koonin, and M. Weiss, "Three-dimensional time-dependent Hartree–Fock calculations: Application to $^{16}O + {}^{16}O$ collisions," *Phys. Rev. C* 17:1682–1699, 1978.

[846] K. Yabana and G. F. Bertsch, "Time-dependent local-density approximation in real time," *Phys. Rev. B* 54:4484–4487, 1996.

[847] O. Sugino and Y. Miyamoto, "Density-functional approach to electron dynamics: Stable simulation under a self-consistent field," *Phys. Rev. B* 59:2579–2586, 1999.

[848] H. Talezer and R. Kosloff, "An accurate and efficient scheme for propagating the time-dependent Schrödinger equation," *J. Chem. Phys.* 81:3967–3971, 1984.

[849] C. Ullrich, *Time-Dependent Density-Functional Theory: Concepts and Applications*, Oxford University Press, Oxford, U.K., 2012.

[850] T. M. Maier, H. Bahmann, A. V. Arbuznikov, and M. Kaupp, "Validation of local hybrid functionals for TDDFT calculations of electronic excitation energies," *J. Chem. Phys.* 144:074106, 2016.

[851] I. Vasiliev, S. Ogut, and J. R. Chelikowsky, "*Ab initio* excitation spectra and collective electronic response in atoms and clusters," *Phys. Rev. Lett.* 82:1919–1922, 1999.

[852] C. Yannouleas and U. Landman, "Molecular dynamics in shape space and femtosecond vibrational spectroscopy of metal clusters," *J. Phys. Chem. A* 102:2505–2508, 1998.

[853] A. Rubio, J. A. Alonso, X. Blase, L. C. Balbas, and S. G. Louie, "*Ab initio* photoabsorption spectra and structures of small semiconductor and metal clusters," *Phys. Rev. Lett.* 77:247–250, 1996.

[854] A. D. Yoffe, "Semiconductor quantum dots and related systems: Electronic, optical, luminescence and related properties of low dimensional systems," *Adv. Phys.* 50:1–208, 2001.

[855] G. Belomoin, A Smith, S. Rao, R. Twesten, J. Therrien, M. Nayfeh, L. Wagner, L. Mitas, and S. Chaieb, "Observation of a magic discrete family of ultrabright Si nanoparticles," *Appl. Phys. Lett* 80:841–843, 2002.

[856] A. Tsolakidis, D. Sanchez-Portal, and R. M. Martin, "Calculation of the optical response of atomic clusters using time-dependent density functional theory and local orbitals," *Phys. Rev. B* 66:235416, 2002.

[857] R. Bauernschmitt, R. Ahlrichs, F. H. Hennrich, and M. M. Kappes, "Experiment versus time dependent density functional theory prediction of fullerene electronic absorption," *J. Am. Chem. Soc.* 120:5052–5059, 1998.

[858] M. W. D. Hanson-Heine, M. W. G., and N. A. Besley, "Assessment of time-dependent density functional theory with the restricted excitation space approximation for excited state calculations of large systems," *Mol. Phys.* 116:1452–1459, 2018.

[859] L. Kronik, R. Stein, S. Refaely-Abramson, and R. Baer, "Excitation gaps of finite-sized systems from optimally tuned range-separated hybrid functionals," *J. Chem. Theory Comput.* 8:1515–1531, 2012.

[860] G. F. Bertsch, J.-I. Iwata, Angel Rubio, and K. Yabana, "Real-space, real-time method for the dielectric function," *Phys. Rev. B* 62:7998–8002, 2000.

[861] J. B. Krieger and G. J. Iafrate, "Time evolution of Bloch electrons in a homogeneous electric field," *Phys. Rev. B* 33:5494–5500, 1986.

[862] R. van Leeuwen, "Key concepts of time-dependent density-functional theory," *Int. J. Mod. Phys. B* 15:1969–2023, 2001.

[863] M. A. L. Marques, A. Castro, and A. Rubio, "Assessment of exchange–correlation functionals for the calculation of dynamical properties of small clusters in time-dependent density functional theory," *J. Chem. Phys.* 115:3006–3014, 2001.

[864] M. Steslicka, "From Tamm to Shockley: An historical comment," *Prog. Surf. Sci.* 42:11–18, 1993.

[865] I. Tamm, "Ueber eine moegliche Art der Elektronenbindung an Kristalloberflaechen," *Z. Phys.* 76:849–850, 1932.

[866] R. De L. Kronig and W. G. Penney, "Quantum mechanics of electrons in crystal lattices," *Proc. R. Soc. A* 130:499–513, 1931.

[867] C. Davisson and L. H. Germer, "Diffraction of electrons by a crystal of nickel," *Phys. Rev.* 30:705–740, 1927.

[868] S. LaShell, B. A. McDougall, and E. Jensen, "Spin splitting of an Au(111) surface state band observed with angle resolved photoelectron spectroscopy," *Phys. Rev. Lett.* 77:3419–3422, 1996.

[869] H. Yan, B. Stadtmuller, N. Haag, S. Jakobs, J. Seidel, D. Jungkenn, S. Mathias, M. Cinchetti, M. Aeschlimann, and C. Felser, "Topological states on the gold surface," *Nat. Commun.* 6:10167, 2015.

[870] E. I. Rashba and V. I. Sheka, "Symmetry of energy bands in crystals of wurtzite type ii. symmetry of bands with spin–orbit interaction included (English translation: Supplemental Material to the paper by G. Bihlmayer, O. Rader, and R. Winkler, Focus on the Rashba effect, *New J. Phys. 17,* 050202 (2015))," *Fiz. Tverd. Tela – Collected Papers (Leningrad)* II:162–176, 1959.

[871] Yu. A. Bychkov and E. I. Rashba, "Properties of a 2d electron gas with a lifted spectrum degeneracy," *Sov. Phys. – JETP Lett.* 39:78–81, 1984.

[872] A. A. Stekolnikov, J. Furthmüller, and F. Bechstedt, "Absolute surface energies of group-IV semiconductors: Dependence on orientation and reconstruction," *Phys. Rev. B* 65:115318, 2002.

[873] S. B. Healy, C. Filippi, P. Kratzer, E. Penev, and M. Scheffler, "Role of electronic correlation in the Si(100) reconstruction: A quantum Monte Carlo study," *Phys. Rev. Lett.* 87:016105, 2001.

[874] C. G. Van de Walle and R. M. Martin, "Theoretical study of Si/Ge interfaces," *J. Vac. Sci. Technol. B* 3(4):1256–1259, 1985.

[875] K. Steiner, W. Chen, and A. Pasquarello, "Band offsets of lattice-matched semiconductor heterojunctions through hybrid functionals and $G_0 W_0$," *Phys. Rev. B* 89:205309, 2014.

[876] W. A. Harrison, E. A. Kraut, J. R. Waldrop, and R. W. Grant, "Polar heterojunction interfaces," *Phys. Rev. B* 18:4402–4410, 1978.

[877] H. Y. Hwang, Y. Iwasa, M. Kawasaki, B. Keimer, N. Nagaosa, and Y. Tokura, "Emergent phenomena at oxide interfaces," *Nat. Mater.* 11:103, 2012, review article.

[878] P. Zubko, S. Gariglio, M. Gabay, P. Ghosez, and J.-M. Triscone, "Interface physics in complex oxide heterostructures," *Annu. Rev. Condens. Matter Phys.* 2:141–165, 2011.

[879] N. C. Bristowe, P. Ghosez, P. B. Littlewood, and E. Artacho, "The origin of two-dimensional electron gases at oxide interfaces: insights from theory," *J. Phys. Condens. Matter* 26:143201, 2014.

[880] L. Bjaalie, B. Himmetoglu, L. Weston, A. Janotti, and C. G. Van de Walle, "Oxide interfaces for novel electronic applications," *New J. Phys.* 16:025005, 2014.

[881] R. Pentcheva and W. E. Pickett, "Electronic phenomena at complex oxide interfaces: insights from first principles," *J. Phys. Condens. Matter* 22:043001, 2010.

[882] T. Rodel, et al., "Universal fabrication of 2d electron systems in functional oxides," *Adv. Mater.* 28:1976–1980, 2016.

[883] L. F. Mattheiss, "Energy bands for $KNiF_3$, $SrTiO_3$, $KMoO_3$, and $KTaO_3$," *Phys. Rev. B* 6:4718–4740, 1972.

[884] Z. Zhong, A. Tóth, and K. Held, "Theory of spin–orbit coupling at $LaAlO_3$/$SrTiO_3$ interfaces and $SrTiO_3$ surfaces," *Phys. Rev. B* 87:161102, 2013.

[885] A. Splendiani, L. Sun, Y. Zhang, T. Li, J. Kim, C.-Y. Chim, G. Galli, and F. Wang, "Emerging photoluminescence in monolayer MoS_2," *Nano Lett.* 10:1271–1275, 2010.

[886] G. Wang, A. Chernikov, M. M. Glazov, T. F. Heinz, X. Marie, T. Amand, and B. Urbaszek, "Colloquium: Excitons in atomically thin transition metal dichalcogenides," *Rev. Mod. Phys.* 90:021001, 2018.

[887] D. Y. Qiu, F. H. da Jornada, and S. G. Louie, "Screening and many-body effects in two-dimensional crystals: Monolayer MoS_2," *Phys. Rev. B* 93:235435, 2016.

[888] F. A. Rasmussen and K. S. Thygesen, "Computational 2d materials database: Electronic structure of transition-metal dichalcogenides and oxides," *J. Phys. Chem. C* 119:13169–13183, 2015.

[889] G. H. Wannier, "The structure of electronic excitations in the insulating crystals," *Phys. Rev.* 52:191–197, 1937.

[890] G. Blount, in *Solid State Physics*, edited by H. Ehrenreich, F. Seitz, and D. Turnbull, Academic, New York, 1962, p. 305.

[891] N. Marzari, A. A. Mostofi, J. R. Yates, I. Souza, and D. Vanderbilt, "Maximally localized Wannier functions: Theory and applications," *Rev. Mod. Phys.* 84:1419–1475, 2012.

[892] W. Kohn, "Analytic properties of Bloch waves and Wannier functions," *Phys. Rev. B* 115:809–821, 1959.

[893] C. Brouder, G. Panati, M. Calandra, C. Mourougane, and N. Marzari, "Exponential localization of Wannier functions in insulators," *Phys. Rev. Lett.* 98:046402, 2007.

[894] W. Kohn, "Construction of Wannier functions and applications to energy bands," *Phys. Rev. B* 7:4388–4398, 1973.

[895] D. W. Bullett, "A chemical pseudopotential approach to covalent bonding. I," *J. Phys. C: Solid State Phys.* 8:2695–2706, 1975.

[896] P. W. Anderson, "Self-consistent pseudopotentials and ultralocalized functions for energy bands," *Phys. Rev. Lett.* 21:13, 1968.

[897] A. K. McMahan, J. F. Annett, and R. M. Martin, "Cuprate parameters from numerical Wannier functions," *Phys. Rev. B* 42:6268, 1990.

[898] I. Schnell, G. Czycholl, and R. C. Albers, "Hubbard-U calculations for Cu from first-principle Wannier functions," *Phys. Rev. B* 65:075103, 2002.

[899] S. F. Boys, "Construction of some molecular orbitals to be approximately invariant for changes from one molecule to another," *Rev. Mod. Phys.* 32:296–299, 1960.

[900] N. Marzari and D. Vanderbilt, "Maximally localized generalized Wannier functions for composite energy bands," *Phys. Rev. B* 56:12847–12865, 1997.

[901] I. Souza, T. J. Wilkens, and R. M. Martin, "Polarization and localization in insulators: generating function approach," *Phys. Rev. B* 62:1666–1683, 2000.

[902] P. L. Silvestrelli, N. Marzari, D. Vanderbilt, and M. Parrinello, "Maximally-localized Wannier functions for disordered systems: Application to amorphous silicon," *Solid State Commun.* 107:7–11, 1998.

[903] G. Berghold, C. J. Mundy, A. H. Romero, J. Hutter, and M. Parrinello, "General and efficient algorithms for obtaining maximally localized Wannier functions," *Phys. Rev. B* 61:10040–10048, 2000.

[904] I. Souza, N. Marzari, and D. Vanderbilt, "Maximally localized Wannier functions for entangled energy bands," *Phys. Rev. B* 65:035109, 2002.

[905] O. K. Andersen, A. I. Liechtenstein, O. Jepsen, and F. Paulsen, "LDA energy bands, low-energy hamiltonians, t', t'', t (k), and J(perpendicular)," *J. Phys. Chem. Solids* 56:1573, 1995.

[906] J. R. Yates, X. Wang, D. Vanderbilt, and I. Souza, "Spectral and Fermi surface properties from Wannier interpolation," *Phys. Rev. B* 75:195121, 2007.

[907] Y.-S. Lee, M. Buongiorno Nardelli, and N. Marzari, "Band structure and quantum conductance of nanostructures from maximally localized Wannier functions: The case of functionalized carbon nanotubes," *Phys. Rev. Lett.* 95:076804, 2005.

[908] L. D. Landau and E. M. Lifshitz, *Electrodynamics of Continuous Media*, Pergamon Press, Oxford, U.K., 1960.

[909] R. P. Feynman, R. B. Leighton, and M. Sands, *Lectures on Physics, Vol. 2*, Addison Wesley Publishing Company, Reading, MA, 1982.

[910] M. E. Lines and A. M. Glass, *Principles and Applications of Ferroelctrics and Related Materials*, Clarendon Press, Oxford, 1977.

[911] R. M. Martin, "Comment on: Calculation of electric polarization in crystals," *Phys. Rev. B* 9:1998, 1974.

[912] A. K. Tagantsev, "Review: Electric polarization in crystals and its response to thermal and elastic perturbations," *Phase Transit.* 35:119, 1991.

[913] D. J. Thouless, M. Kohmoto, M. P. Nightingale, and M. den Nijs, "Quantized Hall conductance in a two-dimensional periodic potential," *Phys. Rev. Lett.* 49:405–408, 1982.

[914] D. J. Thouless, "Quantization of particle transport," *Phys. Rev. B* 27:6083–6087, 1983.

[915] Q. Niu and D. J. Thouless, "Quantised adiabatic charge transport in the presence of substrate disorder and many-body interaction," *J. Phys. A* 17:2453, 1984.

[916] M. L. Cohen and S. G. Louie, *Fundamentals of Condensed Matter Physics*, Cambridge University Press, Cambridge, U.K., 2016.

[917] E. Kaxiras and J. D. Joannopoulos, *Quantum Theory of Materials*, 2nd rev. ed., Cambridge University Press, Cambridge, U.K., 2019.

[918] D. H. Vanderbilt, *Berry Phases in Electronic Structure Theory*, Cambridge University Press, Cambridge, U.K., 2018.

[919] R. Resta, "The insulating state of matter: A geometric approach," *Eur. Phys. J. B* 79:121–137, 2011.

[920] G. Ortiz, I. Souza, and R. M. Martin, "The exchange–correlation hole in polarized dielectrics: Implications for the microscopic functional theory of dielectrics," *Phys. Rev. Lett.* 80:353–356, 1998.

[921] W. Kohn, "Theory of the insulating state," *Phys. Rev.* 133:A171–181, 1964.

[922] R. Resta, "The quantum mechanical position operator in extended systems," *Phys. Rev. Lett.* 80:1800–1803, 1998.

[923] R. Resta and S. Sorella, "Electron localization in the insulating state," *Phys. Rev. Lett.* 82:370–373, 1999.

[924] C. Aebischer, D. Baeriswyl, and R. M. Noack, "Dielectric catastrophe at the Mott transition," *Phys. Rev. Lett.* 86:468–471, 2001.

[925] G. Arlt and P. Quadflieg, "Piezoelectricity in III–V compounds with a phenomenological analysis of the piezoelectric effect," *Phys. Status Solidi* 25:323, 1968.

[926] R. M. Martin, "Comment on: Piezoelectricity under hydrostatic pressure," *Phys. Rev. B* 6:4874, 1972.

[927] D. Vanderbilt, "Berry-phase theory of proper piezoelectric response," *J. Phys. Chem. Solids* 61:147–151, 2000.

[928] C. Kallin and B. I. Halperin, "Surface-induced charge disturbances and piezoelectricity in insulating crystals," *Phys. Rev. B* 29:2175–2189, 1984.

[929] R. Resta, "Theory of the electric polarization in crystals," *Ferroelectrics* 136:51, 1992.

[930] R. Resta, "Towards a quantum theory of polarization in ferroelectrics: The case of $KNbO_3$," *Europhys. Lett.* 22:133–138, 1993.

[931] G. Ortiz and R. M. Martin, "Macroscopic polarization as a geometric quantum phase: Many-body formulation," *Phys. Rev. B* 49:14202–14210, 1994.

[932] X. Gonze, D. C. Allan, and M. P. Teter, "Dielectric tensor, effective charges, and phonons in α-quartz by variational density-functional perturbation theory," *Phys. Rev. Lett.* 68:3603–3606, 1992.

[933] A. Dal Corso and F. Mauri, "Wannier and Bloch orbital computation of the nonlinear susceptibility," *Phys. Rev. B* 50:5756–5759, 1994.

[934] W. Kleemann, F. J. Schäfer, and M. D. Fontana, "Crystal optical studies of spontaneous and precursor polarization in $KNbO_3$," *Phys. Rev. B* 30:1148–1154, 1984.

[935] R. Resta, "Why are insulators insulating and metals conducting?," *J. Phys. Condens. Matter* 14:R625–R656, 2002.

[936] E. K. Kudinov, "Difference between insulating and conducting states," *Sov. Phys. Solid State* 33:1299–1304, 1991, [Fiz. Tverd. Tela 33, 2306 (1991)].

[937] H. B. Callen and T. A. Welton, "Irreversibility and generalized noise," *Phys. Rev.* 83:34–40, 1951.

[938] H. B. Callen and R. F. Greene, "On a theorem of irreversible thermodynamics," *Phys. Rev.* 86:702–710, 1952.

[939] R. Kubo, "A general expression for the conductivity tensor," *Can. J. Phys.* 34:1274, 1956.

[940] P. C. Martin, *Measurement and Correlation Functions*, Gordon and Breach, New York, 1968.

[941] D. R. Penn, "Wave-number-dependent dielectric function of semiconductors," *Phys. Rev.* 128:2093–2097, 1962.

[942] C. Sgiarovello, M. Peressi, and R. Resta, "Electron localization in the insulating state: Application to crystalline semiconductors," *Phys. Rev. B* 64:115202, 2001.

[943] M. Z. Hasan and C. L. Kane, "Colloquium: Topological insulators," *Rev. Mod. Phys.* 82:3045–3067, 2010.

[944] X.-L. Qi and S.-C. Zhang, "Topological insulators and superconductors," *Rev. Mod. Phys.* 83:1057–1110, 2011.

[945] J. K. Asboth, L. Oroszlany, and A. Palyi, *Lecture Notes in Physics*, vol. 919, *A Short Course on Topological Insulators: Band Structure and Edge States in One and Two Dimensions*, Springer, Heidelburg, Germany, 2016.

[946] A. Bernevig, *Topological Insulators and Topological Superconductors*, Princeton University Press, Princeton, NJ, 2013.

[947] A. Bansil, H. Lin, and T. Das, "Colloquium: Topological band theory," *Rev. Mod. Phys.* 88:021004, 2016.

[948] L. Fu, "Topological crystalline insulators," *Phys. Rev. Lett.* 106:106802, 2011.

[949] F. D. M. Haldane, "Nobel lecture: Topological quantum matter," *Rev. Mod. Phys.* 89:040502, 2017.

[950] D. J. Thouless, *Topological Quantum Numbers in Nonrelativistic Physics*, World Scientific, Singapore, 1988.

[951] J. B. Kogut and M. A. Stephanov, *The Phases of Quantum Chromodynamics: From Confinement to Extreme Environments, Cambridge Monographs on Particle Physics, Nuclear Physics and Cosmology*, Cambridge University Press, Cambridge, U.K., 2003.

[952] Frank Wilczek, "Particle physics and condensed matter: the saga continues," *Phy. Scr.* 2016:014003, 2016.

[953] R. Jackiw and C. Rebbi, "Solitons with fermion number 1/2," *Phys. Rev. D* 13:3398–3409, 1976.

[954] W. P. Su, J. R. Schrieffer, and A. J. Heeger, "Solitons in polyacetylene," *Phys. Rev. Lett.* 42:1698–1701, 1979.

[955] A. A. Soluyanov and D. Vanderbilt, "Wannier representation of Z_2 topological insulators," *Phys. Rev. B* 83:035108, 2011.

[956] R. Yu, X.-L. Qi, A. Bernevig, Z. Fang, and X. Dai, "Equivalent expression of Z_2 topological invariant for band insulators using the non-Abelian Berry connection," *Phys. Rev. B* 84:075119, 2011.

[957] D. Gresch, Gabriel Autès, O. V. Yazyev, M. Troyer, D. Vanderbilt, B. A. Bernevig, and Alexey A. Soluyanov, "Z2Pack: Numerical implementation of hybrid Wannier centers for identifying topological materials," *Phys. Rev. B* 95:075146, 2017.

[958] B. Bradlyn1, L. Elcoro, J. Cano1, M. G. Vergniory, Z. Wang, C. Felser, M. I. Aroyo, and B. A. Bernevig, "Topological quantum chemistry," *Nature* 547:298–305, 2017.

[959] C. W. J. Beenakker, "Search for majorana fermions in superconductors," *Ann. Rev. Condens. Matter Phys.* 4:113–136, 2013.

[960] R. S. K. Mong and V. Shivamoggi, "Edge states and the bulk-boundary correspondence in Dirac Hamiltonians," *Phys. Rev. B* 83:125109, 2011.

[961] A. P. Schnyder, S. Ryu, A. Furusaki, and A. W. W. Ludwig, "Classification of topological insulators and superconductors in three spatial dimensions," *Phys. Rev. B* 78:195125, 2008.

[962] X.-L. Qi, T. L. Hughes, and S.-C. Zhang, "Topological field theory of time-reversal invariant insulators," *Phys. Rev. B* 78:195424, 2008.

[963] A. Kitaev, "Periodic table for topological insulators and superconductors," *AIP Conf. Proc.* 1134:22–30, 2009.

[964] S. Ryu, A. P. Schnyder, A. Furusaki, and A. W. W. Ludwig, "Topological insulators and superconductors: Tenfold way and dimensional hierarchy," *New J. Phy.* 12:065010, 2010.

[965] E. J. Mele and M. J. Rice, "Vibrational excitations of charged solitons in polyacetylene," *Phys. Rev. Lett.* 45:926–929, 1980.

[966] M. J. Rice and E. J. Mele, "Elementary excitations of a linearly conjugated diatomic polymer," *Phys. Rev. Lett.* 49:1455–1459, 1982.

[967] S. S. Pershoguba and V. M. Yakovenko, "Shockley model description of surface states in topological insulators," *Phys. Rev. B* 86:075304, 2012.

[968] J. Zak, "Berry's phase for energy bands in solids," *Phys. Rev. Lett.* 62:2747–2750, 1989.

[969] P. Jadaun, D. Xiao, Q. Niu, and K. Banerjee, S, "Topological classification of crystalline insulators with space group symmetry," *Phys. Rev. B* 88:085110, 2013.

[970] A. Alexandradinata, X. Dai, and B. A. Bernevig, "Wilson-loop characterization of inversion-symmetric topological insulators," *Phys. Rev. B* 89:155114, 2014.

[971] X.-L. Qi, Y.-S. Wu, and S.-C. Zhang, "Topological quantization of the spin Hall effect in two-dimensional paramagnetic semiconductors," *Phys. Rev. B* 74:085308, 2006.

[972] L. Fu and C. L. Kane, "Topological insulators with inversion symmetry," *Phys. Rev. B* 76:045302, 2007.

[973] B. A. Bernevig, T. L. Hughes, and S.-C. Zhang, "Quantum spin Hall effect and topological phase transition in HgTe quantum wells," *Science* 314:1757–1761, 2006.

[974] M. König, S. Wiedmann, C. Brüne, A. Roth, H. Buhmann, L. W. Molenkamp, X.-L. Qi, and S.-C. Zhang, "Quantum spin Hall insulator state in HgTe quantum wells," *Science* 318:766–770, 2007.

[975] J. W. Nicklas and J. W. Wilkins, "Accurate electronic properties for (Hg,Cd)Te systems using hybrid density functional theory," *Phys. Rev. B* 84:121308, 2011.

[976] E. O. Kane, "Band structure of indium antimonide," *J. Phy. Chem. of Solids* 1:249–261, 1957.

[977] F. D. M. Haldane, "Model for a quantum Hall effect without Landau levels: Condensed-matter realization of the 'parity anomaly,'" *Phys. Rev. Lett.* 61:2015–2018, 1988.

[978] K. Nakada, M. Fujita, G. Dresselhaus, and M. S. Dresselhaus, "Edge state in graphene ribbons: Nanometer size effect and edge shape dependence," *Phys. Rev. B* 54:17954–17961, 1996.

[979] F. Reis, G. Li, L. Dudy, M. Bauernfeind, S. Glass, W. Hanke, R. Thomale, J. Schäfer, and R. Claessen, "Bismuthene on a SiC substrate: A candidate for a high-temperature quantum spin Hall material," *Science* 357:287–290, 2017.

[980] L. Fu, C. L. Kane, and E. J. Mele, "Topological insulators in three dimensions," *Phys. Rev. Lett.* 98:106803, 2007.

[981] H. B. Nielsen and M. Ninomiya, "Absence of neutrinos on a lattice: (I). Proof by homotopy theory," *Nucl. Phys. B* 185:20–40, 1981.

[982] Y. Xia, D. Qian, D. Hsieh, L. Wray, A. Pal, H. Lin, A. Bansil, D. Grauer, Y. S. Hor, R. J. Cava, and M. Z. Hasan, "Observation of a large-gap topological-insulator class with a single Dirac cone on the surface," *Nat. Phys.* 5:398, 2009.

[983] P. Larson, V. A. Greanya, W. C. Tonjes, Rong Liu, S. D. Mahanti, and C. G. Olson, "Electronic structure of Bi_2X_3 ($X = S, Se, T$) compounds: Comparison of theoretical calculations with photoemission studies," *Phys. Rev. B* 65:085108, 2002.

[984] W. C. Herring, "Accidental degeneracy in the energy bands of crystals," *Phys. Rev.* 52: 365–373, 1937.

[985] H. Weyl, "Elektron und gravitation. I," *Z. Phys.* 56:330–352, 1929.

[986] N. P. Armitage, E. J. Mele, and A. Vishwanath, "Weyl and Dirac semimetals in three-dimensional solids," *Rev. Mod. Phys.* 90:015001, 2018.

[987] M. Zahid Hasan, Su-Yang Xu, Ilya Belopolski, and Shin-Ming Huang, "Discovery of Weyl fermion semimetals and topological Fermi arc states," *Ann. Rev. Condens. Matter Phys.* 8:289–309, 2017.

[988] H. Yan and C. Felser, "Topological materials: Weyl semimetals," *Ann. Rev. Condens. Matter Phys.* 8:337–354, 2017.

[989] A. Vishwanath, "Viewpoint: Where the Weyl things are," *Physics* 8:84–85, 2015.

[990] G. E. Volovik, *The Universe in a Helium Droplet*, Oxford University Press, Oxford, U.K., 2009.

[991] B. Q. Lv, et al., "Experimental discovery of Weyl semimetal TaAs," *Phys. Rev. X* 5:031013, 2015.

[992] S.-Y. Xu, et al., "Discovery of a Weyl fermion semimetal and topological Fermi arcs," *Science* 349:613–617, 2015.

[993] H. Yan and S.-C. Zhang, "Topological materials," *Rep. Prog. Phy.* 75:096501, 2012.

[994] G. C. Evans, *Functionals and Their Applications*, Dover, New York, 1964.

[995] L. D. Landau and E. M. Lifshitz, *Quantum Mechanics: Non-relativistic Theory*, Pergamon Press, Oxford, U.K., 1977.

[996] R. Shankar, *Principles of Quantum Mechanics*, Plenum Publishing, New York, 1980.

[997] C. Kittel, *Quantum Theory of Solids,* 2nd rev. ed., John Wiley & Sons, New York, 1964.

[998] W. Jones and N. H. March, *Theoretical Solid State Physics,* vol. 2, John Wiley & Sons, New York, 1976.

[999] H. Mori, "A continued-fraction representation of the time-correlation functions," *Prog. Theor. Phys.* 34:399, 1965.

[1000] R Kubo, "Statistical-mechanical theory of irreversible processes. I. General theory and simple applications to magnetic and conduction problems," *Rep. Prog. Phys.* 12:570, 1957.

[1001] D. A. Greenwood, "The Boltzmann equation in the theory of electrical conduction in metals," *Proc. Phys. Soc. (London)* 71:585, 1958.

[1002] P. Nozières and D. Pines, "Electron interaction in solids. collective approach to the dielectric constant," *Phys. Rev.* 109:762–777, 1959.

[1003] H. Ehrenreich and M. H. Cohen, "Self-consistent field approach to the many-electron problem," *Phys. Rev.* 115:786–790, 1959.

[1004] S. Doniach and E. H. Sondheimer, *Green's Functions for Solid State Physicists*, W. A. Benjamin, Reading, MA, 1974. Reprinted in Frontiers in Physics Series, no. 44.

[1005] E. P. Wigner, "Über eine Verschärfung des Summensatzes," *Phys. Z.* 32:450, 1931.

[1006] H. Kramers, C. C. Jonker, and T. Koopmans, "Wigners Erweiterung des Thomas-Kuhnschen Summensatzes für ein Elektron in einem Zentralfeld," *Z. Phys.* 80:178, 1932.

[1007] N. Wiser, "Dielectric constant with local field effects included," *Phys. Rev.* 129:62–69, 1963.

[1008] W. Cochran and R. A. Cowley, "Dielectric constants and lattice vibrations," *J. Phys. Chem. Solids* 23:447, 1962.

[1009] R. Zallen, "Symmetry and reststrahlen in elemental crystals," *Phys. Rev.* 173:824–832, 1968.

[1010] R. Zallen, R. M. Martin, and V. Natoli, "Infrared activity in elemental crystals," *Phys. Rev. B* 49:7032–7035, 1994.

[1011] W. F. Cady, *Piezoelectricity*, McGraw-Hill, New York, 1946.

[1012] R. M. Martin, "Piezolectricity," *Phys. Rev. B* 5(4):1607–1613, 1972.

[1013] P. P. Ewald, "Die Berechnung optischer und electrostatischer Gitterpotentiale," *Ann. Phy.* 64:253, 1921.

[1014] H. Kornfeld, "Die Berechnung electrostatischer Potentiale und der Energie von Dipole- und Quadrupolgittern," *Z. Phys.* 22:27, 1924.

[1015] K. Fuchs, "A quantum mechanical investigation of the cohesive forces of metallic copper," *Proc. Roy. Soc.* 151:585, 1935.

[1016] R. A. Coldwell-Horsfall and A. A. Maradudin, "Zero-point energy of an electron lattice," *J. Math. Phys.* 1:395, 1960.

[1017] M. P. Tosi, in *Solid State Physics*, edited by H. Ehrenreich, F. Seitz, and D. Turnbull, Academic, New York, 1964.

[1018] L. M. Fraser, W. M. C. Foulkes, G. Rajagopal, R. J. Needs, S. D. Kenny, and A. J. Williamson, "Finite-size effects and coulomb interactions in quantum Monte Carlo calculations for homogeneous systems with periodic boundary conditions," *Phys. Rev. B* 53:1814, 1996.

[1019] J. E. Lennard-Jones and B. M. Dent, "Cohesion at a crystal surface," *Trans. Faraday Soc.* 24:92–108, 1928.

[1020] P. A. Schultz, "Local electrostatic moments and periodic boundary conditions," *Phys. Rev. B* 60:1551–1554, 1999.

[1021] G. Makov and M. C. Payne, "Periodic boundary conditions in *ab initio* calculations," *Phys. Rev. B* 51:4014–4022, 1995.

[1022] L. N. Kantorovich, "Elimination of the long-range dipole interaction in calculations with periodic boundary conditions," *Phys. Rev. B* 60:15476, 1999.

[1023] A. Sommerfeld, *Mechanics of Deformable Bodies*, Academic Press, New York, 1950.

[1024] M. Born, W. Heisenberg, and P. Jordan, "Zur Quantenmechanik, II," *Z. Phys.* 35:557, 1926.

[1025] B. Finkelstein, "Uber den Virialsatz in der Wellenmechanik," *Z. Phys.* 50:293, 1928.

[1026] J. C. Slater, "The virial and molecular structure," *J. Chem. Phys.* 1:687, 1933.

[1027] E. Schrödinger, "The energy-impulse hypothesis of material waves," *Ann. Phys. (Leipzig)* 82:265, 1927.

[1028] R. P. Feynman, Undergraduate thesis, unpublished, Massachusetts Institute of Technology, 1939.

[1029] P. C. Martin and J. Schwinger, "Theory of many particle systems. I," *Phys. Rev.* 115: 1342–1373, 1959.

[1030] C. Rogers and A. Rappe, "Unique quantum stress fields," *AIP Conf. Proc.* 582, pp. 91–96, 2001.

[1031] N. Chetty and R. M. Martin, "First-principles energy density and its applications to selected polar surfaces," *Phys. Rev. B* 45:6074–6088, 1992.

[1032] N. Chetty and R. M. Martin, "*GaAs* (111) and (-1-1-1) surfaces and the *GaAs/AlAs* (111) heterojunction studied using a local energy density," *Phys. Rev. B* 45:6089–6100, 1992.

[1033] K. Rapcewicz, B. Chen, B. Yakobson, and J. Bernholc, "Consistent methodology for calculating surface and interface energies," *Phys. Rev. B* 57:7281–7291, 1998.

[1034] R. M. Martin, unpublished, 2002.

[1035] A. Savin, "Expression of the exact electron-correlation-energy density functional in terms of first-order density matrices," *Phys. Rev. A* 52:R1805–R1807, 1995.

[1036] M. Levy and A. Gorling, "Correlation-energy density-functional formulas from correlating first-order density matrices," *Phys. Rev. A* 52:R1808–R1810, 1995.

[1037] H. Stoll, E. Golka, and H. Preuss, "Correlation energies in the spin-density functional formalism. II. Applications and empirical corrections," *Theor. Chim. Acta* 55:29, 1980.

[1038] A. D. Becke, "Hartree–Fock exchange energy of an inhomogeneous electron gas," *Int. J. Quantum Chem.* 23:1915, 1983.

[1039] W. L. Luken and J. C. Culbertson, "Localized orbitals based on the Fermi hole," *Theor. Chim. Acta* 66:279, 1984.

[1040] J. F. Dobson, "Interpretation of the Fermi hole curvature," *J. Chem. Phys.* 94:4328–4333, 1991.

[1041] M. H. Cohen, D. Frydel, K. Burke, and E. Engel, "Total energy density as an interperative tool," *J. Chem. Phys.* 113:2990–2994, 2000.

[1042] B. Hammer and M. Scheffler, "Local chemical reactivity of a metal alloy surface," *Phys. Rev. Lett.* 74:3487–3490, 1995.

[1043] M. J. Godfrey, "Stress field in quantum systems," *Phys. Rev. B* 37:10176–10183, 1988.

[1044] A. Filippetti and V. Fiorentini, "Theory and applications of the stress density," *Phys. Rev. B* 61:8433–8442, 2000.

[1045] C. Rogers and A. Rappe, "Geometric formulation of quantum stress fields," *Phys. Rev. B* 65:224117, 2002.

[1046] D. G. Pettifor, "Pressure-cell boundary relation and application to transition-metal equation of state," *Commun. Phys.* 1:141, 1976.

[1047] A. D. Becke and K. E. Edgecombe, "A simple measure of electron localization in atomic and molecular systems," *J. Chem. Phys.* 92:5397–5403, 1990.

[1048] A. Savin, R. Nesper, Steffen Wengert, and T. F. Fssler, "ELF: The Electron Localization Function," *Angew. Chem., Int. Ed.* 36:1808–1832, 1997.

[1049] M. Methfessel and M. van Schilfgaarde, "Derivation of force theorems in density-functional theory: Application to the full-potential LMTO method," *Phys. Rev. B* 48:4937–4940, 1993.

[1050] J. Grafenstein and P. Ziesche, "Andersen's force theorem and the local stress field," *Phys. Rev. B* 53:7143–7146, 1996.

[1051] E. U. Condon and G. H. Shortley, *Theory of Atomic Spectra*, Cambridge University Press, New York, 1935.

[1052] J. A. Gaunt, "Triplets of helium," *Phil. Trans. Roy. Soc. (London)* 228:151–196, 1929.

[1053] B. Numerov, "Note on the numerical integration of $d^2x/dt^2 = f(x,t)$," *Astron. Nachr.* 230:359–364, 1927.

[1054] M. T. Heath, *Scientific Computing: An Introductory Survey*, McGraw-Hill, New York, 1997.

[1055] P. E. Gill, W. Murray, and M. H. Wright, *Practical Optimization*, Academic Press, London, 1981.

[1056] G. Kresse and J. Furthmüller, "Efficient iterative schemes for *ab initio* total-energy calculations using a plane-wave basis set," *Phys. Rev. B* 54:11169–11186, 1996.

[1057] P. Pulay, "Convergence acceleration of iterative sequences. The case of SCF iteration," *Chem. Phys. Lett.* 73:393–397, 1980.

[1058] P. Pulay, "Improved SCF convergence acceleration," *J. Comp. Chem.* 3:556–560, 1982.

[1059] J. H. van Lenthe and P. Pulay, "A space-saving modification of Davidson's eigenvector algorithm," *J. Comp. Chem.* 11:1164–1168, 1990.

[1060] H. Thirring, "Space lattices and specific heat," *Phys. Zeit.* 14:867, 1913.

[1061] C. Lanczos, *Applied Analysis*, Printice Hall, New York, 1956.

[1062] N. I. Akhiezer, *The Classical Moment Problem*, Oliver and Boyd, Edinburgh, 1965.

[1063] H. Roder, R. N. Silver, J. J. Dong, and D. A. Drabold, "Kernel polynomial method for a nonorthogonal electronic-structure calculation of amorphous diamond," *Phys. Rev. B* 55:15382, 1997.

[1064] J. Skilling, in *Maximum Entropy and Bayesian Methods*, edited by J. Skilling, Kluwer, Dordrecht, 1989, p. 455.

[1065] L. R. Mead, "Approximate solution of Fredholm integral equations by the maximum-entropy method," *J. Math. Phys.* 27:2903, 1986.

[1066] S. Goedecker, "Linear scaling electronic structure methods," *Rev. Mod. Phys.* 71:1085–1123, 1999.

[1067] T. A. Arias, "Multiresolution analysis of electronic structure: Semicardinal and wavelet bases," *Rev. Mod. Phys.* 71:267–311, 1999.

[1068] C. G. J. Jacobi, "Über ein leichtes Verfahren die in der Theorie der Säculärstörrungen vorkommenden Gleichungen numerisch aufzulösen," *Crelle's J.* 30:51–94, 1846.

[1069] J. L. Martins and M. L. Cohen, "Diagonalization of large matrices in pseudopotential band-structure calculations: Dual-space formalism," *Phys. Rev. B* 37:6134–6138, 1988.

[1070] C. M. M. Nex, "A new splitting to solve large hermitian problems," *Comp. Phys. Comm.* 53:141, 1989.

[1071] M. P. Teter, M. C. Payne, and D. C. Allan, "Solution of Schrödinger's equation for large systems," *Phys. Rev. B* 40:12255–12263, 1989.

[1072] A. P. Seitsonen, M. J. Puska, and R. M. Nieminen, "Real-space electronic-structure calculations: Combination of the finite-difference and conjugate-gradient methods," *Phys. Rev. B* 51:14057–14061, 1995.

[1073] B. N. Parlett, *The Symmetric Eigenvalue Problem*, Prentice Hall, Engelwood Cliffs, NJ, 1980.

[1074] Y. Saad, *Iterative Methods for Sparse Linear Systems*, 2nd ed., SIAM, Philadelphia, PA, 2003.

[1075] E. R. Davidson, "The iterative calculation of a few of the lowest eigenvalues and corresponding eigenvectors of large real-symmetric matrices," *J. Comp. Phys.* 17:87, 1975.

[1076] C. Lanczos, "An iteration method for the solution of the eigenvalue problem of linear differential and intergral operators," *J. Res. Natl. Bur. Stand.* 45:255, 1950.

[1077] H. Q. Lin and J. E. Gubernatis, "Exact diagonalization methods for quantum systems," *Comp. Phys.* 7:400–407, 1993.

[1078] L.-W. Wang and A. Zunger, "Large scale electronic strucuture calculations using the Lanczos method," *Comp. Mat. Sci.* 2:326–340, 1994.

[1079] E. R. Davidson, in *Methods in Computational Molecular Physics*, edited by H. F. Diercksen and S. Wilson, D. Reidel Publishing Co., Dordrecht, 1983, pp. 95–113.

[1080] E. R. Davidson, "Monster matrices: Their eigenvalues and eigenvectors," *Comp. Phys.* 7:519, 1993.

[1081] A. Booten and H. van der Vorst, "Cracking large scale eigenvalue problems. Part I: Algorithms," *Comp. Phys.* 10:239–242, 1996.

[1082] D. M. Wood and A. Zunger, "A new method for diagonalizing large matrices," *J. Phys. A* 18:1343–1359, 1985.

[1083] H. Kim, B. D. Yu, and J. Ihm, "Modification of the DIIS method for diagonalizing large matrices," *J. Phys. A* 27:1199–1204, 1994.

[1084] I. Stich, R. Car, M. Parrinello, and S. Baroni, "Conjugate gradient minimization of the energy functional: A new method for electronic structure calculation," *Phys. Rev. B* 39:4997, 1989.

[1085] D. M. Bylander, L. Kleinman, and S. Lee, "Self-consistent calculations of the energy bands and bonding properties of $B_{12}C_3$," *Phys. Rev. B* 42:1394–1403, 1990.

[1086] T. A. Arias, M. C. Payne, and J. D. Joannopoulos, "*Ab initio* molecular dynamics: Analytically continued energy functionals and insights into iterative solutions," *Phys. Rev. Lett.* 69:1077–1080, 1992.

[1087] A. Canning, L. W. Wang, A. Williamson, and A. Zunger, "Parallel empirical pseudopotential electronic structure calculations for million atom systems," *J. Comp. Phys.* 160:29, 2000.

[1088] T. Ericsson and A. Ruhe, "The spectral transformation Lanczos method for the numerical solution of large sparse generalized symmetric eigenvalue problems," *Math. Comp.* 35:1251–1268, 1980.

[1089] R. R. Sharma, "General expressions for reducing the Slater–Koster linear combination of atomic orbitals integrals to the two-center approximation," *Phys. Rev. B* 19:2813–2823, 1979.

[1090] C. Cohen-Tannoudji, B. Diu, and F. Laloë, *Quantum Mechanics*, Wiley-Interscience, Paris, 1977.

[1091] P. A. M. Dirac, *The Principles of Quantum Mechanics*, Oxford University Press, Oxford, 1930.

[1092] J.M. Ziman, *Principles of the Theory of Solids*, Cambridge University Press, Cambridge, 1989.

[1093] J. D. Bjorken and S. D. Drell, *Relativistic Quantum Mechanics*, McGraw-Hill, New York, 1964.

[1094] D. D. Koelling and B. N. Harmon, "A technique for relativistic spin-polarized calculations," *J. Phys. C* 10:3107–3114, 1977.

[1095] A. H. MacDonald, W. E. Pickett, and D. Koelling, "A linearised relativistic augmented-plane-wave method utilising approximate pure spin basis functions," *J. Phys. C: Solid State Phys.* 13:2675–2683, 1980.

[1096] Y. Aharonov and D. Bohm, "Further discussion of the role of electromagnetic potentials in the quantum theory," *Phys. Rev.* 130:1625–1632, 1963.

[1097] B. Simon, "Holonomy, the quantum adiabatic theorem, and Berry's phase," *Phys. Rev. Lett.* 51:2167–2170, 1983.

[1098] *Advanced Series in Mathematical Physics*, vol. 5, *Geometric Phases in Physics*, edited by F. Wilczek and A. Shapere, World Prss, Singapore, 1989.

[1099] P. A. M. Dirac, "Quantised singularities in the electromagnetic field," *Proc. R. Soc. A* 133:60–72, 1931.

[1100] R. E. Prange and S. M. Girvin, *The Quantum Hall Effect*, Springer-Verlag, New York, 1990.

[1101] B. I. Halperin, "Quantized Hall conductance, current-carrying edge states, and the existence of extended states in a two-dimensional disordered potential," *Phys. Rev. B* 25:2185–2190, 1982.

[1102] R. B. Laughlin, "Quantized Hall conductivity in two dimensions," *Phys. Rev. B* 23:5632–5633, 1981.

[1103] E. H. Hall, "On a new action of the magnet on electric currents," *Am. J. Math.* 2:287–292, 1879.

[1104] X. Gonze, et al., "Recent developments in the ABINIT software package," *Comput. Phys. Commun.* 205:106–131, 2016.

[1105] S. J. Clark, M. D. Segall, C. J. Pickard, P. J. Hasnip, M. J. Probert, K. Refson, and M. C. Payne, "First principles methods using CASTEP," *Z. Kristallographie* 220:567–570, 2005.

[1106] P. Giannozzi, et al., "QUANTUM ESPRESSO: A modular and open-source software project for quantum simulations of materials," *J. Phys. Condens. Matter* 21:395502, 2009.

[1107] R. Dovesi, et al., "Quantum-mechanical condensed matter simulations with CRYSTAL," *Wiley Interdiscip. Rev. Comput. Mol. Sci.* 8:e1360, 2018.

[1108] A. Castro, H. Appel, M. Oliveira, C. A. Rozzi, X. Andrade, F. Lorenzen, M. A. L. Marques, E. K. U. Gross, and A. Rubio, "OCOTOPUS: A tool for the application of time-dependent density functional theory," *Phys. Stat. Sol. B* 243:2465–2488, 2006.

[1109] D. R. Bowler, R. Choudhury, M. J. Gillan, and T. Miyazaki, "Recent progress with large-scale *ab initio* calculations: the conquest code," *Phys. Stat. Sol. B* 243:989–1000, 2006.

[1110] C.-K. Skylaris, P. D. Haynes, A. A. Mostofi, and M. C. Payne, "Introducing ONETEP: Linear-scaling density functional simulations on parallel computers," *J. Chem. Phys.* 122:084119, 2005.

[1111] P. D. Haynes, A. A. Mostof, C.-K. Skylaris, and M. C. Payne, "ONETEP: Linear-scaling density-functional theory with plane-waves," *J. Phys. Conf. Ser.* 26:143–148, 2006.

[1112] A. A. Mostofi, J. R. Yates, G. Pizzi, Y.-S. Lee, I. Souza, D. Vanderbilt, and N. Marzari, "An updated version of wannier90: A tool for obtaining maximally-localised Wannier functions," *Comput. Phys. Commun.* 185:2309–2310, 2014.

[1113] Y. Wang, J. Lv, L. Zhu, and Y. Ma, "CALYPSO: A method for crystal structure prediction," *Comput. Phys. Commun.* 183(10):2063–2070, 2012.

Index

Printed in the United States
by Baker & Taylor Publisher Services